Health-Related Disorders in Children and Adolescents

Applying Psychology in the Schools Book Series

Assessing Bilingual Children in Context: An Integrated Approach
Edited by Amanda B. Clinton

Autism Spectrum Disorder in Children and Adolescents: Evidence-Based Assessment and Intervention in Schools
Edited by Lee A. Wilkinson

Behavioral Interventions in Schools: Evidence-Based Positive Strategies, Second Edition
Edited by Steven G. Little and Angeleque Akin-Little

Empowered Families, Successful Children: Early Intervention Programs That Work
Susan Epps and Barbara J. Jackson

Empowered Learning in Secondary Schools: Promoting Positive Youth Development Through a Multitiered System of Supports
Cynthia E. Hazel

Enhancing Relationships Between Children and Teachers
Robert C. Pianta

Health-Related Disorders in Children and Adolescents: A Guidebook for Educators and Service Providers, Second Edition
Edited by Michelle M. Perfect, Cynthia A. Riccio, and Melissa A. Bray

Healthy Eating in Schools: Evidence-Based Interventions to Help Kids Thrive
Catherine P. Cook-Cottone, Evelyn Tribole, and Tracy L. Tylka

Implementation of Mental Health Programs in Schools: A Change Agent's Guide
Susan G. Forman

Promoting Mind–Body Health in Schools: Interventions for Mental Health Professionals
Edited by Cheryl Maykel and Melissa A. Bray

Psychoeducational Assessment and Intervention for Ethnic Minority Children: Evidence-Based Approaches
Edited by Scott L. Graves Jr. and Jamilia J. Blake

School-Based Mental Health Services: Creating Comprehensive and Culturally Specific Programs
Bonnie Kaul Nastasi, Rachel Bernstein Moore, and Kristen M. Varjas

School-Centered Interventions: Evidence-Based Strategies for Social, Emotional, and Academic Success
Dennis J. Simon

Self-Regulated Learning Interventions With At-Risk Youth: Enhancing Adaptability, Performance, and Well-Being
Edited by Timothy J. Cleary

Single-Case Intervention Research: Methodological and Statistical Advances
Edited by Thomas R. Kratochwill and Joel R. Levin

Teleconsultation in Schools: A Guide to Collaborative Practice
Aaron J. Fischer and Bradley S. Bloomfield

Testing Accommodations for Students With Disabilities: Research-Based Practice
Benjamin J. Lovett and Lawrence J. Lewandowski

Treatment Integrity: A Foundation for Evidence-Based Practice in Applied Psychology
Edited by Lisa M. Hagermoser Sanetti and Thomas R. Kratochwill

Universal Screening in Educational Settings: Evidence-Based Decision Making for Schools
Edited by Ryan J. Kettler, Todd A. Glover, Craig A. Albers, and Kelly A. Feeney-Kettler

Working With Parents of Aggressive Children: A Practitioner's Guide, Second Edition
Timothy A. Cavell and Lauren B. Quetsch

Working With Parents of Noncompliant Children: A Guide to Evidence-Based Parent Training for Practitioners and Students
Mark D. Shriver and Keith D. Allen

This volume is impressive in its organization, readability, and coverage of a wide range of common and uncommon health conditions. The inclusion of practical, evidence-based medical, psychosocial, and academic interventions is especially useful. This is a highly valuable resource for practitioners, trainers, and students in school psychology and other educational professions.

—**Thomas J. Power, PhD, ABPP,** Professor, School Psychology in Pediatrics and Psychiatry, Children's Hospital of Philadelphia; Perelman School of Medicine at University of Pennsylvania, Philadelphia, PA, United States

This is not just another summary of facts: It is a sourcebook for providers and researchers to further explore topics some have never heard of before. This is what I consider a true contribution to the field of psychology.

—**Elaine Clark, PhD,** Professor, Educational Psychology, University of Utah, Salt Lake City, UT, United States; Fellow, American Psychological Association

The second edition of *Health-Related Disorders in Children and Adolescents* is an outstanding new volume and a worthy tribute to Dr. LeAdelle Phelps's classic text. The tone and focus of the book support the role of psychologists and educators in interdisciplinary coordination and consultation for children and adolescents with medical issues. Drs. Perfect, Riccio, and Bray have brilliantly modernized, reorganized, and updated an important text in pediatric school psychology.

—**Steven R. Shaw, PhD,** Associate Professor, Department of Educational and Counselling Psychology, McGill University, Montreal, QC, Canada

Health-Related Disorders in Children and Adolescents

A Guidebook for Educators and Service Providers

Second Edition

Michelle M. Perfect, Cynthia A. Riccio, and Melissa A. Bray *Editors*

AMERICAN PSYCHOLOGICAL ASSOCIATION

Published by
American Psychological Association
750 First Street, NE
Washington, DC 20002
https://www.apa.org

Order Department
https://www.apa.org/pubs/books
order@apa.org

Typeset in Meridien and Ortodoxa by TIPS Publishing Services, Carrboro, NC

Printer: Gasch Printing, Odenton, MD
Cover Designer: Gwen J. Grafft, Minneapolis, MN

Library of Congress Cataloging-in-Publication Data

CIP Data has been applied for.
Library of Congress Control Number: 2023934120

https://doi.org/10.1037/0000349-000

Printed in the United States of America

10 9 8 7 6 5 4 3 2 1

CONTENTS

CONTRIBUTORS

Keiko Aoyagi, PhD, Portland State University, Portland, OR, United States
Sai Sudha Aravala, MPH, BS, New York University School of Global Public Health, New York City, NY, United States
Megan Aros-O'Malley, PhD, District Medical Group Children's Rehabilitative Services, Phoenix, AZ, United States
Abigail Baxter, PhD, University of South Alabama, Mobile, AL, United States
Aarti P. Bellara, PhD, Western Carolina University, Cullowhee, NC, United States
Savina Maria Bello, MA, University of Arizona, Tucson, AZ, United States
Evelyn Bilias-Lolis, PhD, Fairfield University, Fairfield, CT, United States
Sarah E. Bills, PhD, University of South Carolina, Columbia, SC, and Cincinnati Children's Hospital Medical Center, Cincinnati, OH, United States
Jeff Bostwick, PhD, University of Delaware, Newark, DE, United States
Adeline M. Bray, BS, Touro College of Osteopathic Medicine, Middletown, NY, United States
Clark R. Bray, BSE, University of Connecticut, Storrs, CT, United States
Melissa A. Bray, PhD, University of Connecticut, Storrs, CT, United States
Alyssa M. Bunyea, MA, University of Connecticut, Storrs, CT, United States
Lindsey J. Carnes, PhD, Texas A&M University, College Station, TX, United States
Stihlyn Chamberlain, PhD, University of Arizona, Tucson, AZ, United States
Tiffany Chenneville, PhD, University of South Florida, St. Petersburg, FL, United States

Cindy Chin, MD, University of Arizona, Tucson, AZ, United States
Kelly N. Clark, PhD, Louisiana State University, Baton Rouge, LA, United States
Christine L. Cole, PhD, Lehigh University, Bethlehem, PA, United States
Samantha Coyle, PhD, Montclair State University, Montclair, NJ, United States
Karen Cross, PhD, University of Connecticut, Storrs, CT, United States
Brittany A. Dale, PhD, Ball State University, Muncie, IN, United States
Johanna deLeyer-Tiarks, PhD, School of Psychology, Adelphi University, Garden City, NY, United States
Priscilla H. Duong, PhD, Ann & Robert H. Lurie Children's Hospital of Chicago, Chicago, IL, United States
Stewart W. Ehly, PhD, University of Iowa, Iowa City, IA, United States
Noel Estrada-Hernandez, PhD, CRC, University of Iowa, Iowa City, IA, United States
Allison Fairchild, PhD, University of Arizona, Tucson, AZ, United States
Melissa C. Fleuhr, PsyD, Rutgers University–New Brunswick, New Brunswick, NJ, United States
Susan G. Forman, PhD, Rutgers University–New Brunswick, New Brunswick, NJ, United States
Craig L. Frisby, PhD, (Emeritus) University of Missouri, Columbia, MO, United States
Sara S. Frye, PhD, University of Arizona, Tucson, AZ, United States
Kemesha Gabbidon, PhD, University of South Florida, St. Petersburg, FL, United States
Lauren Gammie, PhD, University of Connecticut, Storrs, CT, United States
Nicholas W. Gelbar, PhD, University of Connecticut, Storrs, CT, United States
Carly B. Gilson, PhD, The Ohio State University, Columbus, OH, United States
Alyssa A. Gonzalez, PhD, Texas A&M University, College Station, TX, United States
Timothy S. Hartshorne, PhD, Central Michigan University, Mount Pleasant, MI, United States
Daphne J. Hill, PhD, Texas A&M University, College Station, TX, United States
Larissa Hoefler, MA, Adelphi University, Garden City, NY, United States
Kandace M. Hoppin, EdD, Towson University, Towson, MD, United States
George W. Hynd, EdD, (Emeritus) University of Georgia, Athens, GA, United States
Melina Islas, PhD, University of Arizona, Tucson, AZ, United States
Randa Jarrar, MD, Phoenix Children's Hospital, Phoenix, AZ, United States
Megan Jeune, PhD, Western Governor's University, Millcreek, UT, United States

Emily M. Jimenez, PhD, Texas A&M University, College Station, TX, United States

Lauren E. Klein, PhD, Department of Educational Psychology, University of Connecticut, Storrs, CT, United States

Heather Kwolek, MA, University of Connecticut, Storrs, CT, United States

Cindy C. Labbe, BSN, BS, RN, University of Connecticut, Storrs, CT, United States

Cynthia K. Lang, PhD, Texas A&M University, College Station, TX, United States

Natalie A. Lárez, MEd, University of Arizona, Tucson, AZ, United States

Michelle Levine-Schmitt, MA, EdM, NCSP, University of Connecticut, Storrs, CT, United States

Meghan Long, BS, University of Connecticut, Storrs, CT, United States

Christine K. Malecki, PhD, Northern Illinois University, DeKalb, IL, United States

Suzanne G. Margiano, PhD, NCSP, Department of Educational Psychology, University of Connecticut, Storrs, CT, United States

Cheryl Maykel, PhD, Rivier University, Nashua, NH, United States

David E. McIntosh, PhD, Ball State University, Muncie, IN, United States

Lorette McWilliams, PhD, School Counseling Department, Assumption University, Worcester, MA, United States

Maria Paula Mello, PhD, BCBA, St. John's University, Queens, NY, United States

Ivette Merced, MA, MA, EdS, NCSP, University of Arizona, Tucson, AZ, United States

Marlena L. Minkos, PhD, University of Connecticut, Storrs, CT, United States

Terry Monkaba, MBA, Williams Syndrome Association, Troy, MI, United States

Linda W. Morse, PhD, (Emerita) Mississippi State University, Mississippi State, MS, United States

Melanie C. Morse, PhD, University of Virginia School of Medicine, Charlottesville, VA, United States

Taylor-Kristen Myers, MAT, University of Arizona, Tucson, AZ, United States

Katherine R. Nelson, MA, SYC, NCSP, University of Connecticut, Storrs, CT, United States

Megan Nickels, PhD, Western Governors University, Salt Lake City, UT, United States

Cassandra Odell, MA, Adelphi University, Garden City, NY, United States

Julia Ogg, PhD, Northern Illinois University, DeKalb, IL, United States

Phyllis S. Ohr, PhD, Hofstra University, Hempstead, NY, United States

Robin Pegg, MEd, COTA/L, ATP, ROH, Grand Rapids Community College, Grand Rapids, MI, United States

Elizabeth Perdue, PhD, LP, LSSP, NCSP, Texas A&M University, College Station, TX, United States
Michelle M. Perfect, PhD, University of Arizona, Tucson, AZ, United States
Alyssa Perri Elias, PsyD, Adelphi University, Garden City, NY, United States
Justina Petrullo, BA, Centenary University, Hackettstown, NJ, United States
Sade S. Porter, PsyD, Rutgers University–New Brunswick, New Brunswick, NJ, United States
Madison Preece, BS, University of Arizona, Tucson, AZ, United States
Sherine D. Presley, MEd, Texas A&M University, College Station, TX, United States
Stevie Puckett-Perez, PhD, ABPP, Children's Health, University of Texas Southwestern, Dallas, TX, United States
Mickey Randolph, PhD, Western Carolina University, Cullowhee, NC, United States
Cynthia A. Riccio, PhD, (Emeritus) Texas A&M University, College Station, TX, United States
Patricia Rice Doran, EdD, Towson University, Towson, MD, United States
Eric L. Robinson, PhD, Baylor University, Waco, TX, United States
Fay Roseman, PhD, West Coast University, Irvine, CA, United States
Lydia Rumpf, BA, Adelphi University, Garden City, NY, United States
David E. Sandberg, PhD, Susan B. Meister Child Health Evaluation and Research Center, Department of Pediatrics, University of Michigan Medical School, Ann Arbor, MI, United States
Maryann Santos, PhD, (Dean Emerita) Purdue University, West Lafayette, IN, United States
Kari A. Sassu, PhD, NCSP, Southern Connecticut State University, New Haven, CT, United States
Ethan J. Schilling, PhD, NCSP, Western Carolina University, Cullowhee, NC, United States
Craig Schramm, MD, University of Connecticut, Storrs, CT, United States
Carissa Scogin, MA, Department of Educational Psychology, University of Connecticut, Storrs, CT, United States
Jeffrey D. Shahidullah, PhD, The University of Texas at Austin, Austin, TX, United States
Agnes Shine, PhD, NCSP, Barry University, Miami Shores, FL, United States
Graciela E. Silva, PhD, MPH, MT, University of Arizona, Tucson, AZ, United States
Krystal T. Simmons, PhD, Texas A&M University, College Station, TX, United States
Lillian J. Slavin, PhD, Nemours Children's Hospital, Wilmington, DE, United States
Jeanette Smith, PhD, Phoenix Children's Hospital, Phoenix, AZ, United States
Anita Sohn McCormick, PhD, Texas A&M University, College Station, TX, United States

Danielle Stern, MA, University of Connecticut, Storrs, CT, United States
Brooke R. Stettler, MA, Montclair State University, Montclair, NJ, United States
Dan Strissel, PhD, Northern Illinois University, DeKalb, IL, United States
Huilin Linda Sun, PhD, Texas A&M University, College Station, TX, United States
Kristina I. Suorsa-Johnson, PhD, Division of Psychiatry and Behavioral Health, Department of Pediatrics, University of Utah Spencer Fox Eccles School of Medicine, Salt Lake City, UT, United States
Kerrilyn Surdi, MA, Hofstra University, Hempstead, NY, United States
Harvey N. Switzky, PhD, (Emeritus) Northern Illinois University, DeKalb, IL, United States
Hiroko Tanaka, PhD, University of Arizona, Banner University Medical Center, Tucson, AZ, United States
Alana E. Telesford, PhD, Child Mind Institute, New York, NY, United States
Lea A. Theodore, PhD, Adelphi University, Garden City, NY, United States
Rebecca J. Tipton-DeClue, PhD, Baylor University, Waco, TX, United States
Jennifer Tucker, PT, DPT, PhD, PCS, University of Central Florida, Orlando, FL, United States
Carolyn Tureaud, BA, University of Arizona, Tucson, AZ, United States
James P. Van Haneghan, PhD, University of South Alabama, Mobile, AL, United States
Chelsea Vaughan, PhD, LSSP, Hill Country Sleep and Behavioral Health, Austin, TX, United States
Elana S. Volfinzon, BS, University of Connecticut, Storrs, CT, United States
Bianca S. Watkins, PhD, Texas A&M University, College Station, TX, United States
Moira Wendel, PhD, Northern Illinois University, DeKalb, IL, United States
Mark Wheeler, MD, University of Arizona, Tucson, AZ, United States
Emily L. Winter, PhD, NCSP, Sasco River Center, Darien, CT, United States
David L. Wodrich, PhD, University of Arizona, Tucson, AZ, United States

SERIES FOREWORD

Outside of their homes, children spend more time in schools than in any other setting. From gun violence tragedies such as Uvalde, Parkland, and Sandy Hook to more hopeful developments such as the movement toward improved mental and physical health and academic achievement, there is an ongoing need for high-quality writing that speaks to ways in which children, families, and communities associated with schools worldwide can be supported through the application of sound psychological research, theory, and practice.

The American Psychological Association (APA) Books Program and APA Division 16 (School Psychology) have partnered to produce the Applying Psychology in the Schools Book Series for over two decades. The mission of this series is to increase the visibility of the science, practice, and policy for children and adolescents in schools and communities. The result has been a robust collection of scholarly work that appeals to psychologists and individuals from all fields who have reason to seek and use what psychology has to offer in schools.

As editors of the second edition of *Health-Related Disorders in Children and Adolescents: A Guidebook for Educators and Service Providers,* Michelle Perfect, Cynthia Riccio, and Melissa Bray have compiled chapters from expert authors that provide educators, parents, service providers, and health care professionals with contemporary research on the prevalence, symptoms, outcomes, educational implications, and intervention of over 60 different pediatric medical conditions. LeAdelle Phelps conceptualized the first edition as a response to the limited information available in 1988 to school personnel about students with chronic illness. Likewise, health care providers needed to be equipped with information about the educational needs of these youth.

Since its initiation, many individuals have made significant contributions to this book series. We would like to acknowledge the dedication of past series editors Sandra L. Christensen, Catherine Christo, Jan Hughes, R. Steve McCallum, David McIntosh, LeAdelle Phelps, Linda Reddy, Susan Sheridan, Christopher H. Skinner, David Shriberg, and Melissa Pearrow. Second, we also thank Linda Malnasi McCarter and the editorial team of APA Books for their work and support, as well as all of the people at APA Books who have worked behind the scenes to bring this book to fruition. Finally, we thank the author teams for their collaborative efforts in writing their respective chapter in *Health-Related Disorders in Children and Adolescents: A Guidebook for Educators and Service Providers.*

The leadership of Division 16 welcomes your comments about this volume and your ideas for other topics you would like to see explored in this series. To share your thoughts, please visit the Division 16 website (https://www.apa.org/about/division/div16).

—*Michelle M. Perfect, PhD*
Series Editor

PREFACE

This book is a revision of my 1998 text titled *Health-Related Disorders in Children and Adolescents*, published by the American Psychological Association.[1] The first edition was very well received by the psychological community. I began with a focus from a school psychology perspective but was uniquely able to provide insight to a myriad of the subdisciplines of psychology. I have devoted much of my career to the area of psychological and physical health, including such areas as genetics, brain physiology, and the immune system, which are presently forthcoming, utilizing experimental methodology, gathering causal data. The recognition that the psyche is integral to physical functioning is not a new concept but one that is becoming more and more important in terms of research and practice in psychology. The first edition of this text included many low-incidence chronic illnesses that affect the social, cognitive, and academic functioning of youth. This revision used stringent criteria in determining which disorders would be included, with experts leading each chapter representing various disciplines in psychology. The update to this text has categorized these inclusions into the major body systems confirmed by medical professionals. It will serve as an empirically supported resource that highlights the connection of the mind and body with implications for early intervention and education. The new editors were carefully chosen to serve, with my input into their selection and the direction of this cutting-edge revised text. Dr. Michelle Perfect, the lead editor, is meticulous in her work, knowledgeable, and dedicated. Dr. Cyndi Riccio, lead editor two, is well known in this area as an expert, persistent, and productive. Dr. Melissa

[1]Professor LeAdelle Phelps dictated this preface, word for word, to Dr. Melissa Bray in September 2019, less than a week before her death.

Bray, last editor, is insightful and well published in the area of mind–body health. I am grateful that they agreed to work together with me to publish this revision.

—Dr. LeAdelle Phelps

Dr. Phelps earned her PhD from the University of Utah. Following her education, she quickly became a leader in school psychology. She was a professor at the University at Buffalo, where she served as director of the Counseling Psychology/School Psychology Program, associate dean for Academic Affairs, and chair of the Department of Counseling, School and Educational Psychology. She had a passion for the integration of physical health and wellness with psychology and education. Throughout her career, she was heavily involved in national leadership and published widely. The first edition of *Health-Related Disorders in Children and Adolescents*, published by the American Psychological Association in 1998, was a bestseller. Dr. Phelps was fully dedicated to contributing to and publishing this new edition.

I

INTRODUCTION

1

Introduction to the Second Edition

Michelle M. Perfect, Cynthia A. Riccio, and Melissa A. Bray

Although estimates vary, as many as one fourth of school-aged students experience some form of a health-related condition—the equivalent of over 15 million individuals under the age of 17 (Van Cleave et al., 2010). One possible explanation for these high rates has been the significant improvements in survival rates for children with chronic illnesses (American Academy of Pediatrics, 2016). By definition, a *health-related condition* occurs when there is a specific set of symptoms, with those symptoms persisting for 3 or more months (Katz et al., 2015). Most practitioners, regardless of their professional orientation, are familiar with disorders like attention-deficit/hyperactivity disorder (ADHD), Down syndrome, and other more frequently encountered health-related chronic conditions.

Over 20 years ago, the first edition of this book, *Health-Related Disorders in Children and Adolescents: A Guidebook for Understanding and Educating* (Phelps, 1998), was published, supplying vital empirical information about medical conditions that had been previously unavailable and providing practical information about how to support these students not only medically but also educationally and social–emotionally. This second edition focuses on disorders with less widespread research and information yet with a prevalence of at least one in 25,000 individuals. In many cases, these less researched conditions co-occur with ADHD or other emotional and behavioral disorders (Pan & Bölte, 2020). Moreover, it is important to note that additional syndromes or disorders may exist or have yet to be identified. Taken together, the conditions selected

https://doi.org/10.1037/0000349-001
Health-Related Disorders in Children and Adolescents: A Guidebook for Educators and Service Providers, Second Edition, M. M. Perfect, C. A. Riccio, and M. A. Bray (Editors)

for inclusion demonstrate the similarities and differences across a range of disorders. With the updated organization and research included here, the second edition may prove helpful for psychologists, medical professionals, educational professionals, and others involved in behavioral health, as well as university training programs.

THE INTEGRATED COLLABORATIVE APPROACH

As noted already, over the past 2 decades, innovative and effective medical treatments have led to increased survival rates, necessitating an updated resource that summarizes the prevailing issues related to health-related conditions, potential accommodations, and needed supports that would allow medically involved students to achieve success. At the same time, there has been growing awareness of the need for coordinated behavioral health services. The educational implications for children with health-related difficulties and the need for collaboration among parents and medical, behavioral health, and educational professionals have been known for some time (Harris, 2009; Power et al., 2003). Reauthorization of the Individuals With Disabilities Education Act (2004) with Other Health Impairment as a disability category cemented the mandate for thoughtful coordination of educational programming, including psychological services, for children with health conditions. Despite the frequency and mandates, however, empirical studies have continued to demonstrate that there are immense unmet needs for children with chronic conditions and their families. For the children, this educational–health care gap exists due to limitations of regulations governing education and lack of research to identify and support the appropriate educational services needed.

School psychologists and other mental health professionals in the schools are in a unique position to take the lead in orchestrating and coordinating school-based services for students. These professionals have knowledge of special education law as well as training and skills in consultation and collaboration among school-based professionals and parents. Although medical professionals have expertise in addressing medical issues, mental health professionals like school psychologists understand the complex nature of cognitive, academic, and psychosocial factors of children with health-related conditions (Root et al., 2016).

This second edition is intended to provide a synergy of scientific underpinnings and practical research-based suggestions. The editors recognize that the book is not exhaustive; not all health conditions are included, and prevalence may vary depending on developmental level. In order to accommodate the number of disorders, chapter content is targeted and specific to the goals of this text: to inform users of the most up-to-date information on symptoms, outcomes, and potential interventions.

ORGANIZATION AND STRUCTURE OF THE CHAPTERS

The etiology of health conditions varies widely but typically involves disruption or dysfunction in one or more body systems. Body systems can be categorized as involving (a) the blood, cardiovascular system, and circulatory system; (b) the respiratory system; (c) the central nervous system; (d) the musculoskeletal system, focusing on bone and muscle; (d) the digestive system; and (e) the endocrine and reproductive systems. In addition, some disorders are best classified by mixed or multiple systems. Where possible, this text organizes disorders on the basis of the primary system or systems involved, with a number of disorders grouped as multiple system disorders. A brief introductory chapter about the body system(s) and a global understanding across the disorders is provided at the beginning of each part, with the following chapters listed alphabetically. All chapters have a similar structure: Etiology; Prevalence and Incidence; Symptoms; Outcomes, organized by Medical, Cognitive/Academic, and Social–Emotional and Behavioral; Interventions, organized by Medical Management, Cognitive/Academic, and Social–Emotional and Behavioral; Conclusion; Resources; and References.

Genetic Etiology

Health-related disorders may be attributable to heritability and genetics such that the presence of the disorder is evident across family members and generations, with specific genes identified. Genes are found in DNA, and for many disorders, atypical series on specific locations on a given specific gene or genes give rise to the disorders. When multiple genes and locations are involved, the extent to which atypical patterns are present determines the symptom presentation and the body system(s) affected. Throughout this text, authors present a summary of information about what is known for each condition or group of disorders regarding genetics and mechanisms that could lead to genetic alteration.

Symptom Presentation

Taken together, the body system(s) involved and the variation in underlying genetic contribution give rise to a range of symptoms. Depending on the disorder, the identification of the problem and subsequent identification of causes may occur as early as in utero, at birth, in early childhood, at school age, or later, depending on when the disorder and its effects manifest. Where there is a positive family history, genetic testing may be done along with routine blood testing at birth. The initial effects and symptom manifestation may affect attainment of even very early developmental milestones or may become more apparent over age. Most often, the disorder or disease manifests before or when the child begins school, leading to identification of the disorder (Bai et al., 2017).

Anticipated Outcomes

Medical outcomes are featured in each chapter for readers to understand the prognosis and health implications of the health conditions. At the same time, cognitive ability and acquisition of academic skills, as well as social–emotional development, may be compromised as the disorder manifests. As children enter school, considering implications for medical, cognitive/academic, and social–emotional factors in a coordinated fashion becomes critical. What is known about cognitive and academic outcomes associated with the disorder is highlighted. Similarly, anticipated social–emotional and behavioral issues associated with the disorder are discussed. Reviewed together, the extent of synergy across medical, cognitive/academic, and social–emotional and behavioral outcomes becomes evident. This speaks to the need for those involved in treating and supporting children with chronic disorders, regardless of their primary professional responsibility, to consider all child-specific facets, as well as the family system.

School-Based Interventions

Within each chapter, evidence-based interventions from a medical, behavioral health, and educational perspective are offered with the caveat that what works best will need to be individually determined as part of each child's medical treatment and educational planning. Medical management may or may not be extensive. Moreover, physical symptoms and medical needs often change over the course of development. Similarly, as the child progresses through school, curricular demands and expectations for independent function shift. Finally, the social and behavioral demands and pressures change. Most importantly, the medical status, cognitive/academic challenges and successes, and social and behavioral difficulties interact, rather than occurring in isolation. Thus, the use of a team approach is emerging as a preferred model, involving service providers from all contexts related to the child. This team includes medical practitioners, educators, and mental health professionals, such as nurses, special and regular education teachers, and psychologists. It also includes consideration of the family context. The child is not the only individual affected by the health-related condition; the family system is challenged as well. Family support is important to the outcomes for these children and can include parent training so that the family system may be empowered to build on strengths and assets.

Summary and Resources

Each disorder-focused chapter ends with a summary paragraph, highlighting the most salient information provided within the chapter. In some cases, the conclusion also identifies areas of additional research. To facilitate further study of the conditions of interest, authors were asked to provide resources that may provide further detail or be appropriate for sharing with parents and other professionals working with that child.

CALL TO ACTION

As mentioned, a significant gap persists between professionals who work with children with chronic health disorders (e.g., medical staff, educators, mental health professionals). Many health care settings have only recently begun to incorporate behavioral health as an integrated service; fewer use an interdisciplinary team that includes school-based staff. Within educational settings, there are already established teams aligned with special education or the Americans With Disabilities Act. The coordination of services to integrate health care and educational teams is a common component across chapters in this text. Bidirectional flow and communication are needed to meet the medical, educational, and social and behavioral needs of children with health-related disorders. Hopefully, as you use this text, you will be energized to work toward a more integrated and collaborative approach to identification, goal determination, intervention and accommodations, and progress monitoring. A more detailed discussion of coordinated care across disorders is provided in Chapter 2 by Forman et al.

RESOURCES

U.S. Department of Education. (2019). *A guide to the individualized education program.* https://www2.ed.gov/parents/needs/speced/iepguide/index.html

Office of Genomics and Precision Public Health. (2021). *Genetics basics.* Centers for Disease Control and Prevention. https://www.cdc.gov/genomics/about/basics.htm

Disability Rights Education & Defense Fund. (n.d.). *A comparison of ADA, IDEA, and Section 504.* https://dredf.org/legal-advocacy/laws/a-comparison-of-ada-idea-and-section-504/

Project Pencil. (2016). *Eight steps to success for teachers of children with chronic illness.* https://projectpencil.com/wp-content/uploads/2016/02/Project_PENCIL_Infographics_8_steps_Teachers.pdf

National Center for Chronic Disease Prevention and Health Promotion. (2022). *Supporting students with chronic health conditions in school-based OST programs.* Centers for Disease Control and Prevention. https://www.cdc.gov/healthyschools/managing_CHC_OST.htm

REFERENCES

American Academy of Pediatrics. (2016). *Percentage of U.S. children who have chronic health conditions on the rise.* Science Daily. https://www.sciencedaily.com/releases/2016/04/160430100357.htm

Americans With Disabilities Act of 1990, 42 U.S.C. § 12101 *et seq.* (1990). https://www.ada.gov/pubs/adastatute08.htm

Bai, G., Herten, M. H., Landgraf, J. M., Korfage, I. J., & Raat, H. (2017). Childhood chronic conditions and health-related quality of life: Findings from a large population-based study. *PLOS ONE, 12*(6), Article e0178539. https://doi.org/10.1371/journal.pone.0178539

Harris, M. S. (2009). School reintegration for children and adolescents with cancer: The role of school psychologists. *Psychology in the Schools, 46*(7), 579–592. https://doi.org/10.1002/pits.20399

Individuals With Disabilities Education Act, 20 U.S.C. § 1400–1415 (2004).

Katz, J., Rosenbloom, B. N., & Fashler, S. (2015). Chronic pain, psychopathology, and *DSM-5* somatic symptom disorder. *Canadian Journal of Psychiatry, 60*(4), 160–167. https://doi.org/10.1177/070674371506000402

Pan, P.-Y., & Bölte, S. (2020). The association between ADHD and physical health: A co-twin control study. *Scientific Reports, 10*(1), Article 22388. https://doi.org/10.1038/s41598-020-78627-1

Phelps, L. (Ed.). (1998). *Health-related disorders in children and adolescents: A guidebook for understanding and educating*. American Psychological Association.

Power, T. J., DuPaul, G. J., Shapiro, E. S., & Kazak, A. E. (2003). *Promoting children's health: Integrating health, school, family, and community systems*. Guilford Press.

Root, M. M., Bray, M. A., Maykel, C., Cross, K., Shankar, N., & Theodore, L. (2016). Students with cancer: Presenting issues and effective solutions. *International Journal of School & Educational Psychology, 4*(1), 25–33. https://doi.org/10.1080/21683603.2016.1130549

Van Cleave, J., Gortmaker, S. L., & Perrin, J. M. (2010). Dynamics of obesity and chronic health conditions among children and youth. *JAMA, 303*(7), 623–630. https://doi.org/10.1001/jama.2010.104

2

Importance of Coordinated Care in Meeting the Needs of Children and Families

Susan G. Forman, Melissa C. Fleuhr, Sade S. Porter, and Jeffrey D. Shahidullah

The provision of social, educational, behavioral health, and physical health services for medically involved children is largely fragmented and not coordinated across the service systems in which children interact—health care, school, and family/community systems (Kuo et al., 2018). Data from a national survey of children's health (Brown et al., 2014) indicated that 41.2% of parents reported having an unmet need for coordinated care of their child's health-related disorder. Further, higher risk for unmet need for coordinated care was associated with having an anxiety disorder, higher parenting stress, lower income, and public or no health insurance.

Information on child and adolescent physical and behavioral health problems has substantially increased in scope and complexity, making it difficult for an individual provider to have all the knowledge needed to diagnose and manage all physical and behavioral health conditions. Adding to this complexity, many children and adolescents have comorbid conditions, increasing the information needed for accurate diagnosis and effective treatment. Many pediatric behavioral health conditions, such as autism spectrum disorder and attention-deficit/hyperactivity disorder, have physical concomitants and consequences. Physical illness can affect school attendance; academic achievement; and relationships with peers, teachers, and family members (Forman & Shahidullah, 2018). Approximately 65% of children with chronic medical conditions have been found to have a clinically significant or diagnosed behavioral health disorder (Glassgow et al., 2018). Thus, assessment of psychosocial functioning is important for the provision of high-quality physical health care, and tracking of

https://doi.org/10.1037/0000349-002
Health-Related Disorders in Children and Adolescents: A Guidebook for Educators and Service Providers, Second Edition, M. M. Perfect, C. A. Riccio, and M. A. Bray (Editors)

physical health is important as part of provision of behavioral health services. Chronic health conditions are increasing in incidence (Perrin et al., 2014) and require long-term services that are also complex and multifaceted.

Monitoring treatment effectiveness is essential in high-quality health care provision and can best be accomplished through coordinated care. Assessment of treatment adherence and progress monitoring toward treatment goals is typically related to child or adolescent functioning in multiple settings, including school and home, indicating the importance of observation and evaluation by parents and multiple professionals in these various settings (Compton et al., 2010).

Health care access patterns indicate that children and adolescents receive care through a number of systems, including primary care practices, subspecialty medical clinics, mental health specialty clinics, schools, and other local and regional organizations that may provide services for special populations (Polaha et al., 2011; Rones & Hoagwood, 2000). Sometimes access patterns are related to the availability of professionals in the community, whereas other times these patterns are related to ease-of-access issues (e.g., transportation, office or service hours, cultural compatibility).

COORDINATION AND BEYOND: DEFINITION

Asarnow and colleagues (2017) described a continuum of collaboration from *coordinated care*, in which professionals practice separately but exchange information, to *collaborative care* based on the chronic care model, in which there is a partnership between behavioral health and primary care clinicians, patients, and families using a shared treatment plan and a care manager and psychiatric consultant are incorporated as part of the health care team. A distinction also has been made between the definitions of communication and collaboration. *Communication* refers to a one-time, unidirectional sharing of information. *Collaboration*, on the other hand, consists of many people working together in an ongoing manner to plan and problem solve to promote positive patient outcomes (Bradley-Klug et al., 2010).

Provision of collaborative care is based on five principles (Ratzliffe et al., 2016). Care is *patient centered*, with providers using a shared care plan. It is *population based;* patients receive care preventively, proactively, and with tracking. Care is *evidence based*, including both psychosocial and medical treatment. Care is *measurement based*, with tracking of treatment effectiveness informing treatment adjustments. Care is *accountable*, with specified treatment targets for patients and use of quality improvement methods to improve health care team functioning (Ratzliffe et al., 2016).

CURRENT STATUS OF COORDINATED AND COLLABORATIVE CARE

Despite the prevalence of comorbid physical and mental health problems, most pediatric generalists and subspecialists do not routinely inquire about, screen for, or refer for most psychosocial concerns (Green et al., 2019; Williams et al., 2005), and they provide information to mental health providers on referred patients less than half the time (Ross et al., 2011).

Primary care is the setting in which children and families typically first present with behavioral, developmental, or emotional concerns, and parents generally view the primary care physician (PCP) as the most common source of assistance for these concerns (Polaha et al., 2011). At the same time, PCPs report a number of barriers that limit their ability to manage behavioral health concerns, including lack of time; problems with reimbursement for these services; lack of training, knowledge, and confidence related to psychosocial issues; and lack of access to specialty mental health clinicians for referral (Horwitz et al., 2015). The school setting also has the potential to serve as a nexus for coordination of physical and behavioral health services. For a number of reasons (e.g., lack of trained personnel, organizational values emphasizing academic performance, Health Insurance Portability and Accountability Act, Family Educational Rights and Privacy Act), schools may lack the capacity to address student physical and behavioral health in a way that is coordinated with providers outside the school system. School personnel have reported problems with accessing pediatric professionals, having different views on child development than physicians, and not having time to engage in collaboration (Bradley-Klug et al., 2013). Likewise, pediatricians generally do not coordinate care with relevant school personnel, and training in school collaboration is not typically emphasized in their medical training (Shahidullah et al., 2019).

In response to federal health care reform and the need for practice redesign, a number of initiatives have developed to foster increased care coordination across systems, such as the integration of behavioral health services within primary care practice. The Patient Protection and Affordable Care Act (ACA) aimed to offer greater access to and better quality of health care by integrating existing systems and providers to deliver comprehensive care within the context of the patient-centered medical home (PCMH) model. The PCMH model emphasizes comprehensive primary care in which services are coordinated across a multidisciplinary health care team while emphasizing continuous communication and information transfer (Braddock et al., 2013). A growing body of research has demonstrated that integrated medical-behavioral care within primary care practices is effective in eliminating or reducing common access barriers, improving health outcomes, reducing health care costs, and enhancing the patient and families' experience of care (e.g., Asarnow et al., 2015; Richardson et al., 2017). An extension of the PCMH, the patient-centered medical home neighborhood (PCMH-N) is a framework that addresses collaboration between PCPs, specialty providers, and other professionals outside of the primary care practice who compose the health care and community service system. Core components of this model include bidirectional communication; consultation; information flow; and development of agreements on communication, coordination, and comanagement (Greene et al., 2016).

A number of other service delivery models have been developed that explicitly emphasize care coordination between the family, school, and primary care practices. The Family Check-Up (Dishion et al., 2014) model is a strengths-based and family-centered intervention that promotes early detection and evidence-based parent management training to prevent disruptive behavior problems. This brief intervention is designed for use within schools and early childhood programs (e.g., Head Start preschools), community mental health programs, and primary care practices. The Partnering to Achieve School Success (PASS; Power et al., 2014) model employs behavioral health clinicians and community partners within primary care practices to deliver brief and tailored interventions to address the unique challenges faced by low-income families when accessing evidence-based treatments. This multimodal treatment consists of evidence-based parenting practices and behavioral support strategies, collaborative care as it relates to conjunctive psychotropic medication, and teacher consultation within the school setting. The PASS model incorporates motivational interviewing during treatment sessions and in-between-session phone calls and problem solving to address barriers to care (Power et al., 2010).

Given the prevalence of comorbid behavioral health conditions in children with physical health disorders, providers and families need to coordinate care between the medical home and behavioral health specialists within the community. Due to the lack of access to child and adolescent psychiatrists, particularly in poor urban and rural underserved areas, a number of coordinated psychiatric service models (Massachusetts Child Psychiatry Access Project; Straus & Sarvet, 2014) and collaborative care models (Richardson et al., 2014) have been developed to improve levels of access, quality, and continuity of evidence-based care. The strength of the coordinated model is that it provides training and offsite consultation to increase the knowledge, skills, and confidence of primary care clinicians in managing psychotropic medications through case-based consultation. The strength of collaborative care models is that they build on coordinated models to include care managers who can provide brief, on-site behavioral health services and help PCPs manage administrative tasks such as administering, scoring, and documenting screening measures.

Borrowing from the idea of off-site behavioral health support in response to the current shortages of school-based professionals with expertise in mental health, an increasing number of programs enhance community capacity to deliver needed behavioral health care through coordination with school-based professionals. For example, a partnership between a public school system and a hospital resulted in the development of the Texas Child Health Access Through Telemedicine (TCHATT; Webb, 2020) program. This program was designed to deliver telemedicine services to public school students experiencing a mental health crisis. TCHATT clinicians and professionals work together to provide rapid assessment, triage, stabilization, and connection to community-based providers using a liaison system led by the on-site school counselor.

TEAMS AND COLLABORATION

Within and across child-serving organizations and systems, teams are vehicles for increasing health care coordination and interprofessional collaboration. Teams have been described as a way of organizing work so that more can be accomplished than by individuals (Bell et al., 2018), and *teamwork* has been defined as "the integration of individuals' efforts toward the accomplishment of a shared goal" (Mathieu et al., 2017, p. 458). The Institute of Medicine (2003) Committee on the Health Professions Education Summit identified the capacity to work in interdisciplinary teams as a core competency that all physical and behavioral health clinicians should possess to ensure continuous and reliable health care.

Effective team functioning in health care involves several strategies and behaviors, such as sharing health goals for the patient, clarifying roles and workflow, building trust among professionals, and strengthening communication. Teams must be successful at both taskwork and teamwork in order to be effective. Taskwork consists of the skills needed to accomplish specific work-related tasks, whereas teamwork consists of interrelated thoughts, feelings, and behaviors of team members that facilitate the coordinated functioning of the team (Driskell et al., 2018).

Professional associations have cited the importance of teamwork in improving health care quality, identifying core competencies that are necessary to support professional engagement in teamwork. The Interprofessional Education Collaborative (IPEC; 2016) identified four broad competency domains for health professionals: (a) working with individuals of other professions; (b) maintaining mutual respect and shared values; (c) using roles and knowledge of multiple professions to address health care of patients and populations; and (d) communicating in a manner that supports a team approach to prevention and treatment and applying relationship-building values and team dynamics principles to the planning, delivery, and evaluation of health care. These competencies are thought to provide the basis for collaboration between all health professionals, with the goal of positive outcomes in individual and population health.

METHODS OF INCREASING COORDINATION AND COLLABORATION

A number of methods support training and uptake of interprofessional collaborative practices and team-based care for professionals working with children with health-related disorders. The development of training competencies necessary for future health service professionals appropriately includes not only discipline-specific professional competencies but also interprofessional competencies that are transdisciplinary and applicable to any provider.

TeamSTEPPS (Agency for Healthcare Research and Quality, 2017) is an evidence-based team training program to improve communication and teamwork skills among professionals. The TeamSTEPPS program provides learning activities for trainees and practitioners, including communication skills, leadership skills, situation monitoring, and mutual support. It has been used across health care institutions and is customizable for use in other service sectors. TEACH Teamwork (Benishek et al., 2016) is a self-guided program for school-based professionals based on TeamSTEPPs.

CONCLUSION

Coordination and collaboration across disciplines and child-serving systems may reduce barriers to and increase the uptake of high-quality health care. Individual/relational factors and structural/organizational factors have been found to affect implementation of coordination and collaboration (Forman et al., 2018). Research is needed to identify evidence-based strategies for increasing coordination and collaboration across professionals and child-serving systems so that goals of improving the quality of individual care, the health of populations, and reducing care costs can be realized.

RESOURCES

Forman, S. G., & Shahidullah, J. D. (Eds.). (2018). *Handbook of pediatric behavioral healthcare: An interdisciplinary collaborative approach.* Springer. https://doi.org/10.1007/978-3-030-00791-1

American Psychological Association. (2015, September 17). *Psychologists in integrated health care: Pediatric primary care* [Video]. YouTube. https://www.youtube.com/watch?v=gd-4daXuTEQ

American Psychological Association. (2015, September 30). *Psychologists in integrated health care: Family medicine* [Video]. YouTube. https://www.youtube.com/watch?v=fH_s8VVJD1s

Agency for Healthcare Research and Quality. (2017). *TeamSTEPPS® 2.0.* https://www.ahrq.gov/teamstepps/about-teamstepps/index.html

American Psychological Association. (2015). *TEACH Teamwork: An evidence-based, self-guided program on how to work effectively in teams.* https://www.apa.org/education/k12/teach-teamwork

REFERENCES

Agency for Healthcare Research and Quality. (2017). *TeamSTEPPS® 2.0.* https://www.ahrq.gov/teamstepps/about-teamstepps/index.html

Asarnow, J. R., Kolko, D. J., Miranda, J., & Kazak, A. E. (2017). The pediatric patient-centered medical home: Innovative models for improving behavioral health. *American Psychologist, 72*(1), 13–27. https://doi.org/10.1037/a0040411

Asarnow, J. R., Rozenman, M., Wiblin, J., & Zeltzer, L. (2015). Integrated medical-behavioral care compared with usual primary care for child and adolescent behavioral health: A meta-analysis. *JAMA Pediatrics, 169*(10), 929–937. https://doi.org/10.1001/jamapediatrics.2015.1141

Bell, S. T., Brown, S. G., Colaneri, A., & Outland, N. (2018). Team composition and the ABCs of teamwork. *American Psychologist, 73*(4), 349–362. https://doi.org/10.1037/amp0000305

Benishek, L. E., Gregory, M. E., Hodges, K., Newell, M., Hughes, A. M., Marlow, S., Lacerenza, C., Rosenfield, S., & Salas, E. (2016). Bringing the science of team training to school-based teams. *Theory Into Practice, 55*(2), 112–119. https://doi.org/10.1080/00405841.2016.1148987

Braddock, C. H., III, Snyder, L., Neubauer, R. L., & Fischer, G. S. (2013). The patient-centered medical home: An ethical analysis of principles and practice. *Journal of General Internal Medicine, 28*(1), 141–146. https://doi.org/10.1007/s11606-012-2170-x

Bradley-Klug, K. L., Jeffries-DeLoatche, K. L., Walsh, A. S. J., Bateman, L. P., Nadeau, J., Powers, D. J., & Cunningham, J. (2013). School psychologists' perceptions of primary care partnerships: Implications for building the collaborative bridge. *Advances in School Mental Health Promotion, 6*(1), 51–67. https://doi.org/10.1080/1754730X.2012.760921

Bradley-Klug, K. L., Sundman, A. N., Nadeau, J., Cunningham, J., & Ogg, J. (2010). Communication and collaboration with schools: Pediatricians' perspectives. *Journal of Applied School Psychology, 26*(4), 263–281. https://doi.org/10.1080/15377903.2010.518583

Brown, N. M., Green, J. C., Desai, M. M., Weitzman, C. C., & Rosenthal, M. S. (2014). Need and unmet need for care coordination among children with mental health conditions. *Pediatrics, 133*(3), e530–e537. https://doi.org/10.1542/peds.2013-2590

Compton, S. N., Walkup, J. T., Albano, A. M., Piacentini, J. C., Birmaher, B., Sherrill, J. T., Ginsburg, G. S., Rynn, M. A., McCracken, J. T., Waslick, B. D., Iyengar, S., Kendall, P. C., & March, J. S. (2010). Child/Adolescent Anxiety Multimodal Study (CAMS): Rationale, design, and methods. *Child and Adolescent Psychiatry and Mental Health, 4*(1), 1. https://doi.org/10.1186/1753-2000-4-1

Dishion, T. J., Brennan, L. M., Shaw, D. S., McEachern, A. D., Wilson, M. N., & Jo, B. (2014). Prevention of problem behavior through annual family check-ups in early childhood: Intervention effects from home to early elementary school. *Journal of Abnormal Child Psychology, 42*(3), 343–354. https://doi.org/10.1007/s10802-013-9768-2

Driskell, J. E., Salas, E., & Driskell, T. (2018). Foundations of teamwork and collaboration. *American Psychologist, 73*(4), 334–348. https://doi.org/10.1037/amp0000241

Family Educational Rights and Privacy Act of 1974, 34 C.F.R. § 99 (2009). https://www.govinfo.gov/app/details/FR-2008-12-09/E8-28864

Forman, S. G., Chaudhuri, A., & Barone, C. (2018). Interprofessional collaboration. In S. G. Forman & J. D. Shahidullah (Eds.), *Handbook of pediatric behavioral healthcare: An interdisciplinary collaborative approach* (pp. 31–43). Springer.

Forman, S. G., & Shahidullah, J. D. (Eds.). (2018). *Handbook of pediatric behavioral healthcare: An interdisciplinary collaborative approach.* Springer. https://doi.org/10.1007/978-3-030-00791-1

Glassgow, A. E., Gerges, M., Martin, M. A., Estrada, I., Issa, Z., Lapin, K., Morell, L., Solis, N., Van Voorhees, B., & Risser, H. J. (2018). Integration of mental health services into an innovative health care delivery model for children with chronic conditions. *Children and Youth Services Review, 95*, 144–151. https://doi.org/10.1016/j.childyouth.2018.10.023

Green, C., Stein, R. E. K., Storfer-Isser, A., Garner, A. S., Kerker, B. D., Szilagyi, M., Hoagwood, K. E., & Horwitz, S. M. (2019). Do subspecialists ask about and refer families with psychosocial concerns? A comparison with general pediatricians. *Maternal and Child Health Journal, 23*(1), 61–71. https://doi.org/10.1007/s10995-018-2594-y

Greene, C. A., Ford, J. D., Ward-Zimmerman, B., Honigfeld, L., & Pidano, A. E. (2016). Strengthening the coordination of pediatric mental health and medical care: Piloting a collaborative model for freestanding practices. *Child and Youth Care Forum, 45*(5), 729–744. https://doi.org/10.1007/s10566-016-9354-1

Health Insurance Portability and Accountability Act of 1996, Pub. L. No. 104-191, 100 Stat. 2548 (1996). https://www.govinfo.gov/app/details/PLAW-104publ191

Horwitz, S. M., Storfer-Isser, A., Kerker, B. D., Szilagyi, M., Garner, A., O'Connor, K. G., Hoagwood, K. E., & Stein, R. E. (2015). Barriers to the identification and management of psychosocial problems: Changes from 2004 to 2013. *Academic Pediatrics, 15*(6), 613–620. https://doi.org/10.1016/j.acap.2015.08.006

Institute of Medicine. (2003). *Health professions education: A bridge to quality*. National Academies Press.

Interprofessional Education Collaborative. (2016). *Core competencies for interprofessional collaborative practice: Report of an expert panel.*

Kuo, D. Z., McAllister, J. W., Rossignol, L., Turchi, R. M., & Stille, C. J. (2018). Care coordination for children with medical complexity: Whose care is it, anyway? *Pediatrics, 141*(Suppl. 3), S224–S232. https://doi.org/10.1542/peds.2017-1284G

Mathieu, J. E., Hollenbeck, J. R., van Knippenberg, D., & Ilgen, D. R. (2017). A century of work teams in the *Journal of Applied Psychology*. *Journal of Applied Psychology, 102*(3), 452–467. https://doi.org/10.1037/apl0000128

Perrin, J. M., Anderson, L. E., & Van Cleave, J. (2014). The rise in chronic conditions among infants, children, and youth can be met with continued health system innovations. *Health Affairs, 33*(12), 2099–2105. https://doi.org/10.1377/hlthaff.2014.0832

Polaha, J., Dalton, W. T., III, & Allen, S. (2011). The prevalence of emotional and behavior problems in pediatric primary care serving rural children. *Journal of Pediatric Psychology, 36*(6), 652–660. https://doi.org/10.1093/jpepsy/jsq116

Power, T. J., Hughes, C. L., Helwig, J. R., Nissley-Tsiopinis, J., Mautone, J. A., & Lavin, H. J. (2010). Getting to first base: Promoting engagement in family-school intervention for children with ADHD in urban, primary care practice. *School Mental Health, 2*(2), 52–61. https://doi.org/10.1007/s12310-010-9029-2

Power, T. J., Mautone, J. A., Marshall, S. A., Jones, H. A., Cacia, J., Tresco, K., Cassano, M. C., Jawad, A. F., Guevara, J. P., & Blum, N. J. (2014). Feasibility and potential effectiveness of integrated services for children with ADHD in urban primary care practices. *Clinical Practice in Pediatric Psychology, 2*(4), 412–426. https://doi.org/10.1037/cpp0000056

Ratzliff, A., Cerimele, J., Katon, W., & Unutzer, J. (2016). Using collaborative care to create effective mental and primary health care teams. In A. Ratzliff, J. Unutzer, W. Katon, & K. A. Stephens (Eds.), *Integrated care: Creating effective mental and primary health care teams* (pp. ix–xiv). Wiley.

Richardson, L. P., Ludman, E., McCauley, E., Lindenbaum, J., Larison, C., Zhou, C., Clarke, G., Brent, D., & Katon, W. (2014). Collaborative care for adolescents with depression in primary care: A randomized clinical trial. *JAMA, 312*(8), 809–816. https://doi.org/10.1001/jama.2014.9259

Richardson, L. P., McCarty, C. A., Radovic, A., & Suleiman, A. B. (2017). Research in the integration of behavioral health for adolescents and young adults in primary care settings: A systematic review. *Journal of Adolescent Health, 60*(3), 261–269. https://doi.org/10.1016/j.jadohealth.2016.11.013

Rones, M., & Hoagwood, K. (2000). School-based mental health services: A research review. *Clinical Child and Family Psychology Review, 3*(4), 223–241. https://doi.org/10.1023/A:1026425104386

Ross, W. J., Chan, E., Harris, S. K., Goldman, S. J., & Rappaport, L. A. (2011). Pediatrician-psychiatrist collaboration to care for children with attention deficit hyperactivity disorder, depression, and anxiety. *Clinical Pediatrics, 50*(1), 37–43. https://doi.org/10.1177/0009922810379499

Shahidullah, J. D., Forman, S. G., Palejwala, M. H., Shafrir, R., Barone, C., Pincus, L. E., Chaudhuri, A., & Lee, E. (2019). National survey of chief pediatric residents' attitudes, practices, and training in collaborating with schools. *Journal of Interprofessional Education & Practice, 15*, 82–87. https://doi.org/10.1016/j.xjep.2019.02.008

Straus, J. H., & Sarvet, B. (2014). Behavioral health care for children: The Massachusetts Child Psychiatry Access Project. *Health Affairs, 33*(12), 2153–2161. https://doi.org/10.1377/hlthaff.2014.0896

Webb, S. (2020, November 14). Houston teens have struggled to cope with COVID: A new state program aims to help. *Houston Chronicle*. https://www.houstonchronicle.com/news/houston-texas/houston/article/houston-teens-struggle-to-cope-with-covid-program-15725648.php

Williams, J., Palmes, G., Klinepeter, K., Pulley, A., & Foy, J. M. (2005). Referral by pediatricians of children with behavioral health disorders. *Clinical Pediatrics, 44*(4), 343–349. https://doi.org/10.1177/000992280504400410

II

BLOOD, CARDIOVASCULAR, AND CIRCULATORY SYSTEM DISORDERS

3

Overview of Circulatory System Disorders

Jeff Bostwick, Clark R. Bray, and Heather Kwolek

Blood, cardiovascular, and circulatory system (BCCS) disorders are a broad category of disorders affecting some of the most important systems in the body. These disorders range from genetic anomalies to structural problems that occur during development to acquired conditions later in life, and they can affect the body at the genetic, cellular, or system level. A few consistent themes emerge in looking at the effects of these disorders in children. Most children with BCCS disorder seem to be at higher potential risk for depression or anxiety, which can be common among children with any serious medical concern. Many of the disorders covered in this chapter can lead to a higher incidence of bleeding, bruising, or injury, indicating a greater need for physical supports for these children. Still, the wide range of possible symptoms and potential problems that children with BCCS disorders might experience speaks to the need for children with BCCS disorders to be treated on an individual basis. The life experience of any two given children with BCCS disorders may be as different as between a child with a BCCS disorder and one without.

BODY SYSTEM INVOLVEMENT AND FUNCTIONING

The circulatory system is composed of the heart, veins, arteries, and capillaries. It is responsible for the movement of nutrients and oxygen-rich blood throughout the body and the carrying of deoxygenated blood back to the lungs. The two subsections of the circulatory system are the *cardiovascular*, or blood-vascular,

https://doi.org/10.1037/0000349-003
Health-Related Disorders in Children and Adolescents: A Guidebook for Educators and Service Providers, Second Edition, M. M. Perfect, C. A. Riccio, and M. A. Bray (Editors)

system and the *lymph-vascular* system (Aaronson et al., 2020). The cardiovascular system is responsible for the circulation of blood, and the lymph-vascular system is responsible for the circulation of lymph throughout nodes, glands, and vessels. Lymph is used to filter toxins out of blood. The circulatory system is a highly regulated and finely tuned system, as it is responsible for the movement of hormones and other substances, and as such, minor blockages, interruptions, and diseases have the distinct ability to cause severe or even fatal issues, such as a myocardial infarction (heart attack) or transient ischemic attack (stroke; Lu et al., 2015). Some of the most common circulatory diseases in adults are high blood pressure, coronary artery disease, and chronic obstructive pulmonary disease (Lu et al., 2015). The most common heart diseases in children and adolescents are ventricular septal defects, tetralogy of Fallot, and transposition of the great arteries (Tom-Revzon, 2007). The common symptoms and complaints of those, regardless of age, with heart and circulatory diseases are shortness of breath; fatigue; weakness; swelling of legs, ankles, and feet; sweating; and reduced ability to exercise (World Health Organization, 2021).

COMMON COMPLAINTS AND INDICATORS OF DYSFUNCTION

BCCS disorders and their corresponding symptoms vary widely. However, some common themes may be found across these disorders. Blood disorders may be associated with excessive bruising, recurrent nosebleeds, anemia, shortness of breath, a fast heartbeat, fatigue, and chronic or recurring infections, depending on the aspect(s) of the blood (red blood cells, white blood cells, or platelets) that are most affected (Kuter, 2021). In some cases, as the disorder progresses, multiple parts of the blood will be affected and individuals may experience many of these symptoms. Common symptoms across cardiovascular and other circulatory disorders may include irregular heartbeat, heart murmurs, a fast or slow heartbeat, shortness of breath, skin discoloration (typically gray or blue) from hypoxic episodes, feeling lightheaded or dizzy, fatigue, and other circulatory challenges. Given the varied nature of the symptoms that may be experienced, it is important to speak to the individual to discover what symptoms they find most challenging and which they would most benefit from support for.

PREVIEW OF MAJOR BLOOD, CARDIOVASCULAR, AND CIRCULATORY SYSTEM CONDITIONS IN PEDIATRICS

Because of the diversity of symptoms that can be experienced across BCCS disorders, an understanding of the features of a child's particular disorder is crucial to providing appropriate supports for that child. The next several chapters, previewed here, detail the symptoms and effects of many of the most common childhood BCCS disorders.

Cardiac Disorders

Though various conditions fall under the label "cardiac disorders," the most common cardiac disorder affecting children is congenital heart disease. *Congenital heart disease* is an umbrella term for a wide variety of specific medical conditions, each of which has its own etiology, symptoms, and treatments. Congenital heart disease occurs when some aspect of the heart is not developed at birth, does not develop typically, is not formed typically, or otherwise does not function correctly. Effects on the child with congenital heart disease and their family change based on severity of the defect, necessary surgery and treatments, individual characteristics, and family resources, among other things. Nevertheless, most children with congenital heart disease survive and even thrive, able to engage in most activities other children their age do. Ehly and Estrada-Hernandez (Chapter 4) review the prevalence and incidence of congenital heart disease; the etiology and symptoms of the most common congenital heart defects; the medical, cognitive, and social–emotional impacts congenital heart disease has on students; and the broader psychosocial implications and their consequences for school-based supports for students.

Childhood Leukemia

Leukemia, a cancer wherein a person produces excessive white blood cells and is unable to protect themselves against diseases, is the most common type of cancer among children. Initially, children may experience very few symptoms, but as the leukemia progresses, they may experience unexplained flulike symptoms, more illnesses and infections than typical, and bleeding problems, among others. Modern treatment typically consists of chemotherapy, which has its own short-term and long-term effects that may substantially affect the child and must be taken into consideration when planning supports. Some adverse effects experienced by children with leukemia include neuropsychological deficits such as in executive functioning, reduced academic achievement, and increased social–emotional challenges. Theodore et al. (Chapter 5) quickly review the etiology, prevalence, and symptoms of leukemia, then examine the physical, cognitive, social–emotional, and behavioral impacts of the cancer and its treatment. They conclude with a review of principles guiding interventions and supports, especially within schools, for children with leukemia.

22q11.2 Deletion Syndrome

The most common of deletion syndromes, *22q11.2 syndrome* is the result of a deletion on chromosome 22. Due to variance in how the gene is specifically affected by the deletion, the syndrome is characterized by great variability in presenting symptoms. Common characteristics are specific facial features; palatal differences; medical challenges affecting, among others, the endocrine, immune, and cardiovascular systems; and psychiatric challenges. Diagnosis often occurs subsequent to identifying associated conditions, especially cardiac disease or neurological conditions such as epilepsy. Duong and Tanaka (Chapter 6) review the etiology and symptoms associated with 22q11.2 deletion syndrome before discussing its developmental impact and intervention considerations given the varied nature of the syndrome.

Hemophilia

Hemophilia (sometimes also spelled haemophilia) is a clotting disorder characterized by below-normal levels of a specific clotting protein (or *factor*) in the blood. The primary symptom of hemophilia is increased bleeding, particularly internal bleeding into joints. This bleeding often results in pain and loss of joint mobility and is usually treated through applying ice and compression to the area. Hemophilia (particularly more severe versions) is often treated preventatively through routine treatment to replace the missing clotting factor.

Though hemophilia does not typically have a direct impact on scholastic performance, it can have indirect impacts. Treatment for hemophilia can be prohibitively expensive, bleeding episodes can result in missed classes or social events, and the stigma of having a bleeding disorder and being treated as different can result in social challenges as well. In Chapter 7, Randolph and Schilling provide more depth about these potential challenges as well as some discussion of the broader social and educational implications of living with hemophilia.

Human Immunodeficiency Virus

The *human immunodeficiency virus* (HIV) is an infection of the CD4-T cells in the body's immune system and is responsible for acquired immune deficiency syndrome (AIDS). HIV can live in the body for years before progressing to AIDS, though the timeline for this progression varies based on treatment and management of the virus. Because of its impact on the central nervous system, children with HIV can experience some developmental delays (particularly children who acquire HIV in utero via mother-to-child transmission); however, children may also present as asymptomatic and with few differences from their peers.

Chenneville and Gabbidon (Chapter 8) detail the range of impacts of HIV and AIDS on childhood and education, as well as describing the ways in which appropriate management of the disease can reduce these impacts. They also include statistics on prevalence across a variety of demographics and suggestions for ways to support children with HIV/AIDS in social, cognitive, academic, and behavioral domains.

Noonan Syndrome

Noonan syndrome is a common genetic disorder that results in abnormal development of various parts of the body due to an inherited genetic mutation. Approximately one in every 1,000 to 2,500 people are born with Noonan syndrome. The developmental abnormalities associated with it include deviations in facial features such as wide-set eyes, cardiovascular issues such as congenital heart disease or valve disorders, growth issues, and learning disabilities. Although there is no cure for Noonan syndrome, advanced medical care is available that can be successfully applied to almost all the related impairments. For example, individuals with Noonan syndrome may undergo surgery to repair heart valves, may take medications to prevent cardiovascular issues from progressing, and may be prescribed growth hormones for slow growth rate. Children with Noonan syndrome have been observed to exhibit some social–emotional behavioral concerns. However, when compared with peers, their mental health functioning is similar, whereas their cognitive and learning problems are more pronounced. Thus, students with Noonan syndrome may reach developmental milestones and achievements later than their peers and most likely will require special education services. Margiano et al. (Chapter 9) cover some implications for children with Noonan syndrome and discuss some school-based interventions and management.

Sickle Cell Anemia

Sickle cell anemia is a hereditary blood disorder where the affected individual's red blood cells are malformed and appear as sickles or crescent moons rather than the typical oval shape. This malformation is due to an abnormality in hemoglobin, a protein found in red blood cells that facilitates the carrying of oxygen throughout the circulatory system. The hemoglobin abnormality can lead to anemia, a lack of healthy red blood cells to carry enough oxygen around the body. Further, the sickle-shaped cells are prone to creating blockages in small blood vessels due to their shape and rigidity.

Morse et al. (Chapter 10) describe sickle cell anemia in more depth and discuss several issues that can affect children with this disorder. For instance, children with sickle cell anemia can also exhibit poor academic achievement that is related to increased absenteeism relative to their peers. They are also more likely to experience restrictions in physical activity, which contributes to increases in anxiety and depression related specifically to academic settings.

HEALTH CARE NEEDS AND MEDICAL SPECIALTIES

The needs of children with BCCS disorders are quite varied. Some such disorders (e.g., hemophilia, HIV/AIDS, leukemia) primarily affect children by interfering with physical activity and require support related principally to increased absenteeism, whereas other disorders (e.g., 22q11.2 deletion syndrome, Noonan syndrome) are more likely to cause a wide array of physical and developmental symptoms, requiring more intensive or varied support. Additionally, due to the potentially severe nature of many BCCS disorders, children with these disorders may be at increased risk for developing anxiety or depression related to their disorder. The diversity of possible concerns for children with BCCS disorders highlights the importance of a highly individualized, team approach to care and support. Children with BCCS disorders are best treated by specialists in their specific disorder or disorders (usually hematologists or cardiovascular pediatric specialists) as well as professionals in related areas, including mental health professionals.

REFERENCES

Aaronson, P. I., Ward, J. P., & Connolly, M. J. (2020). *The cardiovascular system at a glance.* John Wiley & Sons.

Kuter, D. J. (2021). Symptoms of blood disorders. In S. Falk, J. L. Kaplan, R. B. Lynn, and E. Yeh (Eds.), *Merck manual for the consumer.* https://www.merckmanuals.com/home/blood-disorders/symptoms-and-diagnosis-of-blood-disorders/symptoms-of-blood-disorders

Lu, L., Liu, M., Sun, R., Zheng, Y., & Zhang, P. (2015). Myocardial infarction: Symptoms and treatments. *Cell Biochemistry and Biophysics, 72*(3), 865–867. https://doi.org/10.1007/s12013-015-0553-4

Tom-Revzon, C. (2007). Cardiovascular diseases in children. *U.S. Pharmacist, 32*(3), 52–65.

World Health Organization. (2021, June 11). *Cardiovascular diseases (CVDs).* https://www.who.int/news-room/fact-sheets/detail/cardiovascular-diseases-(cvds)

4

Cardiac Disorders

Stewart W. Ehly and Noel Estrada-Hernandez

In the 25 years since the first edition of this book was published, options have expanded for care of children with pediatric cardiology disorders. Even in 2010, Kuch and Orr noted that "advances in cardiology, intensive care, and surgical treatment have led to the survival of children with previously lethal congenital cardiac defects" (p. 13). Success in addressing these defects continues to advance.

PREVALENCE AND INCIDENCE

Children are affected by cardiac disorders in many ways. In the United States, the chance of having a child with a heart defect is approximately one in 100 (Khoshnood et al., 2012). Using data from 2010, Gilboa et al. (2016) estimated that 1 million children live with congenital heart defects in the United States. Congenital heart disease (Jerves et al., 2020) is the most common congenital defect worldwide (8.2/1,000 live births), yet 70% to 90% of these cases are of an unknown underlying etiology.

Congenital abnormalities become obvious in several ways to alert caregivers and physicians to the potential for problems. In previous decades, surgical intervention was often attempted only in older children who had survived the first few years of childhood. Increasingly, with advances in care, earlier interventions have become possible. Triedman and Newburger (2016) argued that although many challenges in the care of infants and children with congenital

https://doi.org/10.1037/0000349-004
Health-Related Disorders in Children and Adolescents: A Guidebook for Educators and Service Providers, Second Edition, M. M. Perfect, C. A. Riccio, and M. A. Bray (Editors)

heart disease exist, accurate diagnosis and effective treatment of even the most complex congenital heart lesions have become standard practice.

Parents often ask pediatricians for information on symptoms related to heart problems. The Children's Hospital of Philadelphia provides a standard symptom list to guide parents toward medical attention (see the link in the Resources section). Infants may have trouble breathing during feeding, display blue gums or tongue, and even pass out. Older toddlers and young children may struggle during activities and easily get out of breath or sweaty. Teens may continue to struggle with activities and have heart palpitations or dizziness and chest pain. All symptoms are of potential concern and should motivate the parent to seek medical attention.

CONDITIONS ASSOCIATED WITH CONGENITAL HEART DISEASE: ETIOLOGY AND SYMPTOMS

The heart is a muscular pump that is responsible for circulating blood. The right and left sides of the organ are separate functional units, each consisting of a filling chamber (atrium) and a much thicker ventricle. The right side receives deoxygenated venous blood returning from the tissues and pumps it into the lungs by the pulmonary arteries. The blood then returns to the left side and is pumped by the left ventricle into the tissues, transported by the aorta and arteries. The category of *cardiac disorders* includes congenital (inborn) lesions, the primary focus of this chapter.

A number of conditions are present in patients with congenital heart disease. Listed are those defects commonly reported for the population of pediatric heart patients. (For extensive documentation on all listed defects, see Allen et al., 2013; Munoz et al., 2010.) Overall, the more severe the impact of the condition at birth, the more critical immediate care is. Although surgical success continues to increase in cardiac care, survival of the individual will depend on the severity of the condition and the level of medical attention that is provided.

Atrial septal defect is a congenital condition that involves a hole in the wall between the two upper chambers of the heart. Small defects may cause no problems, but larger defects can produce damage in the heart and lungs. Openings in the atrial septum at any of three locations can affect the flow of oxygenated blood in the heart. The majority of patients are asymptomatic, although infants will be affected. Without surgical intervention, life expectancy in some patients will be affected; surgery can perform closure of the defect. Operative risk is low, and life expectancy remains normal.

Atrioventricular canal defect is a combination of issues that can produce a defect in the center of the heart organ. The condition is congenital and is associated in many cases with Down syndrome. The defect affects the lungs due to extra blood flowing to them from the heart. Surgery during a child's 1st year may be recommended to repair the defect. Untreated cases can lead to heart failure.

Bicuspid aortic valve is a condition (which can be inherited) associated with a child being born with one less cusp to the aortic valve. This results in narrowing of the aortic valve and reduces the flow of blood from the heart to the body. Other risks may be associated with the condition. A heart murmur may indicate a bicuspid aortic valve. There are multiple surgical options available to treat the condition.

Coarctation of the aorta is the narrowing of the aorta, which can force the heart to pump harder to distribute blood. The condition is generally present at birth, can range from mild to severe, and is often associated with other heart defects. Treatment is generally successful but involves lifelong attention by medical professionals.

Congenital mitral valve anomalies are congenital defects that affect the mitral valve in the heart. Several types exist and can cause problems in the heart's distribution of blood. Additional heart defects are often present. Surgical repair of the mitral valve or replacement of the valve are options. Lifelong care from medical professionals is typically required.

Double-outlet right ventricle is a congenital condition in which abnormal placement of the heart's arteries coincides with a hole between the lower heart chambers (see the discussion of ventricular septal defect). The result of this condition is that oxygen saturations are lower than normal and too much blood may be delivered to the lungs, causing heart failure and growth problems. Surgery early in a child's life may be required.

Ebstein anomaly is a rare congenital condition in which the tricuspid valve does not function correctly. Blood may leak through the valve, affecting functioning. Treatment options include medication and surgery.

Eisenmenger syndrome is a congenital defect that causes a hole between the heart chambers. Problems associated with blood flood can develop and become a life-threatening condition. Treatment procedures, including surgery, are available.

Hypoplastic left heart syndrome is a rare congenital defect in which the left side of the heart does not develop normally. Medication, surgery, and even transplants can be required to address the condition. A mother is at higher risk of having other children with similar or related conditions. Genetic counseling is available.

Kawasaki disease is a condition that affects children, most of whom recover. The disease involves inflammation of the walls of arteries throughout the body and can affect the supply of blood to the heart. The condition is often treatable, especially if a cardiac specialist begins intervention early after onset.

Long QT syndrome is a condition that can involve rapid and irregular heartbeats that can trigger fainting spells and seizures. Due to potential sudden death, treatment is important, generally via medication.

Partial anomalous pulmonary venous return is a congenital defect in which blood from the lungs flows to an incorrect location in the heart. The defect involves some of the pulmonary veins incorrectly being attached to the heart or blood vessels. Treatment, if recommended, can involve surgery. Children will need regular follow-ups to monitor the condition.

Patent ductus arteriosus is a condition that involves an opening between the major blood vessels from the heart. If the opening remains, treatment may be indicated. The goal is to support the flow of blood so that weakening of heart muscles does not occur. Treatment can be provided by medication, catherization, and surgery.

Patent foramen ovale is a hole in the heart at birth that remains open. The condition occurs in 25% of the normal population without complication. Complications, although generally not noticed, can develop over time.

Pulmonary atresia is a congenital defect that is usually diagnosed soon after birth. The valve that pumps blood to the lungs does not form correctly and creates a life-threatening condition. Surgical intervention may be available, with long-term attention to the child's care being necessary. Reducing the potential of the condition centers on recommendations for prenatal care.

Pulmonary atresia with intact ventricular septum and *pulmonary atresia with ventricular septum defect* are conditions typically found at birth with the discovery of heart valve defects. Surgical options are available.

Pulmonary valve stenosis is a condition on or near the valve that affects blood flow. The condition ranges from mild to severe with problems requiring surgery (usually very successful). Severe cases are treated at infancy; all other cases generally are treated with surgery when the child is older.

Tetralogy of Fallot is a rare congenital condition that is caused by four heart defects. A combination of four specific defects in the heart produces obstructions to the flow of blood. Symptoms can include failure to thrive, cyanosis (due to an increased concentration of reduced hemoglobin in capillary circulation), and hypoxic episodes (lack of oxygen supply) that increase in frequency over time, producing death in some cases. Diagnosis is generally early in infancy. Surgical intervention followed by long-term medical care often has very positive results.

Total anomalous pulmonary venous return is a congenital condition that involves incorrect placement of blood vessels between the lungs and heart. Blood flow may be reduced or blocked. Surgical treatment of the young child with routine follow-up will produce benefits to development.

Transposition of the great arteries is a rare congenital defect in which the two main arteries that leave the heart are reversed, which changes the circulation of blood through the body. The defect can be noted prenatally or soon after birth. Corrective surgery is very beneficial, with good long-term results.

Tricuspid atresia is a congenital heart defect in which the tricuspid valve between the two heart chambers does not form, which dramatically affects oxygen throughout the body. Prognosis for an infant will vary, depending on the underlying defects and the degree of pulmonary blood flow. Multiple surgeries are required throughout the lifespan, with routine medical monitoring of the patient's general condition.

Truncus arteriosis is a rare congenital defect in which one blood vessel rather than two blood vessels leads from the heart. A hole between the two lower chambers of the heart usually develops. The result is severe circulatory problems. Surgery is generally successful and often conducted while the infant is young. Because potential complications later in life are not unusual, routine medical attention is important.

Vascular rings, usually present at birth, involve malformation of the aortic arch in the main blood vessel from the heart. Other defects may be present. Surgery can treat the rings to avoid complications. Long-term monitoring and support can be required, with special attention to pulmonary and digestive problems.

Ventricular septal defect (VSD) is a common congenital defect involving a hole in the heart, which causes the heart to pump harder than normal. An opening in the ventricular (lower chamber) septum (dividing wall or partition), VSD can take one of four forms depending on the location of the opening. The majority of defects close before 2 years of age, although some will close as late as 7 years of age. Larger holes may require surgical attention. The defect can run in families and may occur with other genetic conditions.

Wolff-Parkinson-White syndrome is a rare condition, present at birth, in which a rapid heartbeat is caused by an extra electrical pathway within the heart. Although the condition is generally not life threatening, ablation can be used to correct problems in heart rhythm.

IMPACT ON THE STUDENT AND OUTCOMES

Medical

Chronic conditions, like congenital heart diseases, are a common experience for many individuals at different developmental stages. These conditions have the potential to affect one's physical, psychological, educational, vocational, social, and economic functioning (Falvo, 2018). The effects of such conditions are dependent on various aspects of the individual, including but not limited to type and time of diagnosis; whether the condition had been acquired or congenital; gender, age, and family of origin; and other environmental factors and resources. These factors are important in shaping the psychosocial experience of the individual and the road to adjustment and development of the disability identity.

Cognitive/Academic

A number of studies have explored the direct effects of congenital heart disease conditions in the cognitive development of children and adolescents. As noted earlier, studies have produced mixed and inconclusive results (Karsdorp et al., 2007). Some results have suggested that individuals with more severe forms of congenital heart diseases are likely to experience lower levels of cognitive functioning compared with those individuals with less severe forms of similar conditions. Moreover, studies suggest that specifically the areas of verbal IQ (e.g., comprehensive skills) and performance IQ (e.g., an individual's organizational, visualization, and perceptual skills) are affected differently in children across developmental stages. Although research findings presented in this review are not conclusive, they do provide an avenue for the consideration of potential supports for children who are diagnosed with such conditions.

Social-Emotional and Behavioral

Cardiac conditions, especially in children, also have an effect on the family structure and all its members. Research has documented the experiences of parents and siblings in relation to the diagnosis of one of their members' chronic illness. These reactions include but are not limited to shock, mourning, withdrawal from larger family, anxiety, marital distress, economic issues, uncertainty about the future, and concerns related to adequate health care and the competence of the physicians (Ehly, 1998; Seligman, 1993; Smart, 2009). In addition, siblings may experience additional feelings such as abandonment or may resent the extra attention their sibling receives from parents in terms of appointments and care. Many of these reactions are related to the developmental stage of the child who is experiencing the condition. The earlier the developmental stage (e.g., infant, toddler, early childhood), the more likely these sibling reactions are to be experienced. As the individual develops (e.g., early adolescence) and becomes more active in their own care, these feelings are expected to reduce.

Most children with congenital heart diseases are able to be fully active and experience many of the traditional landmarks of human growth and development. Once the medical condition experienced by the child is stabilized, the goal of any intervention is to facilitate or enhance the *quality of life* (QOL). QOL is defined as the individual's conceptualization of their physical, emotional, educational, and social well-being. In other words, QOL is a personal indicator of one's life satisfaction in relation to overall health (Areias et al., 2013).

PSYCHOEDUCATIONAL IMPLICATIONS AND SCHOOL-BASED INTERVENTIONS

Medical and Health Management

As children transition to adolescence and adulthood, some researchers have proposed the development of health-transition programs (Sable et al., 2011). Such programs can provide age-appropriate health education and can help children to develop skills in communication, decision making, self-advocacy, self-care, and empowerment. The goal of such programs is to increase health care participation and overall QOL for these individuals. Overall services and support that are provided to the individual and the family system should monitor and address physical health (e.g., care, puberty); relationships, including family and friends; emotional support (e.g., self-regulation of feelings and emotions related to health condition); development of an appropriate educational and vocational plan, including career selection that considers impact of congenital heart disease; and other personal factors (e.g., appropriate health routine, including exercise, sex role development, independence). As noted earlier, the main goal is to provide support to the individual in a manner that they can effectively manage and successfully increase QOL issues.

Social-Emotional and Behavioral

Researchers have explored the many factors that aid in the adjustment to chronic illness and that improve QOL across the different developmental stages (Falvo, 2018; Smart, 2009). For most children with congenital heart diseases, problems become more apparent when children enter school and are expected to be active physically, perform academically, and have good social relations. For some children, the experience does not normalize (SickKids, 2009). The concern, of course, is that these problems will be internalized and will influence how children live their lives, how they socialize, and how well they cope over time. Researchers have debated, with mixed results and nondefinitive conclusions, whether children who are diagnosed experience psychosocial challenges based on symptoms associated with their cognitive and psychological functioning (Karsdorp et al., 2007). The hypothesis is that these children may develop psychopathology, anxiety, depression, and behavioral problems that interfere with educational attainment and overall QOL factors. Other studies have suggested that severity of the cardiac condition and number of surgeries are factors that will also have an effect on the individual's cognitive and psychological outlook (Areias et al., 2013).

For some children with congenital heart diseases, the experience causes lasting distress. Past experiences, frequent medical appointments, surgeries, and treatment have made children aware of how different their life is. Awareness of physical restrictions, for instance, may produce feelings of isolation, anxiety, internalized feelings (sometimes aggressive), and depression in a child, especially in older children (Karsdorp et al., 2007) who associate playing sports with the most effective way of fitting into a social environment. Such a reaction is important to consider because during most of the early years in school, the feeling of belongingness is based on active play and socialization. Researchers (e.g., Falvo, 2018) have noted that cardiovascular patients might experience symptoms related to posttraumatic stress disorder. Symptoms include intense fear (e.g., of death), sense of loss of control, and nightmares. Any of these symptoms can have a profound effect on the development of emotional and social well-being of the child.

CONCLUSION

The experience of having a chronic illness as a child can cause distress and difficulty. As the child walks through the different developmental stages, it is necessary that supports are provided in the areas of personal care (e.g., learning about things that the child can and cannot do); education (e.g., identifying any potential supports needed to enhance educational attainment); and relationships, including family and friends. In many cases, it is necessary to provide individual emotional support. The goal is to allow the child to express, recognize, and manage the emotional consequences of having a cardiovascular disease.

In early stages of development, it is also important to provide support to the parental system because they are the main source of support to the child. Parental health education, counseling, or guidance will provide good grounds to explore feelings, emotions, and expectations of their child. Within this network of services, parents need to become aware of all necessary supports to address the education, health (including mental health), vocational, and social future needs of the child. When necessary, it is important that parents participate in individual or couples therapy to address any distress that may have an effect in the family system. The overall goal is to instill hope in the parents.

RESOURCES

Children's Hospital of Philadelphia. (n.d.). *Symptoms that might indicate a heart problem.* https://www.chop.edu/conditions-diseases/symptoms-might-indicate-heart-problem

School-Based Health Alliance. (n.d.). *School-based health center playbook on health care transition.* https://tools.sbh4all.org/health-care-transition/health-care-transition-home/

REFERENCES

Allen, H. D., Driscoll, D. J., Shaddy, R. E., & Feltes, T. F. (2013). *Moss and Adam's heart disease in infants, children, and adolescents: Including the fetus and young adult* (8th ed.). Wolters Kluwer.

Areias, M. E. G., Pinto, C. I., Vieira, P. F., Teixeira, F., Coelho, R., Freitas, I., Matos, S., Castro, M., Sarmento, S., Viana, V., Quintas, J., & Areias, J. C. (2013). Long term psychosocial outcomes of congenital heart disease (CHD) in adolescents and young adults. *Translational Pediatrics, 2*(3), 90–98. https://doi.org/10.3978/j.issn.2224-4336.2013.06.02

Ehly, S. W. (1998). Cardiovascular disorders. In L. Phelps (Ed.), *Health-related disorders in children and adolescents: A guidebook for understanding and educating* (pp. 121–130). American Psychological Association. https://doi.org/10.1037/10300-017

Falvo, D. R. (2018). *Medical and psychosocial aspects of chronic illness and disability* (6th ed.). Jones and Bartlett.

Gilboa, S. M., Devine, O. J., Kucik, J. E., Oster, M. E., Riehle-Colarusso, T., Nembhard, W. N., Xu, P., Correa, A., Jenkins, K., & Marelli, A. J. (2016). Congenital heart defects in the United States: Estimating the magnitude of the affected population in 2010. *Circulation, 134*(2), 101–109. https://doi.org/10.1161/CIRCULATIONAHA.115.019307

Jerves, T., Beaton, A., & Kruszka, P. (2020). The genetic workup for structural congenital heart disease. *American Journal of Medical Genetics: Part C, Seminars in Medical Genetics, 184*(1), 178–186. https://doi.org/10.1002/ajmg.c.31759

Karsdorp, P. A., Everaerd, W., Kindt, M., & Mulder, B. J. M. (2007). Psychological and cognitive functioning in children and adolescents with congenital heart disease: A meta-analysis. *Journal of Pediatric Psychology, 32*(5), 527–541. https://doi.org/10.1093/jpepsy/jsl047

Khoshnood, B., Lelong, N., Houyel, L., Thieulin, A.-C., Jouannic, J.-M., Magnier, S., Delezoide, A.-L., Magny, J.-F., Rambaud, C., Bonnet, D., Goffinet, F., & the EPICARD Study Group. (2012). Prevalence, timing of diagnosis and mortality of newborns with congenital heart defects: A population-based study. *Heart, 98*(22), 1667–1673. https://doi.org/10.1136/heartjnl-2012-302543

Kuch, B. A., & Orr, R. A. (2010). Triage and transport of infants and children with cardiac disease. In R. A. Munoz, V. O. Morell, E. M. da Cruz, & C. G. Vetterly (Eds.), *Critical care of children with heart disease: Basic medical and surgical concepts* (pp. 13–22). Springer.

Munoz, R. A., Morell, V. O., da Cruz, E. M., & Vetterly, C. G. (Eds.). (2010). *Critical care of children with heart disease: Basic medical and surgical concepts*. Springer

Sable, C., Foster, E., Uzark, K., Bjornsen, K., Canobbio, M. M., Connolly, H. M., Graham, T. P., Gurvitz, M. Z., Kovacs, A., Meadows, A. K., Reid, G. J., Reiss, J. G., Rosenbaum, K. N., Sagerman, P. J., Saidi, A., Schonberg, R., Shah, S., Tong, E., & Williams, R. G. (2011). Best practices in managing transition to adulthood for adolescents with congenital heart disease: The transition process and medical and psychosocial issues: A scientific statement from the American Heart Association. *Circulation, 123*(13), 1454–1485. https://doi.org/10.1161/CIR.0b013e3182107c56

Seligman, M. (1993). Group work with parents of children with disabilities. *Journal for Specialists in Group Work, 18*(3), 115–126. https://doi.org/10.1080/01933929308413745

SickKids. (2009, December 14). *Social and emotional effects for children with heart disease*. AboutKidsHealth. https://www.aboutkidshealth.ca/Article?contentid=1704&language=English

Smart, J. (2009). *Disability, society, and the individual* (2nd ed.). Pro-Ed.

Triedman, J. K., & Newburger, J. W. (2016). Trends in congenital heart disease: The next decade. *Circulation, 133*(25), 2716–2733. https://doi.org/10.1161/CIRCULATIONAHA.116.023544

5

Childhood Leukemia

Lea A. Theodore, Karen Cross, Lauren Gammie, Marlena L. Minkos, Danielle Stern, and Alyssa Perri Elias

Leukemia, the most common type of cancer among children and adolescents, is a cancer of the white blood cells. Children with a diagnosis of leukemia produce an excessive number of abnormal white blood cells that inundate the child's bloodstream, resulting in the body's inability to protect itself from disease. Leukemia may be classified as either acute or chronic. Acute leukemia, which is considered to be a rapidly developing cancer and the most common cancer among children, may be further divided to include acute lymphoblastic leukemia (ALL) and acute myeloid leukemia (AML), depending on whether lymphocytes or myelocytes are affected. ALL is most frequently diagnosed in children between the ages of 2 and 8 years, although it can be diagnosed at any age. Similarly, AML also can occur at any age but tends to be diagnosed prior to 2 years of age. Chronic leukemia is a slow-developing cancer (National Cancer Institute, 2018).

ETIOLOGY

It is generally accepted that leukemia develops as the result of genetic DNA mutations, causing the rapid development of abnormal cells. Most leukemias result from noninherited genetic mutations and typically develop randomly; however, children who have siblings or an identical twin are at greater risk for developing leukemia than are only children. Other risk factors for childhood leukemia include certain genetic disorders (i.e., Down syndrome, Klinefelter

https://doi.org/10.1037/0000349-005
Health-Related Disorders in Children and Adolescents: A Guidebook for Educators and Service Providers, Second Edition, M. M. Perfect, C. A. Riccio, and M. A. Bray (Editors)

syndrome); exposure to radiation or chemotherapy, perhaps due to previous cancer treatment; or being a recipient of organ transplantations that require medication to suppress the immune system (American Cancer Society, 2019b; Wiemels, 2012).

PREVALENCE AND INCIDENCE

Leukemia, regardless of type, comprises approximately 30% of all childhood cancers, with more than 3,000 children diagnosed each year (Whitehead et al., 2016). Over the past 40 years, there has been an increase of approximately 55% of children being diagnosed with this disorder (Whitehead et al., 2016). Notably, Latinx children experience a higher incidence of leukemia than Caucasians, African Americans, or Asian Americans (Metayer et al., 2016; Whitehead et al., 2016).

SYMPTOMS

Symptoms of leukemia are often insidious, with many children not evidencing any symptoms or warning signs during the early stages of cancer. However, parents should be alert to flulike symptoms, including night sweats, fatigue, and fever, that extend longer than a typical illness. Because children with leukemia have compromised immune systems, they are also at greater risk of infections. Moreover, as the disease advances, both red blood cells and platelets are affected, resulting in anemia and bleeding problems, such as recurrent nosebleeds. Symptoms associated with childhood leukemia include excessive fatigue, swollen lymph nodes, decreased appetite, fever, joint pain, headaches, seizures, coordination and gait issues, vision problems, and difficulty breathing (Barbel & Peterson, 2015).

IMPACT ON THE STUDENT AND OUTCOMES

Medical

Children being treated for leukemia experience both short- and long-term side effects. In the short term, children may lose their hair and experience nausea and vomiting, fatigue, pain, and skin rashes. Long-term side effects, also known as late effects, may occur once a child is in remission and is cancer-free. These effects are most often the result of the treatment, not the cancer. Approximately 70% of children develop late effect symptoms in addition to short-term effects (American Cancer Society, 2019a). The most common late effects experienced by children with leukemia include thyroid problems, typically hypothyroidism, as well as hearing loss, tinnitus, and dizziness. Children also may experience vision problems and dental issues, such as tooth decay and gum disease, and are at greater risk for organ damage to the lungs, liver, heart, and kidneys (Kaspers, 2012). Both chemotherapy and radiation may result in delayed sexual development and/or fertility issues. Given these reproductive risks, physicians often take special measures, such as banking sperm and eggs prior to treatment to ensure survivors have healthy children in the future (Hargreave et al., 2013). Finally, children with leukemia have an increased risk of developing a secondary cancer in the future (Metayer et al., 2016).

In light of the types of impairments evidenced by children with leukemia, psychologists have turned to more comprehensive neuropsychological assessment measures to assess late effects of central nervous system (CNS) chemotherapy treatments, which affect the brain and spinal cord. CNS chemotherapy involves the direct infusion of powerful medications into one's veins that are intended to kill rapidly growing cancer cells. Cancer cells grow and multiply quickly, and the dosage and frequency of chemotherapy are idiosyncratic, based on each child's individual circumstances. Thus, chemotherapy treatment varies; it could be weekly or there may be a break between chemotherapy sessions so that children and adolescents may recover from the adverse side effects. Treatment may be given in outpatient settings, in hospitals or doctor's offices, or at home if taking pills rather than having an infusion. Among children who receive CNS treatments, researchers report poorer performance on measures of attention, perceptual motor skills, and executive functions (Jacola et al., 2016). Although deficits in cognitive flexibility, inattention in conjunction with hyperactivity, and sluggish cognitive tempo may be subtle, neuropsychological deficits are known to contribute to poor academic performance and cannot be ignored.

Cognitive/Academic

As contemporary chemotherapy treatments have replaced cranial radiation therapy, fewer deficits on cognitive measures have been reported. However, findings remain mixed, with significant neurocognitive deficits occurring in 40% to 60% of patients, particularly in executive functioning (Moleski, 2000). Cognitively, children demonstrate deficits of 6 to 8 points on measures of intellectual functioning (Iyer et al., 2015). They also evidence memory impairments, decreased nonverbal skills, and impaired processing speed (Cheung et al., 2017; Jacola et al., 2016). Such deficits may limit a student's ability to efficiently and accurately retain and process information. Children with leukemia also may display impairment in executive functioning skills, including initiation, planning, and organization of tasks (Cheung et al., 2017). Notably, children also may evidence below-average fine motor skills, visuomotor integration, and verbal short-term memory. Impairments in overall cognitive ability, memory, processing speed, executive function, and fine motor skills in turn lead to lower academic achievement. Overall, academic achievement scores approximate one standard deviation lower for children with leukemia, which is the result of treatment and school absences. Mathematics deficits have been noted as a primary area of educational concern. Conklin et al. (2012) reported that as higher doses of CNS treatment are employed, children's reading and spelling scores are adversely affected. Furthermore, children who have received CNS chemotherapy or proton radiation therapy are significantly more likely to receive special education services and are less likely to graduate from high school (Bisen-Hersh et al., 2011).

Social-Emotional and Behavioral

Children diagnosed with leukemia are at increased risk of experiencing adverse social–emotional and behavioral outcomes that could potentially affect their performance in school and long-term adjustment (Brinkman et al., 2016). For example, child and adolescent survivors of leukemia demonstrate deficits in sustained attention, evidence higher rates of externalizing behaviors and increased levels of hyperactive/impulsive behavior and oppositional defiant disorder, and experience difficulty with sleep quality and fatigue symptoms (Liu et al., 2018).

PSYCHOEDUCATIONAL IMPLICATIONS AND SCHOOL-BASED INTERVENTIONS

Medical and Health Management

Psychoeducation for parents, the child, and all team personnel should be provided, as understanding leukemia is critical to helping them understand the presentation and course of the disease, as well as preparing them to deal with treatments and outcomes. Chemotherapy is the primary treatment for childhood leukemia, with radiation, stem cell transplants, and targeted drug therapy (Eryılmaz & Canpolat, 2017). During treatment, children with leukemia often undergo invasive and painful procedures. As a result, interventions should be designed to also assist with pain management and distress. Importantly, mind–body health approaches, including relaxation and guided imagery, desensitization, modeling, distraction, and positive reinforcement, used in combination with cognitive behavioral interventions, have shown to be effective methods for pain management after medical procedures (Kazak & Kunin-Batson, 2001).

Cognitive/Academic

The development of educational treatment plans falls under the purview of Section 504, with a classification of "Other Health Impairment," or OHI. Shortening school days, incorporating rest periods, adjusting the amount of required school work, providing one-to-one instruction and supplemental tutoring, as well as supportive counseling, and modifying the student's dress code (i.e., allowing them to wear a hat) are examples of common services a student with leukemia may benefit from upon returning to school. School absences may be frequent and often unpredictable. Should this occur, homebound accommodations should be provided. Attending school, even part of the day, can improve adjustment, enhance academic achievement, and minimize social isolation. Finally, engaging the child in physical activities may promote friendships, enhance motor skills, and increase the strength and quality of life among children with leukemia (Zupanec et al., 2017). Recommendations from the American Cancer Society (2019b) include but are not limited to the following:

- Students would benefit from extended time on assignments, including tests and written assignments.
- Lengthy projects should be broken down into more manageable segments.
- When completing tasks that require multistep directives, one instruction should be given at a time and/or the student should receive instructions in a written format so that they may be reviewed as necessary.
- Schedule breaks into lengthy study or work times. If a student needs a break, provide them with a "pass" system that may be used to take a short break from class. Further, direct instruction regarding appropriate use of this pass should be discussed prior to use.
- When required to remember rote information (e.g., spelling words), repetition and rehearsal of information would be beneficial.
- Across activities, comprehension should be monitored closely. Attempt to teach concepts and give assignments in smaller units when possible, reviewing frequently.
- Teachers (and parents) should provide clear and concise directions using multiple methods (e.g., oral and written instructions) to ensure understanding as well as have students paraphrase directions and instructions.
- Teachers may consider providing prior warning before calling on students to answer a question in class (e.g., before a specific lesson, teacher may say, "I am going to call on you during this lesson and ask you to tell me about the main idea of this story"). This warning may be faded as the level of comfort with answering orally in class increases.
- Counseling sessions to discuss reintegration and feelings with respect to returning to school, including but not limited to addressing workload and friendships as well as providing coping skills, are recommended.
- To address executive functioning deficits, visual checklists, nonverbal signs, timers, written instructions, and visual labels all serve the function of cueing the student to engage in an expected behavior, self-monitor, or complete tasks according to certain steps. Auditory instructions should be repeated in order to enhance encoding.

Social-Emotional and Behavioral

Children's comfort and feelings of acceptance as they reenter school can be greatly affected by the responses of classmates. The educative inclusion of classmates facilitates their understanding of the disease and provides an opportunity to ask questions they may have. Pairing a student with a buddy will also facilitate acclimation to the school setting. A warm welcome from fellow peers upon the student's reentry to school fosters support for the reintegration process (Suzuki & Kato, 2003). Participation in structured social skills activities at school would be beneficial, as would counseling services, to discuss reintegration issues, coping with leukemia, and other idiosyncratic issues the child may be experiencing.

CONCLUSION

Childhood leukemia, a cancer of the white blood cells, affects children's cognitive, academic, social–emotional, and neuropsychological functioning and has deleterious short- and long-term side effects. Given the serious health and personal risks stemming from childhood leukemia, it is imperative to employ evidence-based interventions to address issues ranging from pain management to coping with the illness, as well as facilitating the transition from hospital to school settings. Thus, a multidisciplinary team, ideally with the school psychologist serving as the point of contact, is imperative for seamless communication among all individuals who work with the child to ensure continuity of care.

RESOURCES

Leukemia and Lymphoma Society. (n.d.). *Patient and caregiver support and counseling: Children and families*. https://www.lls.org/support/other-helpful-organizations/patient-and-caregiver-resources-support-and-counseling/children-and-families

Childhood Leukemia Society. (n.d.). *Resources for families*. https://www.clf4kids.org/forfamilies.php

REFERENCES

American Cancer Society. (2019a, February 12). *Survival rates for childhood leukemias*. https://www.cancer.org/cancer/leukemia-in-children/detection-diagnosis-staging/survival-rates.html

American Cancer Society. (2019b, July 22). *Treating childhood leukemia*. https://www.cancer.org/cancer/leukemia-in-children/treating.html

Barbel, P., & Peterson, K. (2015). Recognizing subtle signs and symptoms of pediatric cancer. *Nursing, 45*(4), 30–37. https://doi.org/10.1097/01.NURSE.0000461852.18315.b5

Bisen-Hersh, E. B., Hineline, P. N., & Walker, E. A. (2011). Disruption of learning processes by chemotherapeutic agents in childhood survivors of acute lymphoblastic leukemia and preclinical models. *Journal of Cancer, 2*, 292–301. https://doi.org/10.7150/jca.2.292

Brinkman, T. M., Li, C., Vannatta, K., Marchak, J. G., Lai, J. S., Prasad, P. K., Kimberg, C., Vuotto, S., Di, C., Srivastava, D., Robison, L. L., Armstrong, G. T., & Krull, K. R. (2016). Behavioral, social, and emotional symptom comorbidities and profiles in adolescent survivors of childhood cancer: A report from the childhood cancer survivor study. *Journal of Clinical Oncology, 34*(28), 3417–3425. https://doi.org/10.1200/JCO.2016.66.4789

Cheung, Y. T., Brinkman, T. M., Mulrooney, D. A., Mzayek, Y., Liu, W., Banerjee, P., Panoskaltsis-Mortari, A., Srivastava, D., Pui, C. H., Robison, L. L., Hudson, M. M., & Krull, K. R. (2017). Impact of sleep, fatigue, and systemic inflammation on neurocognitive and behavioral outcomes in long-term survivors of childhood acute lymphoblastic leukemia. *Cancer, 123*(17), 3410–3419. https://doi.org/10.1002/cncr.30742

Conklin, H. M., Krull, K. R., Reddick, W. E., Pei, D., Cheng, C., & Pui, C. H. (2012). Cognitive outcomes following contemporary treatment without cranial irradiation for childhood acute lymphoblastic leukemia. *Journal of the National Cancer Institute, 104*(18), 1386–1395. https://doi.org/10.1093/jnci/djs344

Eryılmaz, E., & Canpolat, C. (2017). Novel agents for the treatment of childhood leukemia: An update. *OncoTargets and Therapy, 10*, 3299–3306. https://doi.org/10.2147/OTT.S126368

Hargreave, M., Jensen, A., Toender, A., Andersen, K. K., & Kjaer, S. K. (2013). Fertility treatment and childhood cancer risk: A systematic meta-analysis. *Fertility and Sterility, 100*(1), 150–161. https://doi.org/10.1016/j.fertnstert.2013.03.017

Iyer, N. S., Balsamo, L. M., Bracken, M. B., & Kadan-Lottick, N. S. (2015). Chemotherapy-only treatment effects on long-term neurocognitive functioning in childhood ALL survivors: A review and meta-analysis. *Blood, 126*(3), 346–353. https://doi.org/10.1182/blood-2015-02-627414

Jacola, L. M., Edelstein, K., Liu, W., Pui, C. H., Hayashi, R., Kadan-Lottick, N. S., Srivastava, D., Henderson, T., Leisenring, W., Robison, L. L., Armstrong, G. T., & Krull, K. R. (2016). Cognitive, behaviour, and academic functioning in adolescent and young adult survivors of childhood acute lymphoblastic leukaemia: A report from the Childhood Cancer Survivor Study. *The Lancet Psychiatry, 3*(10), 965–972. https://doi.org/10.1016/S2215-0366(16)30283-8

Kaspers, G. J. L. (2012). Pediatric acute myeloid leukemia. *Expert Review of Anticancer Therapy, 12*(3), 405–413. https://doi.org/10.1586/era.12.1

Kazak, A., & Kunin-Batson, A. (2001). Psychological and integrative interventions in pediatric procedure pain. In G. A. Finley & P. J. McGrath (Eds.), *Acute and procedure pain in infants and children* (pp. 77–100). IASP Press.

Liu, W., Cheung, Y. T., Brinkman, T. M., Banerjee, P., Srivastava, D., Nolan, V. G., Zhang, H., Gurney, J. G., Pui, C. H., Robison, L. L., Hudson, M. M., & Krull, K. R. (2018). Behavioral symptoms and psychiatric disorders in child and adolescent long-term survivors of childhood acute lymphoblastic leukemia treated with chemotherapy only. *Psycho-Oncology, 27*(6), 1597–1607. https://doi.org/10.1002/pon.4699

Metayer, C., Dahl, G., Wiemels, J., & Miller, M. (2016). Childhood leukemia: A preventable disease. *Pediatrics, 138*(Suppl 1), S45–S55. https://doi.org/10.1542/peds.2015-4268H

Moleski, M. (2000). Neuropsychological, neuroanatomical, and neurophysiological consequences of CNS chemotherapy for acute lymphoblastic leukemia. *Archives of Clinical Neuropsychology, 15*(7), 603–630. https://doi.org/10.1093/arclin/15.7.603

National Cancer Institute. (2018, October 8). *Cancer in children and adolescents*. https://www.cancer.gov/types/childhood-cancers/child-adolescent-cancers-fact-sheet

Suzuki, L. K., & Kato, P. M. (2003). Psychosocial support for patients in pediatric oncology: The influences of parents, schools, peers, and technology. *Journal of Pediatric Oncology Nursing, 20*(4), 159–174. https://doi.org/10.1177/1043454203254039

Whitehead, T. P., Metayer, C., Wiemels, J. L., Singer, A. W., & Miller, M. D. (2016). Childhood leukemia and primary prevention. *Current Problems in Pediatric and Adolescent Health Care, 46*(10), 317–352. https://doi.org/10.1016/j.cppeds.2016.08.004

Wiemels, J. (2012). Perspectives on the causes of childhood leukemia. *Chemico-Biological Interactions, 196*(3), 59–67. https://doi.org/10.1016/j.cbi.2012.01.007

Zupanec, S., Jones, H., McRae, L., Papaconstantinou, E., Weston, J., & Stremler, R. (2017). A sleep hygiene and relaxation intervention for children with acute lymphoblastic leukemia: A pilot randomized controlled trial. *Cancer Nursing, 40*(6), 488–496. https://doi.org/10.1097/NCC.0000000000000457

6

22q11.2 Deletion Syndrome or DiGeorge Syndrome

Priscilla H. Duong and Hiroko Tanaka

The 22q11.2 deletion syndrome (22q11.2DS) is the most common chromosomal microdeletion disorder and has wide-ranging signs and symptoms that may impact nearly any part of the body. Prior to the discovery of the genetic underpinning of 22q11.2DS and due to its heterogenous presentation (Driscoll et al., 1992), the syndrome was known by many different names based on the presenting clinical symptoms, including DiGeorge syndrome, velocardiofacial syndrome, Shprintzen syndrome, conotruncal anomaly face syndrome, autosomal dominant Opitz G/BBB syndrome, and Cayler cardiofacial syndrome (Cuneo, 2001).

ETIOLOGY

22q11.2DS is a genetic disorder resulting from deletion on the long arm of chromosome 22 near region q11.2. Approximately 90% of 22q11.2DS cases involve de novo nonhomologous meiotic recombination events (Bertrán et al., 2018). However, given that it is a haploinsufficient disorder, an individual with 22q11.2DS has a 50% chance of having an affected child in each pregnancy (Bassett et al., 2011). The syndrome results from hemizygous deletions and recombinations of 22q11.2. While the deletion size does not explain the heterogenous presentation, phenotypic expression of 22q11.2DS may be linked to the deleted region and specific missing genes. For example, the genes *TBX1* and *CRKL* are involved in heart and craniofacial abnormalities, and the genes *COMT*

https://doi.org/10.1037/0000349-006
Health-Related Disorders in Children and Adolescents: A Guidebook for Educators and Service Providers, Second Edition, M. M. Perfect, C. A. Riccio, and M. A. Bray (Editors)

and *PRODH* are associated with schizophrenia (Clelland et al., 2016; Unolt et al., 2018). Whole-genome analyses have also shown altered function in neighboring genes outside the main deletion area, which may contribute to the variety of clinical presentations (Dantas et al., 2019).

PREVALENCE AND INCIDENCE

22q11.2DS is the most common chromosomal microdeletion syndrome, equally affecting male and female individuals as well as racial/ethnic groups, with an incidence of one in 1,000 fetuses and one in 4,000 to 6,000 births (Grati et al., 2015). However, the actual prevalence may be higher given variable phenotypic expression that may lead to underdiagnosis (McDonald-McGinn & Zackai, 2008), and true figures may increase with improved prenatal and newborn screening. Confirmation of 22q11.2DS is most often conducted via fluorescence in situ hybridization.

SYMPTOMS

As previously described, individuals with 22q11.2DS can have varying clinical signs and symptoms impacting many different organ systems that may range from mild functional impact to severe illness. Presenting medical signs/symptoms include cardiovascular disease, immunodeficiency, distinctive physical features (e.g., bulbous nasal tip, abnormalities of the auricular helix of the ear, protuberant ears, eye hooding, epicanthal folds, micrognathia [undersized jaw]), palatal and related defects, gastrointestinal/genitourinary involvement, endocrine involvement, ophthalmologic involvement (e.g., strabismus), orthopedic manifestations (e.g., skeletal abnormalities, short stature, scoliosis, club feet, polydactyly), hematologic/oncologic conditions (e.g., thrombocytopenia, cancers), and renal abnormalities (Bassett et al., 2011; Bertrán et al., 2018; Bohm et al., 2017; Campbell et al., 2018; Homans et al., 2018; McDonald-McGinn et al., 2015; Swillen & McDonald-McGinn, 2015). There is a higher incidence of epilepsy in individuals with 22q11.2DS compared with the general population, with many having seizures in the context of hypocalcemia or brain involvement (Bassett et al., 2011; Hopkins et al., 2018). Additionally, developmental delays (many with neuroradiographic findings) and behavioral/psychiatric concerns are also common (Bohm et al., 2017; Campbell et al., 2018; McDonald-McGinn et al., 2015).

IMPACT ON THE STUDENT AND OUTCOMES

Medical

Given the variability in presentation of 22q11.2DS, a highly individualized approach is necessary. If possible, it is recommended that children with 22q11.2DS receive multidisciplinary care through a clinic that specializes in the syndrome with inclusion of genetic counseling that provides updated information at each life stage. In the most severe cases, there may be fetal loss or infant death (4% mortality rate with median age of 5 months old), with most deaths resulting from severe cardiac disease and associated complications (Campbell et al., 2018). With 60% to 75% of individuals having congenital cardiac anomalies and nearly half of those with moderate or complex presentations, surveillance via echocardiogram is recommended, with regular monitoring and cardiac surgical intervention as indicated (Bassett et al., 2011; Campbell et al., 2018; McDonald-McGinn et al., 2015). Palatal and related disorders are also common, with approximately 75% of individuals presenting with symptoms that may include velopharyngeal insufficiency (causing abnormal nasal airflow during speech), chronic ear infections, and sensorineural and/or conductive hearing loss (Bassett et al., 2011). Although less common, surgical intervention may also be indicated to address palatal abnormalities (e.g., cleft palate) as well as more severe skeletal abnormalities (e.g., cervical cord compression) or gastrointestinal issues (e.g., gastrointestinal tube placement for feeding; Bassett et al., 2011; Homans et al., 2018). Immunodeficiency or allergies affect approximately 75% of individuals with 22q11.2DS, and thus testing may be necessary to define the immune dysfunction (e.g., impaired T cell production, thymic hypoplasia), with monitoring through immunology, rheumatology, otolaryngology, allergy, and respiratory experts (Bassett et al., 2011; Campbell et al., 2018; McDonald-McGinn et al., 2015). In the context of common endocrine (e.g., growth hormone deficiency, hypocalcemia) and gastrointestinal issues (e.g., vomiting, chronic constipation), there are also heightened risks for short stature, weight deficiency, and failure to thrive (Giardino et al., 2014). Thus, monitoring through endocrinology, gastroenterology, and support from a dietician/feeding team may be indicated. While not a comprehensive list, monitoring/surveillance may also be needed through ophthalmology, rheumatology, urology, nephrology, neurology, gynecology, radiology, and hematology/oncology (Bassett et al., 2011; McDonald-McGinn et al., 2015).

Cognitive/Academic

In infancy, it is important to evaluate prelinguistic communication (e.g., eye gaze, facial expression, joint attention, early vocalizations, response to vocalizations) to examine risk for velopharyngeal dysfunction, hearing concerns, and/or autism spectrum disorder (ASD; Solot et al., 2019). As a result of palatal and other neuroanatomical abnormalities, speech difficulties (e.g., hypernasality) and articulation/phonological errors often emerge when children with 22q11.2DS become verbal (Baylis & Shriberg, 2019; Campbell et al., 2018). Hypotonia, or low muscle tone, also contributes to mouth movement difficulties (Baylis & Shriberg, 2019). Developmentally, children with 22q11.2DS are slower to meet motor and language developmental milestones, with the median age for walking and talking at 16 months and 19 months, respectively (Campbell et al., 2018). Most individuals with 22q11.2.DS present with cognitive deficits, with intellectual ability significantly below age expectations (i.e., full-scale IQ averaging 70–76) and 30% of individuals meeting criteria for intellectual disability (Campbell et al., 2018; Moberg et al., 2018). Verbal abilities and nonverbal abilities appear to be impacted relatively equally when individuals with 22q11.2DS are analyzed across the lifespan (Moberg et al., 2018), although some data suggest a discrepancy with relatively stronger verbal abilities at a younger age and decline in verbal skills in adolescence or early adulthood (Moberg et al., 2018; Swillen et al., 2018). Given risk factors for developmental delays, children should undergo developmental assessments to determine needs for outpatient speech and language, occupational, and physical therapies.

Other neuropsychological domains affected may include visuospatial processing, visuomotor coordination, long-term memory, working memory, processing speed, and attention, which are typically one standard deviation below age-expectations (Moberg et al., 2018). Consistent with intellectual ability, individuals with 22q11.2DS demonstrate attenuated academic skills, with a relative strength in word reading and weaknesses in math (particularly math applications), reading comprehension, and higher level written expression (Antshel et al., 2014; De Smedt et al., 2009; Hamsho et al., 2017). Executive functioning weaknesses (including organization and planning) are also very common in individuals with 22q11.2DS, and these executive weaknesses may also underlie academic difficulties involving higher level processing and problem solving (Antshel et al., 2014). Additionally, daily living skills (i.e., adaptive functioning) in individuals with 22q11.2DS are on average affected at the same level as intellectual ability (i.e., approximately two standard deviations below the general population), though intellectual functioning only explains a small portion of the overall variability in daily living skills (Schneider et al., 2014).

Social-Emotional and Behavioral

According to Schneider and colleagues (2014), over half of individuals with 22q11.2DS have a co-occurring psychiatric condition. The conditions most commonly identified during childhood include ASD, attention-deficit/hyperactivity disorder (ADHD), and anxiety disorders. Those with comorbid 22q11.2DS and ADHD more frequently meet criteria for the inattentive subtype, rather than the hyperactive–impulsive or combined types.

About 20% of children with 22q11.2DS receive a comorbid diagnosis of ASD (Campbell et al., 2018). Social deficits are pervasive and are characterized by impaired social communication and social cognition, with relatively spared social motivation and empathy (Angkustsiri et al., 2014). These children have milder social deficits than most other children diagnosed with ASD, but children with 22q11.2DS frequently present with repetitive/restricted behaviors regardless of comorbid ASD diagnosis (Serur et al., 2019).

Per Schneider and colleagues (2014), during adolescence and early adulthood, individuals with 22q11.2DS are at risk for mood disorders and psychosis.

With regard to the latter, individuals with 22q11.2DS have a 30-fold increased risk of developing psychosis, including elevated positive (e.g., delusions, suspiciousness, hallucinations, disorganized thinking), negative (e.g., social anhedonia, avolition, reduced ideational richness, deterioration of role functioning), disorganized (e.g., odd behavior, trouble with focus, problems with hygiene), and general prodromal symptoms (e.g., dysphoric mood, motor disturbance, poor stress tolerance; Shapiro et al., 2011). Some studies have suggested that cognitive decline in verbal intellectual abilities or attention/executive functioning emerges prior to development of psychosis (Chawner et al., 2019).

PSYCHOEDUCATIONAL IMPLICATIONS AND SCHOOL-BASED INTERVENTIONS

Following diagnosis of 22q11.2DS, families of infants are highly encouraged to seek out free early intervention services, which are federally mandated to exist in every state. These services provide support from birth to 3 years old to address motor, cognitive, communication, social–emotional, and adaptive development. After age 3 years old, all states have programs to continue lifelong support via a Division of Developmental Disabilities or similar department (for a complete list, see the National Association of State Directors of Developmental Disabilities Services resource at the end of the chapter). Service eligibility varies state-to-state, and some states have a patchwork of different programs to cover ages 3 to 21 years old. When entering formal schooling, a service plan should be established in the school system to document specific needs of the student. In the public school system, this involves development of an individualized education program (in accordance with the Individuals With Disabilities Education Act) or Section 504 plan (enforced through the Office for Civil Rights). To address the complex academic needs of a student with 22q11.2DS, it will be important for the education team to establish regular communication with the student's family, medical team, and outpatient therapists.

Medical and Health Management

As previously described, there are many medical considerations that may have functional impact in the school environment. These may include medication administration (e.g., antiseizure medications for epilepsy), medical care (e.g., g-tube feedings) needed during the school day, and accommodations to address physical symptoms (e.g., breaks for fatigue). To address muscle weakness (e.g., hypotonia) or motor deficits associated with 22q11.2DS, school-based occupational and physical therapies may be provided when functional academic performance is impacted. Even if regular therapies are not indicated, there may be a need for occupational or physical therapy consultation to support environmental accommodations (e.g., extra time to walk to class, assistive technology for writing assignments, access to a scribe) as well as modifications (e.g., changes to physical education requirements). For students with 22q11.2DS who are deaf or hard of hearing, accommodations and modifications should be made to ensure adequate access to the curriculum, including assistive technology accommodations, access to personal hearing instruments, and modifications of assignments (for a comprehensive list, see the Hands and Voices resource at the end of the chapter). Additionally, if significant surgery or medical absences are anticipated, there should be a plan to accommodate missed attendance, assignments, and tests (e.g., extended deadlines, excusing nonessential academic assignments).

Cognitive/Academic

Given the variable developmental trajectory and possible plateau or decline, individuals with 22q11.2DS will benefit from regular multidisciplinary evaluations to best determine the most appropriate resources and accommodations to support development. An international panel of speech and language therapists and researchers with expertise in 22q11.2DS developed best practice guidelines for the management of individuals with the disorder (Solot et al., 2019). In the toddler to preschool years, there should be monitoring and intervention to address speech sound errors and social communication skills. Specialized speech therapy techniques may be necessary for cleft palate and velopharyngeal dysfunction, while principles of motor learning are recommended for motor speech deficits. In the school-age years, ongoing monitoring and intervention should address speech and language deficits, including expressive and receptive language, pragmatic language use, and misarticulations. Nasopharyngoscopic biofeedback may be useful to target remaining compensatory misarticulations. In the classroom setting, it is important to teach at a verbal level matching the student's skills; using repetition and concrete language are often helpful strategies, but adapted educational materials may also be needed.

Consistent with high comorbidity with ADHD, many of the neuropsychological deficits associated with 22q11.2DS mirror those associated with ADHD, including deficits in attention, processing speed, working memory, and executive functioning (Halperin et al., 2008). Empirical evidence supports implementation of behavioral, academic, and self-regulation interventions to address symptoms of ADHD (DuPaul et al., 2014). Behaviorally, this may include use of differential teacher attention (e.g., verbally praising on-task behavior and ignoring off-task behavior) and use of token reinforcement/response-cost systems (e.g., gaining and losing time to play with a specific toy). Academic strategies include providing clear information about what is to be learned, instructing skills in small incremental steps, continually assessing student understanding, supporting active participation, and implementing accommodations (e.g., extra time to complete tasks). Self-monitoring broadly involves teaching students to consistently identify target behaviors and development of a system to attend and track these behaviors. With older age, there should be a shift to focus on development of executive functioning skills to increase independence, which includes direct instruction for effective notetaking, organizational skills (e.g., time management, organizing materials, organizing thoughts to support written expression), and studying (Evans et al., 2014). With regard to engagement in higher level academic-based linguistic tasks (e.g., writing and reading comprehension), graphic organizers or story maps may be helpful for organizing thoughts. Across recommended interventions, daily report cards (e.g., tracking the frequency with which homework assignments are turned in) and other methods for quantitatively monitoring effectiveness of interventions are used (Dupaul et al., 2014; Evans et al., 2014).

Children with 22q11.2DS typically perform better during the early school years, likely reflecting adequate performance with rote and concrete learning (Kates et al., 2015; Mosheva et al., 2019). As previously discussed, even with relatively preserved intellectual functioning, individuals with 22q11.2DS are at higher risk for learning disabilities. Those identified with a specific learning disability should participate in the general education classroom for most of the day with pull-out academic instruction in the specified subject. It is important that schools employ evidence-based practices for identified learning disabilities, using standardized monitoring to evaluate success of the intervention (for a summary of academic evidence-based practices, see the Iris Center resource at the end of this chapter). Classroom accommodations or modifications may additionally be needed in related subjects. For example, due to deficits associated with a math learning disability, individuals may require additional supports in science, including extra time to complete work, access to a multiplication chart or calculator, or access to a notecard for exams to support multistep problem solving. While cognitive and academic abilities in individuals with 22q11.2DS typically predict educational placement (e.g., general education placement vs. self-contained classroom), employment in adulthood is better predicted by adaptive functioning over cognitive ability (Mosheva et al., 2019). This stresses the importance of integrating adaptive functioning and employment training into the academic curriculum to support gainful employment for adults with 22q11.2DS. In the final years of secondary school (by age 16 or earlier), planning for transition services should be initiated. These services may provide mentoring and support for independent living skills as well as finding jobs and housing (e.g., group homes, supportive housing). Depending on cognitive and adaptive impairment, it may be necessary to appoint a competent adult as legal guardian or to confer power of attorney to make financial and medical decisions.

Social–Emotional and Behavioral

The comorbid psychiatric conditions associated with 22q11.2DS warrant close monitoring with communication between the student's family, school team, and medical team to discuss changes with social–emotional and/or behavioral functioning. This is particularly important during adolescence and early adulthood given concern for psychosis. Outside of school, a student with 22q11.2DS is often followed by psychiatry for pharmacologic management of comorbid psychiatric conditions (e.g., ADHD, schizophrenia, mood disorders). With medication adjustment, daily report cards at school may provide helpful information about efficacy of the medication as well as any adverse side effects.

In addition to pharmacologic management, psychological and behavioral supports are warranted. Children with 22q11.2DS who present with destructive and inappropriate behaviors have been found to be responsive to behavioral interventions based on differential reinforcement in combination with psychotropic medication (Busch et al., 2022). Relatedly, applied behavior analysis is another evidence-based behavioral intervention typically used for those diagnosed with ASD (Kates et al., 2016). While evidence-based psychotherapy approaches like cognitive behavior therapy (CBT) are typically recommended to address mood disorders, such as anxiety and depression, special considerations must be made for individuals with 22q11.2DS given comorbid cognitive and social deficits. Thus, practical adaptations may be made for adolescents with 22q11.2DS to engage in CBT, including shorter sessions, frequent breaks, repetition of concepts, limited use of written materials, explicit use of turn taking, and multiple adult facilitators per CBT group (Fjermestad et al., 2015). In the school setting, involvement of school counselors or social workers is likely helpful for monitoring psychosocial adjustment.

In the case of more severe pathology, such as emergence of schizophrenia, it will be important for students with 22q11.2DS and their families to engage in family therapy with long-term psychoeducation provided to protect against psychotic relapse and rehospitalization (Bustillo et al., 2001). In the school setting, this may be supported through adherence to the student's psychotropic medication regimen as well as monitoring of positive and negative symptoms. Additionally, in high school, the education team should assist the student with finding a supportive vocational environment. Furthermore, some preliminary data suggest that CBT may be used to decrease positive psychotic symptoms (Demily & Franck, 2016).

22q11.2DS is associated with several psychiatric disorders that also involve social functioning deficits, including ASD, ADHD, and schizophrenia. Given social and cognitive deficits, individuals with 22q11.2DS are not just vulnerable for social isolation but also prone to exploitative relationships (Fung et al., 2015). In adulthood, individuals with 22q11.2DS who endorse having friendships were also more likely to have higher adaptive behavior (Mosheva et al., 2019). Taken together, it is essential to support social cognitive and social skills in individuals with 22q11.2DS. Several social skills training and social cognition programs have been found to be effective for improving social behaviors (Bustillo et al., 2001; Shashi et al., 2015). In the school setting, research on academic placement for children with disabilities has demonstrated the importance of opportunities to interact with typically developing peers to support social competence (Fisher & Meyer, 2002). This may be further supported through structured social activities (e.g., peer lunch bunch facilitated by an adult) and addressing social skills through speech and language therapy or counseling services. Furthermore, school staff should monitor for peer conflict and student exploitation, with appropriate intervention.

CONCLUSION

22q11.2DS is a complex and heterogenous disorder, and its management requires a multidisciplinary team approach. As with all children with medical conditions, it is important for educators, medical providers, and therapists to maintain open communication with a child's family for coordination of care. Medical factors as well as social–emotional, behavioral, and cognitive functioning must be carefully monitored to optimize long-term outcomes.

RESOURCES

International 22q11.2 Foundation Inc. http://www.22q.org/

22q Family Foundation. https://22qfamilyfoundation.org/

National Association of State Directors of Developmental Disabilities Services. (2023). *State agencies*. https://www.nasddds.org/state-agencies/

Johnson, C. D. (2014). *EP/504 checklist: Accommodations and modifications for students who are deaf and hard of hearing*. Hands and Voices. https://handsandvoices.org/pdf/IEP_Checklist.pdf

Iris Center. (n.d.). *Evidence-based practice summaries*. https://iris.peabody.vanderbilt.edu/resources/ebp_summaries/

REFERENCES

Angkustsiri, K., Goodlin-Jones, B., Deprey, L., Brahmbhatt, K., Harris, S., & Simon, T. J. (2014). Social impairments in chromosome 22q11.2 deletion syndrome (22q11.2DS): Autism spectrum disorder or a different endophenotype? *Journal of Autism and Developmental Disorders, 44*(4), 739–746. https://doi.org/10.1007/s10803-013-1920-x

Antshel, K., Hier, B., Fremont, W., Faraone, S. V., & Kates, W. (2014). Predicting reading comprehension academic achievement in late adolescents with velo-cardio-facial (22q11.2 deletion) syndrome (VCFS): A longitudinal study. *Journal of Intellectual Disability Research, 58*(10), 926–939. https://doi.org/10.1111/jir.12134

Bassett, A. S., McDonald-McGinn, D. M., Devriendt, K., Digilio, M. C., Goldenberg, P., Habel, A., Marino, B., Oskarsdottir, S., Philip, N., Sullivan, K., Swillen, A., & Vorstman, J. (2011). Practical guidelines for managing patients with 22q11.2 deletion syndrome. *The Journal of Pediatrics, 159*(2), 332–339. https://doi.org/10.1016/j.jpeds.2011.02.039

Baylis, A. L., & Shriberg, L. D. (2019). Estimates of the prevalence of speech and motor speech disorders in youth with 22q11.2 deletion syndrome. *American Journal of Speech-Language Pathology, 28*(1), 53–82. https://doi.org/10.1044/2018_AJSLP-18-0037

Bertrán, M., Tagle, F. P., & Irarrázaval, M. (2018). Psychiatric manifestations of 22q11.2 deletion syndrome: A literature review. *Neurologia, 33*(2), 121–128. https://doi.org/10.1016/j.nrleng.2015.07.014

Bohm, L. A., Zhou, T. C., Mingo, T. J., Dugan, S. L., Patterson, R. J., Sidman, J. D., & Roby, B. B. (2017). Neuroradiographic findings in 22q11.2 deletion syndrome. *American Journal of Medical Genetics: Part A, 173*(8), 2158–2165. https://doi.org/10.1002/ajmg.a.38304

Busch, L., Saini, V., Karim, S., & Jones, R. (2022). Evaluation and maintenance of behavioral interventions for 22q11.2 deletion syndrome. *Developmental Neurorehabilitation, 25*(3), 170–177. https://doi.org/10.1080/17518423.2021.1960919

Bustillo, J. R., Lauriello, J., Horan, W. P., & Keith, S. J. (2001). The psychosocial treatment of schizophrenia: An update. *The American Journal of Psychiatry, 158*(2), 163–175. https://doi.org/10.1176/appi.ajp.158.2.163

Campbell, I. M., Sheppard, S. E., Crowley, T. B., McGinn, D. E., Bailey, A., McGinn, M. J., Unolt, M., Homans, J. F., Chen, E. Y., Salmons, H. I., Gaynor, J. W., Goldmuntz, E., Jackson, O. A., Katz, L. E., Mascarenhas, M. R., Deeney, V. F. X., Castelein, R. M., Zur, K. B., Elden, L., . . . McDonald-McGinn, D. M. (2018). What is new with 22q? An update from the 22q and You Center at the Children's Hospital of Philadelphia. *American Journal of Medical Genetics: Part A, 176*(10), 2058–2069. https://doi.org/10.1002/ajmg.a.40637

Chawner, S. J. R. A., Niarchou, M., Doherty, J. L., Moss, H., Owen, M. J., & van den Bree, M. B. M. (2019). The emergence of psychotic experiences in the early adolescence of 22q11.2 deletion syndrome. *Journal of Psychiatric Research, 109*, 10–17. https://doi.org/10.1016/j.jpsychires.2018.11.002

Clelland, C. L., Drouet, V., Rilett, K. C., Smeed, J. A., Nadrich, R. H., Rajparia, A., Read, L. L., & Clelland, J. D. (2016). Evidence that COMT genotype and proline interact on negative-symptom outcomes in schizophrenia and bipolar disorder. *Translational Psychiatry, 6*(9), Article e891. https://doi.org/10.1038/tp.2016.157

Cuneo, B. F. (2001). 22q11.2 deletion syndrome: DiGeorge, velocardiofacial, and conotruncal anomaly face syndromes. *Current Opinion in Pediatrics, 13*(5), 465–472. https://doi.org/10.1097/00008480-200110000-00014

Dantas, A. G., Santoro, M. L., Nunes, N., de Mello, C. B., Pimenta, L. S. E., Meloni, V. A., Soares, D. C. Q., Belangero, S. N., Carvalheira, G., Kim, C. A., & Melaragno, M. I. (2019). Downregulation of genes outside the deleted region in individuals with 22q11.2 deletion syndrome. *Human Genetics, 138*(1), 93–103. https://doi.org/10.1007/s00439-018-01967-6

Demily, C., & Franck, N. (2016). Cognitive behavioral therapy in 22q11.2 microdeletion with psychotic symptoms: What do we learn from schizophrenia? *European Journal of Medical Genetics, 59*(11), 596–603. https://doi.org/10.1016/j.ejmg.2016.09.007

De Smedt, B., Swillen, A., Verschaffel, L., & Ghesquière, P. (2009). Mathematical learning disabilities in children with 22q11.2 deletion syndrome: A review. *Developmental Disabilities Research Reviews, 15*(1), 4–10. https://doi.org/10.1002/ddrr.44

Driscoll, D. A., Spinner, N. B., Budarf, M. L., McDonald-McGinn, D. M., Zackai, E. H., Goldberg, R. B., Shprintzen, R. J., Saal, H. M., Zonana, J., Jones, M. C., Mascarello, J. T., & Emanuel, B. S. (1992). Deletions and microdeletions of 22q11.2 in velo-cardio-facial syndrome. *American Journal of Medical Genetics, 44*(2), 261–268. https://doi.org/10.1002/ajmg.1320440237

DuPaul, G. J., Gormley, M. J., & Laracy, S. D. (2014). School-based interventions for elementary school students with ADHD. *Child and Adolescent Psychiatric Clinics, 23*(4), 687–697. https://doi.org/10.1016/j.chc.2014.05.003

Evans, S. W., Langberg, J. M., Egan, T., & Molitor, S. J. (2014). Middle school–based and high school–based interventions for adolescents with ADHD. *Child and Adolescent Psychiatric Clinics, 23*(4), 699–715. https://doi.org/10.1016/j.chc.2014.05.004

Fisher, M., & Meyer, L. H. (2002). Development and social competence after two years for students enrolled in inclusive and self-contained educational programs. *Research and Practice for Persons With Severe Disabilities, 27*(3), 165–174. https://doi.org/10.2511/rpsd.27.3.165

Fjermestad, K. W., Vatne, T. M., & Gjone, H. (2015). Cognitive behavioral therapy for adolescents with 22q11.2 deletion syndrome. *Advances in Mental Health and Intellectual Disabilities, 9*(1), 30–39. https://doi.org/10.1108/AMHID-05-2014-0017

Fung, W. L. A., Butcher, N. J., Costain, G., Andrade, D. M., Boot, E., Chow, E. W., Chung, B., Cytrynbaum, C., Faghfoury, H., Fishman, L., García-Miñaúr, S., George, S., Lang, A. E., Repetto, G., Shugar, A., Silversides, C., Swillen, A., van Amelsvoort, T., McDonald-McGinn, D. M., & Bassett, A. S. (2015). Practical guidelines for managing adults with 22q11.2 deletion syndrome. *Genetics in Medicine, 17*(8), 599–609. https://doi.org/10.1038/gim.2014.175

Giardino, G., Cirillo, E., Maio, F., Gallo, V., Esposito, T., Naddei, R., Grasso, F., & Pignata, C. (2014). Gastrointestinal involvement in patients affected with 22q11.2 deletion syndrome. *Scandinavian Journal of Gastroenterology, 49*(3), 274–279. https://doi.org/10.3109/00365521.2013.855814

Grati, F. R., Molina Gomes, D., Ferreira, J. C. P. B., Dupont, C., Alesi, V., Gouas, L., Horelli-Kuitunen, N., Choy, K. W., García-Herrero, S., de la Vega, A. G., Piotrowski, K., Genesio, R., Queipo, G., Malvestiti, B., Hervé, B., Benzacken, B., Novelli, A., Vago, P., Piippo, K., . . . Vialard, F. (2015). Prevalence of recurrent pathogenic microdeletions and microduplications in over 9500 pregnancies. *Prenatal Diagnosis, 35*(8), 801–809. https://doi.org/10.1002/pd.4613

Halperin, J. M., Trampush, J. W., Miller, C. J., Marks, D. J., & Newcorn, J. H. (2008). Neuropsychological outcome in adolescents/young adults with childhood ADHD: Profiles of persisters, remitters and controls. *Journal of Child Psychology and Psychiatry, 49*(9), 958–966. https://doi.org/10.1111/j.1469-7610.2008.01926.x

Hamsho, N., Antshel, K. M., Eckert, T. L., & Kates, W. R. (2017). Childhood predictors of written expression in late adolescents with 22q11.2 deletion syndrome: A longitudinal study. *Journal of Intellectual Disability Research, 61*(5), 501–511. https://doi.org/10.1111/jir.12370

Homans, J. F., Tromp, I. N., Colo, D., Schlösser, T. P., Kruyt, M. C., Deeney, V. F., Crowley, T. B., McDonald-McGinn, D. M., & Castelein, R. M. (2018). Orthopaedic manifestations within the 22q11.2 deletion syndrome: A systematic review. *American Journal of Medical Genetics: Part A, 176*(10), 2104–2120. https://doi.org/10.1002/ajmg.a.38545

Hopkins, S. E., Chadehumbe, M., Blaine Crowley, T., Zackai, E. H., Bilaniuk, L. T., & McDonald-McGinn, D. M. (2018). Neurologic challenges in 22q11.2 deletion syndrome. *American Journal of Medical Genetics: Part A, 176*(10), 2140–2145. https://doi.org/10.1002/ajmg.a.38614

Kates, W. R., Tang, K. L., Antshel, K. M., & Fremont, W. P. (2015). Behavioral and psychiatric phenotypes in 22q11.2 deletion syndrome. *Journal of Developmental and Behavioral Pediatrics, 36*(8), Article 639. https://doi.org/10.1097/DBP.0000000000000210

McDonald-McGinn, D. M., Sullivan, K. E., Marino, B., Philip, N., Swillen, A., Vorstman, J. A., Zackai, E. H., Emanuel, B. S., Vermeesch, J. R., Morrow, B. E., Scambler, P. J., & Bassett, A. S. (2015). 22q11.2 deletion syndrome. *Nature Reviews Disease Primers, 1*(1), 1–19. https://doi.org/10.1038/nrdp.2015.71

McDonald-McGinn, D. M., & Zackai, E. H. (2008). Genetic counseling for the 22q11.2 deletion. *Developmental Disabilities Research Reviews, 14*(1), 69–74. https://doi.org/10.1002/ddrr.10

Moberg, P. J., Richman, M. J., Roalf, D. R., Morse, C. L., Graefe, A. C., Brennan, L., Vickers, K., Tsering, W., Kamath, V., Turetsky, B. I., Gur, R. C., & Gur, R. E. (2018).

Neurocognitive functioning in patients with 22q11.2 deletion syndrome: A meta-analytic review. *Behavior Genetics, 48*(4), 259–270. https://doi.org/10.1007/s10519-018-9903-5

Mosheva, M., Pouillard, V., Fishman, Y., Dubourg, L., Sofrin-Frumer, D., Serur, Y., Weizman, A., Eliez, S., Gothelf, D., & Schneider, M. (2019). Education and employment trajectories from childhood to adulthood in individuals with 22q11.2 deletion syndrome. *European Child & Adolescent Psychiatry, 28*(1), 31–42. https://doi.org/10.1007/s00787-018-1184-2

Schneider, M., Debbané, M., Bassett, A. S., Chow, E. W., Fung, W. L. A., van den Bree, M., Owen, M., Murphy, K. C., Niarchou, M., Kates, W. R., Antshel, K. M., Fremont, W., McDonald-McGinn, D. M., Gur, R. E., Zackai, E. H., Vorstman, J., Duijff, S. N., Klaassen, P. W., Swillen, A., . . . Eliez, S. (2014). Psychiatric disorders from childhood to adulthood in 22q11.2 deletion syndrome: Results from the International Consortium on Brain and Behavior in 22q11.2 Deletion Syndrome. *The American Journal of Psychiatry, 171*(6), 627–639. https://doi.org/10.1176/appi.ajp.2013.13070864

Serur, Y., Sofrin Frumer, D., Daon, K., Sobol-Havia, D., Weinberger, R., Shulman, C., & Gothelf, D. (2019). Psychiatric disorders and autism in young children with 22q11.2 deletion syndrome compared to children with idiopathic autism. *European Psychiatry, 55*, 116–121. https://doi.org/10.1016/j.eurpsy.2018.10.007

Shapiro, D. I., Cubells, J. F., Ousley, O. Y., Rockers, K., & Walker, E. F. (2011). Prodromal symptoms in adolescents with 22q11.2 deletion syndrome and schizotypal personality disorder. *Schizophrenia Research, 129*(1), 20–28. https://doi.org/10.1016/j.schres.2011.03.030

Shashi, V., Harrell, W., Eack, S., Sanders, C., McConkie-Rosell, A., Keshavan, M. S., Bonner, M. J., Schoch, K., & Hooper, S. R. (2015). Social cognitive training in adolescents with chromosome 22q11.2 deletion syndrome: Feasibility and preliminary effects of the intervention. *Journal of Intellectual Disability Research, 59*(10), 902–913. https://doi.org/10.1111/jir.12192

Solot, C. B., Sell, D., Mayne, A., Baylis, A. L., Persson, C., Jackson, O., & McDonald-McGinn, D. M. (2019). Speech-language disorders in 22q11.2 deletion syndrome: Best practices for diagnosis and management. *American Journal of Speech-Language Pathology, 28*(3), 984–999. https://doi.org/10.1044/2019_AJSLP-16-0147

Swillen, A., & McDonald-McGinn, D. (2015). Developmental trajectories in 22q11.2 deletion syndrome. *American Journal of Medical Genetics: Part C. Seminars in Medical Genetics, 169*(2), 172–181. https://doi.org/10.1002/ajmg.c.31435

Swillen, A., Moss, E., & Duijff, S. (2018). Neurodevelopmental outcome in 22q11.2 deletion syndrome and management. *American Journal of Medical Genetics: Part A, 176*(10), 2160–2166. https://doi.org/10.1002/ajmg.a.38709

Unolt, M., Versacci, P., Anaclerio, S., Lambiase, C., Calcagni, G., Trezzi, M., Carotti, A., Crowley, T. B., Zackai, E. H., Goldmuntz, E., Gaynor, J. W., Digilio, M. C., McDonald-McGinn, D. M., & Marino, B. (2018). Congenital heart diseases and cardiovascular abnormalities in 22q11.2 deletion syndrome: From well-established knowledge to new frontiers. *American Journal of Medical Genetics: Part A, 176*(10), 2087–2098. https://doi.org/10.1002/ajmg.a.38662

7

Hemophilia

Mickey Randolph and Ethan J. Schilling

Hemophilia is a rare, sex-linked, recessive blood clotting disorder caused by a chromosomal abnormality affecting approximately 20,000 persons in the United States. Hemophilia primarily affects male individuals and can be characterized as mild, moderate, or severe. Based on the categorization, the impact on an individual and their family will be dramatically different. This chapter discusses the possible impact of hemophilia for children/adolescents and the family and ways to address some of these issues.

ETIOLOGY

Inheritance of hemophilia is X-linked; therefore, male individuals are more typically diagnosed with the disorder. The disorder is characterized by prolonged bleeding episodes due to reduced clotting factor, not more frequent bleeding. The two more common types of hemophilia are hemophilia A, which results from reduced levels of clotting factor VIII, and hemophilia B, which results from reduced clotting factor IX. Both clotting factor VIII and IX are a type of protein needed to form blood clots.

https://doi.org/10.1037/0000349-007
Health-Related Disorders in Children and Adolescents: A Guidebook for Educators and Service Providers, Second Edition, M. M. Perfect, C. A. Riccio, and M. A. Bray (Editors)

PREVALENCE AND INCIDENCE

Hemophilia is considered to be a rare disorder, as it has been diagnosed in approximately 20,000 people in the United States. Hemophilia A is almost 4 times more prevalent than hemophilia B, occurring in one in 6,500 births versus one in 25,000 (Konkle et al., 2017). Both types of hemophilia can be characterized as mild, moderate, or severe. Mild hemophilia is characterized by 6% to 30% of normal levels of clotting factors and represents about 25% of the population diagnosed with hemophilia. Individuals with mild hemophilia are likely to experience bleeds after a serious injury or surgery. Those with moderate hemophilia have 1% to 5% of clotting factor, comprise about 15% of cases, and experience bleeding after injuries or even spontaneous bleeds. Severe hemophilia is characterized by factor levels less than 1% and represents 60% of the cases of hemophilia, with bleeding occurring after injuries or surgeries, spontaneous bleeding (e.g., nosebleeds without any trauma, tooth extractions, some joint bleeds), and bleeding into joints and muscles (leading to acute hemarthrosis and arthropathy). For many with the diagnosis, joint bleeds are accompanied by limited range of motion and chronic pain.

SYMPTOMS

Diagnosis varies as a function of the severity of the disorder, with severe hemophilia being diagnosed as early as infancy (e.g., during a circumcision). Most individuals are diagnosed using special blood coagulation tests to determine how long it takes their blood to clot. Symptomatology for hemophilia is difficult to explicitly generalize, as it depends in large part on the severity of the disorder (mild, moderate, or severe). Early signs of mild hemophilia include excessive bleeding after incidents such as tooth extractions. However, bleeding episodes are infrequent, and most mild cases are not diagnosed until adulthood. Individuals with moderate hemophilia are typically diagnosed before the age of 6 and experience prolonged bleeding episodes on a more regular basis (i.e., monthly or yearly). Severe hemophilia is diagnosed before the age of 2, with the child experiencing routine bleeding episodes, unfortunately with internal and joint bleeding, leading to extreme pain and possible long-term joint damage (Konkle et al., 2017). In general, hemophilia should be investigated as a possible cause if any of the following occur: hemarthrosis, intracranial bleeding, or other unexplained bleeding without a known trauma; menorrhagia; prolonged nosebleed (especially recurrent or bilateral); and prolonged, renewed, or oozing bleeding (Konkle et. al., 2017). The most obvious symptom individuals with hemophilia experience is pain, which is chronic in some cases (Witkop et al., 2016).

IMPACT ON THE STUDENT AND OUTCOMES

Medical

Many of the health concerns associated with hemophilia have been addressed with improved infusion techniques and preventive prophylaxis treatments that maintain a certain level of clotting factor in the blood. However, one persistent problem is the development of *inhibitors*, or antibodies that see an infusion factor (either VIII or IX) as a potential threat to the body and work to remove it before it can stop a bleed. The development of inhibitors requires an individual to seek additional treatment with bypassing agents. *Bypassing agents* are simply drugs that bypass the inhibitor to stop a bleed (e.g., Novo Seven, FEIBA). If a plan to stop an inhibitor is not successful, there is a greater chance of long-term joint damage, hospitalization, or death. Inhibitors are identified through routine lab screenings or when prophylaxis becomes less effective in preventing bleeds. The most common concern for individuals with hemophilia is the continued occurrence of joint bleeds, leading to development of hemophilic arthropathy (the breaking down of cartilage and the lining of the joint). This condition may lead to irreversible joint damage and disability, and although joint replacement is possible, it may not restore full joint movement. Medical prophylaxis has helped address this complication for most individuals with hemophilia (Franchini & Mannucci, 2012).

Cognitive/Academic

Children and adolescents with hemophilia may experience negative school-based outcomes as either a direct or indirect consequence of their disease. Despite the fact that no significant differences in intellectual functioning (i.e., measured IQ) have been found in students with hemophilia in comparison with healthy peers, some past research has indicated that children and adolescents with hemophilia experience poorer academic performance in the form of lower grades across classes (Basu et al., 2010). Furthermore, individuals reporting more than 12 bleeds annually are more likely to experience these academic difficulties than those with milder forms of hemophilia that result in fewer bleeds (Basu et al., 2010).

Some have argued that lower school performance in these students may be due to greater numbers of absences and subsequent lost instructional time due to bleeds and other related aspects of disease management, referred to as "lost days" (Recht et al., 2014). As approximately half of bleeding episodes for students with hemophilia tend to occur during the school day, it is clear how disruptive these episodes can be to a student's learning in the classroom (Recht et al., 2014). Furthermore, families of children and adolescents with hemophilia report that bleeding episodes lasting more than 3 days are often the most disruptive to family and school functioning given the sheer time involved in the management of these bleeds. Despite such difficulties, students with hemophilia generally experience similar or, in some cases, higher high school graduation rates compared with their healthy peers (Drake et al., 2010).

Social-Emotional and Behavioral

Most children and adolescents with hemophilia will need to monitor their physical activity, especially in contact sports where bleeds are more likely. This can become problematic when sports are linked to peer acceptance and male identity in some cultures (Buzzard, 1996). For example, adolescence may represent a particularly challenging time for the individual with hemophilia, given the emphasis on increased physical activity (i.e., organized sports) as an important means of socialization with peers. Adolescents with hemophilia may feel greater resentment for having to sit out of these activities to prevent bleeds (Casey & Brown, 2003). It is important to work with these individuals to find appropriate socialization activities fitting with their own particular interests if higher contact sporting activities are not feasible. Some researchers and practitioners have argued for specific types of physical activity programs to decrease bleeding episodes, emphasizing the benefits of weight-bearing exercise, aerobic exercise, and balancing activities (Philpott et al., 2010).

Other issues to consider when working with an individual with hemophilia include the impact on the family and the impact of the individual's social–emotional development. For families with hemophilia, the change to the family system comes early, as children are typically diagnosed with hemophilia soon after birth or as very young children. When this happens, parents must assume the additional role of "parent of a chronically ill child." Problems may emerge if only one parent takes on this role. Additionally, there may be issues with the spousal subsystem due to the degree that the workload and emotional stress interferes with the couple's ability to spend time together. Siblings may also be affected as more time and attention is spent with the child diagnosed with hemophilia. The system itself may be overburdened by many complications, such as having a bleeding event interrupt or prevent a family plan. The financial aspects of treating this disorder may also serve as a hardship for families, preventing them from allocating money for education, leisure, or simple daily needs (Beeton et al., 2007).

In addition to affecting family functioning, hemophilia has been associated with externalizing, internalizing, and competence problems. In several studies, although individuals with hemophilia scored lower than their peers, norm scores still fell within the average range on the Child Behavior Checklist and Family Assessment Measure (Evans et al., 2000). Other researchers have reported significant differences in these areas, with individuals with hemophilia experiencing more depressive symptoms, greater anxiety, and weaker peer relationships (Casey & Brown, 2003). Generally, individuals with hemophilia report lower perceptions of health-related quality of life and feeling different in comparison with others without a hemophilia diagnosis. These individuals are then at greater risk for the experience of adverse psychological consequences, including feeling resentful toward having to sit out activities that healthy peers are engaging in, feeling isolated or withdrawn from others, and feeling like they have to hide their condition from others (Casey & Brown, 2003). Finally, perhaps as a result of such difficulties, they are more likely to experience lower levels of overall self-esteem at home and at school (Limperg et al., 2018).

PSYCHOEDUCATIONAL IMPLICATIONS AND SCHOOL-BASED INTERVENTIONS

Given the potential challenges, it is important that those involved in the care of children and adolescents with hemophilia are aware of these areas of potential problems and are able to effectively intervene to best assist them in their development. The costs of treating hemophilia are difficult to project. Some costs are direct (the costs of treatment, e.g., clotting factors, prophylaxis), and others are indirect (e.g., medical appointments, time away from work during a bleed, one parent remaining at home to care for the child/adolescent). It is estimated that the direct annual cost of treating hemophilia ranges from $60,000 to $500,000 for prophylaxis treatments to over a million dollars for individuals with inhibitors (Saxena, 2013).

Medical and Health Management

Many of the complications associated with hemophilia in the past (e.g., having an allergic reaction or contracting hepatitis or HIV during blood transfusions) have been decreased or even eliminated as a function of medical advances. For example, development of recombinant clotting factor products in the lab has decreased the need for donations of human plasma, and techniques to test human plasma for certain diseases have improved. Individuals with severe hemophilia are typically placed on preventive prophylaxis treatments, and family members—and the individuals with hemophilia themselves, as they age—can be trained to administer prophylaxis at home. Prophylaxis has significantly decreased the impact of some of the more serious spontaneous or nonspontaneous internal bleeding episodes by maintaining the level of clotting factor in the patient's blood. The long-term prognosis for individuals diagnosed with hemophilia has improved to such an extent that many are now being diagnosed with and having to address other medical issues (e.g., obesity and other aging issues; Baker et al., 2013).

Cognitive/Academic

Cognitive and academic interventions for children with hemophilia may not be required; however, schools may be included in the management of hemophilia by using adaptive physical education practices and educating school personnel on hemophilia (Philpott et al., 2010). In severe cases in which bleeding episodes are not as well controlled, schools may need to provide students with accommodations (e.g., extended time for assignments, supplemental instruction) to account for missed instructional time.

As academic demands increase in the school-age years, it is also important to identify any academic challenges faced by the child. It is important that teachers recognize difficulties when they occur and engage in compensatory strategies in the classroom to account for such deficits. Although special education teachers report being more informed than general education teachers about health conditions, including hemophilia, they are not more confident about meeting the academic needs of these students (Nabors et al., 2008). Therefore, school psychologists and other support staff more knowledgeable about the student's condition and any presenting deficits can then help to educate teachers and other staff about steps they can take to support the student given their current needs.

Social-Emotional and Behavioral

In the preschool years, children and families are usually just starting to adjust to a hemophilia diagnosis and the new demands of disease management. A period of normalization within the child's family can be particularly useful at this early stage and includes making sense of their child's condition and future, incorporating active disease management into daily routines, reassuring each other that things will be okay, and engaging in conversations with others and seeking social support when needed (Emiliani et al., 2011). School psychologists and other mental health professionals can be particularly helpful at this point in encouraging greater access to psychosocial resources (e.g., social support options, supporting counseling for the family) as needed or requested.

In the school-age years, children with hemophilia are often starting to take a more active role in self-management of their condition, including engaging in preventative therapy, bleed recognition, self-infusion of medicine, medicine management, self-care routines, and pain management (Khair et al., 2015). They will likely need assistance in navigating the shift from parental to self-management of hemophilia symptoms, which should involve experiential learning and practicing care skills as well as individualized education on elements required to actively care for the disease (Khair et al., 2015). Encouraging a greater sense of motivation and responsibility around self-management at this point can then help the child with hemophilia feel more competent in coping with disease-related challenges when they arise and have a greater willingness to engage in activities with peers.

As children with hemophilia get older, perceptions of differences with healthy peers often become more apparent. In particular, they may hold a view that their peers do not like them or will exclude them from activities because of their condition (Casey & Brown, 2003). This is why it is vital to ensure that peers are educated about what a hemophilia diagnosis means for the child (i.e., basic disease definitions and any challenges their classmate with hemophilia may face as a result) in a developmentally appropriate way (Casey & Brown, 2003). Support groups for children with hemophilia can also be particularly useful in helping them see that they are not alone in dealing with difficult feelings around their condition; however, it should be recognized that group-based approaches may be overwhelming to some children, in which case an individual approach to support might be more appropriate.

CONCLUSION

In conclusion, though hemophilia is a chronic condition with potentially debilitating symptoms, advances in medical technology and prevention treatments mean most individuals will go on to live long lives. Although this is a medical diagnosis, it is recognized to impact all areas of a person's life and those around them. Families with a member diagnosed with hemophilia are recommended to contact a comprehensive hemophilia treatment center, which can address the diagnosis from a multidisciplinary/comprehensive perspective (i.e., medical, psychosocial, educational, and individualized treatment; Centers for Disease Control and Prevention, 2022).

RESOURCES

Centers for Disease Control and Prevention. (2023). *Hemophilia*. https://www.cdc.gov/ncbddd/hemophilia/

Centers for Disease Control and Prevention. (2022). *Hemophilia treatment centers (HTC)*. https://www.cdc.gov/ncbddd/hemophilia/htc.html

National Hemophilia Foundation. 7 Penn Plaza, Suite 1204, New York, NY 10001; 212-328-3700(P); 212-328-3777(F). https://www.hemophilia.org

KidsHealth. (2020). *Hemophilia*. https://kidshealth.org/en/parents/hemophilia.html

Hemophilia Federation of America. (n.d.). *Back to school*. https://www.hemophiliafed.org/resource/back-to-school/

REFERENCES

Baker, J. R., Riske, B., Drake, J. H., Forsberg, A. D., Atwood, R., Voutsis, M., & Shearer, R. (2013). U.S. Hemophilia Treatment Center population trends 1990–2010: Patient diagnoses, demographics, health services utilization. *Haemophilia, 19*(1), 21–26. https://doi.org/10.1111/j.1365-2516.2012.02915.x

Basu, J., Chowdhury, M. R., & Mitra, A. K. (2010). Cognitive functioning, personality variables, and academic achievement of hemophilic and normal children: A comparative study. *Psychological Studies, 55*(2), 165–171. https://doi.org/10.1007/s12646-010-0021-6

Beeton, K., Neal, D., Watson, T., & Lee, C. A. (2007). Parents of children with haemophilia—A transforming experience. *Haemophilia, 13*(5), 570–579. https://doi.org/10.1111/j.1365-2516.2007.01494.x

Buzzard, B. M. (1996). Sports and hemophilia: Antagonist or protagonist. *Clinical Orthopaedics and Related Research, 328,* 25–30. https://doi.org/10.1097/00003086-199607000-00006

Casey, R. L., & Brown, R. T. (2003). Psychological aspects of hematologic diseases. *Child and Adolescent Psychiatric Clinics of North America, 12*(3), 567–584. https://doi.org/10.1016/S1056-4993(03)00025-7

Centers for Disease Control and Prevention. (2022). *Hemophilia treatment centers (HTC).* https://www.cdc.gov/ncbddd/hemophilia/htc.html

Drake, J. H., Soucie, J. M., Cutter, S. C., Forsberg, A. D., Baker, J. R., & Riske, B. (2010). High school completion rates among men with hemophilia. *American Journal of Preventive Medicine, 38*(4, Suppl.), S489–S494. https://doi.org/10.1016/j.amepre.2009.12.024

Emiliani, F., Bertocchi, S., Potì, S., & Palareti, L. (2011). Process of normalization in families with children affected by hemophilia. *Qualitative Health Research, 21*(12), 1667–1678. https://doi.org/10.1177/1049732311417456

Evans, M., Cottrell, D., & Shiach, C. (2000). Emotional and behavioural problems and family functioning in children with haemophilia: A cross-sectional survey. *Haemophilia, 6*(6), 682–687. https://doi.org/10.1046/j.1365-2516.2000.00416.x

Franchini, M., & Mannucci, P. M. (2012). Past, present and future of hemophilia: A narrative review. *Orphanet Journal of Rare Diseases, 7*(1), Article 24. https://doi.org/10.1186/1750-1172-7-24

Khair, K., Meerabeau, L., & Gibson, F. (2015). Self-management and skills acquisition in boys with haemophilia. *Health Expectations, 18*(5), 1105–1113. https://doi.org/10.1111/hex.12083

Konkle, B. A., Huston, H., & Fletcher, S. N. (2017). Hemophilia B. In M. P. Adam, H. H. Ardinger, R. A. Pagon, S. E. Wallace, L. J. H. Bean, K. Stephens, & A. Amemiya (Eds.), *GeneReviews*. University of Washington. https://www.ncbi.nlm.nih.gov/books/NBK1495/

Limperg, P. F., Haverman, L., Maurice-Stam, H., Coppens, M., Valk, C., Kruip, M. J. H. A., Eikenboom, J., Peters, M., & Grootenhuis, M. A. (2018). Health-related quality of life, developmental milestones, and self-esteem in young adults with bleeding disorders. *Quality of Life Research, 27*(1), 159–171. https://doi.org/10.1007/s11136-017-1696-0

Nabors, L. A., Little, S. G., Akin-Little, A., & Iobst, E. A. (2008). Teacher knowledge of and confidence in meeting the needs of children with chronic medical conditions: Pediatric psychology's contribution to education. *Psychology in the Schools, 45*(3), 217–226. https://doi.org/10.1002/pits.20292

Philpott, J., Houghton, K., & Luke, A. (2010). Physical activity recommendations for children with specific chronic health conditions: Juvenile idiopathic arthritis, hemophilia, asthma and cystic fibrosis. *Paediatrics & Child Health, 15*(4), 213–218. https://doi.org/10.1093/pch/15.4.213

Recht, M., Neufeld, E. J., Sharma, V. R., Solem, C. T., Pickard, A. S., Gut, R. Z., & Cooper, D. L. (2014). Impact of acute bleeding on daily activities of patients with congenital hemophilia with inhibitors and their caregivers and families: Observations from the Dosing Observational Study in Hemophilia (DOSE). *Value in Health, 17*(6), 744–748. https://doi.org/10.1016/j.jval.2014.07.003

Saxena, K. (2013). Barriers and perceived limitations to early treatment of hemophilia. *Journal of Blood Medicine, 4,* 49–56. https://doi.org/10.2147/JBM.S43734

Witkop, M. L., Peerlinck, K., & Luxon, B. A. (2016). Medical co-morbidities of patients with haemophilia: Pain, obesity and hepatitis C. *Haemophilia, 22*(Suppl. 5), 47–53. https://doi.org/10.1111/hae.12996

8

Human Immunodeficiency Virus (HIV)

Tiffany Chenneville and Kemesha Gabbidon

The human immunodeficiency virus (HIV), the virus that causes acquired immune deficiency syndrome (AIDS), is thought to be a mutation of the simian immunodeficiency virus contracted from chimpanzees in Central Africa as early as the late 1800s (Centers for Disease Control and Prevention [CDC], 2018a). Although HIV first existed in the United States in the mid-1970s, it was not identified until the early 1980s, when the first cases appeared. Since then, it has become a global health crisis.

ETIOLOGY

HIV infection occurs when the retrovirus invades one's bloodstream or mucosal membrane. Mucosal membranes line internal organs and other body cavities, including the vagina, urethra, underside of the foreskin, mouth, and rectum. The virus can also enter the bloodstream through a break in the skin, such as a prick with a contaminated needle. HIV operates by infecting specific immune system cells, particularly the CD4-T cells (also known as T helper cells) and macrophages. These immune cells play a critical role in the immune response to a variety of infections. During the early phase of HIV infection, HIV-specific CD4-T cells responding to the virus may be destroyed (CDC, 2018a). Over time, this impairs the immune system, limiting its ability to control the spread of HIV. This also leaves the body vulnerable to opportunistic infections. Currently, the most common ways HIV is spread are through unprotected sexual intercourse;

https://doi.org/10.1037/0000349-008
Health-Related Disorders in Children and Adolescents: A Guidebook for Educators and Service Providers, Second Edition, M. M. Perfect, C. A. Riccio, and M. A. Bray (Editors)

sharing contaminated needles and syringes; and mother-to-child transmission during pregnancy, delivery, or breastfeeding. Sexual intercourse is by far the most common mode of HIV transmission (CDC, 2018a).

PREVALENCE AND INCIDENCE

There are an estimated 38 million people living with HIV worldwide, including 3.4 million youths ages 15 to 24 (Joint United Nations Programme on HIV/AIDS, 2019, 2021). Within the United States, there are currently 1.2 million people living with HIV, with 20% of all new infections occurring among youths (CDC, 2022a, 2022b). Racial, ethnic, and sexual orientation minorities continue to experience high rates of HIV infection. Gay, bisexual, and other men who have sex with men (GBMSM) remain the most affected subpopulation in the United States, accounting for 71% of all new HIV diagnoses in 2020 (CDC, 2020). Among them, Blacks/African Americans (one in two) and Hispanics/Latinos (one in four) experience the highest odds of infection compared with Whites (one in 11; CDC, 2016).

Between 2016 and 2020, HIV trends decreased among GBMSM across racial/ethnic categories generally but remained stable for young GBMSM (ages 13–24; CDC, 2020). Rates among racial/ethnic minorities remain disproportionately high. In 2020, Black/African American GBMSM accounted for 39% of all new HIV diagnoses, followed by Hispanic/Latino GBMSM, who accounted for 31%, and White GBMSM, who accounted for 25% (CDC, 2022b). HIV diagnoses among youth ages 13 to 24 also varied by race and ethnicity; young Black/African American GBMSM accounted for 54% of new cases, young Hispanic/Latino GBMSM accounted for 27%, and young White GBMSM accounted for 14% (CDC, 2022b).

Overall, Blacks/African Americans experience the highest disease burden among any racial or ethnic group. Black/African American men have a higher lifetime risk (one in 20) compared with White men (one in 132; CDC, 2016). Black/African American women also have a higher lifetime risk (one in 48) compared with White women (one in 880). In addition, women who inject drugs have a lifetime risk of one in 23, and men who inject drugs have a risk of one in 36. Geographic distribution of HIV within the United States shows a disproportionate burden of HIV in southern states, which account for 51% of all people with HIV (CDC, 2022b). Globally, Sub-Saharan Africa carries over 70% of the global disease burden (Kharsany & Karim, 2016).

SYMPTOMS

The stages of HIV infection are (a) acute retroviral syndrome, (b) clinical latency period, and (c) AIDS. During the acute retroviral syndrome stage (i.e., acute

HIV infection), some individuals may experience a flulike illness that occurs between Weeks 1 and 4 (CDC, 2018a). During this stage, individuals have a high viral load and are especially contagious. During the clinical latency period (i.e., asymptomatic HIV infection), HIV remains active within the body, reproducing at low levels. There are often no symptoms of illness during this stage. For those who are not receiving treatment, the clinical latency period can last about a decade, although some may transition through stages more rapidly. For those who are receiving care, maintenance at the clinical latency stage may occur for several decades (CDC, 2018a). During the final stage, AIDS, symptoms include chills, fever, sweats, weight loss, swollen lymph nodes, and weakness (CDC, 2018b). Individuals are diagnosed with AIDS when their CD4-T cell count drops below 200 cells/mm^3 or when they develop opportunistic infections, such as candidiasis of the bronchi, trachea, esophagus, or lungs; invasive cervical cancer; coccidioidomycosis; Kaposi sarcoma; pneumocystis carinii pneumonia; and/or HIV-related encephalopathy, among others. Without appropriate treatment, individuals with HIV may survive approximately 3 years in this stage.

IMPACT ON THE STUDENT AND OUTCOMES

The impact of HIV on students is significant. In addition to medical outcomes associated with an HIV diagnosis, which may interfere with school functioning, HIV may affect cognitive functions, deterring academic progress. Further, HIV may be associated with social–emotional and behavioral issues that can affect academic functioning. The medical, cognitive/academic, and social–emotional/behavioral outcomes associated with HIV are described in further detail next.

Medical

In cases where HIV is well managed and asymptomatic, children and adolescents are likely to present with medical outcomes no different from their healthy peers (Reitz & Gallo, 2015), with the exception of the side effects of a drug treatment known as highly active antiretroviral therapy (HAART), which range in severity from mild (e.g., nausea, vomiting, diarrhea, headaches, dry mouth) to life-threatening (e.g., anemia, liver or kidney dysfunction; Bindu & Anusha, 2011). Medical outcomes vary widely in cases of symptomatic or poorly managed HIV and depend on a variety of factors, including, but not limited to, medication adherence, comorbid disease, and time since infection (Martin et al., 2005). Different strains of HIV exist, which also may affect medical outcomes in that certain strains may be resistant to medication. Children and adolescents living with HIV who are symptomatic are at risk for opportunistic infections in addition to general fatigue, diarrhea, weight loss, and fever.

Cognitive/Academic

Children with perinatally acquired HIV (mother-to-child transmission) may experience developmental delays (e.g., cognitive, motor, and language delays) given HIV's effects on the central nervous system. These delays may or may not be long-lasting, with some research suggesting HAART may protect against ongoing neurodevelopmental declines, thus speaking to the need for early identification and treatment (Whitehead et al., 2014). For adolescents who acquire HIV behaviorally, the impact on the central nervous system may result in a deterioration of functioning in areas such as attention, memory, and executive functioning. As Nichols (2017) emphasized, the neurodevelopmental impact of HIV is complicated by a variety of factors, such as the timing of HAART initiation, medication adherence, and the presence of other environmental and developmental risk factors. Neurodevelopmental complications common among children and adolescents living with HIV can result in academic difficulties, which may be exacerbated by frequent absences due to illness or medical appointments, as well as challenges associated with the social–emotional and behavioral outcomes of HIV, as described next.

Social–Emotional and Behavioral

The psychosocial outcomes associated with pediatric and adolescent HIV are numerous. It is well documented that youth living with HIV (YLWH) are at increased risk for mental health problems, including anxiety, depression, and posttraumatic stress disorder. A recent study found that age and education interacted with mental health symptoms such that symptoms of anxiety and depression were more prevalent among older YLWH and symptoms of posttraumatic stress disorder were more prevalent among YLWH with less education (Lynn et al., 2018). There are a variety of reasons for the elevated prevalence of mental health problems, particularly internalizing disorders, among YLWH. In addition to the challenges of living with a chronic health condition, YLWH must contend with the fact that HIV continues to be a stigmatized disease. Fear of ostracism related to HIV may result in social isolation and also may present as a barrier to treatment. YLWH face difficult decisions regarding disclosure, including to whom and when to disclose their HIV status and what to do in the aftermath of disclosure (Marhefka et al., 2017). Medication adherence can also be challenging for YLWH.

Although similarities exist between youths with vertically or perinatally (mother-to-child) and horizontally or behaviorally (person-to-person) acquired HIV, some unique differences between these groups do exist. For example, children with perinatally acquired HIV are faced with the fact their mother has HIV or, in cases of maternal death, may be dealing with issues related to adoption or living in foster care or with other family members. Disclosure for children with perinatally acquired HIV is further complicated by the fact that self-disclosure may result in family disclosure. Meanwhile, adolescents with behaviorally acquired HIV may confront unique issues related to risky behaviors such as substance use and unsafe sex practices. There appears to be a cyclical relationship between risky behavior and behavioral infection whereby the behaviors that put adolescents at risk for HIV then become risk factors for living with HIV. For example, mental health symptoms (e.g., depression, anxiety, stress) may increase HIV risk (Rueda et al., 2016) and also may be exacerbated as a result of an HIV diagnosis. Similarly, substance use may increase risk for contracting HIV, decrease the likelihood of HIV testing, and negatively affect medication adherence (Rueda et al., 2016).

Issues related to medication adherence also may differ between children with perinatally acquired HIV and adolescents with behaviorally acquired HIV for a variety of reasons (Thurston et al., 2017). For example, children born with HIV may face medication fatigue and also may face challenges related to the transition of medication management from parent or caregiver to child. Adolescents who acquire HIV behaviorally may face challenges related to the adjustment of living with a chronic illness and a preoccupation with stigma and, consequently, concerns about privacy. Substance use among adolescents also complicates medication adherence.

PSYCHOEDUCATIONAL IMPLICATIONS AND SCHOOL-BASED INTERVENTIONS

Given the physical, cognitive, and psychosocial outcomes described in this chapter, school-aged children and adolescents living with HIV are likely to present with unique needs in the school setting. As Nickels (2017) noted, students with HIV often are treated differently, and unfairly so, than students with other disabilities or chronic illnesses. School-based professionals, in collaboration with families and health care providers, are in a position to positively influence the physical, cognitive, social, and emotional development of these youths and to help prevent HIV among those at risk. Best practices suggest the need for a multitiered approach for addressing HIV along the prevention-to-treatment continuum (Chenneville, 2014; National Association of School Psychologists, 2019). With a focus on prevention, Tiers 1 and 2 contribute to creating a culture conducive to reducing stigma for YLWH, which is critical. Tier 3 focuses on strategies for addressing the needs of YLWH directly.

Medical and Health Management

The U.S. Department of Health and Human Services (2021, 2023) recommends early initiation of HAART for children and adolescents diagnosed with HIV. Using a combination of three of more drugs, HAART stops the virus from replicating inside the body, which reduces damage to the immune system, thus slowing progression to AIDS. By lowering viral load, HAART can also limit onward HIV transmission to others. Current guidelines suggest regular monitoring via, at minimum, quarterly medical appointments, during which time CD4-T cell count and viral load can be assessed. The most important thing parents, caregivers, and school personnel can do to help YLWH to combat the physical outcomes associated with HIV is to make sure they are managing their disease by regular attendance at doctor's appointments and adherence to medication regimens. For younger children, disease management is primarily the responsibility of parents. Therefore, it is critical for parents to work with medical providers, other caregivers, and school personnel to develop a disease management plan. As children living with HIV age into adolescence, they become increasingly responsible for their own disease management, and adolescents who contract HIV behaviorally often are responsible for their own disease management from the time of diagnosis. Encouragement from parents, caregivers, and school personnel is vital given that social support has been identified as a key factor in successful treatment and retention in medical care. Collaboration between families, schools, and medical providers is recommended.

When HIV is well managed, students living with HIV should not present with attendance problems, with the exception of missing school for quarterly doctor's appointments, and should not have restrictions in physical education or other areas. Poor school attendance and/or restrictions may only apply when YLWH are symptomatic or if HIV has progressed to AIDS. In such cases, educators should communicate with families when there are infectious disease outbreaks within the school to avoid further health complications for YLWH.

Cognitive/Academic

To address the cognitive and academic outcomes associated with HIV, psychoeducational assessments and interventions may be necessary in the school setting. Students living with HIV may be eligible for accommodations in the regular classroom under Section 504 of the Americans With Disabilities Act and/or may require exceptional student education services (e.g., under the Other Health Impairment category or other categories as applicable). Specific accommodations and educational needs will vary depending on the needs of the student. Therefore, individualized accommodation or educational plans that take into account the unique needs of the student are important. YLWH also may require support services in and outside of school (e.g., speech/language therapy, occupational therapy) to maximize functioning.

Pennar et al. (2018) developed an intervention designed to promote resilience and health outcomes to improve neurocognitive resources for YLWH. The intervention showed promise in preliminary studies and might be useful for addressing some of the cognitive issues facing this population. However, the intervention was not school based and did not focus on academic outcomes. As Nichols (2017) highlighted, very few controlled studies of cognitive and academic interventions for YWLH have been conducted. Based on findings from a systematic review of articles addressing the developmental challenges of YLWH, Sherr et al. (2014) concluded there is an urgent need for intervention research to address the unique cognitive and educational needs of this population. Given that specific cognitive and academic interventions are lacking, particularly evidence-based school interventions, it may be necessary to adapt existing evidence-based interventions for the school setting and for YLWH. Originally designed to adapt existing evidence-based HIV-prevention interventions for specific populations, the ADAPT-ITT model proposed by Wingood and DiClemente (2008) includes eight phases and might be useful for adapting existing evidence-based cognitive and academic interventions for YLWH.

Social–Emotional and Behavioral

YLWH may benefit from mental health screening and services within and outside the educational setting. Individual and/or family therapy may be beneficial for some YLWH to address mental health symptoms that may exist (e.g., depression, anxiety, posttraumatic stress) as well as issues YLWH commonly confront, such as disclosure decisions and dating/sexual decision making. Stigma-reduction programs may also be beneficial for addressing both projected, or enacted, and internalized HIV stigma in the school setting. Within this context, assertiveness training and psychoeducation may be helpful.

Because of the stigma associated with HIV, many youths do not disclose their HIV status to schools. Thus, although there are many school-based HIV-prevention programs (see Walsh et al., 2017), intervention studies to address the social–emotional and behavioral needs of YLWH in the school setting are lacking. Therefore, evidence-based interventions established in other settings have to be adapted for the school setting. Walsh et al. (2017) described several evidence-based interventions specifically designed for YLWH, including Health and Wellness Cognitive Behavioral Therapy, a program designed to address depressive symptoms and promote the mental health of YLWH (Kennard et al., 2014); Healthy Choices, a brief motivational interviewing intervention designed to reduce depression, substance use, and risky sexual behaviors among YLWH (Naar-King et al., 2010); and Choosing Life: Empowerment! Action! Results!, a modularized intervention to reduce substance use among YLWH (Rotheram-Borus et al., 2004). Bhana et al.'s (2020) systematic review of mental health interventions for YLWH in low- to middle-income countries revealed three group interventions for YLWH, which might be adapted for the school setting or for high-income countries.

CONCLUSION

Children and adolescents with HIV face a variety of physical, mental, and psychosocial issues that may require intervention. The information presented in this chapter may serve as a resource for psychologists, educators, infectious disease physicians, pediatricians, and families of YLWH to help youths with an HIV diagnosis adjust and thrive.

RESOURCES

Chenneville, T. (Ed.). (2017). *A clinical guide to pediatric HIV: Bridging the gaps between research and practice*. Springer.
National Association of School Psychologists. (2019). *Supporting students living with, affected by, or at risk for HIV* [Position statement].
Health and Human Services Office of Adolescent Health. https://www.hhs.gov/ash/oah/resources-and-training/for-families/index.html
KidsHealth. (2022). *What are HIV and AIDS?* https://kidshealth.org/en/kids/hiv.html

REFERENCES

Americans With Disabilities Act of 1990, 42 U.S.C. § 12101 *et seq.* (1990). https://www.ada.gov/pubs/adastatute08.htm
Bhana, A., Abas, M. A., Kelly, J., van Pinxteren, M., Mudekunye, L. A., & Pantelic, M. (2020). Mental health interventions for adolescents living with HIV or affected by HIV in low- and middle-income countries: Systematic review. *BJPsych Open, 6*(5), Article e104. https://doi.org/10.1192/bjo.2020.67
Bindu, H. A., & Anusha, N. (2011). Adverse effects of highly active anti-retroviral therapy (HAART). *Journal of Antivirals & Antiretrovirals, 3*(4), 60–64. https://doi.org/10.4172/jaa.1000037
Centers for Disease Control and Prevention. (2016). *Lifetime risk of HIV diagnosis in the United States*. https://www.justfacts.com/document/lifetime_risk_hiv.pdf
Centers for Disease Control and Prevention. (2018a). *About HIV AIDS*. https://www.cdc.gov/hiv/basics/whatishiv.html
Centers for Disease Control and Prevention. (2018b). *HIV among U.S. youth 2018*. https://www.cdc.gov/healthyyouth/multimedia/infographics_posters/pdfs/hiv_among_youth_infographic_2018.pdf
Centers for Disease Control and Prevention. (2020). *HIV Surveillance Report, 2020: Vol. 33*. U.S. Department of Health and Human Services. https://www.cdc.gov/hiv/pdf/library/reports/surveillance/cdc-hiv-surveillance-report-2020-updated-vol-33.pdf
Centers for Disease Control and Prevention. (2022a). *Basic statistics*. https://www.cdc.gov/hiv/basics/statistics.html
Centers for Disease Control and Prevention. (2022b). *Special focus profiles*. https://www.cdc.gov/hiv/library/reports/hiv-surveillance/vol-33/content/special-focus-profiles.html
Chenneville, T. (2014). Best practices in responding to HIV in the school setting. In A. Thomas & P. Harrison (Eds.), *Best practices in school psychology* (6th ed., pp. 1389–1402). National Association of School Psychologists.
Joint United Nations Programme on HIV/AIDS. (2019). *Global HIV & AIDS statistics—Fact sheet*. Retrieved November 22, 2022, from https://www.unaids.org/en/resources/fact-sheet
Joint United Nations Programme on HIV/AIDS. (2021). *Young people and HIV*. https://www.unaids.org/sites/default/files/media_asset/young-people-and-hiv_en.pdf
Kennard, B., Brown, L., Hawkins, L., Risi, A., Radcliffe, J., Emslie, G., Mayes, T., King, J., Foxwell, A., Buyukdura, J., Bethel, J., Naar-King, S., Xu, J., Lee, S., Garvie, P., London, C., Tanney, M., & Thornton, S. (2014). Development and implementation of health and wellness CBT for individuals with depression and HIV. *Cognitive and Behavioral Practice, 21*(2), 237–246. https://doi.org/10.1016/j.cbpra.2013.07.003

Kharsany, A. B. M., & Karim, Q. A. (2016). HIV infection and AIDS in Sub-Saharan Africa: Current status, challenges, and opportunities. *The Open AIDS Journal, 10*, 34–48. https://doi.org/10.2174/1874613601610010034

Lynn, C., Bradley-Klug, K., Chenneville, T., St. John Walsh, A., Dedrick, R., & Rodriguez, C. (2018). Mental health screening in integrated care settings: Identifying rates of depression, anxiety, and posttraumatic stress among youth with HIV. *Journal of HIV/AIDS & Social Services, 17*(3), 239–245. https://doi.org/10.1080/15381501.2018.1437585

Marhefka, S. L., Turner, D. E., & Chenneville, T. (2017). HIV disclosure in pediatric populations: Who, what, when to tell, and then what? In T. Chenneville (Ed.), *A clinical guide to pediatric HIV: Bridging the gaps between research and practice* (pp. 189–228). Springer International Publishing.

Martin, L. R., Williams, S. L., Haskard, K. B., & DiMatteo, M. R. (2005). The challenge of patient adherence. *Therapeutics and Clinical Risk Management, 1*(3), 189–199.

Naar-King, S., Parsons, J. T., Murphy, D., Kolmodin, K., Harris, D. R., & the ATN 004 Protocol Team. (2010). A multisite randomized trial of a motivational intervention targeting multiple risks in youth living with HIV: Initial effects on motivation, self-efficacy, and depression. *Journal of Adolescent Health, 46*(5), 422–428. https://doi.org/10.1016/j.jadohealth.2009.11.198

National Association of School Psychologists. (2019). *Supporting students living with, affected by, or at risk for HIV* [Position statement].

Nichols, S. (2017). Developmental considerations for children and youth with HIV. In T. Chenneville (Ed.), *A clinical guide to pediatric HIV: Bridging the gaps between research and practice* (pp. 43–72). Springer International Publishing.

Nickels, M. (2017). Separate and unequal: Students with HIV/AIDS and mathematics education. *Journal of Urban Mathematics Education, 10*(2), 39–51. https://doi.org/10.1007/978-3-319-49704-4

Pennar, A., Naar, S., Woods, S., Nichols, S., Outlaw, A., & Ellis, D. (2018). Promoting resilience through neurocognitive functioning in youth living with HIV. *AIDS Care, 30*(Suppl. 4), 59–64. https://doi.org/10.1080/09540121.2019.1576851

Reitz, M. S., & Gallo, R. C. (2015). Human immunodeficiency viruses. In J. E. Bennett, R. Dolin, & M. J. Blaser (Eds.), *Mandell, Douglas, and Bennett's principles and practice of infectious diseases* (8th ed., pp. 120–133). Elsevier Saunders.

Rotheram-Borus, M. J., Swendeman, D., Comulada, W. S., Weiss, R. E., Lee, M., & Lightfoot, M. (2004). Prevention for substance-using HIV-positive young people: Telephone and in-person delivery. *Journal of Acquired Immune Deficiency Syndromes, 37*(Suppl. 2), S68–S77. https://doi.org/10.1097/01.qai.0000140604.57478.67

Rueda, S., Mitra, S., Chen, S., Gogolishvili, D., Globerman, J., Chambers, L., Wilson, M., Logie, C. H., Shi, Q., Morassaei, S., & Rourke, S. B. (2016). Examining the associations between HIV-related stigma and health outcomes in people living with HIV/AIDS: A series of meta-analyses. *BMJ Open, 6*(7), Article e011453. https://doi.org/10.1136/bmjopen-2016-011453

Sherr, L., Croome, N., Castaneda, K. P., Bradshaw, K., & Romero, R. H. (2014). Developmental challenges in HIV infected children—An updated systematic review. *Children and Youth Services Review, 45*, 74–89.

Thurston, I. B., Decker, K., & Hardin, R. (2017). Antiretroviral medication adherence and disease management in pediatric populations. In T. Chenneville (Ed.), *A clinical guide to pediatric HIV: Bridging the gaps between research and practice* (pp. 163–188). Springer International Publishing.

U.S. Department of Health and Human Services. (2021). *Guidelines for the use of antiretroviral agents in adults and adolescents living with HIV*. https://clinicalinfo.hiv.gov/sites/default/files/guidelines/archive/AdultandAdolescentGL_2021_08_16.pdf

U.S. Department of Health and Human Services. (2023). *Guidelines for the use of antiretroviral agents in pediatric HIV infection*. https://clinicalinfo.hiv.gov/sites/default/files/guidelines/documents/pediatric-arv/guidelines-pediatric-arv.pdf

Walsh, A. S. J., Lynn, C., Wesley, K., O'Leary, K., & Chenneville, T. (2017). HIV prevention and intervention in the school setting. In T. Chenneville (Ed.), *A clinical guide to pediatric HIV: Bridging the gaps between research and practice* (pp. 133–162). Springer International Publishing.

Whitehead, N., Potterton, J., & Coovadia, A. (2014). The neurodevelopment of HIV-infected infants on HAART compared to HIV-exposed but uninfected infants. *AIDS Care, 26*(4), 497–504. https://doi.org/10.1080/09540121.2013.841828

Wingood, G. M., & DiClemente, R. J. (2008). The ADAPT-ITT model: A novel method of adapting evidence-based HIV interventions. *Journal of Acquired Immune Deficiency Syndromes, 47*, S40–S46. https://doi.org/10.1097/QAI.0b013e3181605df1

9

Noonan Syndrome

Suzanne G. Margiano, Lorette McWilliams, Johanna deLeyer-Tiarks, Carissa Scogin, and Lauren E. Klein

Noonan syndrome (NS) is a congenital genetic disorder characterized by a wide range of physical, medical, behavioral, and cognitive characteristics. Also known as familial Turner syndrome and Ullrich–Noonan syndrome, NS has been recognized as a medically classified syndrome since 1963 (Rohrer, 2009). There are numerous and widely varying physical characteristics associated with NS.

ETIOLOGY

As a genetic disorder that interrupts the RAS pathways, NS is referred to as one of the RASopathies (MedlinePlus, 2018). NS etiology relates to gene mutations affecting the RAS-MAPK pathway, which is responsible for cell proliferation, differentiation, and migration (Tafazoli et al., 2018). These mutations cause the genes to be active longer than usual, which produces the volume of symptoms characteristic of NS. Inherited mutations to the *PTPN11* gene account for about half of the cases of NS, and mutations to genes *SOS1*, *RAF1*, and *RIT1* make up about 20% to 25% of cases (MedlinePlus, 2018). For 20% to 30% of the population of individuals with NS, causative mutations remain unidentified (Tafazoli et al., 2018).

Inherited gene mutations associated with NS are dominant and not sex-linked, resulting in one copy of a mutated gene being sufficient to pass on the syndrome and an equal likelihood of inheriting NS across the sexes. Therefore,

https://doi.org/10.1037/0000349-009
Health-Related Disorders in Children and Adolescents: A Guidebook for Educators and Service Providers, Second Edition, M. M. Perfect, C. A. Riccio, and M. A. Bray (Editors)

a child of a parent with NS has a 50% chance of inheritance, whereas a child of parents who do not have NS has less than 1% chance (Allanson & Roberts, 2016). Diagnosis is rendered according to clinical features, but especially given the risk of underdiagnosing in milder presentations, genetic testing can promote accurate determinations (Bhambhani & Muenke, 2014).

PREVALENCE AND INCIDENCE

NS occurs in about one in every 1,000 to 2,500 individuals, with more mild expression in one in 100 (Allanson, 2010). Although NS is often inherited, individuals have been diagnosed due to de novo mutations that occur spontaneously and without inheritance from the parent (Bhambhani & Muenke, 2014; Tafazoli et al., 2018). There is a high degree of variability in NS expression across ethnic groups, though more research is needed to determine the genetic basis in different groups (Tafazoli et al., 2018).

SYMPTOMS

The most common physical features include a distinctive facial appearance with downward slanting and wide-set eyes, drooping eyelids, and a low hairline; low-set or abnormally shaped ears; short stature; concave chest (pectus excavatum); and a webbed, short-appearing neck (Allanson, 2010). Developmental delay; cryptorchidism; and hematologic, lymphatic, and congenital heart defects are also common symptoms found in individuals with NS (Allanson, 2010; Bhambhani & Muenke, 2014). Individuals with NS may experience a mild or severe form of the syndrome, dependent on the number and severity of NS symptoms experienced. Superficial characteristics associated with NS, including the distinctive facial appearance, tend to lessen with age.

IMPACT ON THE STUDENT AND OUTCOMES

Medical

A host of medical conditions are often seen in individuals with NS, though the complete clinical presentation and severity of the associated medical conditions vary from individual to individual. Common medical concomitants of the syndrome include congenital heart defects, blood disorders, delayed puberty, ophthalmological issues, and hearing loss (Allanson, 2010; Cooke et al., 2016; Madan-Khetarpal & Arnold, 2018; Romano et al., 2010). Congenital heart defects, such as pulmonary valve stenosis or hypertrophic cardiomyopathy, are common among those with NS, occurring in up to 50% to 90% of individuals (Allanson, 2010; Allanson & Roberts, 2016). As noted, NS has been associated with slowed growth and delayed puberty, including undescended testes. Associated with these factors, infertility may be present, especially in male patients (Allanson, 2010).

Individuals with NS also may display muscle weakness and skeletal issues such as scoliosis and fragile bones, with associated gross and fine motor coordination difficulties. Additionally, dental/orthodontal irregularities, confounded with muscle weakness, contribute to speech articulation difficulties among children with NS. Ocular dysmorphology (e.g., hypertelorism, ptosis, epicanthal folds) and vision problems (e.g., refractive error, strabismus, nystagmus) are highly prevalent in NS (up to 95% affected), and hearing loss is also quite common (more than 33% affected) and directly resulting from serous otitis media (Allanson, 2010; Bhambhani & Muenke, 2014).

Neurological problems also have been identified, such as central nervous system malformations (e.g., Arnold–Chiari malformation), hydrocephalus, seizures, hypotonia, and laxity or hypermobility of joints, and may manifest in head and neck pain, dizziness, seizures, and balance issues (Allanson, 2010; Bhambhani & Muenke, 2014). Hematologic problems involving coagulation defects are reported in approximately one third of individuals with NS, often reflected in signs of easy bruising or abnormal bleeding, in addition to an increased risk of developing some cancers, such as leukemia (Allanson, 2010; Bhambhani & Muenke, 2014; MedlinePlus, 2018). Further, individuals with NS may experience dermatological issues, such as café au lait spots and lesions (Bhambhani & Muenke, 2014).

Cognitive/Academic

Children with NS may experience developmental delays and reach developmental milestones, such as speaking and walking, later than peers, influenced in part by medical sequelae such as hearing loss, hypotonia, and hyperextensibility (Allanson, 2010). It has been estimated that about one quarter of those living with NS have been diagnosed with intellectual disability (Allanson & Roberts, 2016). Similarly, a strong association has been identified between marked early feeding difficulties and intellectual disability, indicating that symptoms of early "failure to thrive" and reduced oral–motor abilities should be monitored very closely (Allanson, 2010). When not intellectually delayed, the majority of children with NS perform in the low average to average range, though cognitive abilities can range from the low to high range of functioning (Pierpont et al., 2013).

Academic outcomes for children with NS vary, in part as a result of the widely differing symptom profiles comprising the diagnosis (Wingbermuehle et al., 2009). It is estimated that 50% of children with a NS diagnosis have unique learning needs (Pierpont et al., 2009), and up to 40% require special education (Lee et al., 2005; Shaw et al., 2007; van der Burgt et al., 1999).

Communication skills may develop slowly in students diagnosed with NS, reflective of the high prevalence of hearing problems and articulation difficulties associated with physical concomitants of the disorder (Pierpont et al.,

2009). Such difficulties can result in speech or language impairments, and such deficits in areas of communication can necessitate support in the academic areas of reading, writing, and spelling. Writing ability may be further affected by inattention and the higher incidence of fine motor impairment (Pierpont et al., 2009). Though communication difficulties have been observed, Pierpont et al. (2009) found that children with NS performed higher on verbal tasks than nonverbal tasks.

Overall, children with NS tend to exhibit a profile of strengths in verbal comprehension, abstract reasoning, and social cognition, with weaknesses in spatial, perceptual, and planning abilities (Allanson, 2010). Deficits in specific areas of neuropsychological functioning have been documented, including visual processing, verbal long-term memory, language development, and motor skills (Pierpont et al., 2013). There is some evidence that attention and executive functioning are areas of particular challenge for many with NS (Pierpont et al., 2015). Children with NS can present as physically uncoordinated, and up to 50% qualify as having developmental coordination disorder (Lee et al., 2005).

Social-Emotional and Behavioral

Despite common cognitive and learning problems, children with NS exhibit generally typical social interaction skills and self-esteem and have no specific profile of mental or behavioral disorders (Allanson, 2010). There have been very few reports of autistic symptoms, anxiety, severe aggression, or sleep disruption across this population. Behaviorally, no profile of those with NS has emerged; self-esteem appears to be generally comparable to peers (Lee et al., 2005). Overall, there is little data on the psychological health of children and adults with NS, and more research is needed.

PSYCHOEDUCATIONAL IMPLICATIONS AND SCHOOL-BASED INTERVENTIONS

Medical and Health Management

There is no cure for NS; rather, treatments are centered on the individual's particular symptoms and manifestation, often requiring ongoing medical monitoring. Medically, given the frequency of congenital heart disease in NS, a clinical assessment, electrocardiogram, and echocardiogram are recommended for initial cardiological evaluation, with follow-up monitoring and treatment determined by medical findings (Allanson, 2010). Given common neurological problems, low threshold for exploring issues is recommended, with evaluation determined by presenting symptoms and possibly including magnetic resonance imaging, electroencephalogram, or other testing to identify structural anomalies or disorders (Allanson, 2010; Bhambhani & Muenke, 2014). With an extremely high prevalence of ophthalmological problems, thorough early assessment and periodic evaluation are warranted (Allanson, 2010). Vision problems associated with NS are usually treated nonsurgically (e.g., glasses), though surgery may be recommended for cataracts or ptosis. Similarly, hearing testing beginning in infancy and continuing throughout childhood is indicated for individuals with NS, in conjunction with aggressive treatment of ear infections with antibiotics, due to the proportion of children with NS who display hearing difficulties (Allanson, 2010). Routine screenings for hematologic problems and possible further specific testing (e.g., coagulation factors) are recommended (Allanson, 2010). Monitoring for other reported medical problems—dermatological, musculoskeletal, genitourinary, lymphatic—is recommended, with treatment dependent on clinical presentation and evaluation findings (Bhambhani & Muenke, 2014).

Due to the multifaceted nature of NS, consultation among a team of professionals to support psychological, social–emotional, and educational development and progress is warranted. It is essential that appropriate school personnel, such as the school nurse, have ongoing and open communication with the family and medical providers; ongoing medical monitoring among different specialties is expected. Other members of the team would include professionals with various areas of expertise, such as a speech/language pathologist, special education teacher, general education teacher, school psychologist, and school counselor. Time in the classroom, and thus time spent on academic learning and engagement in social interactions, may be adversely affected by time spent in the nurse's office or at medical appointments. These factors will need consideration by the team, and school personnel should monitor and supplement instruction accordingly.

Cognitive/Academic

Screening for eligibility for early intervention services should be initiated as soon as possible. Ongoing vision, hearing, speech and language, and occupational and physical therapy assessments, as well as academic and developmental assessments, should be conducted in consultation with the child's medical team to construct a full picture of the student that includes their strengths as well as needs, with flexibility to meet changing needs over time. Psychoeducational evaluations may be warranted in cases of cognitive and learning difficulties, and individualized education programs may be recommended (Allanson, 2010). The American Academy of Family Physicians recommends developmental assessment annually, beginning after 6 months of age or at time of diagnosis, and baseline neuropsychological assessment upon entering elementary school (Bhambhani & Muenke, 2014).

Social–Emotional and Behavioral

Support for the family system that cares for a child with NS should be considered. Caregivers of children with multiple and ongoing medical needs require resources, and thus the family unit may also need support. Siblings of children with NS may likewise require support. Social support and psychoeducation, often found in support groups and organizations, should be referred to students, their families, and caregivers. Psychiatrists and psychologists can help identify and intervene with anxiety, mood, behavioral, or cognitive problems.

CONCLUSION

NS is a rare genetic disorder with a variety of physical, medical, and developmental characteristics. NS can result from inherited genetic transmission or from spontaneous genetic mutations. Despite the wide range of phenotypic expression, there are some cardinal features associated with NS, such as distinctive facial and physical features and common medical and cognitive manifestations. There is no cure for NS; rather, treatments are centered on the individual's particular symptoms, often requiring continuing medical and educational monitoring and interventions. Ongoing assessments conducted during infancy and early childhood, across multiple affected domains, are strongly recommended.

RESOURCES

New England Regional Genetics Network. (n.d.). *Genetics Education Materials for School Success (GEMSS)*. https://www.gemssforschools.org

MedlinePlus. (2018). *Noonan syndrome*. National Library of Medicine. https://medlineplus.gov/genetics/condition/noonan-syndrome

Genetic and Rare Disease Information Center. (2021). *Noonan syndrome*. National Institutes of Health. https://rarediseases.info.nih.gov/diseases/10955/noonan-syndrome

Noonan Syndrome Foundation. http://www.teamnoonan.org/

MAGIC Foundation. https://www.magicfoundation.org

RASopathies. https://rasopathiesnet.org/

REFERENCES

Allanson, J. E. (2010). Noonan syndrome. In S. B. Cassidy & J. E. Allanson (Eds.), *Management of genetic syndromes* (pp. 569–586). Wiley-Blackwell. https://doi.org/10.1002/9780470893159.ch38

Allanson, J. E., & Roberts, A. E. (2016). Noonan syndrome. In M. P. Adam, G. M. Mirzaa, R. A. Pagon, S. E. Wallace, L. J. H. Bean, K. W. Gripp, & A. Amemiya (Eds.), *GeneReviews*. University of Washington.

Bhambhani, V., & Muenke, M. (2014). Noonan syndrome. *American Family Physician, 89*(1), 37–43.

Cooke, D. W., Divall, S. A., & Radovick, S. (2016). Normal and aberrant growth in children. In S. Melmed, K. S. Polonsky, P. R. Larsen, & H. M. Kronenberg (Eds.), *Williams textbook of endocrinology* (13th ed., pp. 964–1073). Elsevier. https://doi.org/10.1016/B978-0-323-29738-7.00024-1

Lee, D. A., Portnoy, S., Hill, P., Gillberg, C., & Patton, M. A. (2005). Psychological profile of children with Noonan syndrome. *Developmental Medicine and Child Neurology, 47*(1), 35–38. https://doi.org/10.1111/j.1469-8749.2005.tb01037.x

Madan-Khetarpal, S., & Arnold, G. (2018). Genetic disorders and dysmorphic conditions. In B. J. Zitelli, S. C. McIntire, & A. J. Nowalk (Eds.), *Zitelli and Davis' atlas of pediatric physical diagnosis* (7th ed., pp. 1–43). Elsevier.

MedlinePlus. (2018). *Noonan syndrome*. National Library of Medicine. https://medlineplus.gov/genetics/condition/noonan-syndrome

Pierpont, E. I., Pierpont, M. E., Mendelsohn, N. J., Roberts, A. E., Tworog-Dube, E., & Seidenberg, M. S. (2009). Genotype differences in cognitive functioning in Noonan syndrome. *Genes Brain & Behavior, 8*(3), 275–282. https://doi.org/10.1111/j.1601-183X.2008.00469.x

Pierpont, E. I., Tworog-Dube, E., & Roberts, A. E. (2013). Learning and memory in children with Noonan syndrome. *American Journal of Medical Genetics: Part A, 161*(9), 2250–2257. https://doi.org/10.1002/ajmg.a.36075

Pierpont, E. I., Tworog-Dube, E., & Roberts, A. E. (2015). Attention skills and executive functioning in children with Noonan syndrome and their unaffected siblings. *Developmental Medicine and Child Neurology, 57*(4), 385–392. https://doi.org/10.1111/dmcn.12621

Rohrer, T. (2009). Noonan syndrome: Introduction and basic clinical features. *Hormone Research in Paediatrics, 72*(Suppl. 2), 3–7. https://doi.org/10.1159/000243772

Romano, A. A., Allanson, J. E., Dahlgren, J., Gelb, B. D., Hall, B., Pierpont, M. E., Roberts, A. E., Robinson, W., Takemoto, C. M., & Noonan, J. A. (2010). Noonan syndrome: Clinical features, diagnosis, and management guidelines. *Pediatrics, 126*(4), 746–759. https://doi.org/10.1542/peds.2009-3207

Shaw, A. C., Kalidas, K., Crosby, A. H., Jeffery, S., & Patton, M. A. (2007). The natural history of Noonan syndrome: A long-term follow-up study. *Archives of Disease in Childhood, 92*(2), 128–132. https://doi.org/10.1136/adc.2006.104547

Tafazoli, A., Eshraghi, P., Pantaleoni, F., Vakili, R., Moghaddassian, M., Ghahraman, M., Muto, V., Paolacci, S., Golyan, F. F., & Abbaszadegan, M. R. (2018). Novel mutations and their genotype-phenotype correlations in patients with Noonan syndrome, using next-generation sequencing. *Advances in Medical Sciences, 63*(1), 87–93. https://doi.org/10.1016/j.advms.2017.07.001

van der Burgt, I., Thoonen, G., Roosenboom, N., Assman-Hulsmans, C., Gabreels, F., Otten, B., & Brunner, H. G. (1999). Patterns of cognitive functioning in school-aged children with Noonan syndrome associated with variability in phenotypic expression. *The Journal of Pediatrics, 135*(6), 707–713. https://doi.org/10.1016/S0022-3476(99)70089-2

Wingbermuehle, E., Egger, J., van der Burgt, I., & Verhoeven, W. (2009). Neuropsychological and behavioral aspects of Noonan syndrome. *Hormone Research, 72*(Suppl. 2), 15–23. https://doi.org/10.1159/000243774

10

Sickle Cell Anemia

Linda W. Morse, Melanie C. Morse, and Sarah E. Bills

Sickle cell anemia (SCA), the homozygous state for the hemoglobin S gene, is one of the more common and clinically severe hemoglobinopathic abnormalities manifested in various forms of sickle cell disease (SCD). The prevalence of SCD is highest in sub-Saharan Africa, as the distribution of hemoglobin S is highly concentrated in geographic areas where there is a historical incidence of malaria (Rees et al., 2010). Although most common among persons of African descent, this genetic disease affects a number of ethnic groups, including individuals of Mediterranean, Caribbean, South and Central American, East Indian, and Middle Eastern backgrounds (Gustafson et al., 2006; National Heart, Lung, and Blood Institute [NHLBI], 2002). Estimates of the incidence of SCA are approximately one in 365 Black live births; the total is about 100,000 Americans (Centers for Disease Control and Prevention [CDC], 2019). Given this high probability, all 50 states have implemented routine screening for SCD at birth since 2006 (CDC, 2018). Symptoms in newborns do not usually appear until after 6 months of age, and the disease may present with wide variation in symptoms. The body of research related to the treatment of both physical and psychosocial effects of SCD has grown significantly over the past several decades and indicates that the disease often has negative impacts on cognitive and psychosocial development (Armstrong, 2006).

The authors would like to acknowledge the contributions of Agnes E. Shine and Jerry B. Wilson to an earlier version of this chapter.

https://doi.org/10.1037/0000349-010
Health-Related Disorders in Children and Adolescents: A Guidebook for Educators and Service Providers, Second Edition, M. M. Perfect, C. A. Riccio, and M. A. Bray (Editors)

ETIOLOGY

SCDs are classified by genotype, which describes the type of hemoglobin (the oxygen-carrying component of blood) being produced by the two beta globin genes on chromosome 11 and the four alpha globin genes on chromosome 16 (NHLBI, 2002). There are four main forms of SCD: (a) SCA, caused by two abnormal hemoglobin genes in the homozygous condition; (b) sickle β+ thalassemia; (c) hemoglobin sickle cell C disease; and (d) sickle beta^{0} thalassemia (NHLBI, 2002). In addition to these main forms, there are other variations depending on the genotype inherited. Molecular biology techniques are used to establish specific diagnoses.

PREVALENCE

Estimates place the diagnosis of SCD at approximately one out of every 365 Black births and one out of every 16,300 Hispanic American births, with 100,000 total Americans thought to be affected (CDC, 2019). As treatments for SCD are better understood and disseminated, mortality rates continue to improve. Deaths related to SCD among Black children younger than 4 years of age fell by 42% from 1999 to 2002 (CDC, 2019). The median age at death for patients with SCD has been found to be 42 years for women and 38 years for men (Lanzkron et al., 2013).

SYMPTOMS

In SCA, hemoglobin S accounts for approximately 95% of the produced hemoglobin in the blood rather than the normal hemoglobin A. During the deoxygenation of red blood cells, hemoglobin S molecules stick to each sickle-shaped cell rather than the normal rounded doughnut-shaped cells. These sickle-shaped cells become rigid and cause an obstruction as they pass through small blood vessels, resulting in a lack of oxygen and injury to the tissue. The clumping of sickle-shaped cells inside blood vessels can result in occlusion in any organ of the body. An individual may experience symptoms ranging from severe pain to infections, organ damage, or acute chest syndrome due to clogged vessels in the lungs. Armstrong (2006) noted that when sickle hemoglobin is stressed, the resultant occlusion may occur in any organ of the body, resulting in potentially widespread tissue damage. When these sickling episodes occur, a painful crisis may ensue. After repeated episodes, the red blood cells eventually become permanently damaged and cause anemia. Thus, hemolytic anemia and acute vaso-occlusion (i.e., closing or obstruction of the blood vessels) are two of the principle pathophysiological features associated with SCD. Moreover, the effect of complications related to SCD may emerge over time and affect multiple areas of a child's life. For example, a stroke may have lasting consequences, including motor and cognitive impairment, and the possibility of numerous complications exists because no tissue or organ is safe from injury (NHLBI, 2002).

IMPACT ON THE STUDENT AND OUTCOMES

Medical

The severity of the disease is highly variable, affecting some individuals drastically while others maintain a fairly normal life. Physical growth in children is blunted and distorted (i.e., they have spindly arms and legs, poor development, and dental malocclusions, abnormal contact of the upper and lower teeth). Puberty is usually slightly delayed (NHLBI, 2002). Common pain symptoms include muscular, bone, and abdominal pain during pain crises. Depending on the severity of the crisis and the length of the episode (which may last as long as 7–14 days), the child may be hospitalized or treated at home. Pain crises may be treated with over-the-counter medications or opioids (NHLBI, 2002). Boys also may experience priapism, a painful and sustained erection of the penis that may last for several hours. Additionally, children with SCA are frequently at risk for a variety of infections, such as pneumonia, as well as the possibility of stroke. For some, many interacting variables lead to hospitalizations and school absenteeism. SCA also has implications for neurocognitive development due to the possibility of vascular occlusions in the brain, either major (e.g., stroke) or as cumulative small damages over time as a result of the sickling process during pain episodes. Finally, enormous psychosocial pressures face the chronically ill child who knows there is no cure for SCA (NHLBI, 2002).

Cognitive/Academic

With SCA, children may be at risk for impacts on intellectual and neuropsychological functioning as well as academic achievement. Newer studies have suggested that there is a relationship between SCA and lower cognitive performance (Cahill et al., 2019; Kawadler et al., 2016). Steen and colleagues (2005) found lower full-scale IQs in children with SCA even though magnetic resonance imaging did not show cognitive incidents. In a more recent study, Castro and Viana (2019) found that children with SCA had lower Wechsler scores compared with controls. In Day and Chismark's (2006) review of research on the academic and cognitive impact of SCA, half of the studies reviewed found differences in IQ and 71% reported issues with other types of cognition. Additional studies have emphasized the role of central executive functioning (Berkelhammer et al., 2007). For example, Smith and Schatz (2016) assessed school-age children with SCA and found poorer working memory performance. Schatz and colleagues (2001) found that children with SCA who had experienced a cerebral event had higher incidence of retention and use of special services within schools. Taken together, these studies suggest that children with SCA not only have lower IQ scores and neuropsychological functioning but also experience more academic achievement issues than was previously thought.

Social-Emotional and Behavioral

Children with SCA face many potential issues related to their psychosocial development, including learning to cope with their disease, being alienated from other children due to school absenteeism, and feeling different from others. With adolescence comes additional problems related to psychosocial development (Burlew et al., 2000). The adolescent with SCA may have a host of disease-related problems (e.g., priapism; leg ulcers; jaundice; enuresis; difficulties with the femoral head, which may necessitate crutches; residual effects of stroke; pain), making the normal adolescent tasks of identity formation and acceptance much harder.

PSYCHOEDUCATIONAL IMPLICATIONS AND SCHOOL-BASED INTERVENTIONS

Medical and Health Management

One of the major challenges of psychosocial development for children with SCA and their families is the adaptation that must occur throughout the lifespan. Disease management represents a significant stressor for individuals with SCA, who must acquire strategies to prevent and cope with pain crises. In addition, individuals with SCA frequently face personal crises as the disease takes its toll over the lifespan, which significantly affects parent- and child-reported quality of life (Anie, 2005). Youth with SCA should be encouraged to participate in physical activities at school but should be directed to drink ample fluids and take breaks as needed, as dehydration and strenuous physical activity have been linked to an increased risk of disease-related complications (NHLBI, 2002). Extreme heat and cold are also risk factors and should be avoided.

Given these complications, appropriate counseling for families and ongoing, routine medical care is important for managing SCD. Yawn and colleagues (2014) outlined specific treatment recommendations, including daily prophylactic penicillin in young children, annual transcranial doppler examinations (ages 2–16 years), and blood transfusions for children with abnormal doppler scans. Hydroxyurea is often given to individuals with SCD across the lifespan to help manage pain episodes; when such episodes do occur, opioids may be used to manage pain (Yawn et al., 2014).

Cognitive/Academic

Within the school setting, children with SCA should be treated as normally as possible and placed in a regular classroom. It is important to note that, although youth with SCA are at increased risk for cognitive and academic impairments, most children with SCA have normal intelligence and should be able to perform at the same academic level as their peers (NHLBI, 2002). However, school personnel should be informed of the child's condition, and monitoring and screening for any academic difficulties should be implemented (Peterson et al., 2005). High absenteeism caused by infections or pain crises should be expected. Therefore, school personnel should work with parents to plan for absences and arrange appropriate academic supports (e.g., attendance accommodations; Mayes et al., 2011).

Social-Emotional and Behavioral

Emotional difficulties are also an area for concern. In Key and colleagues' (2001) study, adolescents with SCD reported a higher frequency and severity of depressive symptoms when compared with both the normative population as well as adolescents diagnosed with other chronic illnesses (e.g., cystic fibrosis, diabetes). Symptoms of depression and anxiety have been linked to increased hospital admissions and the use of maladaptive coping strategies for pain. Thus, internalizing symptoms should be identified and treated as early as possible (Benton et al., 2007). Youth with SCA should be exposed to positive role models who have coped with the disease and have led successful lives. Career aspirations are important for these youth (NHLBI, 2002). Despite the disease and its implications for a variety of physical and psychological problems, many of these children adjust well, excel academically, and become productive adults. Additionally, many parents may need counseling to help them cope with their own psychological stress, guilt, or tendency to be overly protective (NHLBI, 2002).

CONCLUSION

SCA affects as many as 100,000 Americans (CDC, 2019), with symptoms typically appearing in children after 6 months and resulting in potential significant cognitive/academic and psychosocial issues. Early identification of SCA with the implementation of targeted newborn screening (CDC, 2018), adherence to regularly scheduled vaccinations (e.g., pneumococcal conjugate vaccine; Yanni et al., 2009), and routine monitoring for cerebral infarcts and stroke (NHLBI, 2002) represent advances that contribute to the increased well-being of individuals with SCA. Teachers and psychologists should be aware of possible issues and interventions to alleviate the disease's impact as well as early identification and assessment, including of neuropsychological functioning. Although no cure is available at present, stem cell therapy (Walters, 2015) and gene editing (Demirci et al., 2019) are two promising new techniques. Given advances in the identification and management of SCA, many patients are now living into the 7th and 8th decades (NHLBI, 2002).

RESOURCES

Centers for Disease Control and Prevention. (2022). *What is sickle cell disease?* U.S. Department of Health and Human Services. https://www.cdc.gov/ncbddd/sicklecell/facts.html

Sickle Cell Disease Association of America. http://www.sicklecelldisease.org

REFERENCES

Anie, K. A. (2005). Psychological complications in sickle cell disease. *British Journal of Haematology, 129*(6), 723–729. https://doi.org/10.1111/j.1365-2141.2005.05500.x

Armstrong, F. D. (2006). Cancer and blood disorders in childhood: Biopsychosocial-developmental issues in assessment and treatment. In R. T. Brown (Ed.), *Comprehensive handbook of childhood cancer and sickle cell disease: A biopsychosocial approach* (pp. 17–32). Oxford University Press. https://doi.org/10.1093/oso/9780195169850.003.0006

Benton, T. D., Ifeagwu, J. A., & Smith-Whitley, K. (2007). Anxiety and depression in children and adolescents with sickle cell disease. *Current Psychiatry Reports, 9*(2), 114–121. https://doi.org/10.1007/s11920-007-0080-0

Berkelhammer, L. D., Williamson, A. L., Sanford, S. D., Dirksen, C. L., Sharp, W. G., Margulies, A. S., & Prengler, R. A. (2007). Neurocognitive sequelae of pediatric sickle cell disease: A review of the literature. *Child Neuropsychology, 13*(2), 120–131. https://doi.org/10.1080/09297040600800956

Burlew, K., Telfair, J., Colangelo, L., & Wright, E. C. (2000). Factors that influence adolescent adaptation to sickle cell disease. *Journal of Pediatric Psychology, 25*(5), 287–299.

Cahill, C. R., Leach, J. M., McClure, L. A., Irvin, M. R., Zakai, N. A., Naik, R., Unverzagt, F., Wadley, V. G., Hyacinth, H. I., Manly, J., Judd, S. E., Winkler, C., & Cushman, M. (2019). Sickle cell trait and risk of cognitive impairment in African-Americans: The REGARDS cohort. *eClinicalMedicine, 11*, 27–33. https://doi.org/10.1016/j.eclinm.2019.05.003

Castro, I. P. S., & Viana, M. B. (2019). Cognitive profile of children with sickle cell anemia compared to healthy controls. *Jornal de Pediatria, 95*(4), 451–457. https://doi.org/10.1016/j.jped.2018.04.012

Centers for Disease Control and Prevention. (2018, May). *State-based monitoring for selected hemoglobinopathies*. U.S. Department of Health and Human Services. https://www.cdc.gov/ncbddd/hemoglobinopathies/features/keyfinding-state-based.html

Centers for Disease Control and Prevention. (2019, October). *Data & statistics on sickle cell disease*. U.S. Department of Health and Human Services. https://www.cdc.gov/ncbddd/sicklecell/data.html

Day, S., & Chismark, E. (2006). The cognitive and academic impact of sickle cell disease. *The Journal of School Nursing, 22*(6), 330–335. https://doi.org/10.1177/10598405060220060401

Demirci, S., Leonard, A., Haro-Mora, J. J., Uchida, N., & Tisdale, J. F. (2019). CRISPR/Cas9 for sickle cell disease: Applications, future possibilities, and challenges. In K. Turksen (Ed.), *Cell biology and translational medicine: Vol. 5. Stem cells: Translational science to therapy* (pp. 37–52). Springer. https://doi.org/10.1007/5584_2018_331

Gustafson, K. E., Bonner, M. J., Hardy, K. K., & Thompson, R. J., Jr. (2006). Biopsychosocial and developmental issues in sickle cell disease. In R. T. Brown (Ed.), *Comprehensive handbook of childhood cancer and sickle cell disease: A biopsychosocial approach* (pp. 431–448). Oxford University Press. https://doi.org/10.1093/oso/9780195169850.003.0032

Kawadler, J. M., Clayden, J. D., Clark, C. A., & Kirkham, F. J. (2016). Intelligence quotient in paediatric sickle cell disease: A systematic review and meta-analysis. *Developmental Medicine and Child Neurology, 58*(7), 672–679. https://doi.org/10.1111/dmcn.13113

Key, J. D., Brown, R. T., Marsh, L. D., Spratt, E. G., & Recknor, J. C. (2001). Depressive symptoms in adolescents with a chronic illness. *Children's Health Care, 30*(4), 283–292. https://doi.org/10.1207/S15326888CHC3004_03

Lanzkron, S., Carroll, C. P., & Haywood, C., Jr. (2013). Mortality rates and age at death from sickle cell disease: U.S., 1979–2005. *Public Health Reports, 128*(2), 110–116. https://doi.org/10.1177/003335491312800206

Mayes, S., Wolfe-Christensen, C., Mullins, L. L., & Cain, J. P. (2011). Psychoeducational screening in pediatric sickle cell disease: An evaluation of academic and health concerns in the school environment. *Children's Health Care, 40*(2), 101–115. https://doi.org/10.1080/02739615.2011.566465

National Heart, Lung, and Blood Institute. (2002). The management of sickle cell disease (4th ed., NIH Publication No. 02-2117). National Institutes of Health. https://www.nhlbi.nih.gov/files/docs/guidelines/sc_mngt.pdf

Peterson, C. C., Palermo, T. M., Swift, E., Beebe, A., & Drotar, D. (2005). Assessment of psycho-educational needs in a clinical sample of children with sickle cell disease. *Children's Health Care, 34*(2), 133–148. https://doi.org/10.1207/s15326888chc3402_4

Rees, D. C., Williams, T. N., & Gladwin, M. T. (2010). Sickle-cell disease. *The Lancet, 376*(9757), 2018–2031. https://doi.org/10.1016/S0140-6736(10)61029-X

Schatz, J., Brown, R. T., Pascual, J. M., Hsu, L., & DeBaun, M. R. (2001). Poor school and cognitive functioning with silent cerebral infarcts and sickle cell disease. *Neurology, 56*(8), 1109–1111. https://doi.org/10.1212/WNL.56.8.1109

Smith, K. E., & Schatz, J. (2016). Working memory in children with neurocognitive effects from sickle cell disease: Contributions of the central executive and processing speed. *Developmental Neuropsychology, 41*(4), 231–244. https://doi.org/10.1080/87565641.2016.1238474

Steen, R. G., Fineberg-Buchner, C., Hankins, G., Weiss, L., Prifitera, A., & Mulhern, R. K. (2005). Cognitive deficits in children with sickle cell disease. *Journal of Child Neurology, 20*(2), 102–107. https://doi.org/10.1177/08830738050200020301

Walters, M. C. (2015). Update of hematopoietic cell transplantation for sickle cell disease. *Current Opinion in Hematology, 22*(3), 227–233. https://doi.org/10.1097/MOH.0000000000000136

Yanni, E., Grosse, S. D., Yang, Q., & Olney, R. S. (2009). Trends in pediatric sickle cell disease-related mortality in the United States, 1983–2002. *The Journal of Pediatrics, 154*(4), 541–545. https://doi.org/10.1016/j.jpeds.2008.09.052

Yawn, B. P., Buchanan, G. R., Afenyi-Annan, A. N., Ballas, S. K., Hassell, K. L., James, A. H., Jordan, L., Lanzkron, S. M., Lottenberg, R., Savage, W. J., Tanabe, P. J., Ware, R. E., Murad, M. H., Goldsmith, J. C., Ortiz, E., Fulwood, R., Horton, A., & John-Sowah, J. (2014). Management of sickle cell disease: Summary of the 2014 evidence-based report by expert panel members. *JAMA, 312*(10), 1033–1048. https://doi.org/10.1001/jama.2014.10517

III

CENTRAL NERVOUS SYSTEM DISORDERS

11

Overview of Central Nervous System Disorders in Children

Ivette Merced

The central nervous system (CNS) is a complex system that regulates and coordinates body activities. There are two major divisions of the nervous system: (a) the brain and spinal cord, which make up the CNS; and (b) the peripheral nervous system. The other main organs of the nervous system include the eyes; ears; sensory receptors located in the skin, joints, muscles, and other parts of the body; and sensory organs that regulate taste and smell (Hockenbury & Nolan, 2019).

COMMON COMPLAINTS AND INDICATORS OF DYSFUNCTION

The CNS is vulnerable to various disorders and can be damaged by numerous infections and bodily processes. Some examples include (a) disruptions of blood flow to the brain, (b) cell degeneration, (c) immune system disorders, (d) inborn genetic or metabolic problems, (e) infections, (f) structural defects, (g) toxic exposure or direct effects of drug exposure, (h) trauma, and (i) tumors (Longe, 2021). Though this is not a comprehensive list, it serves to emphasize the complexity of CNS disorders and the array of conditions that can cause damage to the CNS.

This part reviews specific symptomatology for 14 disorders, with symptoms that vary based on the disorder and the individual. The most common signs or symptoms of dysfunction in children include (a) changes in activity, reflexes, or movements; (b) changes in level of consciousness or mood;

https://doi.org/10.1037/0000349-011
Health-Related Disorders in Children and Adolescents: A Guidebook for Educators and Service Providers, Second Edition, M. M. Perfect, C. A. Riccio, and M. A. Bray (Editors)

(c) delays in developmental milestones; (d) increase or lack of growth in head size; (e) lack of coordination; and (f) muscle rigidity, tremors, seizures, wasting, and slurred speech. Older children may report persistent or severe headaches, loss of feeling or tingling, or visual changes (Longe, 2021). The presence of these symptoms and changes in functioning lead to identification of CNS disorders.

CHILDHOOD CENTRAL NERVOUS SYSTEM DISORDERS

Part III discusses 14 childhood CNS disorders and their varying etiologies. Each disorder has its own unique etiology and list of symptoms. A brief description of these disorders is provided here. It is important to remember that each of these disorders is complex and can be caused by multiple factors working in conjunction, with effects on many functional systems.

Childhood-Onset Adrenoleukodystrophy

Adrenoleukodystrophy is a genetic condition that damages the membrane (myelin sheath) that covers nerve cells in the brain and spinal cord. It is caused by a genetic defect on the X chromosome and is noted for causing rapid loss of gray matter, which can cause early death. A child with this condition may experience a range of symptoms, including (a) vision loss, (b) dysphagia (difficulty swallowing), (c) learning disabilities, (d) deafness, (e) seizures, and (f) fatigue (Longe, 2021). The implications for medical, educational, and social/behavioral management are detailed by Switzky and colleagues in Chapter 12.

Agenesis of the Corpus Callosum

Simmons and colleagues (Chapter 13) explore the different causes of *agenesis of the corpus callosum* (AgCC). Although genetic syndromes can be involved in AgCC (e.g., disruption of brain cell migration during fetal development), research also shows that AgCC can be caused by metabolic disorders and fetal alcohol syndrome. Children diagnosed with AgCC may have issues related to feeding; trouble holding their head up, sitting, standing, and walking; and numerous other issues related to physical and mental development (Santo et al., 2012). Considerations for treatment are provided in Chapter 13.

Angelman Syndrome

Angelman syndrome is a neurogenetic syndrome that involves the deletion of maternally transmitted chromosome 15. In Chapter 14, Frye and Fairchild examine the different impacts on a child with Angelman syndrome. Often a child with Angelman syndrome has severe physical and learning disabilities

(Van Buggenhout & Fryns, 2009). Although treatment approaches vary based on the individual, the chapter provides resources and suggestions.

Autism Spectrum Disorder

Although research has not come up with a definitive etiology for *autism spectrum disorder* (ASD), some research has linked both genetic and early environmental factors to ASD. Children with ASD may miss early developmental milestones, present as socially awkward, and have problems with verbal and nonverbal communication (Lai et al., 2014). Alternatively, for high-functioning individuals, the communication and social components may be more apparent over time. Cole and Telesford provide current information on ASD and its potential impacts from medical, educational, and social/behavior perspectives in Chapter 15.

Cerebral Palsy

As explained by Aravala and colleagues (Chapter 16), the etiology of *cerebral palsy* involves disturbance in fetal brain development. Symptoms include physical and motor issues, some of which may be evident at birth, depending on the severity. Though not all children with cerebral palsy have cognitive issues, modifications may be needed to address motor limitations in the school setting. Additionally, children with cerebral palsy often have a treatment team to address motor, speech, and other medical concerns, as well as associated educational and social/behavioral concerns.

Cri du Chat Syndrome

As discussed by Ohr (Chapter 17), *cri du chat syndrome* is a chromosomal disorder most easily identified by the presence of a high-pitched cry similar to the mewing of a cat, microcephaly (small brain), and a host of minor phenotypical anomalies. Intellectual disability and delayed development are evident in early childhood. There is significant genetic variability among individuals with cri du chat syndrome, warranting consideration of treatment on a case-by-case basis. With increases in health care and the availability of early intervention, improved outcomes are being seen. See Chapter 17 for further information, recommendations, and resources.

Down Syndrome

One of the most common CNS disorders, *Down syndrome* (DS) is caused by the addition of a third chromosome 21, or trisomy 21, in some or all DNA. As such, DS can be identified prenatally and is characterized by distinct physical features. Gelbar (Chapter 18) points out that DS is the leading cause of intellectual disability, with educational and social/behavioral implications. Additionally, many individuals with DS are affected by medical issues.

Epilepsy

There are many types of *epilepsy*, as discussed in Chapter 19. In all cases, the diagnosis is made once the child has had two or more seizures not caused by fever. Aros-O'Malley and colleagues review the diverse etiologies, explain the nature of epilepsy, and discuss the relation between the atypical CNS activity and functioning. This includes medical, educational, and social/behavioral implications and treatment with significant differences from individual to individual.

Hereditary Ataxias

Children with *hereditary ataxias* may have poor coordination of movement, unsteady and wide gait, and speech dysarthria (weakness of speech muscles). Hereditary ataxia is considered an autosomal dominant, autosomal recessive, and X-linked disorder in most cases, as discussed in Chapter 20. Myers also reviews the implications on functioning from medical, educational, and social/behavioral perspectives.

Mitochondrial Disorders

Mitochondrial disorders (MDs) are a group of disorders that can manifest in utero during prenatal development and can present into late adulthood. Symptoms of MD can vary depending on which cells have the disrupted mitochondria. A child with MD can show a vast array of symptoms, such as fatigue, seizures, and cognitive disabilities. The impacts and implications of MD are discussed further by Lang and colleagues in Chapter 21.

Pediatric Autoimmune Neuropsychiatric Disorders Associated With Streptococcal Infections and Pediatric Acute-Onset Neuropsychiatric Syndrome

In Chapter 22, Hoppin and Doran discuss *pediatric autoimmune neuropsychiatric disorders associated with streptococcal infections* (PANDAS) and *pediatric acute-onset neuropsychiatric syndrome* (PANS). PANS includes nonstrep and noninfectious causes. Children with PANDAS/PANS can experience obsessive–compulsive behaviors and behavioral dysregulation. These difficulties, as discussed in the chapter, have implications for all areas of functioning and quality of life.

Prader–Willi Syndrome

Prader–Willi syndrome (PWS) affects multiple body systems and is a highly variable genetic disorder. It results from failure of expression of paternally inherited genes in chromosome 15 (see Chapter 14 by Frye and Fairchild for maternal transmission). With PWS, a child may experience a failure to thrive and have a short stature or speech delay. In addition to the medical and educational impacts, Wendel and Ogg (Chapter 23) discuss the social/behavioral issues associated with PWS, including compulsive behavior, self-harm, and aggression.

Rett Syndrome

Rett syndrome is an X-linked neurodevelopmental disorder with impacts on movement, behavior, and cognition. As explained by Gelbar (Chapter 24), many individuals with Rett syndrome have limited communication skills, using their behavior to communicate their needs. Developing any form of purposeful communication is an important part of managing their behavior and fostering all aspects of functioning.

Spina Bifida

Spina bifida is a birth defect associated with vitamin A deficiency in the pregnant mother. In children with spina bifida, the vertebral column often does not close with the spinal cord. A child with spina bifida may have bladder and bowel problems (incontinence); orthopedic malformations, such as problems with knees, hips, or a club foot; paralysis; and other movement-related issues. Roseman and Shine (Chapter 25) discuss the presenting symptoms and the potential effects, depending on the severity, and surgical treatments. Cognitive, educational, and social/behavioral effects and interventions are explored as well.

Williams Syndrome

Williams syndrome is caused by deletion of multiple genes, affecting CNS function and other functional systems. A child with Williams syndrome can have colic or feeding problems, with specific facial features (e.g., small, upturned nose or widely spaced teeth) initially leading to diagnosis. Gilson and colleagues (Chapter 26) provide information on associated disorders (e.g., attention-deficit/hyperactivity disorder, learning disorders) and the impact of short stature and speech delays on educational and social development.

HEALTH CARE NEEDS AND MEDICAL SPECIALTIES

Different kinds of health care professionals can be included in the care of a child with a CNS disorder. For example, neurology is a branch of medicine that manages nervous system disorders. Neurologists often have a primary role in the diagnosis and treatment of CNS disorders. In CNS disorders that involve brain tumors, a pediatric neurosurgeon would be part of the treatment team. Often children with CNS disorders need physical rehabilitative care, and physicians who provide rehabilitative care for children with nervous system disorders are called physical medicine and rehabilitation doctors. In addition, physical therapists, occupational therapists, and speech therapists may be part of the team. In CNS disorders like PANDAS or PANS, a child might also need a psychiatric consult or the services of a behavioral health specialist. In medical settings, teams of medical personnel will work with a child who has a CNS disorder, and the team may include some or all of these specialists as well as neuropsychologists, psychologists, social workers, nurses, and nurse practitioners (Doran et al., 2019).

REFERENCES

Doran, P. D., Amabile, C. L., Tumminaro, T., Korbmacher, H., & Pohlman, D. (2019). *A parents' guide to PANDAS, PANS, and related neuroimmune disorders: Information, support, and advice*. Jessica Kingsley Publishers.

Hockenbury, S. E., & Nolan, S. A. (2019). *Discovering psychology*. Worth Publishers.

Lai, M.-C., Lombardo, M. V., & Baron-Cohen, S. (2014). Autism. *The Lancet, 383*(9920), 896–910. https://doi.org/10.1016/S0140-6736(13)61539-1

Longe, J. L. (2021). *The Gale encyclopedia of medicine* (6th ed.). Gale.

Santo, S., D'Antonio, F., Homfray, T., Rich, P., Pilu, G., Bhide, A., Thilaganathan, B., & Papageorghiou, A. T. (2012). Counseling in fetal medicine: Agenesis of the corpus callosum. *Ultrasound in Obstetrics & Gynecology, 40*(5), 513–521. https://doi.org/10.1002/uog.12315

Van Buggenhout, G., & Fryns, J.-P. (2009). Angelman syndrome (AS, MIM 105830). *European Journal of Human Genetics, 17*(11), 1367–1373. https://doi.org/10.1038/ejhg.2009.67

12

Adrenoleukodystrophy

Harvey N. Switzky, James P. Van Haneghan, and Abigail Baxter

Much regarding adrenoleukodystrophy (X-ALD) has changed in the 25 years since the first edition of this book was published, including substantial increases in understanding the medical aspects of these diseases, their clinical management, and increased patient advocacy and support services throughout the United States and the world. Still, they remain difficult and highly complex disorders for families to navigate and endure. The saga of Augusto and Michaela Odone's quest to save the life of their 5-year-old son Lorenzo, dramatized in the 1992 film *Lorenzo's Oil*, brought X-ALD to the wider audience. X-ALD is a genetic metabolic disease that impairs the white myelin sheath surrounding the nerves of the brain, spinal cord, and peripheral nerves, a process known as *demyelination*, as well as the adrenal cortex and the testis (H. W. Moser, 2006). The myelin sheath permits nerve impulses to be conducted rapidly and efficiently, and as demyelination occurs, nerve functions become erratic, resulting in a variety of physiological and behavioral symptoms: motor dysfunctions involving changes in body tone, gait, and speech; inability to eat; inability to see and hear; deficient memory and attention; unstable emotional behaviors; and inefficient cognitive processing.

ETIOLOGY

X-ALD is caused by mutations in the *ABCD1* gene on the q28 part of the X chromosome, which encodes the membrane protein ALDP involved in the

https://doi.org/10.1037/0000349-012
Health-Related Disorders in Children and Adolescents: A Guidebook for Educators and Service Providers, Second Edition, M. M. Perfect, C. A. Riccio, and M. A. Bray (Editors)

transmembrane transport of very-long-chain fatty acids (VLCFAs), due to impaired peroxisomal VLCFA beta-oxidation. These ALDP defects lead to the characteristic increases in VLCFA levels, the diagnostic disease marker and the cause of demyelination in affected individuals. Molecular mechanisms that are not well understood interact with modifier genes and the environment to induce inflammatory demyelination, neurodegeneration, and also insufficiency in the adrenal glands, causing low levels of cortisone and resulting in Addison's disease, which is associated with fatigue; weight loss; gastrointestinal upset; increased skin pigmentation (bronzing); a general inability to withstand the effects of stress caused by infection, injury, surgery, and fever; and impaired cognitive functioning (Wiesinger et al., 2015).

PREVALENCE AND INCIDENCE

When the father is unaffected and the mother is a carrier, 50% of the daughters are carriers and 50% of the sons are affected by the disorder. If the father is affected and the mother is a carrier, 50% of the daughters are affected and 50% are carriers, whereas only 50% of the sons are affected. Thus, most individuals with X-ALD are male, although a small number are female. X-ALD has been reported in all geographic locations and races, with an approximate incidence ranging from one in 20,000 to one in 40,000 for all male forms (Bezman et al., 2001) and 1.1 in 100,000 for the childhood cerebral form in the United States (H. W. Moser, 2006). X-ALD is usually diagnosed in male individuals by the VLCFA levels in the blood plasma, by magnetic resonance studies of the brain, and by tests of adrenal function. Prenatal screening can be performed at 11 to 13 weeks of pregnancy using chorionic villus sampling or by amniocentesis at 15 to 18 weeks. X-ALD can be detected in female carriers by blood testing and prenatally using amniocentesis and chorionic villus sampling with an incidence of one in 14,000 (H. W. Moser, 2006).

IMPACT ON THE STUDENT AND OUTCOMES

The observed clinical spectrum of X-ALD in male individuals ranges from a rapidly progressing cerebral demyelination of brain function leading to a vegetative state and death within 2 to 3 years of the first symptoms to a very slow decline. Women with X-ALD may develop symptoms by middle age, though cerebral involvement and adrenocortical involvement are rare. The manifestations of X-ALD are highly variable even in family members from the same family in spite of identical *ABCD1* mutations (H. W. Moser, 2006).

There are at least seven major phenotypes of X-ALD distinguished by the rate of progression of the disease, age of onset, part of the nervous system affected, and degree of inflammation (A. B. Moser, 2017; H. W. Moser, 2006; H. W. Moser et al., 2007). Incidences are only approximate.

- Childhood cerebral ALD (CCALD) accounts for 35% to 40% of the cases in the United States. Children develop normally until 4 to 8 years old, with the mean age of onset around 7 years and onset often being misdiagnosed as attention-deficit disorders or learning disabilities. The earliest age of clinical demonstration is 21 months, and onset prior to 3 years is rare. Affected children often show assorted neurological symptoms: focal and generalized seizures, double vision, disordered spatial coordination, hearing impairments, hyperactivity, dementia, poor handwriting, declining school performance, and Addison's disease. This very severe form of X-ALD is associated with almost random degeneration of the white matter of both cerebral hemispheres and severe inflammation of brain neurons. Often adrenal insufficiency is the initial manifestation, with more than 70% of the boys affected. The affected child may show neurological decline leading to a totally helpless vegetative state within 2 to 3 years after diagnosis and death at varying times thereafter. In the vegetative state, the child is bedridden, unable to see or speak, and fed by a nasogastric tube or by a tube directly into the stomach. The child may remain in this state for many years, with a mean age of death at 9 years (H. W. Moser, director, Kennedy-Krieger Institute, personal communication, February 19, 1996).

- Adolescent cerebral ALD (AdolCALD) accounts for less than 5% of the cases in the United States. Children develop normally until 10 to 21 years old. This form has a similar course but often progresses more rapidly, with the mean time between onset and the vegetative state or death around 6 months.

- Adult cerebral ALD (ACALD) accounts for less than 3% of the cases in the United States. It affects individuals over 21 years and is often misdiagnosed as schizophrenia and other psychosis. The disorder resembles CCALD; however, the initial progression is slower. The initial diagnosis is often delayed with no family history or in the absence of Addison's disease.

- Adrenomyeloneuropathy (AMN) accounts for 40% to 45% of the cases in the United States. Individuals develop normally until young adulthood, with the mean age of onset around 27 years. There is progressive stiffening and weakness in the legs often misdiagnosed as multiple sclerosis or hereditary spastic paraparesis. Individuals gradually develop progressive spastic paresis, sensory ataxia, urinary sphincter dysfunction, leg pain, and impotence (H. W. Moser et al., 2007). The disorder is not as devastating as CCALD, with the interval between the development of neurologic symptoms and the vegetative state or death between 13 and 20 years. The two subtypes of AMN are (a) AMN-cerebral, involving demyelination of the brain and resembling CCALD and ACALD, and (b) AMN-pure, with no cerebral involvement, resulting in a more favorable outcome with men sometimes surviving into their 80s. Addison's disease is observed in 70% of the cases of AMN. CCALD and AMN can often co-occur in the same family.

- Adrenal insufficiency-only accounts for 10% of the cases in the United States, which comprises children with Addison's disease but with no or only mildly affected nervous system involvement (e.g., slight to moderate abnormalities on magnetic resonance imaging [MRI] or on neuropsychological testing). However, most children develop X-ALD in adulthood with either the CCALD or AMN form, with the interval between onset of adrenal insufficiency and neurological impairment being highly variable and as long as 32 years. This form is effectively treated with adrenal steroids and is viewed as a relatively treatable form of X-ALD.
- Asymptomatic form accounts for 8% of the cases in the United States consisting of children with the biochemical abnormality of X-ALD, highly elevated saturated VLCFA levels, and no nervous system or adrenal involvement. These cases are only detected because they have a biological relationship with persons having X-ALD, and most diagnoses occur before the child is 7 years old. Currently it is not possible to determine whether a child will develop the CCALD or AMN form, though these children usually will develop full-blown ALD if not treated. Currently there is major progress in treating these children.
- Women with X-ALD consist of half of the carriers of the ALD *ABCD1* gene and have neurological involvement with the mean age of onset in the 40s and 50s. Except for milder clinical symptoms and a slower rate of progression, the disorder resembles AMN but with rarer involvement of the brain or the adrenal glands.

PSYCHOEDUCATIONAL IMPLICATIONS AND SCHOOL-BASED INTERVENTIONS

General supportive care and symptomatic treatment for patients and families by physicians, rehabilitation and social agencies, parent support groups, and schools and teachers are the bedrock for care and treatment. Therapy models for X-ALD are presently under intense scrutiny. Adrenal insufficiency can be treated effectively with adrenal steroids, which are lifesaving.

Medical and Health Management

Diet therapies using Lorenzo's oil (LO) have been attempted, and bone marrow transplants (i.e., hematopoietic stem cell transplantation [HSCT]) and gene therapies are inviting areas of research. Diet therapies are based on the idea of reducing the amount of VLCFAs in the body. Reducing foods containing large amounts of VLCFAs combined with administration of LO (a 4:1 mixture of glycerol triolate and glyceryl trierucate) does indeed normalize the plasma levels of VLCFAs within 4 weeks. However, clinical research has shown that the ingestion of LO *does not significantly* alter the progression of the disease in *symp-*

tomatic individuals with cerebral inflammatory phenotypes (Aubourg et al., 1993; van Geel et al., 1999). In *asymptomatic* boys whose brain MRIs are normal, LO *may have* a preventive effect (H. W. Moser et al., 2005) and a slowing of the progression of the disease in pure AMN forms (Koehler & Sokolowski, 2005). LO therapy may begin at 6 months of age through 10 years in appropriate children (A. B. Moser, 2017).

Bone marrow transplants using suitably matched (human leukocyte antigen-typed) blood (i.e., hematopoietic) stem cells from the bone marrow (HSCT) can produce normal blood cells, which circulate throughout the body and metabolize VLCFAs. Bone marrow derived from donor hematopoietic cells can enter the central nervous system and be transformed into microglial brain cells. Through a poorly understood mechanism, the donor cells provide the entities that can degrade VCLFA and/or prevent CCALD or slow it down (Berger & Gärtner, 2006). Bone marrow transplantation has a relatively high mortality risk but may be useful for children who show evidence of very early cerebral involvement and for whom a well-matched donor is available (Peters et al., 2004).

Mahmood et al. (2007) compared the relative outcomes of the HSCT transplant group versus a comparable group of children who had not been transplanted: Outcomes were best when performed very early in the disease and for those who were least affected. HSCT is strongly recommended for children in the early stages of CCALD but not for those in the more advanced stages or for the children with the asymptomatic form who have a normal MRI (Cartier & Aubourg, 2010; Engelen et al., 2012; Kemper et al., 2017; Miller et al., 2011; H. W. Moser, 2006; Peters et al., 2004; Shapiro et al., 2000). The therapeutic success of bone marrow transplantation has been the replacement of the individual's defective hematopoietic stem cells with genetically normal stem cells from another individual. This strategy is often limited because well-matched donors are difficult to find and provide the Achilles' heel of this intervention.

Gene therapy appears to be the promise of the future, providing the ideal therapy of introducing the normal *ABCD1* gene into the individual's own cells. A viral vector is used to insert a corrected copy of the faulty *ABCD1* gene into the child's stem cells. Often chemotherapy is performed to make room for the genetically altered blood stem cells in the bone marrow, and the altered stem cells are infused back into the child's bloodstream via an intravenous line. Cartier et al. (2009) reported the successful treatment of two 7-year-old boys using gene therapy. Their bone marrow cells were extracted, and a normal copy of the X-ALD gene was inserted into the bone marrow cells using a virus (a lentiviral vector). The boys underwent chemotherapy to eradicate their bone marrow to stop it from producing future gene-deficient stem cells, and then they received an infusion of their own corrected stem cells carrying the normal gene. The boys were followed for 24 and 30 months; 15% of their blood cells demonstrated expression of the normal X-ALD protein, with VLCFA levels reduced by 38% in their blood plasma. Brain MRI scan and psychological cognitive tests showed that progression of the cerebral disease had stopped after 14 to 16 months with the boys remaining stable. The arrest of progressive cerebral demyelization observed was similar to the clinical outcome in HSCT. This study demonstrates that lentiviral-mediated gene therapy of hematopoietic stem cells can provide clinical benefit in X-ALD. A larger study (Eichler et al., 2017) funded by Bluebird Bio, a biotech company based in Cambridge, Massachusetts, known as the STARBEAM study (ALD-102) involved 17 boys aged between 4 and 13 years, median age 6 years, with a median Loes score on MRI of 2 (low neurological involvement) and no clinical signs of cerebral disease on a neurologic function test. They received the Lent-D drug product containing the lentiviral vector and were followed for a median of 29 months (range 22–42 months). On a neurologic function test, 15 of the boys were free of clinical signs of cerebral disease. All the boys were shown to express normal X-ALD proteins, suggesting that Lent-D gene therapy may be a safe and effective alternative to HSCT transplantation in boys with early stage CCALD.

Newborn screening for X-ALD can provide access to the promise of gene therapy before the disease has progressed. In February 2016, X-ALD was added to the Recommended Uniform Screening Panel. At the time of this writing, 12 states test newborns for X-ALD. Identified babies are monitored for adrenal insufficiency, and MRIs will be performed every 6 months to detect changes in cerebral disease. If cerebral disease is present and progressive, the child should be referred for bone marrow transplantation if they have a matching sibling donor, and if no match is found, the child should be referred for *ABCD1* gene therapy (A. B. Moser, 2017).

Social-Emotional and Behavioral

The progressive and devastating breakdown of neurological and behavioral functioning in CCALD leads to considerable stress for families. Parents are profoundly shocked when they begin to realize what is happening to their child. Some parents may break under the strain and withdraw into substance abuse, and cases of child abuse are not uncommon (P. Brazeal, president, United Leukodystrophy Foundation, & R. Brazeal, executive director, United Leukodystrophy Foundation, personal communication, February 15, 1996). A comprehensive management program involving the coordination of medical professionals, counselors, psychologists, social workers, and the school in partnership with the family is essential. Under the provision of the Individuals With Disabilities Education Act, individuals with X-ALD qualify for special services. When medical diagnosis is confirmed, the family and the student need support socially and emotionally. Students and families affected by X-ALD need to believe that they are not alone in facing the uncertainties of this particular disease (P. Brazeal & R. Brazeal, personal communication, February 15, 1996). Family members need to become the best advocates for the child and their condition as they know their child better than anyone, and families have coordinated to form well-organized advocacy groups. It is suggested that families as soon as possible become involved with a parent group, such as those listed in the Resources section. These groups provide practical advice, support, and advocacy.

CONCLUSION

As Dharamsi et al. (2022) reported in a research case study, there is no one clear roadmap for addressing ALD. However, as they noted, a holistic comprehensive approach with a focus on quality of life for the child and the family is crucial to working with families facing this complex degenerative disorder.

RESOURCES

Aidan Jack Seeger Foundation. 70 North 15th St., Brooklyn, NY 11222; 917-750-9390; info@aidanjackseegerfoundation.org. https://www.aldalliance.org/

ALD Connect. 35 Village Road, Suite 100 #353306, Middleton, MA 01949; 617-643-37799; info@aldconnect.org. https://aldconnect.org/

Adrenoleukodystrophy Foundation. 241 Camden St., Slidell, LA 70461; 985-718-4728; information@aldfoundation.org. https://aldfoundation.org/

ALD Life. info@aldlife.org. https://www.alextlc.org/. British charity that provided a series of monographs that provide practical and emotional support for individuals with X-ALD and AMN, which can be retrieved from their website.

Calliope Joy Foundation. PO Box 2866, Bala Cynwyd, PA19004. https://www.thecalliopejoyfoundation.org/. Published an illustrated children's book, *Loie's Disease*, for siblings of children with leukodystrophy.

Fight ALD. PO Box 3318, Vista, CA 92085; info@fightald.org. http://www.fightald.org/

Global Leukodystrophy Initiative. https://glia.org/

Hunters Hope. 21 Princeton Place, Suite 12, PO Box 643, Orchard Park, NY 14127; 716-667-1200. https://www.huntershope.org/

Myelin Project. PO Box 39, Pacific Palisades, CA 90272; 800-869-3546; info@myelin.org. https://www.myelin.org/

National Organization for Rare Disorders. 55 Kenosia Ave, Danbury, CT 06810; 800-999-6673. https://rarediseases.org/

Stop ALD Foundation. 500 Jefferson St. Suite 2000, Houston, TX 77002-7371; 713-756-3232; eve@stopald.org. http://www.stopald.org/

United Leukodystrophy Foundation. 224 North 2nd St. Suite 2, Dekalb, IL 60115; 800-758-5483. https://ulf.org/

World Leukodystrophy Alliance. PO Box 39, Pacific Palisades, CA 90272; 800-869-3546. http://www.leukodystrophyalliance.org/

REFERENCES

Aubourg, P., Adamsbaum, C., Lavallard-Rousseau, M. C., Rocchiccioli, F., Cartier, N., Jambaqué, I., Jakobezak, C., Lemaitre, A., Boureau, F., Wolf, C., & Bougneres, P.-F. (1993). A two-year trial of oleic and erucic acids ("Lorenzo's oil") as treatment for adrenomyeloneuropathy. *The New England Journal of Medicine, 329*(11), 745–752. https://doi.org/10.1056/NEJM199309093291101

Berger, J., & Gärtner, J. (2006). X-linked adrenoleukodystrophy: Clinical, biochemical and pathogenetic aspects. *Biochimica et Biophysica Acta, 1763*(12), 1721–1732. https://doi.org/10.1016/j.bbamcr.2006.07.010

Bezman, L., Moser, A. B., Raymond, G. V., Rinaldo, P., Watkins, P. A., Smith, K. D., Kass, N. E., & Moser, H. W. (2001). Adrenoleukodystrophy: Incidence, new mutation rate, and results of extended family screening. *Annals of Neurology, 49*(4), 512–517. https://doi.org/10.1002/ana.101

Cartier, N., & Aubourg, P. (2010). Hematopoietic stem cell transplantation and hematopoietic stem cell gene therapy in X-linked adrenoleukodystrophy. *Brain Pathology, 20*(4), 857–862. https://doi.org/10.1111/j.1750-3639.2010.00394.x

Cartier, N., Hacein-Bey-Abina, S., Bartholomae, C. C., Veres, G., Schmidt, M., Kutschera, I., Vidaud, M., Abel, U., Dal-Cortivo, L., Caccavelli, L., Mahlaoui, N., Kiermer, V., Mittelstaedt, D., Bellesme, C., Lahlou, N., Lefrère, F., Blanche, S., Audit, M., Payen, E., . . . Aubourg, P. (2009). Hematopoietic stem cell gene therapy with a lentiviral vector in X-linked adrenoleukodystrophy. *Science, 326*(5954), 818–823. https://doi.org/10.1126/science.1171242

Dharamsi, M. S., Mejia, A. A., & De Vargas, C. (2022). Comprehensive care to improve quality of life: A case of childhood adrenoleukodystrophy. *HCA Healthcare Journal of Medicine, 3*(4), 257–262. https://doi.org/10.36518/2689-0216.1441

Eichler, F., Duncan, C., Musolino, P. L. Orchard, P. J., De Oliveira, S., Thrasher, A. J., Armant, M., Dansereau, C., Lund, T. C., Miller, W. P., Raymond, G. V., Sankar, R., Shah, A. J., Sevin, C., Gaspar, H. B., Gissen, P., Amartino, H., Bratkovic, D., Smith, N. J. C., . . . Williams, D. A. (2017). Hematopoietic stem-cell gene therapy for cerebral adrenoleukodystrophy. *The New England Journal of Medicine, 377*(17), 1630–1638. https://doi.org/10.1056/NEJMoa1700554

Engelen, M., Kemp, S., de Visser, M., van Geel, B. M., Wanders, R. J. A., Aubourg, P., & Poll-The, B. T. (2012). X-linked adrenoleukodystrophy (X-ALD): Clinical presentation and guidelines for diagnosis, follow-up and management. *Orphanet Journal of Rare Diseases, 7*(1), Article 51. https://doi.org/10.1186/1750-1172-7-51

Kemper, A., Brosco, J., Comeau, A. Green, N. S., Grosse, S. D., Jones, E., Kwon, J. M., Lam, W. K. K., Ojodu, J., Prosser, L. A., & Tanksley, S. (2017). Newborn screening for X-linked adrenoleukodystrophy: Evidence summary and advisory committee recommendation. *Genetics in Medicine, 19*(1), 121–126. https://doi.org/10.1038/gim.2016.68

Koehler, W., & Sokolowski, P. (2005). Clinical phenotypes, diagnosis and treatment of adulthood X-linked adrenoleukodystrophy. In J. Berger, S. Stoeckler, & W. Koehler (Eds.), *Understanding and treating adrenoleukodystrophy: Present state and future perspectives* (pp. 28–60). SPS Verlagsgesellschaft.

Mahmood, A., Raymond, G. V., Dubey, P., Peters, C., & Moser, H. W. (2007). Survival analysis of haematopoietic cell transplantation for childhood cerebral X-linked adrenoleukodystrophy: A comparison study. *Lancet Neurology, 6*(8), 687–692. https://doi.org/10.1016/S1474-4422(07)70177-1

Miller, W. P., Rothman, S. M., Nascene, D., Kivisto, T., DeFor, T. E., Zieger, R. S., Eisengart, J., Leiser, K., Raymond, G., Lund, T. C., Tolar, J., & Orchard, P. J. (2011). Outcomes after allogeneic hematopoietic cell transplantation for childhood cerebral adrenoleukodystrophy: The largest single-institution cohort report. *Blood, 118*(7), 1971–1978. https://doi.org/10.1182/blood-2011-01-329235

Moser, A. B. (2017, August 18). *Newborn screening for X-linked adrenoleukodystrophy (X-ALD)* [Paper presentation]. 2017 Alabama Newborn Screening Conference, Prattville, AL, United States.

Moser, H. W. (2006). Therapy of X-linked adrenoleukodystrophy. *NeuroRx, 3*(2), 246–253. https://doi.org/10.1016/j.nurx.2006.01.004

Moser, H. W., Mahmood, A., & Raymond, G. V. (2007). X-linked adrenoleukodystrophy. *Nature Clinical Practice Neurology, 3*(3), 140–151. https://doi.org/10.1038/ncpneuro0421

Moser, H. W., Raymond, G. V., Lu, S. E., Muenz, L. R., Moser, A. B., Xu, J., Jones, R. O., Loes, D. J., Melhem, E. R., Dubey, P., Bezman, L., Brereton, N. H., & Odone, A. (2005). Follow-up of 89 asymptomatic patients with adrenoleukodystrophy treated with Lorenzo's oil. *Archives of Neurology, 62*(7), 1073–1080. https://doi.org/10.1001/archneur.62.7.1073

Peters, C., Charnas, L. R., Tan, Y., Ziegler, R. S., Shapiro, E. G., DeFor, T., Grewal, S. S., Orchard, P. J., Abel, S. L., Goldman, A. I., Ramsay, N. K. C., Dusenbery, K. E., Loes, D. J., Lockman, L. A., Kato, S., Aubourg, P. R., Moser, H. W., & Krivit, W. (2004). Cerebral X-linked adrenoleukodystrophy: The international hematopoietic cell transplantation experience from 1982 to 1999. *Blood, 104*(3), 881–888. https://doi.org/10.1182/blood-2003-10-3402

Shapiro, E., Krivit, W., Lockman, L., Jambaqué, I., Peters, C., Cowan, M., Harris, R., Blanche, S., Bordigoni, P., Loes, D., Ziegler, R., Crittenden, M., Ris, D., Berg, B., Cox, C., Moser, H., Fischer, A., & Aubourg, P. (2000). Long-term effect of bone-marrow transplantation for childhood-onset cerebral X-linked adrenoleukodystrophy. *The Lancet, 356*(9231), 713–718. https://doi.org/10.1016/S0140-6736(00)02629-5

van Geel, B. M., Assies, J., Haverkort, E. B., Koelman, J. H., Verbeeten, B., Jr., Wanders, R. J., & Barth, P. G. (1999). Progression of abnormalities in adrenomyeloneuropathy and neurologically asymptomatic X-linked adrenoleukodystrophy despite treatment with "Lorenzo's oil." *Journal of Neurology, Neurosurgery, and Psychiatry, 67*(3), 290–299. https://doi.org/10.1136/jnnp.67.3.290

Wiesinger, C., Eichler, F. S., & Berger, J. (2015). The genetic landscape of X-linked adrenoleukodystrophy: Inheritance, mutations, modifier genes, and diagnosis. *The Application of Clinical Genetics, 8*, 109–121. https://doi.org/10.2147/TACG.S49590

13

Agenesis of the Corpus Callosum

Krystal T. Simmons, Bianca S. Watkins, and Sherine D. Presley

Agenesis of the corpus callosum (AgCC) is a rare congenital disorder in which the corpus callosum does not develop properly. The *corpus callosum* is a band of nerves that serves as a bridge of communication between the left and right hemispheres of the brain. *Agenesis* refers to the absence or failure of a body part to develop. AgCC is characterized as complete agenesis, partial agenesis, hypoplasia (underdeveloped corpus callosum), or dysgenesis (malformation).

ETIOLOGY

The etiology of AgCC development is unknown in most cases. There are many genetic factors associated with AgCC, but there is no single cause. A structural diagnosis is typically confirmed through magnetic resonance imaging, along with prenatal genetic testing and routine sonograms. Up to 45% of cases have been linked to identifiable causes with specific genetic syndromic diagnosis (Schell-Apacik et al., 2008). Some genetic syndromes with identified genes include Andermann (*KCC3* axonopathy) and MASA (*L1CAM*) syndromes. Andermann syndrome presents with progressive neuropathy, cognitive impairment, and dementia (Schell-Apacik et al., 2008). MASA syndrome features include hydrocephalus, aphasia, adducted thumbs, spastic paraplegia, and intellectual disability (Demyanenko et al., 1999). AgCC genetic syndromes that are seen consistently but currently do not have identified genes are Aicardi,

https://doi.org/10.1037/0000349-013
Health-Related Disorders in Children and Adolescents: A Guidebook for Educators and Service Providers, Second Edition, M. M. Perfect, C. A. Riccio, and M. A. Bray (Editors)

acrocallosal, and Vici syndromes (Edwards et al., 2014). Chromosomal abnormalities are seen in approximately 17% of AgCC cases (Glass et al., 2008). AgCC can also result from metabolic and environmental factors, such as antenatal infections (intrauterine), prenatal alcohol exposure, and maternal phenylketonuria (Palmer & Mowat, 2014).

PREVALENCE AND INCIDENCE

In the general population, the birth prevalence of AgCC is estimated to be 1.8 per 10,000 live births, with a higher prevalence in male children (Glass et al., 2008) and rates of 2% to 3% in children with a neurodevelopmental disability (Sotiriadis & Makrydimas, 2012). AgCC prevalence has been found to be lower in infants of Asian mothers and higher in infants of Black mothers compared with White and U.S.-born Latina mothers (Glass et al., 2008).

SYMPTOMS

Co-occurring medical and behavioral diagnoses generate the spectrum of AgCC symptoms. Brown and Paul (2019) identified three core syndromes that are interrelated because of AgCC: "(1) reduced interhemispheric transfer of sensory-motor information; (2) reduced cognitive processing speed; and (3) deficits in complex reasoning and novel problem-solving" (p. 2). A common neurological issue is seizures, which usually have an early onset, though AgCC does not necessarily cause seizures (Unterberger et al., 2016). Approximately 60% to 80% of individuals with AgCC were reported to have developmental delays, especially in gross and fine motor skills such as clumsiness, delayed walking, and dexterity (Tu et al., 2009). Language delays and difficulty with interpersonal skills, understanding social cues, metaphors, humor, and emotional reciprocity are prevalent (Brown et al., 2021; Lau et al., 2013; Tu et al., 2009). Increased sensitivity to touch or lowered pain perception is also common (Doherty et al., 2006). Visual impairments such as nystagmus and strabismus are also associated with symptoms of AgCC (Whitman et al., 2016).

IMPACT ON THE STUDENT AND OUTCOMES

AgCC is a heterogeneous condition with a favorable prognosis overall (Sotiriadis & Makrydimas, 2012). The condition does not worsen in complete agenesis because the brain pathway fibers cannot deteriorate or regenerate. There is no cure or standard course of treatment for AgCC, and mixed research findings and small sample sizes make it difficult to generalize outcomes.

Medical

Impairments to the corpus callosum, which is the largest connective neural pathway in the brain, yield a broad spectrum of health conditions. Close to half of individuals with AgCC experience at least one seizure or are diagnosed with a seizure disorder, along with reports of headaches (Doherty et al., 2006). Most medical treatment involves the management of symptoms and seizures. Sleep disturbances, such as decreased sleep duration, bedtime resistance, sleep anxiety, parasomnias, narcolepsy, night wakings, sleep-disordered breathing, and daytime sleepiness are associated with AgCC (Yates et al., 2018). Research has also shown AgCC co-occurring with bowel and bladder control difficulty (Doherty et al., 2006), feeding (e.g., sucking, chewing, reflux) difficulties in infants (Samanta, 2016), and hearing difficulty (Doherty et al., 2006). Parents experience emotions ranging from anger to denial because of the medical demands needed to care for a child with AgCC. It is important for parents to engage in self-care, seek early intervention, and find a primary physician who understands their child's diagnosis (National Organization for Disorders of the Corpus Callosum [NODCC], 2019a).

Cognitive/Academic

Cognitive abilities vary broadly, ranging from an intellectual developmental disorder classification to above-average cognitive functioning. Those with insignificant brain abnormalities other than AgCC have minimal cognitive and neurological deficits (Brown & Paul, 2019), with possible improvement in intellectual functioning as they age (Siffredi et al., 2013). An individual's cognitive ability may not inform the core syndromes of AgCC but may moderate adaptive skills and abilities to engage in complex tasks (Brown & Paul, 2019).

There is evidence that children with AgCC have strengths in basic reading, spelling, nonverbal skills, and everyday behavioral regulation (Siffredi et al., 2018). Studies show that individuals with AgCC have difficulties with inattention, language, and visual and spatial reasoning; however, most studies drawing these conclusions lacked robust methodological designs (Siffredi et al., 2013). The Siffredi et al. (2013) systematic review also revealed that individuals with AgCC had impairments in math and pragmatic language, with mixed findings related to executive functioning and memory.

Hemispheric pathway disruptions make it difficult for one to understand skills essential for advanced communication, establishing language, and communication delays. Children with AgCC use cognitive strategies to encode and retrieve verbal information that differs from typically developing peers (Siffredi et al., 2018). Difficulty with nonliteral language, such as proverb comprehension, which is unrelated to basic language skills, is a more common language deficit symptomatic of AgCC (Rehmel et al., 2016).

Social-Emotional and Behavioral

AgCC has been associated with deficits in social skills, such as humor, sarcasm, social cues, self-perception, and emotionality (Brown et al., 2021; Renteria-Vazquez et al., 2022). The corpus callosum is an instrumental pathway for facilitating complex emotional processing but is not essential for understanding basic emotional responses. The right hemisphere typically processes primary emotions (e.g., anger) and not social emotions. Further, studies and neuroimaging show a reliance on the right hemisphere for language acquisition by those with AgCC, which accounts for the communication variances affecting socialization skills (Lau et al., 2013). Social difficulties continue into adulthood. Adults with primary AgCC (normal intelligence) may have difficulty anticipating social and emotional outcomes, especially as problems increase in complexity (Young et al., 2019). Pragmatic language skills, semantic development, and nonverbal expression have shown links to right hemispheric functioning and further associations to autism spectrum disorder (ASD). ASD is a developmental condition that has multiple etiologies, including AgCC. Comorbid rates of ASD in individuals with AgCC range from 9.5% to 33% (Lau et al., 2013).

PSYCHOEDUCATIONAL IMPLICATIONS AND SCHOOL-BASED INTERVENTIONS

Empirical support for school-based AgCC interventions is limited, and due to the spectrum of outcomes, treatment focuses on the early identification of associated symptoms and conditions necessitating interventions to meet unique needs. Getting an evaluation by a multidisciplinary team to determine specialized school instruction is an essential first step. The NODCC (2019b) provides parents with a professional communication packet to distribute and educate others regarding their child's strengths and struggles.

Medical and Health Management

Providing the school with an organized medical history is important. Along with a psychoeducational evaluation, this history will help determine the student's present levels of performance, which inform physical, cognitive, academic, language, and behavioral intervention needs. A school health care plan in collaboration with primary care providers should be implemented, including safety planning such as identifying symptoms of a potential medical emergency (e.g., seizure). Other safety accommodations may account for toileting, feeding, and transportation assistance. School nurses are good partners for monitoring health needs and medication management within the school setting. Typical medication treatment will relate to comorbid health conditions such as asthma or seizures. Medical conditions comprising physical disabilities may require adapted physical education or assistive technology devices.

Sensory and Motor

In an international survey, 90% of parents indicated their child with AgCC received some form of therapy, with speech, physical (PT), and occupational (OT) therapies being the most reported forms of therapeutic services (Schilmoeller & Schilmoeller, 2000). Speech therapy will aid in language development, whereas PT and OT will promote the use of an activity to build motor coordination, self-care, and emotion-regulation skills. Consider safety planning for those with less pain sensitivity, as they are susceptible to injury and undetected illness. Children with visual impairments would benefit from low vision rehabilitation services aimed at improving adaptive behavior functioning (Elsman et al., 2019). Effective services may include sports and physical training, engagement in trail-following tasks, and providing low vision devices to improve gross motor, fine motor, and developmental skills, respectively (Elsman et al., 2019).

Cognitive/Academic

Adhering to consistent neurocognitive reevaluations through the medical provider and school (e.g., triennial full and individual evaluations) is important as cognitive demands increase with age, which may create subtle neuropsychological changes (Guadarrama-Ortiz et al., 2020). Inclusive placement is another key factor for improving academic outcomes. Placement decisions based more on unique learning needs and less on sociocultural variables and capacity limitations can lead to greater academic, communication, and social outcomes (Agran et al., 2020). Strategic placement decisions and scheduling are important because it is very common for children with AgCC to have difficulty with change (Tu et al., 2009). Therefore, predictability in the learning environment and alerting the student to changes in advance will aid in meeting academic goals. A common learning pattern for students with AgCC is a fluctuation in learning rate and recall of materials. The callosal absence affects memory and learning, so an emphasis on encoding when teaching information may be most appropriate (Erickson et al., 2014). Erickson and colleagues (2014) found that issues with verbal learning and memory were less related to inattention, retention, and retrieval and that compensatory reorganization can foster learning and memory skills. Further, understanding the hemispheric dominance of those with AgCC can inform academic intervention approaches. For example, when intervening with early readers, Mather (2022) suggested that an overreliance on phonological processing may not be beneficial to those with AgCC. Typically, AgCC does not affect interhemispheric communication via the anterior commissure. The anterior temporal lobe (ATL) directly connects to the anterior commissure, which can serve as a pathway for bilateral visual information and whole-word reading. If the ATL is intact, those with AgCC would likely rely on semantic rather than phonological processing to aid in reading comprehension and, conversely, those without the ATL access may demonstrate good decoding proficiency but poor reading comprehension. Overall, instruction should be specific to the student's strengths and abilities.

Social-Emotional and Behavioral

Monitor potential maladaptive responses to AgCC symptoms (e.g., difficulty establishing healthy peer relationships), and if negative emotional symptoms develop, such as depression and anxiety, the support of a school mental health professional may be warranted. Applied behavior analysis techniques (e.g., prompting and reinforcement), antecedent-based intervention, differential reinforcement, and video modeling are evidence-based practices with the most support for social communication, social interaction, and adaptive behavior skill development (Wong et al., 2015). For those with significant intellectual impairment, skills-based (e.g., self-management) and support-based interventions (e.g., peer training) can be effective when general and special educators collaborate and identify a specific social skill to target (Carter & Hughes, 2005). Another common behavior exhibited by children with AgCC is inattention. Typical interventions for inattentive behaviors include training with extensive practice and daily performance feedback of skills (Evans et al., 2018). If behavioral problems persist, the multidisciplinary team may develop a behavior management plan to address specific issues. Last, conduct transition planning and teach self-advocacy skills early to prepare students with AgCC for adulthood and independent living. Develop transition plans that are unique to the individual by engaging in strengths-based assessments to leverage outcomes, obtaining input from multiple informants (e.g., caregivers and teachers), and maintaining high expectations, as all of these factors can influence student outcomes (Carter et al., 2014).

CONCLUSION

It is important to remember that there are people with AgCC who have normal cognitive abilities and successful academic performance. It is common to focus unintentionally on limitations, so consider formulating recommended accommodations from a strengths-based perspective. Parents and educators should advocate for inclusion opportunities where appropriate. School personnel and treating physicians should be in close communication with parents to ensure interventions occur consistently across settings. For all the recommendations provided, parents and educators should refer to federal and state laws for additional guidance on implementation.

RESOURCES

National Organization for Disorders of the Corpus Callosum (NODCC). PMB 363, 18032-C Lemon Drive, Yorba Linda, CA 92886; 714-747-0063; info@nodcc.org. https://nodcc.org/

University of California San Francisco (UCSF), Fetal Treatment Center. 1855 4th Street, 2nd Floor, Room A-2432, San Francisco, CA 94158-2549; 1-800-RX-FETUS (1-800-793-3887). https://fetus.ucsf.edu/agenesis-corpus-callosum

National Institutes of Health (NIH), National Center for Advancing Translational Sciences (NCATS), Genetic and Rare Diseases Information Center (GARD). Genetic and Rare Diseases Information Center (GARD), PO Box 8126, Gaithersburg, MD 20898; toll-free: 1-888-205-2311. https://rarediseases.info.nih.gov/diseases/1535/corpus-callosum-agenesis

REFERENCES

Agran, M., Jackson, L., Kurth, J. A., Ryndak, D., Burnette, K., Jameson, M., Zagona, A., Fitzpatrick, H., & Wehmeyer, M. (2020). Why aren't students with severe disabilities being placed in general education classrooms: Examining the relations among classroom placement, learner outcomes, and other factors. *Research and Practice for Persons With Severe Disabilities, 45*(1), 4–13. https://doi.org/10.1177/1540796919878134

Brown, W. S., Burnett, K. A., Vaillancourt, A., & Paul, L. K. (2021). Appreciation of social norms in agenesis of the corpus callosum. *Archives of Clinical Neuropsychology, 36*(7), 1367–1373. https://doi.org/10.1093/arclin/acab003

Brown, W. S., & Paul, L. K. (2019). The neuropsychological syndrome of agenesis of the corpus callosum. *Journal of the International Neuropsychological Society, 25*(3), 324–330. https://doi.org/10.1017/S135561771800111X

Carter, E. W., Brock, M. E., & Trainor, A. A. (2014). Transition assessment and planning for youth with severe intellectual and developmental disabilities. *The Journal of Special Education, 47*(4), 245–255. https://doi.org/10.1177/0022466912456241

Carter, E. W., & Hughes, C. (2005). Increasing social interaction among adolescents with intellectual disabilities and their general education peers: Effective interventions. *Research and Practice for Persons With Severe Disabilities, 30*(4), 179–193. https://doi.org/10.2511/rpsd.30.4.179

Demyanenko, G. P., Tsai, A. Y., & Maness, P. F. (1999). Abnormalities in neuronal process extension, hippocampal development, and the ventricular system of L1 knockout mice. *The Journal of Neuroscience, 19*(12), 4907–4920. https://doi.org/10.1523/JNEUROSCI.19-12-04907.1999

Doherty, D., Tu, S., Schilmoeller, K., & Schilmoeller, G. (2006). Health-related issues in individuals with agenesis of the corpus callosum. *Child: Care, Health and Development, 32*(3), 333–342. https://doi.org/10.1111/j.1365-2214.2006.00602.x

Edwards, T. J., Sherr, E. H., Barkovich, A. J., & Richards, L. J. (2014). Clinical, genetic and imaging findings identify new causes for corpus callosum development syndromes. *Brain, 137*(6), 1579–1613. https://doi.org/10.1093/brain/awt358

Elsman, E. B. M., Al Baaj, M., van Rens, G. H. M. B., Sijbrandi, W., van den Broek, E. G. C., van der Aa, H. P. A., Schakel, W., Heymans, M. W., de Vries, R., Vervloed, M. P. J., Steenbergen, B., & van Nispen, R. M. A. (2019). Interventions to improve functioning, participation, and quality of life in children with visual impairment: A systematic review. *Survey of Ophthalmology, 64*(4), 512–557. https://doi.org/10.1016/j.survophthal.2019.01.010

Erickson, R. L., Paul, L. K., & Brown, W. S. (2014). Verbal learning and memory in agenesis of the corpus callosum. *Neuropsychologia, 60*, 121–130. https://doi.org/10.1016/j.neuropsychologia.2014.06.003

Evans, S. W., Owens, J. S., Wymbs, B. T., & Ray, A. R. (2018). Evidence-based psychosocial treatments for children and adolescents with attention deficit/hyperactivity disorder. *Journal of Clinical Child & Adolescent Psychology, 47*(2), 157–198. https://doi.org/10.1080/15374416.2017.1390757

Glass, H. C., Shaw, G. M., Ma, C., & Sherr, E. H. (2008). Agenesis of the corpus callosum in California 1983–2003: A population-based study. *American Journal of Medical Genetics: Part A, 146A*(19), 2495–2500. https://doi.org/10.1002/ajmg.a.32418

Guadarrama-Ortiz, P., Choreño-Parra, J. A., & de la Rosa-Arredondo, T. (2020). Isolated agenesis of the corpus callosum and normal general intelligence development during postnatal life: A case report and review of the literature. *Journal of Medical Case Reports, 14*(1), Article 28. https://doi.org/10.1186/s13256-020-2359-2

Lau, Y. C., Hinkley, L. B., Bukshpun, P., Strominger, Z. A., Wakahiro, M. L., Baron-Cohen, S., Allison, C., Auyeung, B., Jeremy, R. J., Nagarajan, S. S., Sherr, E. H., & Marco, E. J. (2013). Autism traits in individuals with agenesis of the corpus callosum. *Journal of Autism and Developmental Disorders, 43*(5), 1106–1118. https://doi.org/10.1007/s10803-012-1653-2

Mather, D. S. (2022). Preventing children from developing dyslexia: A premature writing hypothesis. *Perceptual and Motor Skills, 129*(3), 468–487. https://doi.org/10.1177/00315125221075001

National Organization for Disorders of the Corpus Callosum. (2019a). *Newly diagnosed.* https://nodcc.org/newly-diagnosed/

National Organization for Disorders of the Corpus Callosum. (2019b). *Parent to professional communication packet.* https://nodcc.org/resources/parent-professional-communication/

Palmer, E., & Mowat, D. (2014). Agenesis of the corpus callosum: A clinical approach to diagnosis. *American Journal of Medical Genetics: Part C, Seminars in Medical Genetics, 166*(2), 184–197. https://doi.org/10.1002/ajmg.c.31405

Rehmel, J. L., Brown, W. S., & Paul, L. K. (2016). Proverb comprehension in individuals with agenesis of the corpus callosum. *Brain and Language, 160,* 21–29. https://doi.org/10.1016/j.bandl.2016.07.001

Renteria-Vazquez, T., Brown, W. S., Kang, C., Graves, M., Castelli, F., & Paul, L. K. (2022). Social inferences in agenesis of the corpus callosum and autism: Semantic analysis and topic modeling. *Journal of Autism and Developmental Disorders, 52*(2), 569–583. https://doi.org/10.1007/s10803-021-04957-2

Samanta, D. (2016). Severe developmental delay and complete agenesis of corpus callosum in a Noonan syndrome patient with SOS1 mutation. *Acta Neurologica Belgica, 116*(2), 223–224. https://doi.org/10.1007/s13760-015-0526-9

Schell-Apacik, C. C., Wagner, K., Bihler, M., Ertl-Wagner, B., Heinrich, U., Klopocki, E., Kalscheuer, V. M., Muenke, M., & von Voss, H. (2008). Agenesis and dysgenesis of the corpus callosum: Clinical, genetic and neuroimaging findings in a series of 41 patients. *American Journal of Medical Genetics: Part A, 146A*(19), 2501–2511. https://doi.org/10.1002/ajmg.a.32476

Schilmoeller, G., & Schilmoeller, K. (2000). Filling the void: Facilitating family support through networking for children with a rare disorder. *Family Science Review, 13,* 224–233.

Siffredi, V., Anderson, V., Leventer, R. J., & Spencer-Smith, M. M. (2013). Neuropsychological profile of agenesis of the corpus callosum: A systematic review. *Developmental Neuropsychology, 38*(1), 36–57. https://doi.org/10.1080/87565641.2012.721421

Siffredi, V., Anderson, V., McIlroy, A., Wood, A. G., Leventer, R. J., & Spencer-Smith, M. M. (2018). A neuropsychological profile for agenesis of the corpus callosum? Cognitive, academic, executive, social, and behavioral functioning in school-age children. *Journal of the International Neuropsychological Society, 24*(5), 445–455. https://doi.org/10.1017/S1355617717001357

Sotiriadis, A., & Makrydimas, G. (2012). Neurodevelopment after prenatal diagnosis of isolated agenesis of the corpus callosum: An integrative review. *American Journal of Obstetrics and Gynecology, 206*(4), 337.e1–337.e5. https://doi.org/10.1016/j.ajog.2011.12.024

Tu, S., Doherty, D., Schilmoeller, K. J., & Schilmoeller, G. L. (2009). Agenesis of the corpus callosum: A literature review. *International Review of Research in Mental Retardation, 38,* 171–193. https://doi.org/10.1016/S0074-7750(08)38007-0

Unterberger, I., Bauer, R., Walser, G., & Bauer, G. (2016). Corpus callosum and epilepsies. *Seizure, 37,* 55–60. https://doi.org/10.1016/j.seizure.2016.02.012

Whitman, M. C., Andrews, C., Chan, W.-M., Tischfield, M. A., Stasheff, S. F., Brancati, F., Ortiz-Gonzalez, X., Nuovo, S., Garaci, F., MacKinnon, S. E., Hunter, D. G., Grant, P. E., & Engle, E. C. (2016). Two unique *TUBB3* mutations cause both CFEOM3 and malformations of cortical development. *American Journal of Medical Genetics: Part A, 170*(2), 297–305. https://doi.org/10.1002/ajmg.a.37362

Wong, C., Odom, S. L., Hume, K. A., Cox, A. W., Fettig, A., Kucharczyk, S., Brock, M. E., Plavnick, J. B., Fleury, V. P., & Schultz, T. R. (2015). Evidence-based practices for children, youth, and young adults with autism spectrum disorder: A comprehensive review. *Journal of Autism and Developmental Disorders, 45*(7), 1951–1966. https://doi.org/10.1007/s10803-014-2351-z

Yates, J. F., Troester, M. M., & Ingram, D. G. (2018). Sleep in children with congenital malformations of the central nervous system. *Current Neurology and Neuroscience Reports, 18*(7), Article 38. https://doi.org/10.1007/s11910-018-0850-6

Young, C. M., Folsom, R. C., Paul, L. K., Su, J., Mangum, R. W., & Brown, W. S. (2019). Awareness of consequences in agenesis of the corpus callosum: Semantic analysis of responses. *Neuropsychology, 33*(2), 275–284. https://doi.org/10.1037/neu0000512

14

Angelman Syndrome

Sara S. Frye and Allison Fairchild

Angelman syndrome was first described by Harry Angelman in 1965 based on his observations of several children with similar behavioral and developmental profiles, including severe intellectual disability, facial abnormalities, ataxia, epilepsy, and frequent periods of laughter (Dan, 2009). Since then, research has provided insight into the implications of the syndrome, which tend to be widespread and lifelong, as well as what supports and services are necessary to address the unique needs of individuals with Angelman syndrome.

ETIOLOGY

The etiology of Angelman syndrome is genetic in nature and most commonly caused by the deletion or dysfunction of the maternal chromosome 15. Developmental and physical markers associated with Angelman syndrome may be apparent as early as 6 months, but other symptoms are not detectable until the child is older. Given the rarity of the condition and potential delay in full presentation, accurate diagnosis of Angelman syndrome may be delayed in some cases.

PREVALENCE AND INCIDENCE

Angelman syndrome is considered to be relatively rare, occurring in about one in every 15,000 individuals worldwide. Data suggest that it is equally present in all

https://doi.org/10.1037/0000349-014
Health-Related Disorders in Children and Adolescents: A Guidebook for Educators and Service Providers, Second Edition, M. M. Perfect, C. A. Riccio, and M. A. Bray (Editors)

ethnic groups and genders (Margolis et al., 2015). Although Angelman syndrome is a genetic condition, it is not typically inherited, and there is generally no family history. The genetic abnormalities that lead to the condition usually take place in the early stages of pregnancy due to random events that cause deletions or errors in the genetic code. The abnormalities in genetic coding responsible for the disorder are very rarely passed from parent to child. Once the condition is suspected, genetic testing is often conducted to confirm the diagnosis.

SYMPTOMS

Angelman syndrome is defined as a severe neurodevelopmental condition characterized by intellectual disability, speech impairment, motor dysfunction, seizures, and behavioral characteristics such as a happy disposition (Williams et al., 2006). Physical markers of the disorder are often present, including craniofacial abnormalities. Microcephaly (i.e., small head circumference) and/or a flat head is common, as well as a prominent chin, deeply set eyes, and a wide-set mouth with protruding tongue (Clayton-Smith & Laan, 2003). In addition, individuals with Angelman syndrome generally exhibit significant delays in developmental milestones, as opposed to regression (e.g., having a skill then losing it), that cause functional impairments.

IMPACT ON THE STUDENT AND OUTCOMES

Medical

Neurological effects of Angelman syndrome are generally widespread. Developmental motor impairment generally starts at birth. Motor milestones are typically delayed, but most patients (90%) are eventually able to learn to walk independently (Williams et al., 2010). Individuals generally exhibit impaired coordination (i.e., ataxia), which may include increased motor activity, jerky movements, tremors in the extremities, and unsteady or abnormal gait. In addition, seizures occur in more than 80% of children and approximately 40% of adults with Angelman syndrome (Margolis et al., 2015). Abnormalities in electroencephalography findings are also common. Sleep problems are experienced by about 35% of those with the condition. Issues include difficulties initiating and maintaining sleep, frequent awakenings, decreased need for sleep, circadian rhythm problems, and nightmares/night terrors (Spruyt et al., 2018). Gastrointestinal and oral-motor problems (e.g., feeding problems, trouble sucking or swallowing, excessive drooling, reflux) are also sometimes present and may require treatment. Incontinence is often an issue for younger individuals with Angelman syndrome, but this may resolve with intervention by adulthood. The more severe gene deletions are also associated with pigmentation problems in the hair and skin (Williams et al., 2010). Despite the physiological and neurological implications of the disorder, life expectancy is normal.

Cognitive/Academic

Developmental delays are typically observed early in the developmental period in individuals with Angelman syndrome. However, the severity of such deficits may be hard to quantify. Psychoeducational assessment often proves difficult due to profound speech difficulties, short attention span, and other factors. Despite these difficulties, assessment practices still typically reveal profound deficits in overall cognitive abilities. Research has estimated that most individuals with Angelman syndrome function in the 2- to 2.5-year-old range (Williams et al., 2010). The most severe developmental delays tend to appear in individuals who have the most common type of chromosome deletion of the maternal chromosome 15q11-13, which affects 70% of those with Angelman syndrome (Clayton-Smith & Laan, 2003). The presence of uncontrolled seizures also contributes to more severe cognitive deficits. Adaptive functioning is also significantly impaired across domains, including difficulties with daily living skills (Micheletti et al., 2016). In addition, children with Angelman syndrome typically have difficulty initiating and sustaining attention, which affects their ability to function in a classroom setting. This can also have an impact on levels of engagement and motivation. Stereotypies, such as hand flapping, are often present and can be distracting to the individual and others around them. Significant challenges with speech and language are also central to those with this condition, which has profound implications for academic functioning. Individuals with Angelman syndrome are mostly nonverbal and do not develop expressive speech or are limited to only a few words. This may be due to a combination of factors, including cognitive reasons (e.g., intellectual disability) and physical issues (e.g., impaired motor planning, protruding tongue). However, receptive language is generally more developed than expressive language (Williams et al., 2006). Most individuals are able to understand simple commands that have to do with their daily routine (Clayton-Smith & Laan, 2003). Despite lacking verbal language, some individuals may learn to communicate using gestures and/or communication devices (Micheletti et al., 2016). Though the level of impairment is somewhat variable, most individuals with Angelman syndrome, particularly those with large gene deletions, are highly dependent on others while completing school, use very simple communication aids to express basic needs, and require high levels of support to participate in instructional activities. However, individuals with smaller deletions may be able to exhibit varying levels of independence in certain contexts. Relative strengths of individuals with Angelman syndrome are in nonverbal reasoning skills and nonverbal social interactions.

Social-Emotional and Behavioral

The unique behavioral characteristics of Angelman syndrome are often what cause clinicians to initially consider the diagnosis (Clayton-Smith & Laan, 2003). Individuals with Angelman syndrome are easily excitable and may present with an overly happy demeanor. Periods of excessive smiling and laughter are hallmark and may be spontaneous or unprovoked. Although the cause of frequent laughter in Angelman syndrome is not known, neuroimaging studies have suggested that patients with Angelman syndrome may have some abnormalities within the humor processing pathway in the brain (Williams et al., 2009). Repetitive behaviors (e.g., hand flapping) and abnormal sensory interests (e.g., licking or mouthing objects) are also common in individuals with Angelman syndrome, which can be mistaken for other neurodevelopmental conditions such as autism spectrum disorder (Williams et al., 2009). Self-injurious behavior has also been reported, as well as aggressiveness toward others, such as pulling at people or hair (Adams et al., 2011). In addition, hyperactivity and a short attention span are frequently present, which can exacerbate functional impairments (Horsler & Oliver, 2006). Although there is overlap between Angelman syndrome and autism spectrum disorder, individuals with Angelman syndrome are often very social and interested in interacting with others. In fact, the desire for social interaction is considered to be a relative strength in these individuals. However, speech and language impairment can make aspects of social interaction difficult.

PSYCHOEDUCATIONAL IMPLICATIONS AND SCHOOL-BASED INTERVENTIONS

There is currently no cure for Angelman syndrome. Treatment involves management of the neurological, behavioral, and physical manifestations of the disorder.

Medical and Health Management

The medical and health needs of individuals with Angelman syndrome are typically addressed through individualized interventions and services. Treatment of seizures may involve the use of anticonvulsant medication, which can lead to undesirable side effects. At school, individualized health care plans should be in place to ensure the safety of the student, such as how to respond in the event of a seizure or instructions on the administration of medication during the school day. Sleep problems may be treated with pharmacological intervention, such as supplemental melatonin, or behavioral sleep interventions. Fatigue may be present due to sleep disturbance and thus require accommodations, such as frequent breaks. Speech therapy is typically needed to address the severe language difficulties associated with the condition. Speech and language therapy should emphasize the use of nonverbal communication, such as instructing the individuals in the use of assistive communication devices. Some research has suggested that the use of sign language may not be effective in this population due to motor difficulties that may cause distortion of desired signs and hand movements. However, those with strong motor control may benefit from learning signs. A more common communication method is the use of gestures or communication boards (Williams et al., 2010). Mobility issues can be addressed with physical therapy, and occupational therapy can help with fine and oral motor control issues. Individuals may also require help with adaptive skills, such as dressing themselves and using feeding utensils. Physical limitations can be accommodated in the classroom (e.g., mobility devices, providing extra space, limiting physical obstructions) and when the child is required to move between locations. Depending on the severity of these impairments, individuals may require both school-based and outpatient services (Margolis et al., 2015).

Cognitive/Academic

As a result of the significant developmental concerns associated with Angelman syndrome, students are in need of specialized educational services. This often involves early intervention services, which then transition into school-based services. Given the developmental delays associated with the syndrome, special education services that are typically provided to students with other developmental delays are likely appropriate. Students will require an individualized education program (IEP) that outlines placement, as well as necessary services, modifications, and accommodations. Intellectual disabilities are a hallmark feature of the disorder, and therefore students may be placed into self-contained classrooms depending on the severity of the cognitive deficits. However, inclusion in the general education classroom is recommended when appropriate, such as for electives. Limited research exists for how students with Angelman syndrome are serviced within the school environment. However, one study indicated that a majority of parents of children with Angelman syndrome (78%) favored inclusion in the general education classroom (Leyser & Kirk, 2011). Depending on the level of impairment, students may need assistance from a one-to-one aide or paraprofessional. Additional services, such as adapted physical education classes and behavioral interventions, may be necessary on a case-by-case basis to allow students to participate in general education (Williams et al., 2010). Individuals with Angelman syndrome will be in need of ongoing supports throughout their lifetimes. Therefore, a well-developed transition plan should be implemented to ensure continuation of services once the individual enters adulthood. Transition plans should be based on the individual's needs, strengths, and preferences and include specific postsecondary goals that address the need for adult services, vocational training, and independent living.

Social–Emotional and Behavioral

Despite the characterization of individuals with Angelman syndrome as being overly happy, many experience difficulties with behavior and emotion regulation (Horsler & Oliver, 2006). Attention problems and hyperactivity are common and can be especially problematic in the classroom setting. Some problems can be addressed with accommodations such as allowing for preferential seating, frequent movement breaks, and use of fidget devices. For other behaviors, functional behavioral assessments can be useful in determining the function of problematic behaviors and developing effective behavior plans. Behavioral modification strategies, such as positive reinforcement, can be helpful in eliminating or reducing problematic behaviors (Williams et al., 2010). In addition, accommodations and recommendations such as following routines, providing cues for transitions, and using positive reinforcement to promote desired behaviors should be included in behavior plans when appropriate. Generally, behavioral difficulties, such as hyperactivity, improve as the individual ages (Clayton-Smith & Laan, 2003). More intensive interventions may be required to address behaviors that are socially disruptive or pose a danger to the individual (e.g., self-injurious). It is important to take the individual's overall level of cognitive functioning into consideration when setting expectations. Clinicians are also encouraged to consider the impact of factors such as sleep disturbance and communication difficulties, which can have behavioral implications. In addition, speech and language impairments are often a source of frustration for these individuals and can lead to behavioral outbursts. Thus, interventions aimed at improving communication may also lead to improvements in mood and/or behavior. The desire for social interaction is considered a relative strength for individuals with Angelman syndrome. Parents and teachers can help foster relationships and related outcomes by providing secure environments with consistent behavioral interventions (Williams et al., 2010). Having strong and supportive relationships can help motivate individuals with Angelman syndrome to work toward improving their communication skills, which can have widespread benefits.

CONCLUSION

As Angelman syndrome first becomes apparent in the developmental period, identification and implementation of early intervention services is critical. Regardless of when the diagnosis is obtained, individuals with Angelman syndrome typically require intensive supports throughout their lifetimes. Thus, there is often a need for coordination of services and involvement of a variety of professionals, such as physicians, school psychologists, occupational and physical therapists, speech therapists, school nurses, and other support staff. Implementation of appropriate interventions and services is critical to ensuring the individual is able to function at their full potential.

RESOURCES

Angelman Syndrome Foundation. 75 Executive Drive, Suite 327, Aurora, IL 60504. https://www.angelman.org

National Institutes of Health (NIH) Genetics Home Reference. 9000 Rockville Pike, Bethesda, MD 20892. https://ghr.nlm.nih.gov

National Organization for Rare Disorders (NORD). 55 Kenosia Avenue, Danbury, CT 06810. https://rarediseases.org

Hewitt, J. (2011). *Angelman syndrome: Causes, tests, and treatments* (M. Gabata, Ed.). CreateSpace Independent Publishing Platform.

REFERENCES

Adams, D., Horsler, K., & Oliver, C. (2011). Age related change in social behavior in children with Angelman syndrome. *American Journal of Medical Genetics: Part A, 155*(6), 1290–1297. https://doi.org/10.1002/ajmg.a.33964

Clayton-Smith, J., & Laan, L. (2003). Angelman syndrome: A review of the clinical and genetic aspects. *Journal of Medical Genetics, 40*(2), 87–95. https://doi.org/10.1136/jmg.40.2.87

Dan, B. (2009). Angelman syndrome: Current understanding and research prospects. *Epilepsia, 50*(11), 2331–2339. https://doi.org/10.1111/j.1528-1167.2009.02311.x

Horsler, K., & Oliver, C. (2006). The behavioural phenotype of Angelman syndrome. *Journal of Intellectual Disability Research, 50*(1), 33–53. https://doi.org/10.1111/j.1365-2788.2005.00730.x

Leyser, Y., & Kirk, R. (2011). Parents' perspectives on inclusion and schooling of students with Angelman syndrome: Suggestions for educators. *International Journal of Special Education, 26*(2), 79–91.

Margolis, S. S., Sell, G. L., Zbinden, M. A., & Bird, L. M. (2015). Angelman syndrome. *Neurotherapeutics, 12*(3), 641–650. https://doi.org/10.1007/s13311-015-0361-y

Micheletti, S., Palestra, F., Martelli, P., Accorsi, P., Galli, J., Giordano, L., Trebeschi, V., & Fazzi, E. (2016). Neurodevelopmental profile in Angelman syndrome: More than low intelligence quotient. *Italian Journal of Pediatrics, 42*(1), Article 91. https://doi.org/10.1186/s13052-016-0301-4

Spruyt, K., Braam, W., & Curfs, L. M. (2018). Sleep in Angelman syndrome: A review of evidence. *Sleep Medicine Reviews, 37*, 69–84. https://doi.org/10.1016/j.smrv.2017.01.002

Williams, C. A. (2005). Neurological aspects of the Angelman syndrome. *Brain & Development, 27*(2), 88–94. https://doi.org/10.1016/j.braindev.2003.09.014

Williams, C. A., Driscoll, D. J., & Dagli, A. I. (2010). Clinical and genetic aspects of Angelman syndrome. *Genetics in Medicine, 12*(7), 385–395. https://doi.org/10.1097/GIM.0b013e3181def138

Williams, C. A., Peters, S. U., & Calculator, S. N. (2009). *Facts about Angelman syndrome*. Angelman Syndrome Foundation. https://www.angelman.org/wp-content/uploads/2019/12/facts_about_as_2009_3-19-10.pdf

15

Autism

Christine L. Cole and Alana E. Telesford

Autism spectrum disorder (ASD) is a neurodevelopmental condition characterized by differences in social communication and social interaction and the presence of intense interests or repetitive behaviors (American Psychiatric Association, 2013). The fifth edition of the *Diagnostic and Statistical Manual of Mental Disorders* (*DSM-5*) described these traits on a continuum defined by the level of support required to address functional needs, ranging from "requiring support" (Level 1) to "requiring very substantial support" (Level 3; American Psychiatric Association, 2013, p. 52). Of note, the level of support needs for an individual on the spectrum may vary across settings (e.g., minimal to no support required in one environment and substantial supports required in another). Thus, autistic children and youth have a diverse presentation of social, behavioral, and language profiles.

ETIOLOGY

There is no single factor that contributes to the development of autistic characteristics. Most scientists agree that genetics, environmental factors, and their interactions play a role, but causal mechanisms are poorly understood (Bölte et al., 2019). Although research findings indicate that parents of an autistic child are more likely to have another child on the spectrum (Ozonoff et al., 2011), the specific genetic risk factors remain difficult to identify (Tordjman et al., 2014). ASD tends to occur more often in children with another genetic or

https://doi.org/10.1037/0000349-015
Health-Related Disorders in Children and Adolescents: A Guidebook for Educators and Service Providers, Second Edition, M. M. Perfect, C. A. Riccio, and M. A. Bray (Editors)

chromosomal condition such as fragile X syndrome or tuberous sclerosis (Zecavati & Spence, 2009), and genetic mutations may increase the risk of ASD (Jónsson et al., 2017). Other possible prenatal, perinatal, and postnatal environmental factors currently being explored include in utero exposure to antiepileptic or other medications, viral infections, parental immigration, and environmental toxins such as air pollution (Rubenstein et al., 2019). It is difficult, however, to establish whether these environmental factors simply co-occur with ASD or contribute to the development of autism traits (Tordjman et al., 2014). The Study to Explore Early Development, funded by the Centers for Disease Control and Prevention (CDC; 2019), is currently the largest multiyear research project in the United States to help identify factors that increase the likelihood of developing ASD.

PREVALENCE AND INCIDENCE

Tracking ASD prevalence poses unique challenges because of the changing diagnostic criteria, heterogeneity of symptoms, and lack of biological diagnostic markers (Baio et al., 2018). Thus, autism identification in children relies exclusively on caregiver report of symptoms and professional observations (American Psychiatric Association, 2013). For several decades, the CDC has tracked the prevalence of ASD among children across 11 sites in the United States. Recent estimates indicate one in 54 children aged 8 have been identified as being on the autism spectrum, which is approximately 175% higher than (2.8 times) the first estimates reported by the Autism and Developmental Disabilities Monitoring Network in 2000 and 2002. Though ASD occurs across all racial, ethnic, gender, and socioeconomic groups, it is currently 4.3 times more likely to be identified in boys than in girls (Maenner et al., 2020).

SYMPTOMS

Differences in social communication and interaction exhibited by children and youth on the spectrum may include social withdrawal or aloofness; stereotyped, delayed, or nonexistent verbal language; differences in nonverbal communication (e.g., variable use of eye contact and gestures); and/or difficulties modulating social behaviors across contexts. Verbally fluent children may not engage in reciprocal social conversation, or their speech may exhibit echolalia, pronoun reversal, or repetitive phrases or vocalizations (Boucher, 2012). Behavioral traits may include stimming (e.g., hand flapping, body rocking, toe walking), strict adherence to routines and/or excessive resistance to change, highly focused interests, over- or underreactivity to sensory input, and/or fascination with the movement of objects (e.g., spinning) or specific parts of objects (e.g., hinged lid; American Psychiatric Association, 2013).

The diverse presentation of ASD can make identification difficult. Some children show features of ASD in early infancy, such as limited eye contact, variable responsiveness to their name, or inconsistent joint attention with others. Other children meet all developmental milestones during the first few months or years of life and later become withdrawn, rigid about daily activities, or hyper- or hyposensitive to sensory input (Baio et al., 2018). An additional challenge is distinguishing the characteristics of ASD from other conditions (Kang et al., 2020); for example, rigidity, repetitive behavior, and social difficulties are also characteristic of anxiety and obsessive-compulsive disorders. Though autism traits are typically present by age 2, they might not be recognized as ASD until they begin to interfere with the social, educational, or other life demands of early childhood, such as dressing oneself and following daily routines (American Psychiatric Association, 2013). Although there is an increased awareness of ASD characteristics, and early diagnosis is a major public health goal, the median age of identification has remained stable over the past 20 years, typically ranging from 29 to 46 months (Maenner et al., 2020).

IMPACT ON THE CHILD AND OUTCOMES

The presence of autism often involves additional medical concerns, co-occurring cognitive and/or academic issues, and/or social–emotional and behavioral difficulties, which may require intervention or supports.

Medical

Children on the spectrum often have co-occurring medical concerns, particularly affecting the immune and digestive systems (Buie et al., 2010). Though physiological symptoms vary in their characteristics and severity (Vargason et al., 2019), common co-occurring conditions include epilepsy or seizure disorders, sleep difficulties, and issues with gastrointestinal and immune functioning (e.g., chronic constipation, eosinophilic esophagitis; Tye et al., 2019). High rates of medical comorbidity typically result in high mortality rates, high health care expenditures, and difficulty accessing coordinated medical care (Thom et al., 2019). Education may be most directly affected by students' sleep disturbances, seizures, food selectivity/sensitivity, and other gastrointestinal issues, which can result in increased school avoidance or negative school experiences.

Cognitive and Academic

Childhood intellectual ability and early language development predict outcomes for children on the spectrum (Gillespie-Lynch et al., 2012). Research has indicated that school-age youth who have higher cognitive abilities and language development are more likely to have better outcomes later in life (Howlin et al.,

2013); individuals with co-occurring intellectual impairments are likely to have significantly poorer life skills (Howlin et al., 2014).

Social–Emotional and Behavioral

A major marker of ASD is the presence of differences in social communication, which may include difficulties with social conversation, emotion recognition, and emotional and behavioral self-regulation (American Psychiatric Association, 2013). Long-term social–emotional and behavioral outcomes in adolescence and adulthood are highly variable, with some individuals requiring less support over time, others requiring more intensive support, and many continuing at stable levels (Howlin et al., 2013). The degree of social–emotional and behavioral support needed appears to be dependent on a combination of factors, including the level of cognitive functioning, language development, co-occurring psychopathology, and access to support services (Levy & Perry, 2011).

PSYCHOEDUCATIONAL IMPLICATIONS AND SCHOOL-BASED SUPPORTS

Due to potential co-occurring medical conditions, collaboration and communication across medical/school professionals and families are particularly important to facilitate optimal health and academic outcomes for students on the spectrum (McClain et al., 2020). Families, school team members, and clinical care providers are encouraged to use a "strengths, challenges, and interventions" approach to guide treatment planning. In this approach, individual strengths and areas of difficulty are identified and recommendations are developed that build on the individual's unique strengths and utilize them to address areas of need.

Pharmacological Intervention

Medication has not been found to effectively treat central characteristics of ASD; however, psychotropic medications may help students benefit from academic, social, and behavioral supports by reducing co-occurring emotional and behavioral symptoms (Myers & Johnson, 2007). Antipsychotics, serotonin-reuptake inhibitors, and stimulant medications are sometimes used to treat aggression, self-injury, repetitive behavior, sleep disturbance, mood concerns, hyperactivity, and/or inattention (McPheeters et al., 2011). A synthesis of the research literature determined there is insufficient empirical support for pharmacological intervention as an evidence-based treatment for youth with ASD (McPheeters et al., 2011), emphasizing the need for nonpharmacological supports.

Cognitive and Academic

The core symptoms associated with ASD can make it difficult for some students on the spectrum to function within a typical classroom environment without appropriate supports (Yianni-Coudurier et al., 2008). The Individuals With Disabilities Education Improvement Act (2004) requires that students' needs be addressed in the least restrictive classroom environment; thus, behavioral, emotional, and academic supports can be provided in the general education setting, in a specialized education setting, or both. For students whose needs can be met in the general education setting, cooperative learning groups, peer tutoring, multimodal instruction, and classwide positive behavior management strategies help to facilitate supportive inclusion (Ferraioli & Harris, 2011). Children on the spectrum with limited expressive language often benefit from school-based speech and language therapies delivered in an individualized or group format (Chenausky et al., 2016; Tager-Flusberg & Kasari, 2013). Students on the spectrum who have difficulties making inferences, attending to relevant text cues, or understanding novel words in context may also benefit from Tier 2 or Tier 3 supports within a multitiered system of supports model to improve reading comprehension (Turner et al., 2017).

Social-Emotional and Behavioral

Behavioral interventions that utilize antecedent–behavior–consequence contingencies have been found to effectively reduce challenging behaviors (e.g., self-injury, aggression) and teach adaptive skills (Reichow & Volkmar, 2010). Traditional applied behavior analysis (ABA) teaches children new skills in highly structured settings (e.g., ABA centers, classrooms, home sessions) through repeated presentation of small units of information (Weitlauf et al., 2014). Historically, young children on the spectrum were encouraged to receive intensive ABA therapy (e.g., 25–40 hours per week) to promote attention, language, cognition, and adaptive skills (Hagopian et al., 2015; Weitlauf et al., 2014). Recently, the field has shifted to utilizing alternative or complementary approaches to ABA. Naturalistic developmental behavioral interventions are delivered in the contexts in which children exhibit target skills (e.g., home, school, community) and use antecedents, prompts, and reinforcers that occur naturally in the child's environment to shape adaptive behaviors (Reichow & Volkmar, 2010). Interest in parent management training has also increased in recent years (Bearss et al., 2018). Parent management training interventions utilize direct instruction, role play, and supervised practice to teach caregivers to become agents of behavior change (Ingersoll & Wainer, 2013; Postorino et al., 2017; Scahill et al., 2016). Self-management strategies teach youth with ASD to apply behavior change principles to their own actions (Shapiro & Cole, 1994). Self-monitoring, goal setting, self-evaluating, and self-reinforcement teaches individuals to regulate their own behavior (Briesch & Chafouleas,

2009), thus promoting the generalizability of adaptive skills across settings (Cooper et al., 2020).

Cognitive behavior therapy (CBT) has been found to successfully address symptoms of anxiety in youth with ASD (Storch et al., 2013). Modifications to traditional CBT methods, such as adjusting the presentation of material (e.g., adding visual cues; National Autism Center, 2015) and emphasizing caregiver involvement (Wood et al., 2015), have been shown to increase the effectiveness of CBT for autistic youth. The role of the family in CBT is to foster the child's independence in managing anxiety by creating structured practice opportunities to use coping skills at home and to provide reinforcement to the child for participating in practice sessions and/or using target skills in vivo (Wood et al., 2015).

Peer training or peer-mediated intervention can be used to support social functioning. Typically, these approaches teach neurotypical peers to interact with youth on the spectrum to support the acquisition of a more diverse range of social skills and increase the frequency of target skills (Chan et al., 2009). Peer-mediated strategies teach peers to model prosocial behaviors and/or cue the child on the spectrum when to engage in specific social skills (National Autism Center, 2015). Peer training is a naturalistic intervention in which skill instruction, practice, and prompting occurs in the contexts where the target skills are required (e.g., small group activities, recess, lunch). Peer training promotes social communication, joint attention, play, school readiness, and academic skills for children and youth, ages 3 to 14 years (Sam & AFIRM Team, 2015).

CONCLUSION

ASD is a lifelong neurodevelopmental condition that can affect many aspects of a person's life. To address the needs of children and youth on the spectrum, supports must be available in home, school, clinic, and community settings to promote behavioral, social–emotional, academic, and adaptive functioning. The academic, social, and emotional functioning of autistic children and youth improves when evidence-based supports are delivered consistently and with high fidelity across relevant settings. Thus, all stakeholders are responsible for delivering appropriate supports, evaluating the impact of these supports on the individual's functioning, and making modifications as needed.

RESOURCES

Johnson, C. R., Butter, E. M., & Scahill, L. (2018). *Parent training for autism spectrum disorder: Improving the quality of life for children and their families*. American Psychological Association.

Goldstein, S., & Ozonoff, S. (Eds.). (2018). *Assessment of autism spectrum disorder* (2nd ed.). Guilford Press.

National Autism Center. (2015). *National Standards Project, Phase 2*. https://nationalautismcenter.org/national-standards/phase-2-2015/

REFERENCES

American Psychiatric Association. (2013). *Diagnostic and statistical manual of mental disorders* (5th ed.). https://doi.org/10.1176/appi.books.9780890425596

Baio, J., Wiggins, L., Christensen, D. L., Maenner, M. J., Daniels, J., Warren, Z., Kurzius-Spencer, M., Zahorodny, W., Robinson Rosenberg, C., White, T., Durkin, M. S., Imm, P., Nikolaou, L., Yeargin-Allsopp, M., Lee, L. C., Harrington, R., Lopez, M., Fitzgerald, R. T., Hewitt, A., . . . Dowling, N. F. (2018). Prevalence of autism spectrum disorder among children aged 8 years—Autism and Developmental Disabilities Monitoring Network, 11 sites, United States, 2014. *Morbidity and Mortality Weekly Report: Surveillance Summaries, 67*(6), 1–23. https://doi.org/10.15585/mmwr.ss6706a1

Bearss, K., Burrell, T. L., Challa, S. A., Postorino, V., Gillespie, S. E., Crooks, C., & Scahill, L. (2018). Feasibility of parent training via telehealth for children with autism spectrum disorder and disruptive behavior: A demonstration pilot. *Journal of Autism and Developmental Disorders, 48*(4), 1020–1030. https://doi.org/10.1007/s10803-017-3363-2

Bölte, S., Girdler, S., & Marschik, P. B. (2019). The contribution of environmental exposure to the etiology of autism spectrum disorder. *Cellular and Molecular Life Sciences, 76*(7), 1275–1297. https://doi.org/10.1007/s00018-018-2988-4

Boucher, J. (2012). Research review: Structural language in autistic spectrum disorder—Characteristics and causes. *Journal of Child Psychology and Psychiatry, 53*(3), 219–233. https://doi.org/10.1111/j.1469-7610.2011.02508.x

Briesch, A. M., & Chafouleas, S. M. (2009). Review and analysis of literature on self-management interventions to promote appropriate classroom behaviors (1988–2008). *School Psychology Quarterly, 24*(2), 106–118. https://doi.org/10.1037/a0016159

Buie, T., Campbell, D. B., Fuchs. G. J., III, Furuta, G. T., Levy, J., Vandewater, J., Whitaker, A. H., Atkins, D., Bauman, M. L., Beaudet, A. L., Carr, E. G., Gershon, M. D., Hyman, S. L., Jirapinyo, P., Jyonouchi, H., Kooros, K., Kushak, R., Levitt, P., Levy, S. E., . . . Winter, H. (2010). Evaluation, diagnosis, and treatment of gastrointestinal disorders in individuals with ASDs: A consensus report. *Pediatrics, 125*(Suppl. 1), S1–S18. https://doi.org/10.1542/peds.2009-1878C

Centers for Disease Control and Prevention. (2019). *Research on autism spectrum disorder: Study to Explore Early Development (SEED)*. U.S. Department of Health and Human Services. https://www.cdc.gov/ncbddd/autism/seed.html

Chan, J. M., Lang, R., Rispoli, M., O'Reilly, M., Sigafoos, J., & Cole, H. (2009). Use of peer-mediated interventions in the treatment of autism spectrum disorders: A systematic review. *Research in Autism Spectrum Disorders, 3*(4), 876–889. https://doi.org/10.1016/j.rasd.2009.04.003

Chenausky, K., Norton, A., Tager-Flusberg, H., & Schlaug, G. (2016). Auditory-motor mapping training: Comparing the effects of a novel speech treatment to a control treatment for minimally verbal children with autism. *PLOS ONE, 11*(11), Article e0164930. https://doi.org/10.1371/journal.pone.0164930

Cooper, J. O., Heron, T. E., & Heward, W. L. (2020). *Applied behavior analysis* (3rd ed.). Pearson Education.

Ferraioli, S. J., & Harris, S. L. (2011). Effective educational inclusion of students on the autism spectrum. *Journal of Contemporary Psychotherapy, 41*(1), 19–28. https://doi.org/10.1007/s10879-010-9156-y

Gillespie-Lynch, K., Sepeta, L., Wang, Y., Marshall, S., Gomez, L., Sigman, M., & Hutman, T. (2012). Early childhood predictors of the social competence of adults with autism. *Journal of Autism and Developmental Disorders, 42*(2), 161–174. https://doi.org/10.1007/s10803-011-1222-0

Hagopian, L. P., Hardesty, S. L., & Gregory, M. (2015). *Overview and summary of scientific support for applied behavior analysis*. Kennedy Krieger Institute. https://www.kennedykrieger.org/sites/default/files/library/documents/patient-care/centers-and-programs/down-syndrome-clinic-and-research-center/aba-scientific-support-9-2015.pdf

Howlin, P., Moss, P., Savage, S., & Rutter, M. (2013). Social outcomes in mid- to later adulthood among individuals diagnosed with autism and average nonverbal IQ as children. *Journal of the American Academy of Child & Adolescent Psychiatry, 52*(6), 572–581. https://doi.org/10.1016/j.jaac.2013.02.017

Howlin, P., Savage, S., Moss, P., Tempier, A., & Rutter, M. (2014). Cognitive and language skills in adults with autism: A 40-year follow-up. *Journal of Child Psychology and Psychiatry, 55*(1), 49–58. https://doi.org/10.1111/jcpp.12115

Individuals With Disabilities Education Improvement Act Amendments of 2004, 11 Stat. 37 U.S.C. § 1401 (2004). https://sites.ed.gov/idea/statute-chapter-33/subchapter-i/1401

Ingersoll, B., & Wainer, A. (2013). Initial efficacy of project ImPACT: A parent-mediated social communication intervention for young children with ASD. *Journal of Autism and Developmental Disorders, 43*(12), 2943–2952. https://doi.org/10.1007/s10803-013-1840-9

Jónsson, H., Sulem, P., Kehr, B., Kristmundsdottir, S., Zink, F., Hjartarson, E., Hardarson, M. T., Hjorleifsson, K. E., Eggertsson, H. P., Gudjonsson, S. A., Ward, L. D., Arnadottir, G. A., Helgason, E. A., Helgason, H., Gylfason, A., Jonasdottir, A., Jonasdottir, A., Rafnar, T., Frigge, M., . . . Stefansson, K. (2017). Parental influence on human germline de novo mutations in 1,548 trios from Iceland. *Nature, 549*(7673), 519–522. https://doi.org/10.1038/nature24018

Kang, E., Gadow, K. D., & Lerner, M. D. (2020). Atypical communication characteristics, differential diagnosis, and the autism spectrum disorder phenotype in youth. *Journal of Clinical Child and Adolescent Psychology, 49*(2), 251–263. https://doi.org/10.1080/15374416.2018.1539912

Levy, A., & Perry, A. (2011). Outcomes in adolescents and adults with autism: A review of the literature. *Research in Autism Spectrum Disorders, 5*(4), 1271–1282. https://doi.org/10.1016/j.rasd.2011.01.023

Maenner, M. J., Shaw, K. A., Baio, J., Washington, A., Patrick, M., DiRienzo, M., Christensen, D. L., Wiggins, L. D., Pettygrove, S., Andrews, J. G., Lopez, M., Hudson, A., Baroud, T., Schwenk, Y., White, T., Rosenberg, C. R., Lee, L. C., Harrington, R. A., Huston, M., . . . Dietz, P. M. (2020). Prevalence of autism spectrum disorder among children aged 8 years—Autism and Developmental Disabilities Monitoring Network, 11 sites, United States, 2016. *Morbidity and Mortality Weekly Report Surveillance Summaries, 69*(4), 1–12. https://doi.org/10.15585/mmwr.ss6904a1

McClain, M. B., Shahidullah, J. D., Mezher, K. R., Haverkamp, C. R., Benallie, K. J., & Schwartz, S. E. (2020). School-clinic care coordination for youth with ASD: A national survey of school psychologists. *Journal of Autism and Developmental Disorders, 50*(9), 3081–3091. https://doi.org/10.1007/s10803-019-03985-3

McPheeters, M. L., Warren, Z., Sathe, N., Bruzek, J. L., Krishnaswami, S., Jerome, R. N., & Veenstra-VanderWeele, J. (2011). A systematic review of medical treatments for children with autism spectrum disorders. *Pediatrics, 127*(5), e1312–e1321. https://doi.org/10.1542/peds.2011-0427

Myers, S. M., Johnson, C. P., & the Council on Children With Disabilities. (2007). Management of children with autism spectrum disorders. *Pediatrics, 120*(5), 1162–1182. https://doi.org/10.1542/peds.2007-2362

National Autism Center. (2015). *National Standards Project, Phase 2.* https://nationalautismcenter.org/national-standards/phase-2-2015/

Ozonoff, S., Young, G. S., Carter, A., Messinger, D., Yirmiya, N., Zwaigenbaum, L., Bryson, S., Carver, L. J., Constantino, J. N., Dobkins, K., Hutman, T., Iverson, J. M., Landa, R., Rogers, S. J., Sigman, M., & Stone, W. L. (2011). Recurrence risk for autism spectrum disorders: A Baby Siblings Research Consortium study. *Pediatrics, 128*(3), e488–e495. https://doi.org/10.1542/peds.2010-2825

Postorino, V., Sharp, W. G., McCracken, C. E., Bearss, K., Burrell, T. L., Evans, A. N., & Scahill, L. (2017). A systematic review and meta-analysis of parent training for disruptive behavior in children with autism spectrum disorder. *Clinical Child and Family Psychology Review, 20*(4), 391–402. https://doi.org/10.1007/s10567-017-0237-2

Reichow, B., & Volkmar, F. R. (2010). Social skills interventions for individuals with autism: Evaluation for evidence-based practices within a best evidence synthesis framework. *Journal of Autism and Developmental Disorders, 40*(2), 149–166. https://doi.org/10.1007/s10803-009-0842-0

Rubenstein, E., Young, J. C., Croen, L. A., DiGuiseppi, C., Dowling, N. F., Lee, L. C., Schieve, L., Wiggins, L. D., & Daniels, J. (2019). Brief report: Maternal opioid prescription from preconception through pregnancy and the odds of autism spectrum disorder and autism features in children. *Journal of Autism and Developmental Disorders, 49*(1), 376–382. https://doi.org/10.1007/s10803-018-3721-8

Sam, A., & AFIRM Team. (2015). *Peer-mediated instruction and intervention.* National Professional Development Center on Autism Spectrum Disorder, FPG Child Development Center, University of North Carolina. http://afirm.fpg.unc.edu/peer-mediated-instruction-and-intervention

Scahill, L., Bearss, K., Lecavalier, L., Smith, T., Swiezy, N., Aman, M. G., Sukhodolsky, D. G., McCracken, C., Minshawi, N., Turner, K., Levato, L., Saulnier, C., Dziura, J., & Johnson, C. (2016). Effect of parent training on adaptive behavior in children with autism spectrum disorder and disruptive behavior: Results of a randomized trial. *Journal of the American Academy of Child & Adolescent Psychiatry, 55*(7), 602–609. https://doi.org/10.1016/j.jaac.2016.05.001

Shapiro, E. S., & Cole, C. L. (1994). *Behavior change in the classroom: Self-management interventions.* Guilford Press.

Storch, E. A., Arnold, E. B., Lewin, A. B., Nadeau, J. M., Jones, A. M., De Nadai, A. S., Mutch, P. J., Selles, R. R., Ung, D., & Murphy, T. K. (2013). The effect of cognitive-behavioral therapy versus treatment as usual for anxiety in children with autism spectrum disorders: A randomized, controlled trial. *Journal of the American Academy of Child & Adolescent Psychiatry, 52*(2), 132–142. https://doi.org/10.1016/j.jaac.2012.11.007

Tager-Flusberg, H., & Kasari, C. (2013). Minimally verbal school-aged children with autism spectrum disorder: The neglected end of the spectrum. *Autism Research, 6*(6), 468–478. https://doi.org/10.1002/aur.1329

Thom, R. P., McDougle, C. J., & Hazen, E. P. (2019). Challenges in the medical care of patients with autism spectrum disorder: The role of the consultation-liaison psychiatrist. *Psychosomatics, 60*(5), 435–443. https://doi.org/10.1016/j.psym.2019.04.003

Tordjman, S., Somogyi, E., Coulon, N., Kermarrec, S., Cohen, D., Bronsard, G., Bonnot, O., Weismann-Arcache, C., Botbol, M., Lauth, B., Ginchat, V., Roubertoux, P., Barburoth, M., Kovess, V., Geoffray, M.-M., & Xavier, J. (2014). Gene × environment interactions in autism spectrum disorders: Role of epigenetic mechanisms. *Frontiers in Psychiatry, 5,* Article 53. https://doi.org/10.3389/fpsyt.2014.00053

Turner, H., Remington, A., & Hill, V. (2017). Developing an intervention to improve reading comprehension for children and young people with autism spectrum disorder. *Educational and Child Psychology, 34*(2), 13–26.

Tye, C., Runicles, A., Whitehouse, A. J. O., & Alvares, G. A. (2019). Corrigendum: Characterizing the interplay between autism spectrum disorder and comorbid medical conditions: An integrative review. *Frontiers in Psychiatry, 10*, Article 438. https://doi.org/10.3389/fpsyt.2019.00438

Vargason, T., Frye, R. E., McGuinness, D. L., & Hahn, J. (2019). Clustering of co-occurring conditions in autism spectrum disorder during early childhood: A retrospective analysis of medical claims data. *Autism Research, 12*(8), 1272–1285. https://doi.org/10.1002/aur.2128

Weitlauf, A. S., McPheeters, M. L., Peters, B., Sathe, N., Travis, R., Aiello, R., Williamson, E., Veenstra-VanderWeele, J., Krishaswami, S., Jerome, R., & Warren, Z. (2014). *Therapies for children with autism spectrum disorder: Behavioral interventions update* (AHRQ Publication No. 14-EHC036-EF). Agency for Healthcare Research and Quality. https://europepmc.org/article/nbk/nbk241444

Wood, J. J., Ehrenreich-May, J., Alessandri, M., Fujii, C., Renno, P., Laugeson, E., Piacentini, J. C., De Nadai, A. S., Arnold, E., Lewin, A. B., Murphy, T. K., & Storch, E. A. (2015). Cognitive behavioral therapy for early adolescents with autism spectrum disorders and clinical anxiety: A randomized, controlled trial. *Behavior Therapy, 46*(1), 7–19. https://doi.org/10.1016/j.beth.2014.01.002

Yianni-Coudurier, C., Darrou, C., Lenoir, P., Verrecchia, B., Assouline, B., Ledesert, B., Michelon, C., Pry, R., Aussilloux, C., & Baghdadli, A. (2008). What clinical characteristics of children with autism influence their inclusion in regular classrooms? *Journal of Intellectual Disability Research, 52*(10), 855–863. https://doi.org/10.1111/j.1365-2788.2008.01100.x

Zecavati, N., & Spence, S. J. (2009). Neurometabolic disorders and dysfunction in autism spectrum disorders. *Current Neurology and Neuroscience Reports, 9*(2), 129–136. https://doi.org/10.1007/s11910-009-0021-x

16

Cerebral Palsy

Sai Sudha Aravala, Adeline M. Bray, and Karen Cross

A common neuromusculoskeletal disease among children is cerebral palsy (CP). CP is identified as a neuromuscular condition in that it incorporates both muscular and neurological complications (Gormley, 2001). It is most common among children and most often identified during the early childhood years, including at the time of birth. There is significant heterogeneity in symptomatology across individuals, as CP occurs on a continuum with mild to severe effects on overall functioning (Centers for Disease Control and Prevention [CDC], 2018).

ETIOLOGY

At the neurological level, what manifests as CP results from atypical brain development, particularly affecting the motor and vestibular (balance) systems (Riccio et al., 2010). Some interference in neural development occurs to alter the typical trajectory either prior to birth (prenatally), during the birthing process (perinatally), or within 1 month of birth (postnatally). Most often the damage occurs during the prenatal or perinatal periods. When it does occur postnatally (i.e., acquired CP), the damage is usually in association with a head injury or infection soon after birth (CDC, 2018).

In terms of prenatal and perinatal causes, there is a high prevalence of CP among those born prematurely. New evidence indicates a possible genetic factor in 14% of cases (Schaefer, 2008). An estimated 5% to 10% of the reported

https://doi.org/10.1037/0000349-016
Health-Related Disorders in Children and Adolescents: A Guidebook for Educators and Service Providers, Second Edition, M. M. Perfect, C. A. Riccio, and M. A. Bray (Editors)

cases are said to stem from prenatal hypoxia or early damage to the brain due to a decrease in oxygen levels (Meberg & Broch, 2004). Although this is a common occurrence, there are many other factors involved in the neonatal and perinatal periods (Meberg & Broch, 2004). CP can also manifest due to intrapartum complications as well as intrauterine pathologies (Stavsky et al., 2017). CP is subtyped as spastic, nonspastic, or other, with overlap with ataxia (i.e., loss of balance and coordination) across subtypes. Of those with CP, the majority (77.4%) are identified to have the spastic subtype (Christensen et al., 2014).

PREVALENCE AND INCIDENCE

CP has a worldwide prevalence of four per 1,000 live births (CDC, 2018). The Autism and Developmental Disabilities Monitoring Network reported that the prevalence of CP ranged from 3.1 to 3.6 per 1,000 in the United States (Christensen et al., 2014). Gender and race differences were found; boys and those who identify as Black, non-Hispanics are more likely to be identified with CP (Christensen et al., 2014; Maenner et al., 2012).

SYMPTOMS

The clinical signs and symptoms of CP emerge prior to age 2 and are validated via various imaging methods and neurological examinations (for a review, see Novak et al., 2017). Spastic symptoms refer to experiencing problems in movements. Children with spastic CP may evidence jerky or exaggerated reflexes and irregular posturing. Within the nonspastic subtype, some children with CP evidence dysfunctions such as tremors, hyper- and hypotonia, and slow movements (athetoid CP). Others exhibit hypotonia (i.e., loss of muscle firmness and strength) on its own (Cerebral Palsy Guide, 2022). In addition, some individuals with CP may experience choreoathetosis (i.e., involuntary movements, twisting or writhing movements). Although the motor difficulties continue across the lifespan, in high-income countries like the United States, most (greater than 66%) with CP will be able to walk and talk (Novak et al., 2017).

IMPACT ON THE STUDENT AND OUTCOMES

Medical

CP is classified as a lifelong disability. Those with more severe motor impairment are subject to paralysis, known as quadriplegia, significantly reducing their mobility (CDC, 2018). Further, in some cases, this severity of CP can lead to seizures and problems with speech, vision, and hearing (CDC, 2018). Many children with CP develop gastroesophageal reflux disease (GERD), and Liptak and Accardo (2004) reported 59% of deaths related to CP were due to problems with GERD. Further complications include a high co-occurrence of epilepsy (41.0%) among those with CP (Christensen et al., 2014).

Cognitive/Academic

Approximately 25% of students with CP present with intellectual disabilities, and half exhibit learning problems (Lai & Yang, 2011). For those with normal intellectual abilities, the learning difficulties likely stem from impaired neurocognitive functioning, including issues with short-term memory and executive functioning (Straub & Obrzut, 2009). Deficits in executive functioning are associated with damage to the prefrontal cortex. Children with CP also struggle with slower response time, inattention, and relative inability to effectively use compensatory strategies (Beckung & Hagberg, 2002; Straub & Obrzut, 2009).

Academically, children with CP have demonstrated poor arithmetic skills (e.g., van Rooijen et al., 2012). Difficulties in math were related to nonverbal intelligence, word decoding, and fine motor skills, particularly the latter two (e.g., van Rooijen et al., 2012, 2015). Related to the arithmetic deficits were impairments in executive functioning and working memory (Jenks et al., 2009; van Rooijen et al., 2015). Deficits in executive functioning emerged even for children with CP who did not have impairments in speech or language (Sakash et al., 2018). Consistent with word-decoding ability associated with math skill acquisition, children with CP may encounter difficulty with reading and spelling, particularly related to visual processes (Critten et al., 2019).

Social-Emotional and Behavioral

Children with CP tend to struggle socially in some regard, often dealing with issues of social isolation (Liptak & Accardo, 2004; Nadeau & Tessier, 2006; Sakash et al., 2018; Sigurdardottir et al., 2010). Nadeau and Tessier (2006) found that female children with CP had decreased social status and suffered more socially compared with their male counterparts with CP. Liptak and Accardo (2004) also identified gender differences, with female children having fewer reciprocated friendships. Further, there is evidence to suggest that children with CP are victimized by their peers, verbally and physically (Nadeau & Tessier, 2006). Social–emotional issues are not limited to social impairment. Sakash and colleagues (2018) linked the social impairment to deficits in executive function; however, it should be noted that co-occurring autism spectrum disorder has been identified in up to 6.9% of those with CP (Christensen et al., 2014). Sigurdardottir and colleagues (2010) found that, compared with children without CP, children with CP evidenced more emotional and behavioral problems, except for somatic complaints. Other researchers have found high levels of depression (Sienko, 2018).

PSYCHOEDUCATIONAL IMPLICATIONS AND SCHOOL-BASED INTERVENTIONS

Medical and Health Management

Common treatments for CP address mobility and reduce spasticity. Physical therapy is another possible intervention that can help children diagnosed with CP gain mobility, as are yoga (Oppenheim, 2009) and aqua therapy (Kelly & Darrah, 2005).

Medication (e.g., botulinum toxin) also may be an option to relax muscles (Ade-Hall & Moore, 2000; Krigger, 2006). Surgery involving selective dorsal rhizotomy is another form of treatment, which involves cutting the dorsal rootlets from L1 and L2 of the spinal cord to reduce or potentially eliminate spasticity (Krigger, 2006). As noted, children with CP often present with GERD, epilepsy, scoliosis, and other medical complications, including sleep issues (Novak et al., 2017). For this reason, medical follow-up and ongoing communication with school personnel is important.

Cognitive/Academic

Children with CP often require communication support from speech and language pathologists due to the motor issues associated with speech production. For children with severe language impairments or complex communication needs, speech and language pathologists utilize alternative augmentative communication devices (Bourke-Taylor et al., 2018). Physical and occupational therapists can work with teachers to provide various low-cost assistive technologies (e.g., pencil grips, weighted pens and pencils, slant boards, mouth sticks). Further, adjustable positioning equipment provides access to classroom activities like writing, painting, drawing, and using computers (da Silva et al., 2018). Other approaches include mouth- or head-controlled joysticks, wrist splints, forearm supports, robotic arms, and slip-on keyboard aids. Windows and Mac OS preferences may be programmed to adjust the time a key is held down before it repeats the letter. Systems to support access to computers, though more expensive, allow access to the full curriculum (Morris, 2006).

Given the likelihood of academic difficulties, even with normal or better intellectual ability, routine standardized assessment or benchmarking to monitor and address difficulties in skill acquisition may be appropriate. Research highlights the importance of word-decoding ability, not only in reading and writing but also in early math skill acquisition (see van Rooijen et al., 2012). In addition, visual spatial skills may be of concern. Modifications to the educational process may also be considered (Jenks et al., 2010). Teachers may have expectations for a child with CP that do not take into account that, despite motor difficulties, some individuals with CP have cognitive ability within the average range or higher.

Social–Emotional and Behavioral

School psychologists and other mental health professionals need to address the high prevalence of depression that occurs in adolescents with CP (Sienko, 2018). Given the potential for social–emotional and behavioral difficulties, preventive actions and monitoring of overall psychosocial functioning may be appropriate. Consequently, a multidisciplinary approach in schools to meet the needs of children with CP enhances not only the educational attainment of the child but also the overall well-being of the child and family. Given evidence of social impairment and victimization, school policies on bullying should be well-implemented and students with CP provided with opportunities to gain social competence.

CONCLUSION

As CP presents with varying symptoms, degrees of physical impairment, and comorbidities, the educational needs of children with CP vary greatly and require an individualized approach to intervention. Thus, a multidisciplinary team consisting of administrators, general education teachers, special education teachers, school nurses, school psychologists, and support services must work alongside families and medical personnel to meet the child's individual needs. The unique challenges of raising a child with CP include consideration of the psychological well-being of the child and family. Dependency of children with CP on family resources also increases the financial and emotional burdens placed on the caregivers (Bourke-Taylor et al., 2010). In addressing the needs of the child with CP, consideration of parental functioning and support services is important.

RESOURCES

Centers for Disease Control and Prevention. (2018). *Cerebral palsy*. U.S. Department of Health and Human Services. https://www.cdc.gov/ncbddd/cp/index.html

National Institute of Neurological Disorders and Stroke. (2022). *Cerebral palsy: Hope through research*. National Institutes of Health. https://www.ninds.nih.gov/Disorders/Patient-Caregiver-Education/Hope-Through-Research/Cerebral-Palsy-Hope-Through-Research

Cerebral Palsy Guide. (2022). *Cerebral palsy symptoms*. https://www.cerebralpalsyguide.com/cerebral-palsy/symptoms/

REFERENCES

Ade-Hall, R. A., & Moore, A. P. (2000). Botulinum toxin type A in the treatment of lower limb spasticity in cerebral palsy. *Cochrane Database of Systemic Reviews*. https://doi.org/10.1002/14651858.CD001408

Beckung, E., & Hagberg, G. (2002). Neuroimpairments, activity limitations, and participation restrictions in children with cerebral palsy. *Developmental Medicine and Child Neurology, 44*(5), 309–316. https://doi.org/10.1111/j.1469-8749.2002.tb00816.x

Bourke-Taylor, H., Howie, L., & Law, M. (2010). Impact of caring for a school-aged child with a disability: Understanding mothers' perspectives. *Australian Occupational Therapy Journal, 57*(2), 127–136. https://doi.org/10.1111/j.1440-1630.2009.00817.x

Bourke-Taylor, H. M., Cotter, C., Lalor, A., & Johnson, L. (2018). School success and participation for students with cerebral palsy: A qualitative study exploring multiple perspectives. *Disability and Rehabilitation, 40*(18), 2163–2171. https://doi.org/10.1080/09638288.2017.1327988

Centers for Disease Control and Prevention. (2018). *Cerebral palsy*. U.S. Department of Health and Human Services. https://www.cdc.gov/ncbddd/cp/index.html

Cerebral Palsy Guide. (2022). *Cerebral palsy symptoms*. https://www.cerebralpalsyguide.com/cerebral-palsy/symptoms/

Christensen, D., Van Naarden Braun, K., Doernberg, N. S., Maenner, M. J., Arneson, C. L., Durkin, M. S., Benedict, R. E., Kirby, R. S., Wingate, M. S., Fitzgerald, R., & Yeargin-Allsopp, M. (2014). Prevalence of cerebral palsy, co-occurring autism spectrum disorders, and motor functioning—Autism and Developmental Disabilities Monitoring Network, USA, 2008. *Developmental Medicine & Child Neurology, 56*(1), 59–65. https://doi.org/10.1111/dmcn.12268

Critten, V., Messer, D., & Sheehy, K. (2019). Delays in the reading and spelling of children with cerebral palsy: Associations with phonological and visual processes. *Research in Developmental Disabilities, 85*, 131–142. https://doi.org/10.1016/j.ridd.2018.12.001

da Silva, A. P., Bulle Oliveira, A. S., Pinheiro Bezerra, I. M., Pedrozo Campos Antunes, T., Guerrero Daboin, B. E., Raimundo, R. D., Dos Santos, V. R., & de Abreu, L. C. (2018). Low cost assistive technology to support educational activities for adolescents with cerebral palsy. *Disability and Rehabilitation: Assistive Technology, 13*(7), 676–682. https://doi.org/10.1080/17483107.2017.1369590

Gormley, M. E., Jr. (2001). Treatment of neuromuscular and musculoskeletal problems in cerebral palsy. *Pediatric Rehabilitation, 4*(1), 5–16. https://doi.org/10.1080/13638490151068393

Jenks, K. M., de Moor, J., & van Lieshout, E. C. (2009). Arithmetic difficulties in children with cerebral palsy are related to executive function and working memory. *Journal of Child Psychology and Psychiatry, 50*(7), 824–833. https://doi.org/10.1111/j.1469-7610.2008.02031.x

Jenks, K. M., de Moor, J., van Lieshout, E. C., & Withagen, F. (2010). Quality of arithmetic education for children with cerebral palsy. *International Journal of Rehabilitation Research, 33*(1), 19–25. https://doi.org/10.1097/MRR.0b013e32832d21b1

Kelly, M., & Darrah, J. (2005). Aquatic exercise for children with cerebral palsy. *Developmental Medicine and Child Neurology, 47*(12), 838–842. https://doi.org/10.1111/j.1469-8749.2005.tb01091.x

Krigger, K. W. (2006). Cerebral palsy: An overview. *American Family Physician, 73*(1), 91–100. https://www.aafp.org/afp/2006/0101/p91.html

Lai, M. C., & Yang, S. N. (2011). Perinatal hypoxic-ischemic encephalopathy. *Journal of Biomedicine and Biotechnology, 2011*, Article 609813. https://doi.org/10.1155/2011/609813

Liptak, G. S., & Accardo, P. J. (2004). Health and social outcomes of children with cerebral palsy. *The Journal of Pediatrics, 145*(2, Suppl.), S36–S41. https://doi.org/10.1016/j.jpeds.2004.05.021

Maenner, M. J., Benedict, R. E., Arneson, C. L., Yeargin-Allsopp, M., Wingate, M. S., Kirby, R. S., Van Naarden Braun, K., & Durkin, M. S. (2012). Children with cerebral palsy: Racial disparities in functional limitations. *Epidemiology, 23*(1), 35–43 https://doi.org/10.1097/EDE.0b013e31823a4205

Meberg, A., & Broch, H. (2004). Etiology of cerebral palsy. *Journal of Perinatal Medicine, 32*(5), 434–439. https://doi.org/10.1515/JPM.2004.143

Morris, R. J. (2006). The use of computer technology for people having a disability. In R. J. Morris (Ed.), *Disability research and policy: Current perspectives* (pp. 81–96). Routledge. https://doi.org/10.4324/9781410615763-11

Nadeau, L., & Tessier, R. (2006). Social adjustment of children with cerebral palsy in mainstream classes: Peer perception. *Developmental Medicine and Child Neurology, 48*(5), 331–336. https://doi.org/10.1017/S0012162206000739

National Institute of Neurological Disorders and Stroke. (2022). *Cerebral palsy: Hope through research*. National Institutes of Health. https://www.ninds.nih.gov/Disorders/Patient-Caregiver-Education/Hope-Through-Research/Cerebral-Palsy-Hope-Through-Research

Novak, I., Morgan, C., Adde, L., Blackman, J., Boyd, R. N., Brunstrom-Hernandez, J., Cioni, G., Damiano, D., Darrah, J., Eliasson, A. C., de Vries, L. S., Einspieler, C., Fahey, M., Fehlings, D., Ferriero, D. M., Fetters, L., Fiori, S., Forssberg, H., Gordon, A. M., . . . Badawi, N. (2017). Early, accurate diagnosis and early intervention in cerebral palsy: Advances in diagnosis and treatment. *JAMA Pediatrics, 171*(9), 897–907. https://doi.org/10.1001/jamapediatrics.2017.1689

Oppenheim, W. L. (2009). Complementary and alternative methods in cerebral palsy. *Developmental Medicine and Child Neurology, 51*(Suppl. 4), 122–129. https://doi.org/10.1111/j.1469-8749.2009.03424.x

Riccio, C. A., Sullivan, J. R., & Cohen, M. J. (2010). *Neuropsychological assessment and intervention for childhood and adolescent disorders*. Wiley. https://doi.org/10.1002/9781118269954

Sakash, A., Broman, A. T., Rathouz, P. J., & Hustad, K. C. (2018). Executive function in school-aged children with cerebral palsy: Relationship with speech and language. *Research in Developmental Disabilities, 78*, 136–144. https://doi.org/10.1016/j.ridd.2018.05.015

Schaefer, G. B. (2008). Genetics considerations in cerebral palsy. *Seminars in Pediatric Neurology, 15*(1), 21–26. https://doi.org/10.1016/j.spen.2008.01.004

Sienko, S. E. (2018). An exploratory study investigating the multidimensional factors impacting the health and well-being of young adults with cerebral palsy. *Disability and Rehabilitation, 40*(6), 660–666. https://doi.org/10.1080/09638288.2016.1274340

Sigurdardottir, S., Indredavik, M. S., Eiriksdottir, A., Einarsdottir, K., Gudmundsson, H. S., & Vik, T. (2010). Behavioural and emotional symptoms of preschool children with cerebral palsy: A population-based study. *Developmental Medicine and Child Neurology, 52*(11), 1056–1061. https://doi.org/10.1111/j.1469-8749.2010.03698.x

Stavsky, M., Mor, O., Mastrolia, S. A., Greenbaum, S., Than, N. G., & Erez, O. (2017). Cerebral palsy—Trends in epidemiology and recent development in prenatal mechanisms of disease, treatment, and prevention. *Frontiers in Pediatrics, 5*, Article 21. https://doi.org/10.3389/fped.2017.00021

Straub, K., & Obrzut, J. E. (2009). Effects of cerebral palsy on neuropsychological function. *Journal of Developmental and Physical Disabilities, 21*(2), 153–167. https://doi.org/10.1007/s10882-009-9130-3

van Rooijen, M., Verhoeven, L., Smits, D.-W., Ketelaar, M., Becher, J. G., & Steenbergen, B. (2012). Arithmetic performance of children with cerebral palsy: The influence of cognitive and motor factors. *Research in Developmental Disabilities, 33*(2), 530–537. https://doi.org/10.1016/j.ridd.2011.10.020

van Rooijen, M., Verhoeven, L., & Steenbergen, B. (2015). From numeracy to arithmetic: Precursors of arithmetic performance in children with cerebral palsy from 6 till 8 years of age. *Research in Developmental Disabilities, 45–46*, 49–57. https://doi.org/10.1016/j.ridd.2015.07.001

17

Cri du Chat Syndrome

Phyllis S. Ohr

Cri du chat ("cat's cry" in French) syndrome is a congenital, neurodevelopmental disorder that results from variable deletions of a region on the short arm of chromosome 5 (5P). The size of the 5P deletion can vary from the entire short arm to only 5P15. The condition was first described by Lejeune et al. (1963), who reported the presence of a high-pitched cry similar to the mewing of a cat, significant mental retardation, microcephaly, and a host of minor phenotypical anomalies in three unrelated children.

ETIOLOGY

Although the constellation of symptoms was described in multiple studies from the 1970s to the late 1990s, research over the past 20 years suggests greater phenotype variability as identified by significant advances in molecular genetic techniques. Specifically, the use of sophisticated methods has enabled researchers to better determine cognitive, learning, social, emotional, and behavioral outcomes of cri du chat syndrome and other genetic disorders (Cornish & Bramble, 2002; Pituch et al., 2010). Given the variability in deletion size and type, identifying phenotypic subsets is informative for both diagnosis and prognosis (Cerruti Mainardi, 2006). The improvements in technology have also enabled investigators to distinguish between deletions that result in the severe disability characteristic of cri du chat syndrome and deletions that result in milder presentations, which are associated with better prognosis.

https://doi.org/10.1037/0000349-017
Health-Related Disorders in Children and Adolescents: A Guidebook for Educators and Service Providers, Second Edition, M. M. Perfect, C. A. Riccio, and M. A. Bray (Editors)

Nguyen and colleagues (2015) contributed information from a cohort of 286 individuals with 5P deletions comprising a 5P Minus Family Database. According to Nguyen et al., deletions occur spontaneously very early in embryonic development and for unknown reasons, with most (80%–90%) related to sperm formation, parents who typically have normal chromosomes, and a low familial probability of the birth of another child with cri du chat syndrome. Nguyen et al. also noted the finding in the literature of nonsymptomatic family members, including parents and siblings, with the same deletion.

PREVALENCE AND INCIDENCE

One of the first epidemiological studies addressing the prevalence of cri du chat syndrome estimated the number of newborns with this disorder to be approximately one in 50,000, making this one of the more common deletion syndromes in humans (Niebuhr, 1978). This early extensive characterization of 331 cases of cri du chat syndrome by Niebuhr (1978) cited the prevalence among those with intellectual disability to be as high as one in 350. Subsequent estimates showed a greater prevalence at one in 37,000 live births, with a range from one in 15,000 to 50,000. (Cerruti Mainardi, 2006). Although cri du chat syndrome affects female children more often than male children, the prevalence among ethnicities or geographical locations has not been noted, nor are there associations with specific prenatal events or parental age (Rodríguez-Caballero et al., 2010).

SYMPTOMS

Typically, individuals with cri du chat syndrome present with a distinct high-pitched monotone cry at birth due to anatomical and/or structural neurological alterations. The cry, which becomes less pronounced as the child grows older, is considered diagnostic of this syndrome because it is not associated with any other chromosomal disorder and is seen at a high frequency in people with the cri du chat syndrome (Cerruti Mainardi, 2006; Niebuhr, 1978; Rodríguez-Caballero et al., 2010). Additional characteristic clinical findings vary with age and encompass a wide spectrum of craniofacial dysmorphia, neurological abnormalities, cardiovascular defects, limb abnormalities, and dermatoglyphics (Niebuhr, 1978). Distinctive facial features may include an abnormally round or plump (moon) face, which often becomes elongated and narrow with advancing age. Other characteristics include microcephaly, a broad nasal bridge, hypertelorism (widely spaced eyes), epicanthal folds, low-set ears, dental malocclusion, and micrognathia (abnormally small jaw), as well as hearing and vision difficulties (Nguyen et al., 2015; Niebuhr, 1978; Rodríguez-Caballero et al., 2010). Clearly there is a wide spectrum of phenotypic features, which present with much variability that is attributed to differences in genotype, specifically the degree and location of the 5P deletion, as well as environmental factors, which have also yielded variability in presentation and outcome in other domains, such as intelligence.

IMPACT ON THE STUDENT AND OUTCOMES

As with many individuals with chromosomal atypicalities, individuals with cri du chat face numerous medical challenges. Infants may display low birth weight and growth deficiencies due to feeding challenges associated with neurodevelopmental anomalies, such as low muscle tone. The presence of cleft lip and palate, congenital heart defects, and scoliosis, as well as delays in gross and fine motor skills, persist throughout childhood and broadly affect functioning.

Cerruti Mainardi (2006) reported on a genotype–phenotype relationship study characterizing 80 Italian individuals with cri du chat syndrome using array comparative genome hybridization. Specifically, two genes that have been mapped to the "critical regions" in cri du chat syndrome are potentially involved in brain development, and their deletion may be associated with variability in intellectual impairment. Cornish and Bramble (2002) noted that individuals with 5P deletions outside the critical region may present with the characteristic cry but not cognitive limitations and stress that a milder presentation with a more optimistic developmental prognosis should be differentiated from the typical cri du chat phenotype associated with the more guarded outcome.

Cognitive/Academic

Although the second most prevalent characteristic of cri du chat syndrome is cognitive limitation, evidence suggests that the IQ scores of these individuals can vary from being profoundly impaired to functioning in the normal range of intellectual ability, depending on the size and region of deletion.

Variability in the degree of deficit in language ability, adaptive skills, and motor development also contributes to diverse levels of intellectual disability. Cornish and Bramble (2002) suggested that the addition of standardized neuropsychological measures to assess intelligence since the late 1990s has clarified patterns in cognitive functioning that differentiate typical from atypical presentations of cri du chat syndrome. In individuals with more guarded prognoses, intellectual functioning is signified by serious deficit (predominantly below average to very below average functioning); language delay is noted, with significant impairment in expressive language and at least mild receptive language delay; and learning disability is moderate to severe. Individuals with a more optimistic diagnosis are characterized by cognitive skills within normal limits, some reduced expressive verbal skills but strengths in nonverbal ability, and learning difficulties rather than documented learning disability.

Social-Emotional and Behavioral

Maladaptive behaviors of individuals with cri du chat syndrome were described in the early research of Wilkins et al. (1980) and Carlin (1990). Almost half of the children exhibited hyperactivity, a short attention span, low tolerance for frustration, self-stimulation, self-harming behaviors, and aggression toward others, with some of these behaviors observed before 1 year of age. Subsequent research confirmed many of the these presentations and also revealed that hyperactivity is a significant behavioral concern, with frequency cited as high as 80% to 90% and criteria for attention-deficit/hyperactivity disorder met by 70% of individuals (Cornish & Bramble, 2002). Attachment to objects and sensitivity to sensory stimuli were also determined to be highly prevalent. Cornish and Bramble (2002) noted several social strengths among individuals with cri du chat syndrome, including social interaction skills and positive demeanor.

Moss and colleagues (2013) also confirmed strengths in the nonverbal and social behavior of children with cri du chat syndrome in their evaluation of autism spectrum disorder (ASD) and several genetically defined syndromes potentially associated with ASD. According to Moss et al., individuals with cri du chat syndrome evidenced fewer ASD characteristics compared with individuals with Cornelia de Lange syndrome. Individuals with cri du chat syndrome demonstrated appropriate social interaction skills and positive affect during conditions of high social attention, suggesting enjoyment of engagement with others, and they increased their social approaches during periods of low attention to gain adult contact.

Teixeira and colleagues (2011) observed and counted adaptive and maladaptive behaviors in 10 children and adolescents with cri du chat syndrome as they engaged in a 20-minute cognitive task. Repetitive movements were observed at the highest rate of frequency, followed by aggressiveness, obsessive attachment to objects, self-harm behavior, and disruptive behavior. A noted strength was rule-following behavior. It was recommended that psychoeducational interventions and parent training aimed at stimulating the repertoire of adaptive behaviors be incorporated into treatment programs for youth with cri du chat syndrome.

PSYCHOEDUCATIONAL IMPLICATIONS AND SCHOOL-BASED INTERVENTIONS

Prior to the 1990s, individuals with cri du chat did not have access to psychoeducational, family, or systematic medical care, which contributed to poor outcomes. It is now recognized that infant intervention, early education, and home-rearing improve prognosis. Professionals have noted the variability of development in several domains, which is likely due to increases in home care as well as availability of early intervention (Albano et al., 2013; Cerruti Mainardi, 2006; Cornish & Bramble, 2002; Nguyen et al., 2015; Rodríguez-Caballero et al., 2010).

Medical and Health Management

Nguyen et al. (2015) reported that those children receiving early intervention sat up, walked independently, dressed themselves, and were toilet trained earlier than those children without interventions. Cerruti Mainardi (2006) also reported that home-reared patients who underwent early educational treatments demonstrated improved prognosis.

Treatment for those with cri du chat syndrome should use a multifaceted team approach focused on individualized needs as determined by a comprehensive evaluation to determine the symptom presentation of each child, adolescent, or adult. For individuals with medical needs, surgical interventions may be necessary to treat a variety of symptoms potentially associated with cri du chat syndrome, including cleft lip and palate, congenital heart defects, and scoliosis. Physical and occupational therapy can address delays in gross and fine motor skills, and audiologists and speech therapists can address communication and expressive language delays using strategies of nonverbal communication, an area of strength for many individuals with cri du chat, and teaching alternatives such as sign language. For children, treatment for growth and feeding concerns can be addressed not only medically but also by developing behavioral plans that incorporate family participation.

Cognitive/Academic

Given the cognitive, language, and learning characteristics associated with cri du chat syndrome, it is extremely probable that most children will require educational intervention (Cochran et al., 2019). Developing an individualized education program will enable the prioritizing of educational goals for each child. This is best approached through collaboration between school personnel, family members, and other professionals (i.e., outside therapists). It has been suggested that individualized education program goals should reflect parent priorities for the child's learning and development. Pituch et al. (2010) surveyed parents of children with cri du chat syndrome to identify the educational priorities that parents have for their children. With respect to high-priority skills rated by the parents, communication was deemed important, particularly listening and responding appropriately to the teacher, asking for information when needed, and following directions. Schwartzman et al. (2021) recently determined that pivotal response treatment, an evidence-based behavioral intervention based on applied behavior analysis principles, improved social communication skills in children with developmental disorders, including children with cri du chat.

Social-Emotional and Behavioral

According to Pituch et al. (2010), parents also prioritized concerns regarding their child's inability to describe their feelings, wants, and needs. Addressing the psychological needs (i.e., emotional, behavioral, and social) of children with cri du chat and their families should be an essential component of a treatment plan.

Several psychological concerns clearly would benefit from behavioral and parenting interventions. For example, hyperactivity, distractibility, disruptive behaviors, and aggression characteristic of some individuals with cri du chat syndrome would be responsive to applied behavior analysis as well as parent psychoeducation and parent support groups (Ajitkumar et al., 2022; Sarimski, 2003). In addition, anxiety symptoms, obsessiveness, sensory sensitivities, self-injurious behavior, and stereotypical behaviors are also present in some children (Moss et al., 2009; Richards et al., 2009; Sarimski, 2003). Behavioral and cognitive behavioral approaches, including psychoeducation, teaching coping and distress tolerance skills, and implementing anxiety management techniques, have been utilized to address internalizing concerns. Specifically, Moskowitz et al. (2017) suggested using a multicomponent behavioral and cognitive behavioral intervention plan to address diverse problematic behaviors.

Parental psychological well-being should also be addressed (Ajitkumar et al., 2022). Griffith et al. (2011) found that parents of children with cri du chat syndrome reported clinical levels of anxiety and depression. Interventions to address parent and child needs within the family context, especially for younger children, would thus be both interventive and preventive. For example, parent–child interaction therapy is an evidence-based treatment for families with young children that addresses both parent and child concerns and has been effectively utilized with children with developmental disabilities (McDiarmid & Bagner, 2005).

CONCLUSION

Due to advances in technology in the past 20 years, neurological, cognitive, academic, social, emotional, and behavioral outcomes are more predictable for individuals with significant genetic variability in cri du chat syndrome. Environmental variability also has significant effects, as increases in health care and the availability of early intervention have contributed greatly to improved outcomes.

RESOURCES

Genetic Rare Diseases Information Center. (2021). *Cri du chat syndrome*. National Center for Advancing Translational Sciences. https://rarediseases.info.nih.gov/diseases/6213/cri-du-chat-syndrome

MedlinePlus. (2022). *Cri-du-chat syndrome*. National Library of Medicine. https://medlineplus.gov/genetics/condition/cri-du-chat-syndrome/

Five P Minus Society. https://fivepminus.org

REFERENCES

Ajitkumar, A., Jamil, R. T., & Mathai, J. K. (2022). *Cri du chat syndrome*. StatPearls Publishing.

Albano, S., Piccardi, L., Pizzamiglio, M. R., Volpe, C., & D'Amico, S. (2013). Narrative discourse and sociocognitive abilities of a child with cri-du-chat syndrome. *The Journal of Genetic Psychology, 174*(1), 51–72. https://doi.org/10.1080/00221325.2011.639409

Carlin, M. E. (1990). The improved prognosis in cri-du-chat syndrome. In W. I. Fraser (Ed.), *Key issues in mental retardation research: Proceedings of 8th Congress of the International Association for the Scientific Study of Mental Deficiency* (pp. 64–73). Routledge.

Cerruti Mainardi, P. (2006). Cri du chat syndrome. *Orphanet Journal of Rare Diseases, 1*(1), Article 33. https://doi.org/10.1186/1750-1172-1-33

Cochran, L., Welham, A., Oliver, C., Arshad, A., & Moss, J. F. (2019). Age-related behavioural change in Cornelia de Lange and cri du chat syndromes: A seven year follow-up study. *Journal of Autism and Developmental Disorders, 49*(6), 2488–2491. https://doi.org/10.1007/s10803-019-04031-y

Cornish, K., & Bramble, D. (2002). Cri du chat syndrome: Genotype–phenotype correlations and recommendations for clinical management. *Developmental Medicine and Child Neurology, 44*(7), 494–497. https://doi.org/10.1111/j.1469-8749.2002.tb00312.x

Griffith, G. M., Hastings, R. P., Oliver, C., Howlin, P., Moss, J., Petty, J., & Tunnicliffe, P. (2011). Psychological well-being in parents of children with Angelman, Cornelia de Lange and cri du chat syndromes. *Journal of Intellectual Disability Research, 55*(4), 397–410. https://doi.org/10.1111/j.1365-2788.2011.01386.x

Lejeune, J., LaFourcade, J., Berger, R., Vialatte, J., Boeswillwald, M., Seringe, P., & Turpin, R. (1963). Trois cas de la deletion partielle du bras court du chromosome 5 [Three cases of partial deletion of the short arm of a 5 chromosome]. *Comptes Rendus Hebdomadaire des Seances de l'Academie des Sciences: D. Sciences Naturelles, 257*, 3098–3102.

McDiarmid, M. D., & Bagner, D. M. (2005). Parent child interaction therapy for children with disruptive behavior and developmental disabilities. *Education & Treatment of Children, 28*(2), 130–141.

Moskowitz, L. J., Walsh, C. E., Mulder, E., McLaughlin, D. M., Hajcak, G., Carr, E. G., & Zarcone, J. R. (2017). Intervention for anxiety and problem behavior in children with autism spectrum disorder and intellectual disability. *Journal of Autism and Developmental Disorders, 47*(12), 3930–3948. https://doi.org/10.1007/s10803-017-3070-z

Moss, J., Howlin, P., Hastings, R. P., Beaumont, S., Griffith, G. M., Petty, J., Tunnicliffe, P., Yates, R., Villa, D., & Oliver, C. (2013). Social behavior and characteristics of autism spectrum disorder in Angelman, Cornelia de Lange, and cri du chat syndromes. *American Journal on Intellectual and Developmental Disabilities, 118*(4), 262–283. https://doi.org/10.1352/1944-7558-118.4.262

Moss, J., Oliver, C., Arron, K., Burbidge, C., & Berg, K. (2009). The prevalence and phenomenology of repetitive behavior in genetic syndromes. *Journal of Autism and Developmental Disorders, 39*(4), 572–588. https://doi.org/10.1007/s10803-008-0655-6

Nguyen, J. M., Qualmann, K. J., Okashah, R., Reilly, A., Alexeyev, M. F., & Campbell, D. J. (2015). 5p deletions: Current knowledge and future directions. *American Journal of Medical Genetics: Part C, Seminars in Medical Genetics, 169*(3), 224–238. https://doi.org/10.1002/ajmg.c.31444

Niebuhr, E. (1978). The cri du chat syndrome: Epidemiology, cytogenetics, and clinical features. *Human Genetics, 44*(3), 227–275. https://doi.org/10.1007/BF00394291

Pituch, K. A., Green, V. A., Didden, R., Whittle, L., O'Reilly, M. F., Lancioni, G. E., & Sigafoos, J. (2010). Educational priorities for children with cri-du-chat syndrome. *Journal of Developmental and Physical Disabilities, 22*(1), 65–81. https://doi.org/10.1007/s10882-009-9172-6

Richards, C., Moss, J., O'Farrell, L., Kaur, G., & Oliver, C. (2009). Social anxiety in Cornelia de Lange syndrome. *Journal of Autism and Developmental Disorders, 39*(8), 1155–1162. https://doi.org/10.1007/s10803-009-0730-7

Rodríguez-Caballero, A., Torres-Lagares, D., Rodríguez-Pérez, A., Serrera-Figallo, M. A., Hernández-Guisado, J. M., & Machuca-Portillo, G. (2010). Cri du chat syndrome: A critical review. *Medicina Oral, Patologia Oral y Cirugia Bucal, 15*(3), e473–e478. https://doi.org/10.4317/medoral.15.e473

Sarimski, K. (2003). Early play behaviour in children with 5p- (cri-du-chat) syndrome. *Journal of Intellectual Disability Research, 47*(2), 113–120. https://doi.org/10.1046/j.1365-2788.2003.00448.x

Schwartzman, J. M., Strong, K., Ardel, C. M., Schuck, R. K., Millan, M. E., Phillips, J. M., Hardan, A. Y., & Gengoux, G. W. (2021). Language improvement following pivotal response treatment for children with developmental disorders. *American Journal on Intellectual and Developmental Disabilities, 126*(1), 45–57. https://doi.org/10.1352/1944-7558-126.1.45

Teixeira, M. C., Emerich, D. R., Orsati, F. T., Rimério, R. C., Gatto, K. R., Chappaz, I. O., & Kim, C. A. (2011). A description of adaptive and maladaptive behaviour in children and adolescents with cri-du-chat syndrome. *Journal of Intellectual Disability Research, 55*(2), 132–137. https://doi.org/10.1111/j.1365-2788.2010.01377.x

Wilkins, L. E., Brown, J. A., & Wolf, B. (1980). Psychomotor development in 65 home-reared children with cri-du-chat syndrome. *The Journal of Pediatrics, 97*(3), 401–405. https://doi.org/10.1016/S0022-3476(80)80189-2

18

Down Syndrome

Nicholas W. Gelbar

Down syndrome (also known as trisomy 21) is the leading known cause of intellectual disability (Presson et al., 2013; Shin et al., 2009). It was first described by an English physician, J. L. H. Down (1866), who characterized children with intellectual disabilities and the distinguishing facial features of the disorder. After the 1959 discovery by a French geneticist that Down syndrome was linked to an extra copy of the 21st chromosome being present in the body cells, the disorder also became known as trisomy 21 (Lejeune et al., 1959). Down syndrome was thus the first form of intellectual disability with a clear genetic origin, though research is still discovering how trisomy 21 shapes brain development and leads to intellectual disability.

PREVALENCE AND INCIDENCE

Down syndrome is estimated to affect approximately eight to 12 out of 10,000 individuals or 0.08% to 0.12% of the population (Presson et al., 2013; Shin et al., 2009). The prevalence increased by 31% from 1979 to 2003 (Shin et al., 2009). However, more recent evidence suggests that this study may have overestimated the prevalence (Presson et al., 2013). Data indicate that male individuals may be slightly more likely to be born with Down syndrome than female individuals (ratio of 1.15 to 1; Shin et al., 2009). The only reported risk factor for Down syndrome is maternal age at pregnancy (Presson et al., 2013).

https://doi.org/10.1037/0000349-018
Health-Related Disorders in Children and Adolescents: A Guidebook for Educators and Service Providers, Second Edition, M. M. Perfect, C. A. Riccio, and M. A. Bray (Editors)

ETIOLOGY

Down syndrome is not an inherited disorder (American Academy of Pediatrics [AAP] Committee on Genetics, 2001). The vast majority of individuals with Down syndrome (approximately 95%) have a complete extra copy of the 21st chromosome, the shortest chromosome, in all of their cells. Approximately 1% to 2% of individuals with Down syndrome exhibit *mosaicism*, in which most of their cells have an extra copy of the 21st chromosome but some of their cells do not have the extra copy (AAP Committee on Genetics, 2001; Chapman & Hesketh, 2000). Those individuals with mosaicism may have slightly milder presentation but may still experience intellectual disability and the other health impairments described subsequently (Hultén et al., 2013). Finally, a small number of individuals (approximately 3%–4%) have a partial copy of the 21st chromosome translocated with another chromosome (most often the 14th chromosome), which appears to be phenotypically identical to the full trisomy 21 (AAP Committee on Genetics, 2001). Approximately 25% of these translocations are inherited, and the parent carries a balanced translocation while the individual with Down syndrome has an unbalanced translocation of the 21st chromosome (Shapiro, 2003).

SYMPTOMS

Similar to other genetically based disorders, Down syndrome presents with incredible variation across individuals. One researcher recently noted, "It remains startling that despite the common theme of trisomy 21, the differences between individuals are often striking, particularly cognitive functions that emerge throughout brain development, organization, and maturation" (Capone, 2020, p. 93). The one unifying manifestation across all individuals with Down syndrome is the presence of intellectual disability, though there is variation in the severity, as individuals with Down syndrome have IQs that range from 30 to 70 with mean IQ of 50 (Capone, 2020).

IMPACT ON THE STUDENT AND OUTCOMES

Down syndrome leads to a variety of medical, cognitive, academic, social, emotional, and behavioral outcomes.

Medical

The genetic impact of trisomy 21 does not just influence brain development but leads to a myriad of disruptions to the development of multiple organ systems that can have important medical/health implications. Individuals with Down syndrome are more likely to experience epilepsy compared with the general population (Arya et al., 2011), with seizures often presenting in early childhood. Trisomy 21 also can cause structural abnormalities in the breathing and gastrointestinal systems (Hamilton et al., 2016). The malformations in the airways coupled with immunodeficiencies (Ram & Chinen, 2011) mean that individuals with Down syndrome are at much higher risk for infections in the lungs, throat, or ears (Venail et al., 2004) and/or sleep apnea (Shott et al., 2006). Upper airway malformations also can lead to cardiovascular difficulties (Watts & Vyas, 2013). Further, hearing impairments/deafness and speech delays are common in this population (Austeng et al., 2013). In addition, individuals with Down syndrome are more likely than the general population to be born with heart malformations (McGrath et al., 2011), but these are often remedied surgically early in life. Down syndrome has been linked to problems with vision and thyroid regulation. Further, individuals with Down syndrome are more likely to have low muscle tone (AAP Committee on Genetics, 2001) and to be overweight/obese (Bertapelli et al., 2016).

Cognitive/Academic

Beginning early in life, individuals with Down syndrome start experiencing delays in reaching developmental milestones and learning (Chapman & Hesketh, 2000). They meet early speech developmental milestones on time but have difficulty transitioning from babbling to intelligible speech (Chapman & Hesketh, 2000). They initially meet early motor milestones on time but are slower to meet later motor milestones, which is likely a consequence of their low muscle tone (Lott, 2012). Individuals with Down syndrome demonstrate better visual memory and phonological retrieval skills but poorer verbal memory skills compared with children with other intellectual disabilities (Conners et al., 2011).

Social-Emotional and Behavioral

Research from the 1990s indicated that individuals with Down syndrome appeared to be at lower risk for engaging in challenging behaviors compared with other individuals with intellectual disabilities (Chapman & Hesketh, 2000). This fostered the belief that their behavioral and social skills were more developed relative to their peers with intellectual disabilities. More recent research has indicated that individuals with Down syndrome are more likely to engage in inattentive, oppositional, or impulsive behaviors compared with typically developing peers (Lott, 2012). Additional research has shown that although individuals with Down syndrome may be social, they still have difficulties engaging in appropriate, sustained interpersonal interactions (Marchal et al., 2016). Further, in the late 1990s, research indicated that some individuals with Down syndrome also met the diagnostic criteria for autism spectrum disorder (Dressler et al., 2011) and that these individuals had greater social and behavioral difficulties compared with other individuals with Down syndrome. Currently, it is estimated that up to 18% of individuals with Down syndrome also have autism spectrum disorder (DiGuiseppi et al., 2010).

PSYCHOEDUCATIONAL IMPLICATIONS AND SCHOOL-BASED INTERVENTIONS

The variation in presentation of Down syndrome leads to a need for highly individualized education programs.

Medical and Health Management

Individuals with Down syndrome are often involved with multiple specialists outside of school. The potential presence of the previously mentioned health risk factors means that individuals with Down syndrome may have more absences from school than other children, which may impact their educational progress. Their educational programs will need to consider this potential for absences and thus are likely to require the provision of extended school year services as well as homebound tutoring if students are absent from school for extended periods of time.

Their medical complexity also will require the support of an individualized health plan in addition to their individualized education program, and thus, the school nurse will be a key member of their school team. Due to their potential difficulties with obesity coupled with low muscle tone, the school programs for individuals with Down syndrome should include curricula that promote both healthy eating and exercise. Individuals with Down syndrome should be encouraged to get involved with extracurricular opportunities, such as inclusive sporting events like the Special Olympics. The AAP Committee on Genetics (2001) provided a complete discussion of the medical management needs of individuals with Down syndrome.

Cognitive/Academic

Browder et al. (2014) created a comprehensive guide to developing programming for individuals with severe disabilities that can serve as an excellent resource. The key message from Browder and colleagues is the necessity of providing highly individualized programming. Some individuals with Down syndrome will be able to be educated primarily in regular education settings with a gradual increase in the amount of curriculum modifications that are necessary. Others will require more specialized instruction in self-contained settings.

In addition, services/accommodations for those presenting with difficulties with expressive language skills and/or pragmatic language skills should be addressed through specific direction instruction. Learning to read can be particularly challenging for individuals with Down syndrome (Felix et al., 2017), but research has demonstrated the efficacy of using systematic, direct approaches for teaching reading skills to individuals with Down syndrome by specifically teaching phonemic awareness (Lemons et al., 2018). It is suggested that school teams explore potential assistive technology options (e.g., text-to-speech software) to further support language and literacy skills of individuals with Down syndrome.

Social-Emotional and Behavioral

As previously mentioned, contemporary research has questioned the notion that individuals with Down syndrome are less likely to engage in challenging behaviors. Consequently, proactive behavior management strategies to address any behavioral difficulties will likely be needed. This would involve conducting functional behavior assessment/analysis to inform the development of individualized behavior intervention plans. In addition, individuals with Down syndrome will require research-based interventions to provide intensive social skills instruction and assistance in developing their understanding of pragmatic language. In schools, this would involve participation in groups run by the school psychologist and/or speech-language pathologist. Individuals with Down syndrome may benefit from peer mentoring programs where they are paired with same-age peers who help them to develop social competencies.

CONCLUSION

Similar to the presentation of other genetic syndromes, individuals with Down syndrome display a variety of strengths and needs that vary from individual to individual. School-based personnel will need to coordinate with outside providers, as individuals with Down syndrome can have medically complicated needs. This coordination and individualization are necessary to ensure that individuals with Down syndrome achieve the best possible quality of life.

RESOURCES

Centers for Disease Control and Prevention. (2022). *Facts about Down syndrome.* U.S. Department of Health and Human Services. https://www.cdc.gov/ncbddd/birthdefects/downsyndrome.html

National Down Syndrome Society. (n.d.). *About Down syndrome.* https://www.ndss.org/about-down-syndrome/down-syndrome/

Mayo Clinic. (2018). *Down syndrome.* https://www.mayoclinic.org/diseases-conditions/down-syndrome/symptoms-causes/syc-20355977

REFERENCES

American Academy of Pediatrics Committee on Genetics. (2001). Health supervision for children with Down syndrome. *Pediatrics, 107*(2), 442–449. https://doi.org/10.1542/peds.107.2.442

Arya, R., Kabra, M., & Gulati, S. (2011). Epilepsy in children with Down syndrome. *Epileptic Disorders, 13*(1), Article 1. https://doi.org/10.1684/epd.2011.0415

Austeng, M. E., Akre, H., Falkenberg, E. S., Øverland, B., Abdelnoor, M., & Kværner, K. J. (2013). Hearing level in children with Down syndrome at the age of eight. *Research in Developmental Disabilities, 34*(7), 2251–2256. https://doi.org/10.1016/j.ridd.2013.04.006

Bertapelli, F., Pitetti, K., Agiovlasitis, S., & Guerra-Junior, G. (2016). Overweight and obesity in children and adolescents with Down syndrome—Prevalence, determinants, consequences, and interventions: A literature review. *Research in Developmental Disabilities, 57,* 181–192. https://doi.org/10.1016/j.ridd.2016.06.018

Browder, D. M., Wood, L., Thompson, J., & Ribuffo, C. (2014). *Evidence-based practices for students with severe disabilities* (Document No. IC-3). University of Florida, Collaboration for Effective Educator, Development, Accountability, and Reform Center. http://ceedar.education.ufl.edu/tools/innovation-configurations/

Capone, G. T. (2020). Current research approaches to Down syndrome: Translational research perspectives. *American Journal on Intellectual and Developmental Disabilities, 125*(2), 93–96. https://doi.org/10.1352/1944-7558-125.2.93

Chapman, R. S., & Hesketh, L. J. (2000). Behavioral phenotype of individuals with Down syndrome. *Mental Retardation and Developmental Disabilities Research Reviews, 6*(2), 84–95. https://doi.org/10.1002/1098-2779(2000)6:2<84::AID-MRDD2>3.0.CO;2-P

Conners, F. A., Moore, M. S., Loveall, S. J., & Merrill, E. C. (2011). Memory profiles of Down, Williams, and fragile X syndromes: Implications for reading development. *Journal of Developmental and Behavioral Pediatrics, 32*(5), 405–417. https://doi.org/10.1097/DBP.0b013e3182168f95

DiGuiseppi, C., Hepburn, S., Davis, J. M., Fidler, D. J., Hartway, S., Lee, N. R., Miller, L., Ruttenber, M., & Robinson, C. (2010). Screening for autism spectrum disorders in children with Down syndrome: Population prevalence and screening test characteristics. *Journal of Developmental and Behavioral Pediatrics, 31*(3), 181–191. https://doi.org/10.1097/DBP.0b013e3181d5aa6d

Down, J. L. H. (1866). Observations on an ethnic classification of idiots. *London Hospital Clinical Lectures and Reports, 3,* 259–262.

Dressler, A., Perelli, V., Bozza, M., & Bargagna, S. (2011). The autistic phenotype in Down syndrome: Differences in adaptive behaviour versus Down syndrome alone and autistic disorder alone. *Functional Neurology, 26*(3), 151–158.

Felix, V. G., Mena, L. J., Ostos, R., & Maestre, G. E. (2017). A pilot study of the use of emerging computer technologies to improve the effectiveness of reading and writing therapies in children with Down syndrome. *British Journal of Educational Technology, 48*(2), 611–624. https://doi.org/10.1111/bjet.12426

Hamilton, J., Yaneza, M. M. C., Clement, W. A., & Kubba, H. (2016). The prevalence of airway problems in children with Down's syndrome. *International Journal of Pediatric Otorhinolaryngology, 81,* 1–4. https://doi.org/10.1016/j.ijporl.2015.11.027

Hultén, M. A., Jonasson, J., Iwarsson, E., Uppal, P., Vorsanova, S. G., Yurov, Y. B., & Iourov, I. Y. (2013). Trisomy 21 mosaicism: We may all have a touch of Down syndrome. *Cytogenetic and Genome Research, 139*(3), 189–192. https://doi.org/10.1159/000346028

Lejeune, J., Turpin, R., & Gautier, M. (1959). Le mongolisme, premier exemple d'aberration autosomique humaine [Mongolism: The first example of human autosomal aberration]. *Annales de Génétique, 1*(4), 1–49.

Lemons, C. J., King, S. A., Davidson, K. A., Puranik, C. S., Al Otaiba, S., & Fidler, D. J. (2018). Personalized reading intervention for children with Down syndrome. *Journal of School Psychology, 66,* 67–84. https://doi.org/10.1016/j.jsp.2017.07.006

Lott, I. T. (2012). Neurological phenotypes for Down syndrome across the life span. In M. Dierssen & R. De La Torre (Eds.), *Down syndrome: From understanding neurobiology to therapy* (pp. 101–121). Elsevier. https://doi.org/10.1016/B978-0-444-54299-1.00006-6

Marchal, J. P., Maurice-Stam, H., Houtzager, B. A., Rutgers van Rozenburg-Marres, S. L., Oostrom, K. J., Grootenhuis, M. A., & van Trotsenburg, A. S. P. (2016). Growing up with Down syndrome: Development from 6 months to 10.7 years. *Research in Developmental Disabilities, 59*, 437–450. https://doi.org/10.1016/j.ridd.2016.09.019

McGrath, R. J., Stransky, M. L., Cooley, W. C., & Moeschler, J. B. (2011). National profile of children with Down syndrome: Disease burden, access to care, and family impact. *The Journal of Pediatrics, 159*(4), 535–540.e2. https://doi.org/10.1016/j.jpeds.2011.04.019

Presson, A. P., Partyka, G., Jensen, K. M., Devine, O. J., Rasmussen, S. A., McCabe, L. L., & McCabe, E. R. (2013). Current estimate of Down syndrome population prevalence in the United States. *The Journal of Pediatrics, 163*(4), 1163–1168. https://doi.org/10.1016/j.jpeds.2013.06.013

Ram, G., & Chinen, J. (2011). Infections and immunodeficiency in Down syndrome. *Clinical and Experimental Immunology, 164*(1), 9–16. https://doi.org/10.1111/j.1365-2249.2011.04335.x

Shapiro, B. L. (2003). Down syndrome and associated congenital malformations. In G. Lubec (Ed.), *Advances in Down syndrome research* (pp. 207–214). Springer. https://doi.org/10.1007/978-3-7091-6721-2_18

Shin, M., Besser, L. M., Kucik, J. E., Lu, C., Siffel, C., Correa, A., & the Congenital Anomaly Multistate Prevalence and Survival Collaborative. (2009). Prevalence of Down syndrome among children and adolescents in 10 regions of the United States. *Pediatrics, 124*(6), 1565–1571. https://doi.org/10.1542/peds.2009-0745

Shott, S. R., Amin, R., Chini, B., Heubi, C., Hotze, S., & Akers, R. (2006). Obstructive sleep apnea: Should all children with Down syndrome be tested? *Archives of Otolaryngology—Head & Neck Surgery, 132*(4), 432–436. https://doi.org/10.1001/archotol.132.4.432

Venail, F., Gardiner, Q., & Mondain, M. (2004). ENT and speech disorders in children with Down's syndrome: An overview of pathophysiology, clinical features, treatments, and current management. *Clinical Pediatrics, 43*(9), 783–791. https://doi.org/10.1177/000992280404300902

Watts, R., & Vyas, H. (2013). An overview of respiratory problems in children with Down's syndrome. *Archives of Disease in Childhood, 98*(10), 812–817. https://doi.org/10.1136/archdischild-2013-304611

19

Epilepsy

Megan Aros-O'Malley, David L. Wodrich, and Randa Jarrar

Epilepsy is defined by an enduring tendency to have unprovoked seizures. Importantly, epilepsy is heterogeneous, with many different causes and presentations. The specific epilepsy type is associated with seizure presentation and, to some extent, cognitive and learning effects, plus treatment regime.

ETIOLOGY

Although an extensive epilepsy classification system exists (see the International League Against Epilepsy; https://www.ilae.org/guidelines/definition-and-classification), a subclassification involving etiology is especially noteworthy: epilepsy due to known, underlying causes (e.g., neurological condition, genetic or metabolic error, traumatic brain injury) versus epilepsy with an unknown cause. Children with epilepsy of known etiology more commonly have cognitive impairment than counterparts whose epilepsy is of unknown etiology (Berg et al., 2008). This makes sense as the former group have epilepsy as part of a pervasive, complex condition (e.g., tuberous sclerosis, Angelman syndrome). This distinction is especially important for school-based practitioners, as rates of intellectual disability are greater for those with epilepsy with a known etiology (Wodrich et al., 2006).

https://doi.org/10.1037/0000349-019
Health-Related Disorders in Children and Adolescents: A Guidebook for Educators and Service Providers, Second Edition, M. M. Perfect, C. A. Riccio, and M. A. Bray (Editors)

PREVALENCE AND INCIDENCE

Epilepsy is the most common childhood neurological condition—affecting an estimated six in 1,000 children worldwide—and is the third most common chronic illness affecting children. A recent meta-analysis of international studies indicates that prevalence is slightly higher for male individuals and peaks in adolescence and early adulthood (Fiest et al., 2017). No consistent racial or ethnic differences in epilepsy have been found. However, lower income is associated with a higher incidence of epilepsy in all racial and ethnic groups (Fiest at al., 2017).

SYMPTOMS

An important subclassification regarding symptoms involves focal versus generalized epilepsy. *Focal epilepsy* denotes seizures that originate in a part of one of the hemispheres, whereas *generalized epilepsy* denotes seizures that involve bilateral networks. Focal seizures therefore may be less obvious (e.g., changes confined to motor movements, limited sensory symptoms, with or without retained awareness). On the other hand, generalized seizures are typically more noticeable and involve loss of awareness, generalized shaking, and possibly loss of continence.

IMPACT ON THE STUDENT AND OUTCOMES

Epilepsy impacts students in many ways, including associated medical treatment, cognitive and academic functioning, and social–emotional and behavioral functioning.

Medical

All cases of epilepsy, regardless of subtype, are likely to be treated with antiepileptic drugs (AEDs). Different AEDs are more effective for certain types of epilepsy (i.e., generalized vs. focal), but overall, 60% to 70% of children with epilepsy become seizure free with use of one AED (Sarhan et al., 2015). Their treatment benefits notwithstanding, AEDs may compromise cognitive functioning (Titus & Thio, 2009). Moreover, cognitive risks grow when multiple AEDs are needed (Titus & Thio, 2009). Common AED side effects include general cognitive slowing; drowsiness; lethargy; disturbances in language, memory, and executive functioning (i.e., attention, concentration, and working memory); irritability; and hyperactivity (Hermann et al., 2010).

Cognitive/Academic

Epilepsy can be associated with direct cognitive impairment (i.e., arising from the medical condition itself). Paralleling the findings cited in this chapter, Berg et al. (2008) found that 84.8% of children with epilepsy with an unknown cause had IQs equal to or greater than 80, but the rate was just 35.7% for peers with a known etiology. However, even among those with unknown etiology, cognitive difficulties sometimes exist. For example, one study found that 12% of youth with new-onset epilepsy of unknown etiology demonstrated assorted cognitive impairments (i.e., verbal, perceptual, speed, attention, executive functioning). Moreover, another 44% of the youth evidenced mild, but significant, differences from healthy controls across all these domains (Hermann et al., 2016). Another study found that children with recent-onset epilepsy of unknown etiology had significantly lower overall IQs than their parents and healthy cousins (Walker et al., 2013). This study is important as it helps control for the direct effect of genetic factors on cognitive functioning.

Attention is one aspect of neurocognitive functioning that appears to be especially vulnerable among children with epilepsy. Several studies have found that approximately one third of this population meet criteria for attention-deficit/hyperactivity disorder (ADHD; Reilly et al., 2013). Furthermore, in contrast to the general population, in which combined presentation of ADHD (inattention and hyperactivity/impulsivity) is predominant, children with epilepsy show more circumscribed difficulties with inattention (Reilly et al., 2013). Even when their symptoms do not warrant a diagnosis of ADHD, children with epilepsy still show increased difficulty with focus and concentration (Williams, 2004).

Although attention appears to be especially compromised with epilepsy, other neurocognitive domains (e.g., memory, processing speed, executive functioning) are frequently affected as well. Specific neurocognitive deficits may depend on the location of the seizure foci. For example, temporal lobe seizure foci may predict memory and language production problems (Rzezak et al., 2007). Other studies, however, have found seizure foci to be an unreliable predictor of difficulties (Bhise et al., 2010). This suggests that all students with epilepsy, regardless of the location of their seizure foci, are at risk for various neurocognitive problems.

Besides direct, epilepsy-related cognitive difficulties, indirect effects also exist. Specifically, seizures sometimes recur throughout the day, disrupting attention, memory, and learning (Wodrich et al., 2006). Moreover, many neurocognitive processes (e.g., attention, processing speed, memory) are likely to be compromised during the postictal (postseizure) period, during which the overt seizure has stopped but the brain has not yet returned to baseline. Last, as previously mentioned, AEDs can also have a negative impact on specific neurocognitive functions as well as overall IQ. A study found that children with epilepsy who underwent brain surgery and subsequently stopped or reduced AED use had postoperative IQ improvement, with 23% of youth improving by 10 or more IQ points (Boshuisen et al., 2015).

Given the heightened neurocognitive risks with epilepsy, it is understandable that students with epilepsy are also at greater risk for learning problems at school. Indeed, rates of specific learning disabilities (SLDs) have been found to be higher compared with healthy peers. In addition, academic underachievement has been documented across all academic areas, including math, writing, and reading (Williams, 2004). For example, one study found that approximately one half (41%–62%) of intellectually intact students with epilepsy had an SLD in at least one academic area. Moreover, seizure control was unrelated to a diagnosis of SLD (Fastenau et al., 2008). This study is important because it demonstrates that even children with well-controlled epilepsy encounter higher than expected risk of learning disabilities. Furthermore, it indicates that the heterogeneity of co-occurring learning problems mirrors the diverse nature of epilepsy itself.

Social–Emotional and Behavioral

Children with epilepsy are also at higher risk for social–emotional difficulties. Indeed, rates of bullying have been found to be higher for these children (42%) than for children with another chronic health condition (chronic kidney disease; 21%) as well as for healthy peers (18%; Hamiwka et al., 2009). Moreover, in a meta-analysis that compared social competence among children with nine different chronic illnesses and healthy children, those with neurological disorders (including epilepsy) were found to have the poorest social competence of any group (Martinez et al., 2011).

The precise causes of social–emotional difficulties among children with epilepsy are not fully understood. One possibility concerns underlying brain dysfunction that causes both the epilepsy and psychological condition. Another possibility is the stigma associated with epilepsy. This perceived stigma may promote social isolation, peer rejection, low self-esteem, and avoidance of age-appropriate activities (Funderburk et al., 2007). Feelings of lost control over the unpredictability of epilepsy and negative attitude toward illness also may contribute to the development of psychopathology (Ekinci et al., 2009). Davies et al. (2003) found that 37% of children with epilepsy developed a psychological condition (e.g., depression, anxiety) compared with only 11% of children with diabetes and 9% of healthy children. Similarly, Lossius et al. (2006) noted rates of 30% to 40%. These studies suggest that approximately one third of children with epilepsy experience a comorbid psychological condition. This is concerning as psychological disorders, such as depression and anxiety, threaten a child's overall quality of life (Ekinci et al., 2009).

PSYCHOEDUCATIONAL IMPLICATIONS AND SCHOOL-BASED INTERVENTIONS

Unfortunately, there is a dearth of research examining the effectiveness of epilepsy-specific interventions for home and schools. Considering this reality, several intuitively plausible and logically derived interventions follow.

Medical and Health Management

As discussed, AEDs are the primary treatment for epilepsy. When AEDs prove ineffective, other treatments may be considered, including the ketogenic diet (high fat diet), neurostimulation, and brain surgery.

With any intervention, a key tenet is collaboration among school-based professionals, clinic-based professionals, and families. A school psychologist, social worker, or school nurse may be uniquely poised to help. They can, for example, coordinate communication among families, teachers, and medical professionals and can consult with teachers to help monitor academic progress. Indeed, consistent communication among stakeholders can help ensure that important information is shared and that all parties are informed of successes, challenges, and progress. For example, when parents or clinic-based professionals communicate AED changes to school professionals, teachers can be used as important informants who can help monitor neurocognitive changes, but only if channels of communication have been established.

Cognitive/Academic

Regarding neurocognitive risks, a thorough assessment may be an important initial step. Indeed, in-depth, comprehensive evaluations that measure intelligence, achievement, neurocognitive processes (e.g., attention, memory), and social–emotional functioning can be paramount in early detection of problems as well as in pinpointing strengths and weaknesses (Buelow & McNelis, 2002). Furthermore, assessments can be useful for tracking cognitive changes over time; they may also help clarify if changes are due to medications, seizures, or both. In addition, if school support is needed, assessment is a necessary precursor to determining special education (in most cases) and/or Section 504 plan eligibility.

Knowledge of strengths and weaknesses may also enable formulation of targeted classroom interventions. For example, recognition that an attention problem exists may indicate need for extended time, redirection, or one-to-one instruction. Interventions that address attention and other specific neurocognitive processes (e.g., memory, language) have been well-documented in the literature and logically could be used in cases of epilepsy. Monitoring of the intervention by collecting data is recommended in order to ensure that progress is being made.

Teacher knowledge appears to be another important factor in supporting students with epilepsy at school. Research indicates that teachers, both in general and those currently teaching a child with epilepsy, have striking epilepsy knowledge gaps (e.g., only 15% knew about attention risk, 7% knew about depressive feelings risk; Wodrich et al., 2011). Understandably, it is challenging to support a student without knowledge of associated risks. In this regard, psychoeducation for teachers may be vital.

Social–Emotional and Behavioral

In terms of social–emotional functioning, individual counseling and/or group social skills programs may be useful for children with epilepsy. Specifically, cognitive behavioral therapy has well-documented effectiveness for a variety of psychological conditions (e.g., depression, anxiety). One study looking specifically at cognitive behavioral therapy with epilepsy found that children felt more socially competent after receiving therapy (Lewis et al., 1990). Moreover, family support also appears to be beneficial. For example, programs that address family communication plus epilepsy education have been found to be effective in reducing family stress, which otherwise fuels depression and low self-esteem among children with epilepsy (Rodenburg et al., 2005).

CONCLUSION

Epilepsy is a common disease that manifests as recurrent seizures. Children with epilepsy face a variety of challenges. Neurocognitive processes, academic achievement, and social–emotional functioning appear to be especially affected. Although a dearth of formal epilepsy-specific intervention research exists, interventions and supports can logically be developed through assessment of a student's strengths and weaknesses. Interventions that include academic supports to address neurocognitive difficulties, social–emotional interventions, teacher psychoeducation, and communication between stakeholders appear to be especially important.

RESOURCES

EdMedKids. (n.d.). *A teacher's guide to instructing chronically ill students.* The University of Arizona. https://www.edmedkids.arizona.edu

Epilepsy Foundation. http://www.epilepsy.com/

Epilepsy Foundation. (2014). *What can parents do to prepare for school?* http://www.epilepsy.com/article/2014/8/what-can-parents-do-prepare-school

REFERENCES

Berg, A. T., Langfitt, J. T., Testa, F. M., Levy, S. R., DiMario, F., Westerveld, M., & Kulas, J. (2008). Global cognitive function in children with epilepsy: A community-based study. *Epilepsia, 49*(4), 608–614. https://doi.org/10.1111/j.1528-1167.2007.01461.x

Bhise, V. V., Burack, G. D., & Mandelbaum, D. E. (2010). Baseline cognition, behavior, and motor skills in children with new-onset, idiopathic epilepsy. *Developmental Medicine and Child Neurology, 52*(1), 22–26. https://doi.org/10.1111/j.1469-8749.2009.03404.x

Boshuisen, K., van Schooneveld, M. M., Uiterwaal, C. S. P. M., Cross, J. H., Harrison, S., Polster, T., Daehn, M., Djimjadi, S., Yalnizoglu, D., Turanli, G., Sassen, R., Hoppe,

C., Kuczaty, S., Barba, C., Kahane, P., Schubert-Bast, S., Reuner, G., Bast, T., Strobl, K., . . . Braun, K. P. J. (2015). Intelligence quotient improves after antiepileptic drug withdrawal following pediatric epilepsy surgery. *Annals of Neurology, 78*(1), 104–114. https://doi.org/10.1002/ana.24427

Buelow, J. M., & McNelis, A. (2002). Should every child with epilepsy undergo a neuropsychological evaluation? *Epilepsy & Behavior, 3*(3), 210–213. https://doi.org/10.1016/S1525-5050(02)00024-0

Davies, S., Heyman, I., & Goodman, R. (2003). A population survey of mental health problems in children with epilepsy. *Developmental Medicine and Child Neurology, 45*(5), 292–295. https://doi.org/10.1111/j.1469-8749.2003.tb00398.x

Ekinci, O., Titus, J. B., Rodopman, A. A., Berkem, M., & Trevathan, E. (2009). Depression and anxiety in children and adolescents with epilepsy: Prevalence, risk factors, and treatment. *Epilepsy & Behavior, 14*(1), 8–18. https://doi.org/10.1016/j.yebeh.2008.08.015

Fastenau, P. S., Shen, J., Dunn, D. W., & Austin, J. K. (2008). Academic underachievement among children with epilepsy: Proportion exceeding psychometric criteria for learning disability and associated risk factors. *Journal of Learning Disabilities, 41*(3), 195–207. https://doi.org/10.1177/0022219408317548

Fiest, K. M., Sauro, K. M., Wiebe, S., Patten, S. B., Kwon, C. S., Dykeman, J., Pringsheim, T., Lorenzetti, D. L., & Jetté, N. (2017). Prevalence and incidence of epilepsy: A systematic review and meta-analysis of international studies. *Neurology, 88*(3), 296–303. https://doi.org/10.1212/WNL.0000000000003509

Funderburk, J. A., McCormik, B. P., & Austin, J. K. (2007). Does attitude toward epilepsy mediate the relationship between perceived stigma and mental health outcomes in children with epilepsy? *Epilepsy and Behavior, 11*(1), 71–76. https://doi.org/10.1016/j.yebeh.2007.04.006

Hamiwka, L. D., Yu, C. G., Hamiwka, L. A., Sherman, E. M., Anderson, B., & Wirrell, E. (2009). Are children with epilepsy at greater risk for bullying than their peers? *Epilepsy & Behavior, 15*(4), 500–505. https://doi.org/10.1016/j.yebeh.2009.06.015

Hermann, B., Meador, K. J., Gaillard, W. D., & Cramer, J. A. (2010). Cognition across the lifespan: Antiepileptic drugs, epilepsy, or both? *Epilepsy & Behavior, 17*(1), 1–5. https://doi.org/10.1016/j.yebeh.2009.10.019

Hermann, B. P., Zhao, Q., Jackson, D. C., Jones, J. E., Dabbs, K., Almane, D., Hsu, D. A., Stafstrom, C. E., Koehn, M. A., Seidenberg, M., & Rathouz, P. J. (2016). Cognitive phenotypes in childhood idiopathic epilepsies. *Epilepsy & Behavior, 61*, 269–274. https://doi.org/10.1016/j.yebeh.2016.05.013

Lewis, M. A., Salas, I., de la Sota, A., Chiofalo, N., & Leake, B. (1990). Randomized trial of a program to enhance the competencies of children with epilepsy. *Epilepsia, 31*(1), 101–109. https://doi.org/10.1111/j.1528-1157.1990.tb05367.x

Lossius, M. I., Clench-Aas, J., van Roy, B., Mowinckel, P., & Gjerstad, L. (2006). Psychiatric symptoms in adolescents with epilepsy in junior high school in Norway: A population survey. *Epilepsy & Behavior, 9*(2), 286–292. https://doi.org/10.1016/j.yebeh.2006.06.018

Martinez, W., Carter, J. S., & Legato, L. J. (2011). Social competence in children with chronic illness: A meta-analytic review. *Journal of Pediatric Psychology, 36*(8), 878–890. https://doi.org/10.1093/jpepsy/jsr035

Reilly, C., Kent, E., & Neville, B. G. R. (2013). Review: Psychopathology in childhood epilepsy. *Child and Adolescent Mental Health, 18*(2), 65–75. https://doi.org/10.1111/j.1475-3588.2012.00648.x

Rodenburg, R., Stams, G. J., Meijer, A. M., Aldenkamp, A. P., & Deković, M. (2005). Psychopathology in children with epilepsy: A meta-analysis. *Journal of Pediatric Psychology, 30*(6), 453–468. https://doi.org/10.1093/jpepsy/jsi071

Rzezak, P., Fuentes, D., Guimarães, C. A., Thome-Souza, S., Kuczynski, E., Li, L. M., Franzon, R. C., Leite, C. C., Guerreiro, M., & Valente, K. D. (2007). Frontal lobe dysfunction in children with temporal lobe epilepsy. *Pediatric Neurology, 37*(3), 176–185. https://doi.org/10.1016/j.pediatrneurol.2007.05.009

Sarhan, E. M., Walker, M. C., & Selai, C. (2015). Evidence for efficacy of combination antiepileptic drugs in treatment of epilepsy. *Journal of Neurology Research, 5*(6), 267–276. https://doi.org/10.14740/jnr356w

Titus, J. B., & Thio, L. L. (2009). The effects of antiepileptic drugs on classroom performance. *Psychology in the Schools, 46*(9), 885–891. https://doi.org/10.1002/pits.20428

Walker, N. M., Jackson, D. C., Dabbs, K., Jones, J. E., Hsu, D. A., Stafstrom, C. E., Sheth, R. D., Koehn, M. A., Seidenberg, M., & Hermann, B. P. (2013). Is lower IQ in children with epilepsy due to lower parental IQ? A controlled comparison study. *Developmental Medicine and Child Neurology, 55*(3), 278–282. https://doi.org/10.1111/dmcn.12040

Williams, J. (2004). Seizure disorders. In R. T. Brown (Ed.), *Handbook of pediatric psychology in school settings* (pp. 221–239). Erlbaum.

Wodrich, D. L., Jarrar, R., Buchhalter, J., Levy, R., & Gay, C. (2011). Knowledge about epilepsy and confidence in instructing students with epilepsy: Teachers' responses to a new scale. *Epilepsy & Behavior, 20*(2), 360–365. https://doi.org/10.1016/j.yebeh.2010.12.002

Wodrich, D. L., Kaplan, A. M., & Deering, W. M. (2006). Children with epilepsy in school: Special service usage and assessment practices. *Psychology in the Schools, 43*(2), 169–181. https://doi.org/10.1002/pits.20123

20

Hereditary Ataxia

Taylor-Kristen Myers

Hereditary ataxia is a cluster of degenerative genetic disorders that adversely impact the nervous system due to deterioration of the cerebellum (Bird, 2018). The cerebellum is vital for all regulation of movement. Ataxias involve genetic disruptions of neurological networking systems that primarily connect the cerebellum, basal ganglia, and cerebral cortex structures of the brain (Bostan et al., 2013). Genetic disruptions of these brain structures can variably affect the physical, emotional, and cognitive abilities of an individual.

ETIOLOGY

Ataxia typically refers to impaired balance or coordination within the human body. Hereditary ataxias may be inherited through a variety of modes, including autosomal recessive cerebellar ataxia (ARCA), autosomal dominant cerebellar ataxia (ADCA), X-linked ataxia (fragile X syndrome), and mitochondrial ataxia (Friedreich's ataxia; Pavone et al., 2017). ARCAs are the most frequent type of hereditary ataxias found among children, where onset occurs prior to the age of 20 years old. They are divided into three classes distinguished by age of onset and etiology (Fogel, 2012). Prevalent and well-known ARCAs include the following:

- Class II: Early-onset ataxias, namely, ataxia telangiectasia (A-T), which is characterized by an onset before age 5 and symptoms affecting both sensory and motor circuits of the cerebellum (Fogel, 2012)

https://doi.org/10.1037/0000349-020
Health-Related Disorders in Children and Adolescents: A Guidebook for Educators and Service Providers, Second Edition, M. M. Perfect, C. A. Riccio, and M. A. Bray (Editors)

- Class III: Adolescent-onset ataxias, with the most prevalent being autosomal recessive ataxia with oculomotor apraxia Type 2 with onset in early to mid-adolescence

ADCAs are rarer and distinguished as spinocerebellar ataxias (SCAs) with typical onset in adulthood. However, some subtypes do present in childhood (see Table 20.1). With such variation among SCAs, there are several proposed etiologies that entail abnormal expression of genetic sequencing (Fogel, 2012).

PREVALENCE AND INCIDENCE

Based on systematic review, overall prevalence of individual ataxias ranges between 0.1 and 10 occurrences in 100,000 persons. Estimates across summed hereditary ataxias in Europe reach prevalence levels as high as 14 in 100,000 (Musselman et al., 2014). Incidence of ARCAs is approximated at four cases in 100,000 persons worldwide and has a prevalence of one in 40,000 to one in 100,000. Prevalence of all types of ADCA is estimated at one in 37,000 worldwide, whereas the overall prevalence of SCAs is one in 33,000 to one in 50,000 (Ruano et al., 2014).

TABLE 20.1. Most Common Autosomal Dominant Ataxias in Children: Onset, Causation, and Presentation

Type	Onset	Causation	Presentation
Dentatorubral pallido-luysian atrophy	Onset ranging from 8 to 60 years old	*ATN1* gene mutation	Chorea, seizures, dementia, myoclonus; often confused with Huntington disease
Spinocerebellar ataxia type 2	Onset ranging from 10 to 60 years old	*ATXN2* gene mutation	Slow saccadic eye movements, peripheral neuropathy, decreased deep tendon reflexes, dementia
Spinocerebellar ataxia type 7	Onset ranging from 6 months to 60 years old	*ATXN7* gene mutation	Visual loss with retinopathy
Spinocerebellar ataxia type 18	Onset ranging from 12 to 25 years old	Responsible gene unidentified	Ataxia with early sensory/motor neuropathy, nystagmus, dysarthria, decreased tendon reflexes, muscle weakness, atrophy, fasciculations, Babinski responses
Spinocerebellar ataxia type 21	Onset ranging from 6 to 30 years old	Responsible gene unidentified	Mild cognitive impairment, tremors, bradykinesia, rigidity
Spinocerebellar ataxia type 28	Onset ranging from 12 to 36 years old	*AFG3L2* gene mutation	Nystagmus, ophthalmoparesis, ptosis, increased tendon reflexes; found in two Italian families
Spinocerebellar ataxia type 29	Onset in early childhood	*ITPR1* gene mutation	Learning deficits, delayed speech, dysarthria, dysmetria

SYMPTOMS

Hereditary ataxia is characterized by slow, progressively impaired functioning of coordinated movement, speech, and balance. Due to improper coordination of the front and back regions of the cerebellum, tasks that demand motor skills and planning are highly affected (Olivito et al., 2018). Additionally, symptoms can extend to include spastic posturing of extremities, eye muscle impairments that limit range of motion, neuropathy (weakness, numbness, and/or pain in the hands and feet), and varying degrees of cognitive and behavioral functioning (Jayadev & Bird, 2013). A-T complications can manifest in other health-related symptoms, including telangiectasia of the conjunctivae (dilated blood vessels next to the mucous membrane covering the surface of the eye and inner surface of the eyelids); hypotonia (low muscle tone); frequent infections from depressed immune system; and an increased risk for leukemia, lymphoma, and breast cancer (Jayadev & Bird, 2013). ADCA SCAs are characterized by uncoordinated gait, movements, and imbalance, as well as impaired neurological processes, including head waddling, other limb movement abnormalities, tremors, seizures, nystagmus (shaky eyes), dysarthria (slowed/slurred speech), and intellectual disability (Pavone et al., 2017).

IMPACT ON THE STUDENT AND OUTCOMES

Medical

Health and medical implications for children with hereditary ataxia are important to note, as there can be high comorbidity of disease due to the extensive and integrative impact of neurological processing within the human body. Autoimmune neurological disorders, lung disease, cancer, and visual impairment are among some of the correlated medical conditions associated with hereditary ataxia. Opsoclonus-myoclonus syndrome, a rare autoimmune neurological disorder, may co-occur with hereditary ataxia. The disorder is characterized by inexplicable staggering and falling, drooling, speech issues, low muscle tone, opsoclonus (rapid, multidirectional eye movement), myoclonus (body jerks), and inability to sleep (Tate et al., 2005). Lung disease has also been found to occur commonly among patients with A-T. Symptoms of lung disease include persistent cough, trouble breathing, recurrent respiratory infections, chest pain, and bodily fatigue. Thus, complications of the respiratory system have been found to be a main contributor of death among those diagnosed with A-T (McGrath-Morrow et al., 2010). Furthermore, just like individuals with two copies of the mutated *ATM* gene associated with A-T, single carriers exhibit increased risks of developing cancer, particularly breast cancer even among adolescent girls (Swift et al., 1987). Additionally, retinal abnormalities in the form of light sensitivity and up to partial or full vision loss are possible for children with hereditary ataxia (Gouw et al., 1994).

Cognitive/Academic

For students diagnosed with hereditary ataxias, it is crucial to consider the cognitive impairments they may face. Academic performance can be severely affected by both the severity of ataxia and the localization of cerebellar deterioration present within the brain (Olivito et al., 2018; Schmahmann, 2019). Specifically, young children may have difficulty initiating language, weakened verbal fluency, and decreased word and story retrieval, as well as impaired abilities in sequencing, planning, and maintaining verbal sets (Schmahmann, 2004). As the cognitive demands of coursework progress, academic tasks that rely heavily on various types of recall, including both immediate and delayed; verbal memory; or logical and orientation-based thinking may become extremely difficult for the student affected by hereditary ataxia (Ma et al., 2014).

Social-Emotional and Behavioral

Behavioral adaptive functionality and activities of daily life can be severely affected by hereditary ataxia. Impaired motor skills, adaptation, and motor sequence learning can negatively affect how students plan, coordinate, and execute their behavioral tasks. Hereditary ataxia effects on social and emotional components are far-reaching. Impairments are seen in areas of social cognition, emotional attribution, and emotional regulation. Research into the social/emotional functioning of students with hereditary ataxia from a neurological framework has assisted in explaining the underlying causation of impaired regulation of emotion seen in some children (Hoche et al., 2016). Cortical impairment to specific areas of the cerebellum can have a myriad of attached complications, including increased irritability, impulsive actions, decreased inhibitions, lability of affect (intense, cyclical bouts of inconsolable crying to uncontrollable fits of laughter), and poor attentional and behavioral modulation (Schmahmann, 2004). Damage in other regions of the cerebellum can produce symptoms of regressive personality changes, apathy, and withdrawal (Schmahmann, 2004). Social and emotional impairments of students with hereditary ataxia can be mistaken for autism spectrum or psychosis spectrum disorders (Schmahmann, 2004).

PSYCHOEDUCATIONAL IMPLICATIONS AND SCHOOL-BASED INTERVENTIONS

Medical and Health Management

For all types and classes of hereditary ataxias, symptomatic therapies such as physical, occupational, and speech therapies are the most effective forms of treatment, as they help to counteract progressive loss of function and maintain some level of performance. As there are no specific treatments to cure hereditary ataxia, symptomatic treatment is most recommended. Schools should provide varied methods of intensive rehabilitative services (Braga Neto et al., 2016). Predominantly, physical therapy is most effective in increasing the use and maintenance of activities of daily life as well as relieving ataxic symptoms. Mobility adaptive devices and physical accommodations both in the classroom and around campus can be made to ensure students have equitable access to a free and public education within the least restrictive environment. Gait complications can be assisted by use of canes, crutches, walkers, and wheelchairs. Adaptive seating, modified playground equipment, and accessible entryways can be useful as well (Bird, 2018; Jayadev & Bird, 2013). Additionally, unconventional forms of therapies, including relaxation and biofeedback, sportive exercise, virtual reality rehabilitation, and physiotherapy, have been found, depending on form, severity, and stage of ataxia, to have a limited but practical positive effect and could be implemented in a complementary manner to more traditional forms of therapy (Braga Neto et al., 2016). Occupational therapy servicing may lead to improvements in fine motor skills and help assuage depressive symptoms linked to lower levels of global functioning (Braga Neto et al., 2016). In certain cases, specialized mechanical devices may aid with tasks that include handwriting, scribing, buttoning, or utensil use (Fogel, 2012; Jayadev & Bird, 2013). As some students diagnosed with hereditary ataxia may also be taking medications that assist with impaired mobility, a qualified health professional should be staffed to monitor medication. Additionally, due to common symptoms of pain, cramps, spasticity, anxiety, and depression experienced by students, pain and psychiatric medication management at school should be considered and available, if necessary.

Cognitive/Academic

Disabilities in cognition and academic ability will vary in degree of severity. Within the classroom, accommodations and modifications should be implemented to help foster learning in a safe and unpressured environment. Use of visual/written scripts to help students tangibly sequence their class expectations and schedule, shortened or extended time for assignments, and explorative and interactive play can expand students' cognitive ability while maintaining varied levels of support (Ganz, 2007). Speech therapy should be provided when the student has difficulties in communication, swallowing, or feeding capability. Additionally, exploration of alternate modes of communication, such as sign language, computer devices, and augmentative and alternative communication (AAC) devices, can be beneficial depending on the severity of dysarthria the student presents with. AAC devices can be aided or unaided, with the latter only requiring the students' body to generate the communication (e.g., gestures, finger spelling) and the former needing transmission such as computer-generated speech devices (Beukelman & Mirenda, 2013).

Social-Emotional and Behavioral

Facilitated, intentional interactions that build interpersonal skills and give students with hereditary ataxia the opportunity to explore and engage with their environment are important. Behavioral and social interventions should be tailored to reduce both noncompliant behaviors and those that interfere with establishing and maintaining positive relationships while simultaneously increasing the likelihood of alternative functional behaviors. Inclusive environments, usage of applied behavior analysis techniques, and psychosocial skills trainings can be useful. Within the classroom, noise and other stimulation should be reduced as much as possible. Task analysis procedures and behavioral systems that incorporate redirection, reteaching, and positive reinforcement should also be used (Aggarwal et al., 2013). Additionally, psychological counseling and therapeutic-based interventions, such as parent management training and cognitive behavior therapy, are useful to assist with mood stabilization and decreasing some forms of anger, depression, irritability, and aggressive behaviors (Sukhodolsky et al., 2016). Stakeholders should be aware of and sensitive to the fact that affected mood can also cause decline in cognitive and motor functioning, potentially compounding symptomatic effects of those with hereditary ataxia (Marvel & Paradiso, 2004).

CONCLUSION

The psychoeducational impact of students living with hereditary ataxia presents a dire need to implement effective accommodations that ensure quality instruction, best fitted for their unique needs. Hereditary ataxia is categorized as both chronic and progressive; thus, generalizable prognosis is unclear. However, occupational, physical, and speech therapeutic interventions are effective for managing symptoms (Fogel, 2012). A multifaceted, student-centered team should integrate efforts of family, school, and health professionals to coordinate rehabilitative services in conjunction with academic, social/behavioral, and medical supports in order to best serve these students.

RESOURCES

American Society for Experimental Neurotherapeutics. 230 Kings Highway East, Suite 245, Haddonfield, NJ 08033; 833-273-6800. https://www.asent.org/

Ataxia Telangiectasia Children's Project. 5300 W. Hillsboro Boulevard, Suite 105, Coconut Creek, FL 33073; 800-543-5728. https://www.atcp.org/

National Ataxia Foundation. 2600 Fernbrook Lane, Suite 119, Minneapolis, MN 55447; 763-553-0020. http://www.ataxia.org

National Organization for Rare Diseases. 55 Kenosia Avenue, Danbury, CT 06810; 203-744-0100. https://rarediseases.org/

SCASource. https://scasource.net/

REFERENCES

Aggarwal, R., Guanci, N., & Appareddy, V. (2013). Issues in treating patients with intellectual disabilities. *Psychiatric Times Special Reports: Cultural Psychiatry, 30*(8). https://www.psychiatrictimes.com/view/issues-treating-patients-intellectual-disabilities

Beukelman, D. R., & Mirenda, P. (2013). *Augmentative & alternative communication: Supporting children and adults with complex communication needs* (4th ed.). Paul H. Brookes Publishing.

Bird, T. D. (2018). Hereditary ataxia overview. In M. P. Adam, G. M. Mirzaa, R. A. Pagon, S. E. Wallace, L. J. H. Bean, K. W. Gripp, & A. Amemiya (Eds.), *GeneReviews*. University of Washington.

Bostan, A. C., Dum, R. P., & Strick, P. L. (2013). Cerebellar networks with the cerebral cortex and basal ganglia. *Trends in Cognitive Sciences, 17*(5), 241–254. https://doi.org/10.1016/j.tics.2013.03.003

Braga Neto, P., Pedroso, J. L., Kuo, S. H., Marcondes, C. F., Jr., Teive, H. A., & Barsottini, O. G. (2016). Current concepts in the treatment of hereditary ataxias. *Arquivos de Neuro-Psiquiatria, 74*(3), 244–252. https://doi.org/10.1590/0004-282X20160038

Fogel, B. L. (2012). Childhood cerebellar ataxia. *Journal of Child Neurology, 27*(9), 1138–1145. https://doi.org/10.1177/0883073812448231

Ganz, J. B. (2007). Using visual script interventions to address communication skills. *Teaching Exceptional Children, 40*(2), 54–58. https://doi.org/10.1177/004005990704000207

Gouw, L. G., Digre, K. B., Harris, C. P., Haines, J. H., & Ptacek, L. J. (1994). Autosomal dominant cerebellar ataxia with retinal degeneration: Clinical, neuropathologic, and genetic analysis of a large kindred. *Neurology, 44*(8), 1441–1447. https://doi.org/10.1212/WNL.44.8.1441

Hoche, F., Guell, X., Sherman, J. C., Vangel, M. G., & Schmahmann, J. D. (2016). Cerebellar contribution to social cognition. *Cerebellum, 15*(6), 732–743. https://doi.org/10.1007/s12311-015-0746-9

Jayadev, S., & Bird, T. D. (2013). Hereditary ataxias: Overview. *Genetics in Medicine, 15*(9), 673–683. https://doi.org/10.1038/gim.2013.28

Ma, J., Wu, C., Lei, J., & Zhang, X. (2014). Cognitive impairments in patients with spinocerebellar ataxia types 1, 2 and 3 are positively correlated to the clinical severity of ataxia symptoms. *International Journal of Clinical and Experimental Medicine, 7*(12), 5765–5771. https://www.ncbi.nlm.nih.gov/pmc/articles/PMC4307551/

Marvel, C. L., & Paradiso, S. (2004). Cognitive and neurological impairment in mood disorders. *Psychiatric Clinics of North America, 27*(1), 19–36. https://doi.org/10.1016/S0193-953X(03)00106-0

McGrath-Morrow, S. A., Gower, W. A., Rothblum-Oviatt, C., Brody, A. S., Langston, C., Fan, L. L., Lefton-Greif, M. A., Crawford, T. O., Troche, M., Sandlund, J. T., Auwaerter, P. G., Easley, B., Loughlin, G. M., Carroll, J. L., & Lederman, H. M. (2010). Evaluation and management of pulmonary disease in ataxia-telangiectasia. *Pediatric Pulmonology, 45*(9), 847–859. https://doi.org/10.1002/ppul.21277

Musselman, K. E., Stoyanov, C. T., Marasigan, R., Jenkins, M. E., Konczak, J., Morton, S. M., & Bastian, A. J. (2014). Prevalence of ataxia in children: A systematic review. *Neurology, 82*(1), 80–89. https://doi.org/10.1212/01.wnl.0000438224.25600.6c

Olivito, G., Lupo, M., Iacobacci, C., Clausi, S., Romano, S., Masciullo, M., Molinari, M., Cercignani, M., Bozzali, M., & Leggio, M. (2018). Structural cerebellar correlates of cognitive functions in spinocerebellar ataxia type 2. *Journal of Neurology, 265*(3), 597–606. https://doi.org/10.1007/s00415-018-8738-6

Pavone, P., Praticò, A. D., Pavone, V., Lubrano, R., Falsaperla, R., Rizzo, R., & Ruggieri, M. (2017). Ataxia in children: Early recognition and clinical evaluation. *Italian Journal of Pediatrics, 43*(1), Article 6. https://doi.org/10.1186/s13052-016-0325-9

Ruano, L., Melo, C., Silva, M. C., & Coutinho, P. (2014). The global epidemiology of hereditary ataxia and spastic paraplegia: A systematic review of prevalence studies. *Neuroepidemiology, 42*(3), 174–183. https://doi.org/10.1159/000358801

Schmahmann, J. D. (2004). Disorders of the cerebellum: Ataxia, dysmetria of thought, and the cerebellar cognitive affective syndrome. *The Journal of Neuropsychiatry and Clinical Neurosciences, 16*(3), 367–378. https://doi.org/10.1176/jnp.16.3.367

Schmahmann, J. D. (2019). The cerebellum and cognition. *Neuroscience Letters, 688*, 62–75. https://doi.org/10.1016/j.neulet.2018.07.005

Sukhodolsky, D. G., Smith, S. D., McCauley, S. A., Ibrahim, K., & Piasecka, J. B. (2016). Behavioral interventions for anger, irritability, and aggression in children and adolescents. *Journal of Child and Adolescent Psychopharmacology, 26*(1), 58–64. https://doi.org/10.1089/cap.2015.0120

Swift, M., Reitnauer, P. J., Morrell, D., & Chase, C. L. (1987). Breast and other cancers in families with ataxia-telangiectasia. *The New England Journal of Medicine, 316*(21), 1289–1294. https://doi.org/10.1056/NEJM198705213162101

Tate, E. D., Allison, T. J., Pranzate, M. R., & Verhu, S. J. (2005). Neuroepidemiologic trends in 105 U.S. cases of pediatric opsoclonus-myoclonus syndrome. *Journal of Pediatric Oncology Nursing, 22*(1), 8–19. https://doi.org/10.1177/1043454204272560

21

Mitochondrial Disorders

Cynthia K. Lang, Alyssa A. Gonzalez, and Cynthia A. Riccio

Mitochondria are a type of organelle, or organized structure, within living cells responsible for processing oxygen and converting food into energy. Mitochondria are responsible for the production of the body's required energy, adenosine triphosphate, through the process of oxidative phosphorylation (Thornton et al., 2014). *Mitochondrial disorders* or myopathies are chronic and progressive inherited diseases that affect the mitochondria's ability to produce the required amount of energy for proper bodily functioning. In individuals with mitochondrial disorders, the process of oxidative phosphorylation has been disrupted.

ETIOLOGY

Primary mitochondrial disorders are inherited when one or both genes responsible for mitochondrial function have mutated, evidenced by failure of mitochondrial DNA. The mitochondria contain their own DNA, and mutations at this level are solely inherited from the mother in mitochondrial inheritance (Saneto & Sedensky, 2013). In contrast to primary genetic mitochondrial disorder, secondary mitochondrial disorder occurs as a result of other disorders, such as cancer and diabetes. Over time, expression of genes associated with mitochondrial disorders declines consistently with typical aging (Bishop et al., 2010).

https://doi.org/10.1037/0000349-021
Health-Related Disorders in Children and Adolescents: A Guidebook for Educators and Service Providers, Second Edition, M. M. Perfect, C. A. Riccio, and M. A. Bray (Editors)

PREVALENCE

Mitochondrial disorders affect about one in 5,000 individuals and can manifest at any age, with newborns as well as adults exhibiting symptoms of the disease (Schaefer et al., 2004). The disorder can affect many organs and cells, including the heart, brain, and skeletal muscles (Smeitink et al., 2006), and can result in epilepsy, visual impairment, behavioral difficulties, cognitive impairments, movement disorders, and episodic encephalopathy (Finsterer, 2006).

SYMPTOMS

Mitochondrial disorders share similar symptoms with many common disorders and are often misdiagnosed. Symptoms of the disease include vision and/or hearing problems; muscle weakness; low muscle tone; heart, kidney, brain, and liver diseases; gastrointestinal disorders; diabetes; movement disorders; dementia; lactic acidosis; and respiratory problems (Thornton et al., 2014). Misdiagnoses include somatoform disorder, psychiatric disorders, multiple sclerosis, chronic fatigue, and fibromyalgia. It can take many years to reach a diagnosis of a mitochondrial disorder based on symptom presentation.

There are different forms of mitochondrial disorders, including myopathic and systemic encephalomyopathic forms. Myopathic forms affect skeletal muscle only, whereas encephalomyopathic forms affect a wide range of organs, such as the nervous system, heart, kidney, and liver. Mitochondrial diseases, particularly the encephalomyopathic forms, are an important cause of short stature and reduction of body mass index in children and adolescents (Castro-Gago et al., 2011). Some syndromes considered mitochondrial disorders include Barth syndrome, chronic progressive external ophthalmoplegia, Kearns–Sayre syndrome, and Pearson syndrome (National Institute of Neurological Disorders and Stroke, 2018).

IMPACT ON THE STUDENT AND OUTCOMES

Medical

Individuals with mitochondrial disorders typically present with a wide range of symptoms, and children affected by these diseases usually require individualized care that often involves the management of more than one condition (Sofou, 2013). The complexity of pediatric mitochondrial diseases and the impact on the child's body are some of the main challenges for both the child and primary caregivers of children affected. There are many moving pieces to medically caring for a child with these conditions, as the average child with a mitochondrial disorder has six organs affected and visits seven specialist doctors for the purposes of medical management. Additionally, a survey found that about 50% of children in this disease group were hospitalized within the previous year (Senger et al., 2016).

Cognitive/Academic

Children with mitochondrial disorders often display significant delays in cognition and psychomotor areas (Eom & Lee, 2017). Results have shown that children with mitochondrial disorders with seizures and an early onset of the disease display poorer cognitive functioning compared with those with mitochondrial disorders without seizures. Mild levels of verbal intellectual impairment on verbal measures and performance have been found in this population. Students may evidence learning disabilities, language impairment, and difficulties with attention and concentration (Schreiber, 2012). Further, students may experience difficulties with executive functioning. They may have difficulty beginning tasks; shifting from one task to another; controlling their emotions; planning and organizing; and taking in information, holding it in immediate awareness, and manipulating the information (Schreiber, 2012).

Social-Emotional and Behavioral

There is a high comorbidity of mitochondrial disease and depressive symptoms, which are believed to be directly associated with the disorder rather than a reaction to the poor physical condition that mitochondrial disease patients are often in (Yu et al., 2005). Major depression may be the first indicator of mitochondrial disease in the adult population (Fattal et al., 2007). The interaction between contextual and genetic characteristics of children with a mitochondrial disease can lead to severe levels of depressive symptoms in this population (Koene et al., 2009).

There is a strong link between mitochondrial disorders and autism spectrum disorder (Haas, 2010). For example, 5% of the autism spectrum population experience mitochondrial disorder in contrast to only 0.01% of the general population (Rossignol & Frye, 2012). Individuals with comorbid autism spectrum disorder and mitochondrial disorder may experience more severe difficulties; however, this is not always the case, as overall impairment depends on the severity of each disorder. Behavioral difficulties expressed by individuals with comorbid autism spectrum disorder include difficulties with social skills and understanding others' perspectives, as well as stereotypical repetitive behaviors (e.g., flapping arms, rocking, pacing) that may further impede their socialization (Haas, 2010).

Other behavioral problems are often associated with psychomotor, cognitive, or language impairment. These may include difficulties with communication, deficits in self-regulation, withdrawal, deficits in attentional control, and feeding and elimination disorders (Feldman et al., 2000) resulting in high levels of parental stress (Sofou, 2013), as well as difficulty with management in the school setting.

PSYCHOEDUCATIONAL IMPLICATIONS AND SCHOOL-BASED INTERVENTIONS

Schools need to be prepared to provide supports to address the myriad physical/medical issues as well as cognitive, academic, social–emotional, and behavioral concerns. Without intervention, these difficulties may prevent individuals with mitochondrial disorders from reaching their potential and limit future success and educational attainment. Provision of services either through a 504 plan or, if more severely affected, in special education, may be appropriate.

Medical and Health Management

Pediatric mitochondrial diseases can produce a wide range of deficits and difficulties that are present or develop over time as the disease progresses. Traditional medical approaches are the standard of care; however, alternative therapies may prove beneficial for this population (Millhouse-Flourie, 2004). These may include physical, occupational, respiratory, speech, equine, and pet therapy in order to improve psychoeducational functioning outcomes.

Health impairments often include physical limitations for the child; physical therapy can assist the child's functioning in this realm through the teaching of new skills to compensate for diminished functioning in certain areas. Specific physical therapy interventions might include thermotherapy, such as heating packs or shortwave diathermy, and cryotherapy, such as ice, gel packs, or utilization of a cold whirlpool (Majkowski & Gill, 2008).

Additionally, occupational therapy can be provided to the child to support problem-solving, perceptual, and abstract-reasoning skills. Specific interventions can include facilitating the development of appropriate sensory integration and motor planning skills and structuring or modifying the student's environment to support sensory, motor, motor planning, and self-regulatory capacities and needs (Smith Roley et al., 2015).

Adaptive resources to help the child with difficult everyday tasks such as eating or dressing also can be provided. Further, when mitochondrial dysfunction interrupts higher cortical function, language disorders may result. In such cases, speech therapy can be an additional support provided to the child to improve functioning (Millhouse-Flourie, 2004). These supports often can be provided in a nonmedical setting (e.g., home, school), which will impose less stress on the child.

Cognitive/Academic

As noted, children and adults with mitochondrial disease often exhibit cognitive deficits, academic deficits, or both. These can include deficits in metacognition, components of executive functioning, and impairments in grades if cognitive and executive functioning deficits reduce one's ability to attend to and engage with the learning material. School-based interventions for executive functioning have been found to be effective in improving cognitive and academic functioning (e.g., Otero et al., 2014). Specific to academic skills, self-regulated strategy development is an overarching approach to improve academic outcomes (e.g., Limpo & Alves, 2014). Similarly, cognitive rehabilitation therapy has been found to be effective in addressing inattention, working memory, and executive function with other populations (e.g., Shaw, 2016) and could be helpful for children with mitochondrial disorders as well.

To address global academic concerns and take into consideration physical limitations, accommodations may include extra time on tests or assignments, oral administration of tests, preferential seating, speech-to-print technology, and a notetaker, which can be incorporated not only in the K–12 setting but in the higher education setting as well (Hart et al., 2010). Additionally, modifications and accommodations can include shortening assignments as well as receiving one-to-one or small-group instruction to promote growth in academic areas.

Social–Emotional and Behavioral

For social–emotional and behavioral concerns, interventions to address depression and anxiety, as well as self-regulation, aggression, and social skills, may be appropriate. As with improving academic functioning, school-based programs that address executive functioning have been found to have positive effects (e.g., Frank et al., 2021). Programs specifically addressing depressive symptoms may be most effective with children with mitochondrial disorders. These include school-based mindfulness programs specific to depression (e.g., Van der Gucht et al., 2017) as well as more general school-based mindfulness programs addressing cognitive and social–emotional development (e.g., McKeering & Hwang, 2019; Schonert-Reichl et al., 2015).

Evidence-based programs should be selected based on the targeted behavior, the goal, the child's level of functioning, and the ability of the parent or teacher to implement same. The 504 plan or individualized education program will need to include a behavioral intervention plan if typical classroom management strategies are not successful. For emotional supports or social skills intervention, related services personnel (i.e., school psychologists) may be involved in meeting the needs of the child with mitochondrial disease.

Physical, cognitive, and psychosocial factors affect not only the child but the parents as well; therefore, supports are needed to help parents manage their children's and their own mental health. The rare and severe nature of mitochondrial diseases, along with their unpredictability, presents unique challenges for parents of children affected (Senger et al., 2016). Further, there is a relationship between a child's health and the psychological functioning of the child's parents within a family unit (Williams et al., 2002). Thus, the role of caregivers is crucial and needs to be part of the conceptualization when considering the impact of the disease not only on the child but also on the family unit.

CONCLUSION

Early intervention, including developing an intervention or treatment plan that involves the child's medical doctor, parents, and appropriate school personnel to carry out such an intervention, would serve to best support the child's needs across settings. Accommodations in the school, home, and medical setting will need to be individualized, as this disease and its symptomatology present differently across individuals. Further, services and supports should be extended to the family members or caregivers, as well as the child with pediatric mitochondrial disease. With mitochondrial disorders, as with any progressive disorder, it is important for there to be frequent monitoring and adjustments made to the plan.

RESOURCES

Cincinnati Children's Hospital. (n.d.). *Human genetics*. https://www.cincinnatichildrens.org/research/divisions/h/genetics

mitoACTION. http://www.mitoaction.org/mito-faq

National Institute of Neurological Disorders and Stroke. (2018). *Mitochondrial myopathy fact sheet*. National Institutes of Health. https://www.ninds.nih.gov/Disorders/Patient-Caregiver-Education/Fact-Sheets/Mitochondrial-Myopathy-Fact-Sheet

REFERENCES

Bishop, N. A., Lu, T., & Yankner, B. A. (2010). Neural mechanisms of ageing and cognitive decline. *Nature, 464*(7288), 529–535. https://doi.org/10.1038/nature08983

Castro-Gago, M., Gómez-Lado, C., Pérez-Gay, L., Eirís-Puñal, J., & Novo-Rodríguez, M. (2011). Growth in children and adolescents with mitochondrial diseases. *Journal of Pediatric Neurology, 9*(4), 435–439.

Eom, S., & Lee, Y. M. (2017). Preliminary study of neurodevelopmental outcomes and parenting stress in pediatric mitochondrial disease. *Pediatric Neurology, 71*, 43–49.e1. https://doi.org/10.1016/j.pediatrneurol.2017.01.019

Fattal, O., Link, J., Quinn, K., Cohen, B. H., & Franco, K. (2007). Psychiatric comorbidity in 36 adults with mitochondrial cytopathies. *CNS Spectrums, 12*(6), 429–438. https://doi.org/10.1017/S1092852900015303

Feldman, M. A., Hancock, C. L., Rielly, N., Minnes, P., & Cairns, C. (2000). Behavior problems in young children with or at risk for developmental delay. *Journal of Child and Family Studies, 9*(2), 247–261. https://doi.org/10.1023/A:1009427306953

Finsterer, J. (2006). Central nervous system manifestations of mitochondrial disorders. *Acta Neurologica Scandinavica, 114*(4), 217–238. https://doi.org/10.1111/j.1600-0404.2006.00671.x

Frank, J. L., Broderick, P. C., Oh, Y., Mitra, J., Kohler, K., Schussler, D. L., Geier, C., Roeser, R. W., Berrena, E., Mahfouz, J., Levitan, J., & Greenberg, M. T. (2021). The effectiveness of a teacher-delivered mindfulness-based curriculum on adolescent social–emotional and executive functioning. *Mindfulness, 12*(5), 1234–1251. https://doi.org/10.1007/s12671-021-01594-9

Haas, R. H. (2010). Autism and mitochondrial disease. *Developmental Disabilities Research Reviews, 16*(2), 144–153. https://doi.org/10.1002/ddrr.112

Hart, D., Grigal, M., & Weir, C. (2010). Expanding the paradigm: Postsecondary education options for individuals with autism spectrum disorder and intellectual disabilities. *Focus on Autism and Other Developmental Disabilities, 25*(3), 134–150. https://doi.org/10.1177/1088357610373759

Koene, S., Kozicz, T. L., Rodenburg, R. J. T., Verhaak, C. M., de Vries, M. C., Wortmann, S., van de Heuvel, L., Smeitink, J. A., & Morava, E. (2009). Major depression in adolescent children consecutively diagnosed with mitochondrial disorder. *Journal of Affective Disorders, 114*(1–3), 327–332. https://doi.org/10.1016/j.jad.2008.06.023

Limpo, T., & Alves, R. A. (2014). Implicit theories of writing and their impact on students' response to a SRSD intervention. *The British Journal of Educational Psychology, 84*(4), 571–590. https://doi.org/10.1111/bjep.12042

Majkowski, G. R., & Gill, N. W. (2008). Physical therapy modalities. In P. H. Seidenberg & A. Beutler (Eds.), *The sports medicine resource manual* (pp. 453–464). Elsevier.

McKeering, P., & Hwang, Y.-S. (2019). A systematic review of mindfulness-based school interventions with early adolescents. *Mindfulness, 10*(4), 593–610. https://doi.org/10.1007/s12671-018-0998-9

Millhouse-Flourie, T. J. (2004). Physical, occupational, respiratory, speech, equine and pet therapies for mitochondrial disease. *Mitochondrion, 4*(5–6), 549–558. https://doi.org/10.1016/j.mito.2004.07.013

National Institute of Neurological Disorders and Stroke. (2018). *Mitochondrial myopathy fact sheet*. National Institutes of Health. https://www.ninds.nih.gov/Disorders/Patient-Caregiver-Education/Fact-Sheets/Mitochondrial-Myopathy-Fact-Sheet

Otero, T. M., Barker, L. A., & Naglieri, J. A. (2014). Executive function treatment and intervention in schools. *Applied Neuropsychology: Child, 3*(3), 205–214. https://doi.org/10.1080/21622965.2014.897903

Rossignol, D. A., & Frye, R. E. (2012). Mitochondrial dysfunction in autism spectrum disorders: A systematic review and meta-analysis. *Molecular Psychiatry, 17*(3), 290–314. https://doi.org/10.1038/mp.2010.136

Saneto, R. P., & Sedensky, M. M. (2013). Mitochondrial disease in childhood: mtDNA encoded. *Neurotherapeutics, 10*(2), 199–211. https://doi.org/10.1007/s13311-012-0167-0

Schaefer, A. M., Taylor, R. W., Turnbull, D. M., & Chinnery, P. F. (2004). The epidemiology of mitochondrial disorders—Past, present and future. *Biochimica et Biophysica Acta, 1659*(2–3), 115–120. https://doi.org/10.1016/j.bbabio.2004.09.005

Schonert-Reichl, K. A., Oberle, E., Lawlor, M. S., Abbott, D., Thomson, K., Oberlander, T. F., & Diamond, A. (2015). Enhancing cognitive and social–emotional development through a simple-to-administer mindfulness-based school program for elementary school children: A randomized controlled trial. *Developmental Psychology, 51*(1), 52–66. https://doi.org/10.1037/a0038454

Schreiber, H. (2012). Pilot study on executive function and adaptive skills in adolescents and young adults with mitochondrial disease. *Journal of Child Neurology, 27*(12), 1506–1516. https://doi.org/10.1177/0883073812442589

Senger, B. A., Ward, L. D., Barbosa-Leiker, C., & Bindler, R. C. (2016). Stress and coping of parents caring for a child with mitochondrial disease. *Applied Nursing Research, 29*, 195–201. https://doi.org/10.1016/j.apnr.2015.03.010

Shaw, D. R. (2016). A systematic review of pediatric cognitive rehabilitation in the elementary and middle school systems. *NeuroRehabilitation, 39*(1), 119–123. https://doi.org/10.3233/NRE-161343

Smeitink, J. A., Zeviani, M., Turnbull, D. M., & Jacobs, H. T. (2006). Mitochondrial medicine: A metabolic perspective on the pathology of oxidative phosphorylation disorders. *Cell Metabolism, 3*(1), 9–13. https://doi.org/10.1016/j.cmet.2005.12.001

Smith Roley, S., Bissell, J., & Frolek Clark, G. (2015). Occupational therapy for children and youth using sensory integration theory and methods in school-based practice.

The American Journal of Occupational Therapy, 69(Suppl. 3), 1–20. https://doi.org/10.5014/ajot.2015.696S04

Sofou, K. (2013). Mitochondrial disease: A challenge for the caregiver, the family, and society. *Journal of Child Neurology, 28*(5), 663–667. https://doi.org/10.1177/0883073813481622

Thornton, B., Cohen, B., Copeland, W., & Maria, B. L. (2014). Mitochondrial disease: Clinical aspects, molecular mechanisms, translational science, and clinical frontiers. *Journal of Child Neurology, 29*(9), 1179–1207. https://doi.org/10.1177/0883073814537379

Van der Gucht, K., Takano, K., Kuppens, P., & Raes, F. (2017). Potential moderators of a school-based mindfulness program on symptoms of depression in adolescents. *Mindfulness, 8*(3), 797–806. https://doi.org/10.1007/s12671-016-0658-x

Williams, P. D., Williams, A. R., Graff, J. C., Hanson, S., Stanton, A., Hafeman, C., Liebergen, A., Leuenberg, K., Setter, R. K., Ridder, L., Curry, H., Barnard, M., & Sanders, S. (2002). Interrelationships among variables affecting well siblings and mothers in families of children with a chronic illness or disability. *Journal of Behavioral Medicine, 25*(5), 411–424. https://doi.org/10.1023/A:1020401122858

Yu, Y. W., Tsai, S. J., Hong, C. J., Chen, T. J., Chen, M. C., & Yang, C. W. (2005). Association study of a *monoamine oxidase A* gene promoter polymorphism with major depressive disorder and antidepressant response. *Neuropsychopharmacology, 30*(9), 1719–1723. https://doi.org/10.1038/sj.npp.1300785

22

Pediatric Autoimmune Neuropsychiatric Disorders Associated With Streptococcal Infections and Pediatric Acute-Onset Neuropsychiatric Syndrome

Kandace M. Hoppin and Patricia Rice Doran

In the mid-1990s, researchers at the National Institute of Mental Health (NIMH) identified a link between recent streptococcal infection and the development of neuropsychiatric symptoms such as separation anxiety, tics, behavioral regression, rage, restricted eating, and obsessive–compulsive disorder (OCD; Swedo et al., 1998).

ETIOLOGY

Research has found that in pediatric autoimmune neuropsychiatric disorders associated with streptococcal infections (PANDAS) and pediatric acute-onset neuropsychiatric syndrome (PANS), exposure to an infection or other agent that activates the immune system creates an immune response that goes awry, causing autoantibodies (or immune cells) to attack brain cells instead (Chang et al., 2015; Platt et al., 2017). The resulting inflammation causes obsessions, compulsions, hallucinations, restricted eating, motor difficulties and tics, behavioral challenges, and other symptoms. PANDAS and PANS typically have a distinct onset (Chang et al., 2015); however, if symptoms are mild at first, parents and clinicians may initially overlook the change in behavior as part of typical development (Rice Doran, 2016b).

https://doi.org/10.1037/0000349-022
Health-Related Disorders in Children and Adolescents: A Guidebook for Educators and Service Providers, Second Edition, M. M. Perfect, C. A. Riccio, and M. A. Bray (Editors)

PREVALENCE AND INCIDENCE

Clear data on incidence and prevalence for PANDAS and PANS are difficult to find, as the research on the condition is relatively new and diagnostic guidelines were only finalized in 2015 (Chang et al., 2015). Scientists at the NIMH have estimated that up to one in 200 children, or 5% to 10% of those with OCD, may have PANDAS (NIMH, n.d.; Westly, 2009), based on clinic records and empirical evidence. The inclusion of a code for PANDAS in the newest revision of the World Health Organization's (2019) *International Statistical Classification of Diseases and Related Health Problems* (*ICD-11*) will help to provide more comprehensive data on incidence and prevalence.

SYMPTOMS

Both PANDAS and PANS are characterized by the rapid onset or intensification of obsessive–compulsive symptoms, anxiety, or restricted eating, in addition to additional cognitive, behavioral, and motor symptoms. Obsessive symptoms might include obsessive thoughts related to contamination and germs, worries about food or choking, fears about harming others, and preoccupations with numbers or patterns. Compulsive symptoms may include behaviors such as frequent handwashing, excessive double-checking, repetitively touching certain things, and insistence on a certain order of events. At times, obsessions and compulsions may escalate and present as challenging behavior if students are prevented from completing a ritual or acting on a compulsion. Additional cognitive, behavioral, and motor symptoms may include motor tics (involuntary movements; e.g., blinking, shoulder shrugging, facial grimacing) and/or vocal tics (sounds uttered unintentionally; e.g., throat clearing, grunting, coughing), oppositional behavior, rage, fine motor impairments, changes in school performance, and sleep disturbances (Chang et al., 2015).

Diagnostic criteria for PANDAS are "the presence of OCD or tics; symptoms evident between age 3 and puberty; acute onset and episodic (relapsing–remitting) course; association with Group A Streptococcus; association with neurological abnormalities" (PANDAS Physicians Network [PPN], 2018, para. 2). Diagnostic criteria for PANS are

> abrupt, acute, dramatic onset of obsessive-compulsive disorder or severely restricted food intake; concurrent presence of additional neuropsychiatric symptoms with accompanying symptoms from two of the following categories: anxiety, emotional lability and/or depression, irritability, aggression, and/or severe oppositional behaviors, behavioral (developmental) regression, sudden deterioration in school performance, motor or sensory abnormalities, and somatic signs and symptoms, including sleep disturbances, enuresis, or urinary frequency. Symptoms are not better explained by a known neurologic or medical disorder. (PPN, 2018, para. 2)

Both disorders typically follow a relapsing–remitting pattern with many episodes occurring during or after infection (Chang et al., 2015; Murphy et al., 2012). Episodes during which PANDAS and PANS symptoms flare up are often referred to as flares or exacerbations (Murphy et al., 2012; Theinemann, 2016). Treatments may include antibiotic therapy to treat or prevent infection; cognitive behavior therapy; selective serotonin reuptake inhibitors; and/or immunomodulatory therapies, such as intravenous immunoglobulin, plasmapheresis, or steroids (NIMH, n.d.). As described in the following section, impact on the affected child can be significant, with symptoms disrupting many or most daily activities.

IMPACT ON THE STUDENT AND OUTCOMES

Medical

PANDAS and PANS are complex neurological disorders, and their medical impact is significant. The diagnosis process is also extensive; PANDAS and PANS are diagnoses of exclusion, and thus, a comprehensive evaluation is needed to eliminate disorders that present with similar symptoms (Chang et al., 2015). Children with PANDAS and PANS may have multifaceted medical needs, including urinary issues, irregular sleep patterns, disordered eating, motor atypicalities, vascular or cardiac issues, and immune-system irregularities (Swedo et al., 2012). These needs often require care from multiple specialists, including rheumatologists, cardiologists, neurologists, infectious disease specialists, mental health clinicians, and psychiatrists, as well as speech, occupational, and physical therapists (Theinemann, 2016). In response to the multidimensional needs that students with PANDAS and PANS often exhibit, a number of interdisciplinary centers of excellence have been established at universities around the country, including Stanford (Lucille Packard Hospital), Harvard (Massachusetts General), and University of Arizona (Steele Center). The multifaceted medical needs of students with PANDAS and PANS often have significant impact on attendance, service delivery, and academic performance in the school setting (Hoppin, 2016; Rice Doran, 2016a), as is discussed more fully in the following sections.

Cognitive/Academic

Studies have suggested cognitive and academic impact both during actively symptomatic periods (Lewin et al., 2011) and up to several years postinfection (Pawela et al., 2017). In particular, areas of impact include visuospatial processing (Lewin et al., 2011); executive functioning (Pawela et al., 2017); and fine motor skills, including writing and drawing (Chang et al., 2015). Frequent absences (due to medical issues, doctor's appointments, and school avoidance or phobia) may further complicate students' ability to complete work and meet curriculum benchmarks, necessitating additional support and accommodations.

Social-Emotional and Behavioral

PANDAS and PANS may affect the child's peer relationships and result in decreased socialization due to reduced school attendance (Rice Doran & O'Hanlon, 2015). Additionally, peers may not be aware of, or understand, the child's diagnosis or needs (Rice Doran, 2016b). Children with PANDAS/PANS may experience depression and/or emotional lability, causing exaggerated changes in their mood and expressions of intense emotions or feelings (e.g., uncontrollable laughing or crying, heightened irritability or temper), often at inappropriate times (Swedo et al., 2012). Children themselves may be frightened or confused as a result of these symptoms (Chang et al., 2015); the rapid onset of illness and resulting changes in their own behavior and emotional state may cause additional distress.

Behavioral changes in the child with PANDAS or PANS may be dramatic, and these behavioral symptoms may wax and wane in conjunction with their treatment status, stress level, and exposure to illness. When an attempt is made to alter their involuntary behavior symptoms, children may try to modify their own behavior—expending large amounts of time and energy trying to suppress obsessive–compulsive rituals, experiencing high levels of stress, anxiety, and fatigue—which comes at a great cost for the child (Hoppin, 2016). Additionally, children experiencing obsessive-compulsive symptoms may feel isolated from their peers, partly because their compulsive behavior leaves them little time to interact or socialize. They may avoid social settings as they are worried or anxious that others may notice these behaviors (Bernstein et al., 2010), and families may experience challenges participating in activities as well (Tona et al., 2017). Parents whose children have PANDAS and PANS also have reported a deterioration of community and family social participation during exacerbations, as well as decreased socialization as a family (Tona et al., 2017); these parents are at risk for emotional difficulties and frequently experience fear and isolation (McClelland et al., 2015). Families of children with PANS demonstrate greater caregiver burden than families of individuals with Alzheimer's disease (Farmer et al., 2018).

PSYCHOEDUCATIONAL IMPLICATIONS AND SCHOOL-BASED INTERVENTIONS

Medical and Health Management

Educators should be aware that PANDAS and PANS may have a significant impact on a student's attendance. Separation anxiety is a symptom of PANDAS (NIMH, n.d.), and students with PANDAS or PANS may have trouble coming to school, or attending for a full day, during exacerbations. During the process of diagnosis and initial treatment, students will likely miss school for specialist appointments, which may include visits to psychiatrists, neurologists, behavioral therapists, or immunologists. Students who undergo immune-based therapies may miss additional days or weeks of school. Further, students with PANDAS and PANS are considered immunocompromised, so they may also need to be out of school if there is danger of being exposed to illness, such as during outbreaks of strep or flu (Theinemann, 2016).

Planning for possible attendance issues should be an essential element of school discussions and should be addressed with understanding. Flexibility is needed, as attendance patterns may change throughout the school year based on the health of the student with PANDAS or PANS. Understanding on the part of school personnel and assistance teams requires taking into consideration the child's current symptoms and health needs, rather than simply prioritizing daily attendance. School personnel can also support families by maintaining communication and notifying families regarding any illnesses in the classroom/school so that they can take precautions as needed.

Cognitive/Academic

Research indicates that academic challenges for children with PANDAS and PANS commonly include visuospatial processing, math, and executive functioning (Lewin et al., 2011). Challenges related to attention, processing, and response time may cause additional academic difficulties and can result in students being misidentified or labeled as having attention-deficit/hyperactivity disorder (Rice Doran, 2015; Tona & Posner, 2011). Students with PANDAS and PANS may also experience difficulty with writing—in terms of organization and in terms of motor skills (Swedo et al., 2012; Tona et al., 2017). Parents of children with PANDAS or PANS often report abrupt deterioration in their children's handwriting (Tona & Posner, 2011).

A wide range of academic accommodations and supports may be helpful for students with PANDAS and PANS. It is crucial for school personnel to engage in ongoing communication with the family to help identify and monitor symptoms of PANDAS/PANS in the school setting and determine what academic supports are needed as well as when and how to best implement them. School personnel should work to create safe, supportive, and responsive classroom environments where expectations are clear, and flexible options are provided for assignments and activities (Hoppin, 2016). Parents of students with PANDAS/PANS have reported their children benefit from extended time for in-class assignments as well as flexible deadlines (including reduction or elimination of homework during symptomatic periods), writing accommodations (keyboard, laptop, specially designed writing tools, scribe or speech-to-text software, graphic organizers), math accommodations (calculator, manipulatives), frequent breaks, sensory supports (special seating, lighting, fidget tools), adapted or modified tasks, and advanced planning and supports during health-related absences (Candelaria Greene, 2016; Rice Doran, 2016a; Rice Doran & O'Hanlon, 2015).

Social-Emotional and Behavioral

Children with PANDAS and PANS often exhibit obsessive-compulsive symptoms (Chang et al., 2015), which may manifest in the school setting as repetitive handwashing, fixations such as repeating activities, needing to have things complete and exactly right before the next task, preoccupation with specific numbers or objects, reliance on rituals, or outbursts when a routine or compulsion is disrupted (Jenike & Boaz, 2012). Depression, agitation, feelings of shame, anxiety, and stress (due to their time-consuming rituals) can contribute to social, emotional, and behavioral difficulties for these students at school (Hoppin, 2016). Students with PANDAS and PANS might also demonstrate sensory issues, which can at times be confused with compulsions, such as the need to touch or mouth objects (Swedo et al., 2012). Other observable behaviors in students with PANDAS and PANS might include motor or vocal tics and/or unusual movements. At times, students' tics may be so severe or incessant that they make it difficult for the student to function in the classroom (Murphy et al., 2010; Swedo et al., 2012). Although these are involuntary, educators may mistake tics for generalized fidgetiness or attempts at disruptive behavior (Rice Doran, 2015). Thus, monitoring of behavioral symptoms at school and communication with the family is imperative. Additionally, students with PANDAS and PANS may experience sudden outbursts of unprovoked rage, aggression, and/or oppositional behaviors at school. These behavior outbursts can be in strong contrast to their typical disposition and demeanor, and the student may feel out of control and unable to explain this sudden behavior and emotions (PPN, 2018). Allowing these students time to deescalate and also discuss their feelings and emotions related to an outburst can help educators more proactively identify potential triggers in the school environment. School personnel should be mindful of the ways these strong emotions may affect both students and the family members who are supporting them.

Students experiencing behavioral and emotional symptoms of PANDAS and PANS may not respond to the traditional use of positive and negative consequences to alter motivation and reduce negative behaviors. School personnel should understand that these students' behaviors are often neurologically based and are not voluntary; students with PANDAS and PANS often cannot explain these behaviors and actively try to relieve the intense feelings that trigger them (PPN, 2018). Behavior plans and supports need to consider that the student cannot suppress these behaviors consistently, even if they are highly motivated to do so. Rather than focusing on reducing behaviors, school personnel should focus on interventions and strategies that can help reduce the feelings, emotions, and triggers that lead to certain behaviors (Hoppin, 2016). School personnel can support students with PANDAS and PANS by creating safe, supportive, and responsive classroom environments where triggers are reduced and positive reinforcement is utilized; these interventions can support all learners and reduce possibility of disruptive outbursts from students with PANDAS or PANS as well as others. School support teams should also engage in ongoing communication and collaboration with the family to help identify and monitor emotional and behavioral symptoms of PANDAS and PANS. Additionally, parents of students with PANDAS and PANS have reported their children benefited from the use of "safe spaces" where they are able to calm down during episodes of rage or extreme anxiety (Rice Doran & O'Hanlon, 2015).

CONCLUSION

It is important for school personnel to keep in mind the ways that PANDAS and PANS symptoms may change over time and may overlap with common symptoms of other disorders. Combined with the episodic nature of PANDAS and PANS, this may make it challenging for school teams to evaluate students for accommodations, services, and supports under Section 504 or through an individualized education program (Individuals With Disabilities Education Improvement Act, 2006; U.S. Department of Education, 2013). However, careful attention to symptoms (including awareness of the difference between challenging behaviors and neurological symptoms such as tics), collaboration with families and with health care and mental health care providers, and differentiation between behaviors and neurological symptoms when appropriate can help teams to serve this population effectively.

RESOURCES

Candelaria Greene, J. (2016). *PANS, CANS, and automobiles: A comprehensive reference guide for helping students with PANDAS and PANS*. First Edition Design Publishing. https://doi.org/10.21899/978-1506901879

Maloney, B. (2010). *Saving Sammy: A mother's fight to cure her son's OCD*. Crown Publishing Group.

Rice Doran, P. (Ed.). (2016). *PANDAS and PANS in school settings: A handbook for educators*. Jessica Kingsley Publishers.

National Institute of Mental Health. (n.d.). *Research conducted at NIMH (intramural research program)*. https://www.nimh.nih.gov/research/research-conducted-at-nimh

National Institute of Mental Health. (2019). *PANDAS—Questions and answers* (NIH Publication No. 19-MH-8092). https://www.nimh.nih.gov/health/publications/pandas/index.shtml

PANDAS Physicians Network. https://www.pandasppn.org/

PANDAS Network. http://pandasnetwork.org

Magnoli, C. (Director). (2018). *Stolen childhood* [Film]. Novaturient Productions. https://www.stolenchildhood.ca/

Sorel, T. (Director). (2017). *My kid is not crazy* [Film]. 4theKids Films. https://mykidisnotcrazy.com

REFERENCES

Bernstein, G. A., Victor, A. M., Pipal, A. J., & Williams, K. A. (2010). Comparison of clinical characteristics of pediatric autoimmune neuropsychiatric disorders associated with streptococcal infections and childhood obsessive-compulsive disorder. *Journal of Child and Adolescent Psychopharmacology, 20*(4), 333–340. https://doi.org/10.1089/cap.2010.0034

Candelaria Greene, J. (2016). *PANS, CANS, and automobiles: A comprehensive reference guide for helping students with PANDAS and PANS*. First Edition Design Publishing. https://doi.org/10.21899/978-1506901879

Chang, K., Frankovich, J., Cooperstock, M., Cunningham, M. W., Latimer, M. E., Murphy, T. K., Pasternack, M., Thienemann, M., Williams, K., Walter, J., Swedo, S. E., & the PANS Collaborative Consortium. (2015). Clinical evaluation of youth with pediatric acute-onset neuropsychiatric syndrome (PANS): Recommendations from the 2013 PANS Consensus Conference. *Journal of Child and Adolescent Psychopharmacology, 25*(1), 3–13. https://doi.org/10.1089/cap.2014.0084

Farmer, C., Thienemann, M., Leibold, C., Kamalani, G., Sauls, B., & Frankovich, J. (2018). Psychometric evaluation of the Caregiver Burden Inventory in children and adolescents with PANS. *Journal of Pediatric Psychology, 43*(7), 749–757. https://doi.org/10.1093/jpepsy/jsy014

Hoppin, K. M. (2016). Emotional and behavioral impact of PANDAS/PANS: Considerations for planning and practice. In P. Rice Doran (Ed.), *PANDAS and PANS in school settings: A handbook for educators* (pp. 115–126). Jessica Kingsley Publishing.

Individuals With Disabilities Education Improvement Act, 34 C.F.R. § 300 *et seq.* (2006). https://sites.ed.gov/idea/files/finalregulations.pdf

Jenike, M., & Boaz, S. (2012). *Sudden and severe onset OCD (PANS/PANDAS)—Practical advice for practitioners and parents*. International OCD Foundation. https://iocdf.org/pandas/

Lewin, A. B., Storch, E. A., Mutch, P. J., & Murphy, T. K. (2011). Neurocognitive functioning in youth with pediatric autoimmune neuropsychiatric disorders associated with streptococcus. *The Journal of Neuropsychiatry and Clinical Neurosciences, 23*(4), 391–398. https://doi.org/10.1176/jnp.23.4.jnp391

McClelland, M., Crombez, M. M., Crombez, C., Wenz, C., Lisius, M., Mattia, A., & Marku, S. (2015). Implications for advanced practice nurses when pediatric autoimmune neuropsychiatric disorders associated with streptococcal infections (PANDAS) is suspected: A qualitative study. *Journal of Pediatric Health Care, 29*(5), 442–452. https://doi.org/10.1016/j.pedhc.2015.03.005

Murphy, T. K., Kurlan, R., & Leckman, J. (2010). The immunobiology of Tourette's disorder, pediatric autoimmune neuropsychiatric disorders associated with streptococcus, and related disorders: A way forward. *Journal of Child and Adolescent Psychopharmacology, 20*(4), 317–331. https://doi.org/10.1089/cap.2010.0043

Murphy, T. K., Storch, E. A., Lewin, A. B., Edge, P. J., & Goodman, W. K. (2012). Clinical factors associated with pediatric autoimmune neuropsychiatric disorders associated with streptococcal infections. *The Journal of Pediatrics, 160*(2), 314–319. https://doi.org/10.1016/j.jpeds.2011.07.012

National Institute of Mental Health. (n.d.). *Research conducted at NIMH (intramural research program)*. https://www.nimh.nih.gov/research/research-conducted-at-nimh

PANDAS Physicians Network. (2018). *PANDAS diagnostic criteria*. https://www.pandasppn.org/ppn-pandas-diagnostic-guidelines/

Pawela, C., Brunsdon, R. K., Williams, T. A., Porter, M., Dale, R. C., & Mohammad, S. S. (2017, April). The neuropsychological profile of children with basal ganglia encephalitis: A case series. *Developmental Medicine and Child Neurology, 59*(4), 445–448. https://doi.org/10.1111/dmcn.13351

Platt, M. P., Agalliu, D., & Cutforth, T. (2017). Hello from the other side: How autoantibodies circumvent the blood–brain barrier in autoimmune encephalitis. *Frontiers in Immunology, 8*, Article 442. https://doi.org/10.3389/fimmu.2017.00442

Rice Doran, P. (2015). Sudden behavioral changes in the classroom: What educators need to know about PANDAS and PANS. *Beyond Behavior, 24*(1), 31–37. https://doi.org/10.1177/107429561502400106

Rice Doran, P. (2016a). Collaborative planning for students with PANDAS and PANS. In P. Rice Doran (Ed.), *PANDAS and PANS in school settings: A handbook for educators* (pp. 124–147). Jessica Kingsley Publishing.

Rice Doran, P. (2016b). What are PANDAS and PANS, and why do educators need to know? In P. Rice Doran (Ed.), *PANDAS and PANS in school settings: A handbook for educators* (pp. 21–37). Jessica Kingsley Publishing.

Rice Doran, P., & O'Hanlon, E. (2015, April 8–11). *Families' experiences with PANDAS and related disorders* [Poster presentation]. Council for Exceptional Children Annual Convention, San Diego, CA, United States.

Swedo, S., Leckman, J., & Rose, N. (2012). From research subgroup to clinical syndrome: Modifying the PANDAS criteria to describe PANS (pediatric acute-onset neuropsychiatric syndrome). *Pediatrics & Therapeutics, 2*(2), Article 113. https://doi.org/10.4172/2161-0665.1000113

Swedo, S. E., Leonard, H. L., Garvey, M., Mittleman, B., Allen, A. J., Perlmutter, S., Lougee, L., Dow, S., Zamkoff, J., & Dubbert, B. K. (1998). Pediatric autoimmune neuropsychiatric disorders associated with streptococcal infections: Clinical description of the first 50 cases. *The American Journal of Psychiatry, 155*(2), 264–271. https://doi.org/10.1176/ajp.155.2.264

Theinemann, M. (2016). Medical history and context of PANDAS and PANS. In P. Rice Doran (Ed.), *PANDAS and PANS in school settings: A handbook for educators* (pp. 115–126). Jessica Kingsley Publishing.

Tona, J., & Posner, T. (2011, November). Pediatric autoimmune neuropsychiatric disorders: A new frontier for occupational therapy intervention. *OT Practice*, 14–22.

Tona, J. T., Bhattacharjya, S., & Calaprice, D. (2017). Impact of PANS and PANDAS exacerbations on occupational performance: A mixed-methods study. *The American Journal of Occupational Therapy, 71*(3), P1–P9. https://doi.org/10.5014/ajot.2017.022285

U.S. Department of Education. (2013). *Protecting students with disabilities: Frequently asked questions about Section 504 and the education of students with disabilities*. http://www2.ed.gov/about/offices/list/ocr/504faq.html

Westly, E. (2009, January 1). From throat to mind: Strep today, anxiety later? *Scientific American*. http://www.scientificamerican.com/article/from-throat-to-mind/

World Health Organization. (2019). *International statistical classification of diseases and related health problems* (11th ed.). https://icd.who.int/

23

Prader–Willi Syndrome

Moira Wendel and Julia Ogg

Prader–Willi syndrome (PWS) is a complex genomic condition affecting multiple systems of the body and is marked by distinct physical attributes and a number of behavioral abnormalities. The syndrome is characterized by excessive hunger, obesity, and behavioral issues such as compulsivity, emotional health issues, and intellectual disability (Cassidy et al., 2012).

ETIOLOGY

The etiology of PWS is rarely hereditary and is often caused by a random mutation resulting in a failure of genetic expression from the paternally inherited chromosome 15. This is most often due to a partial or complete deletion of paternal chromosome 15 (65%–75% of cases), but in the minority of cases (20%–30%) the mother contributes two chromosome 15s (termed uniparental disomy [UPD]), or in very rare cases (1%–3%), part of chromosome 15 has been incorrectly placed (imprinting defect; Cassidy et al., 2012). Some instances of PWS due to imprinting defects are heritable, but the vast majority of causes (more than 96%) are due to random genetic mutation in which there is no family history of the condition. Though individuals with PWS often display similar traits and symptoms due to the disease, severity of symptomatology and impairment vary.

https://doi.org/10.1037/0000349-023
Health-Related Disorders in Children and Adolescents: A Guidebook for Educators and Service Providers, Second Edition, M. M. Perfect, C. A. Riccio, and M. A. Bray (Editors)

PREVALENCE AND INCIDENCE

PWS has a prevalence rate between one in 15,000 and one in 25,000 and affects male and female individuals equally (Cassidy et al., 2012). PWS affects approximately 350,000 to 400,000 individuals worldwide.

SYMPTOMS

As a multisystem disorder, PWS disrupts several primary systems of the body, which indirectly impact other bodily functions, causing a complex and varied range of symptoms that are manifested in individuals on a case-by-case basis. Most symptoms, including the key symptom of overeating (hyperphagia), are due to hypothalamic dysregulation. Specific symptoms related to hypothalamic dysregulation are altered perception and regulation of temperature, high pain threshold, and obstructed breathing during sleep (Angulo et al., 2015). Circadian rhythm disruption due to hypothalamic dysregulation causes sleep disturbance and excessive daytime sleepiness, which ultimately disrupts focus, energy, and neurocognitive functioning. Also related to the hypothalamus is endocrine dysfunction, which causes issues such as growth hormone dysfunction, hypothyroidism, and central adrenal insufficiency (Crinò et al., 2018). Other common symptoms and conditions include respiratory issues, scoliosis, deficits in visual acuity, osteopenia/osteoporosis (common in adults), dry mouth, skin picking, and bruising easily (Cassidy et al., 2012).

Those with PWS often share a common phenotype, although the characteristics can vary. Growth hormone deficiency causes short stature, with untreated individuals reaching a height of about five feet tall. Underdeveloped reproductive systems in both male and female individuals due to lack of sex hormones (hypogonadism) result in delayed and incomplete puberty and, in most cases, infertility (Angulo et al., 2015). Distinct facial features, such as narrow forehead, almond-shaped eyes, narrow nasal bridge, thin upper lip, and turned-down corners of the mouth, may be evident at birth or emerge in childhood. Pale skin and light blonde hair are characteristic for those with the type of PWS that is caused by chromosomal deletion.

Perhaps the most challenging and problematic symptom of PWS is overeating and obesity. The prevalence of overweight status or obesity in adolescents is around 40% and reaches to over 80% in adults (Crinò et al., 2018). Five nutritional phases have been identified, starting with poor feeding in infancy (Phase 1) and transforming into the final phase by middle childhood, in which individuals seldom feel full and have ravenous hunger due to excessive hunger-related hormones. Lack of satiation, particularly in middle childhood and adolescence, causes overeating, preoccupation with food, and impulsive food-related behaviors. Food-seeking behaviors are common, such as eating inedible materials, hoarding or foraging for food, stealing or sneaking food, and stealing money for food. Youth with PWS also demonstrate a higher than typical threshold for vomiting, which means that gorging on food is less likely to be stopped due to sickness. Health complications related to obesity are significant. Up to 25% of individuals with PWS will develop Type 2 diabetes in their lifetime (Cassidy et al., 2012).

IMPACT ON THE STUDENT AND OUTCOMES

Medical

The outcomes for youth with PWS manifest differently across the lifespan with three distinct stages: prenatal and infancy, childhood, and adolescence/adulthood. Several abnormal developmental characteristics are evident at birth; infants are smaller than their siblings and have poor reflexes, underdeveloped genitals, and failure to thrive (Cassidy et al., 2012). Hypotonia, or low muscle tone, is characteristic in infancy and often persists throughout life. Feeding in infancy and weight gain is inhibited due to poor suck reflex. However, a switch from poor feeding and low weight to excessive weight gain occurs when children are between 2 and 4 years old, although their appetite may have not yet increased (Crinò et al., 2018). Weight gain during this stage is not due to excess calories but to other hormonal and physiological abnormalities that contribute to fat storage. Those with PWS must eat below the typical recommended calorie intake for their age to abate weight gain throughout their life.

The symptomatology of PWS changes dramatically as childhood approaches. Between 4 and 8 years old, children develop excessive hunger (hyperphagia) that further contributes to obesity. Several physical health issues emerge in adolescence and adulthood as well. Underdeveloped reproductive systems in both male and female individuals due to lack of sex hormones (hypogonadism) result in delayed and incomplete puberty and often infertility (Cassidy et al., 2012). Notable medical concerns in childhood include skin picking, visual acuity deficits, respiratory issues, and high pain threshold. Risks related to obesity peak in adulthood and are the main causes of death. If weight is not moderated, individuals may develop diabetes, gastric problems, sleep apneas, cardiovascular problems, and heart failure, which may result in a shortened lifespan (McCandless & Committee on Genetics, 2011). Additionally, risk of death by choking is a concern throughout life (Crinò et al., 2018).

Cognitive/Academic

Developmental delays are common among youth with PWS; early language and motor development milestones are reached at double the typical age on average (Cassidy et al., 2012). Most individuals with PWS experience cognitive impairment, with the average IQ falling between 60 and 70. The impairment in school is often great, and most youth have severe learning difficulties and struggle to perform academically (Cassidy et al., 2012). Some authors have reported that youth with PWS have relative strengths in reading and long-term memory, with relative weaknesses in the areas of expressive language and short-term auditory memory (Chedd et al., 2006). Most youth with PWS experience speech and language delays and deficits; however, the degree of impairment can vary from children who are nonverbal to those who may develop typical speech and language skills by adulthood.

Social-Emotional and Behavioral

In contrast to the happy temperament of their toddler selves, a majority of children will develop problem behaviors such as compulsivity, temper tantrums, and stubbornness in early childhood. Changes in routine and transitions become difficult, and food-related behaviors are a major concern at this stage. Many of the behavioral symptoms of PWS have been compared with those of autism spectrum disorder (Cassidy et al., 2012); individuals with PWS may have social–emotional skill impairments, including difficulty with social cues, repetitive behaviors, irritability, adherence to rituals, and difficulty with transitions. These challenges can make it difficult for youth with PWS to maintain friendships.

In adolescence and adulthood, the risk for developing behavioral and mental health disorders increases (Cassidy et al., 2012). Affected teenagers often experience similar changes and insecurities as their peers, but problems unique to those with PWS compound adolescent challenges (McCandless & Committee on Genetics, 2011). Specifically, adolescents with PWS are at increased risk for developing obsessive-compulsive disorder, and compulsive behaviors such as smoking often emerge. In addition, mental health concerns such as depression and anxiety often increase during this period, which may manifest as changes in behavior or behavior problems (Goldstone et al., 2008). Psychiatric illness occurs in 10% to 20% of individuals by young adulthood, and 5% to 10% experience psychosis (Cassidy & Driscoll, 2009). Although elevated risk for psychiatric concerns is present for all youth with PWS, there is evidence that one genetic subtype of PWS in particular (UPD) puts youth at elevated risk for more severe and chronic mental health concerns. In one study, 65% with UPD developed a psychiatric disorder, compared with 28% with deletion. In addition, the severity of symptoms was worse in individuals with UPD (Soni et al., 2007).

PSYCHOEDUCATIONAL IMPLICATIONS AND SCHOOL-BASED INTERVENTIONS

Although most cases of PWS are now diagnosed within the first few months of life, it is critical to educate school staff about the manifestations of the disorder. Psychoeducational implications with regard to physical health, academics, mental and behavioral health, and family functioning for youth with PWS are outlined in the following sections.

Medical and Health Management

The primary medical treatment for PWS is growth hormone treatment, which supports more typical growth patterns among individuals with PWS and helps to prevent obesity (Cassidy et al., 2012); however, growth hormones do not alleviate excessive appetite, and no current treatments are available to regulate appetite. Hyperphagia and food-related behaviors are unique aspects of PWS that are particularly challenging for caregivers (Crinò et al., 2018). Management and restriction of food intake is a primary intervention for PWS (Cassidy et al., 2012), and it is essential that members of the team are on the same page regarding the importance of consistency in the student's dietary plan. Thus, in the school setting it is important that school professionals are cognizant of the food sensitivities of youth with PWS and that multiple school personnel are aware of the issues. For example, school professionals should be aware of the frequency of food-related behavior problems, such as eating nonfood items, stealing food, stealing money to buy food, elopement to obtain food, and temper tantrums about food. Strategies to address these concerns involve limiting access or visual reminders of food, including limiting exposure to food (e.g., removing candy sitting on the teacher's desk), using highly structured routines and increased supervision, and planning for special and holiday events at school involving food (McCandless & Committee on Genetics, 2011). In addition, given the increased threat of choking, staff should be trained in the Heimlich maneuver.

Observational studies indicate that youth with PWS engage in less physical activity than their peers (Bellicha et al., 2021); however, participation in a physical activity program results in increased activity levels and improved physical capacity (Eiholzer et al., 2003). Thus, daily physical activity with muscle training is recommended to address muscle tone and obesity issues common among youth with PWS (Cassidy et al., 2012). However, it should be considered that youth with PWS often have low muscle tone, which may make physical tasks difficult. Thus, a child with PWS will need consultation and supports for physical activities through a physical or occupational therapist.

There are several additional health concerns related to PWS that may be supported by school professionals. Individuals with PWS often experience higher rates of daytime sleepiness, and increasing activity and structured activities may prevent or lessen these symptoms (Angulo et al., 2015). Medications have been used to reduce daytime sleepiness (i.e., modafinil; Driscoll et al., 2017). Another common concern noted among youth with PWS is skin picking, and behavior management strategies in the school setting could be used to address this concern, such as identifying the antecedents of skin picking (e.g., boredom, presence of a lesion) as well as replacement behaviors (e.g., holding something in the hands; Goldstone et al., 2008). In addition, medications have been used to address skin picking (e.g., N-acetylcysteine, topiramate) in this population (Driscoll et al., 2017). Finally, due to underdeveloped reproductive systems, delayed or incomplete puberty is often observed and may further differentiate youth with PWS from their peers. Youth with PWS can be treated with sex hormones, and sex education should occur with consideration of contraception (Cassidy et al., 2012).

Cognitive/Academic

Youth with PWS typically present with a variety of school-related concerns, and the heterogeneous nature of this disorder necessitates individual evaluation and intervention development. Thus, a functional assessment to determine contributions to the problem behavior may be important to inform a behavior intervention plan. Often, individualized services through an individualized education program are warranted. In addition, given the similarities in symptoms demonstrated by youth with PWS and those diagnosed with autism spectrum disorders, strategies used to address these concerns in children with autism could be used to address concerns in PWS (see Chapter 15 by Cole and Telesford). This may include social skills training, visual cues, and individualized academic instruction (Cassidy et al., 2012). In addition, speech and language therapy is indicated to address deficits and delays often found with regard to both articulation and language-related impairments.

Social-Emotional and Behavioral

In younger children, behavioral concerns such as tantrums are common, particularly around food-related conflict and frustrations. Structured classroom management systems that include antecedent supports (e.g., visual reminders of expected behavior, removal of triggering items when possible) as well as consequence-based strategies (e.g., reinforcement for desired behavior) can support positive behaviors. Research on several applied behavior analysis strategies, including differential reinforcement and stimulus control procedures, has demonstrated efficacy in reducing food-stealing behaviors in youth with PWS (Lambert et al., 2019; Maglieri et al., 2000; Page et al., 1983). In addition, supporting youth with PWS in practicing developmentally appropriate social skills is important. This may come through explicit social skill training and role playing.

In adolescence, mental health concerns such as obsessive-compulsive disorder, depression, anxiety, and psychosis frequently emerge for youth with PWS. As youth with PWS reach this age, school professionals can provide parents and other caregivers with information on the early signs of mental health problems so early interventions can be implemented. In addition, school-based treatments for these mental health concerns can be provided. Medications for mental health concerns, including depression, obsessive-compulsive disorder, and skin picking, have been used effectively with individuals with PWS. In particular, selective serotonin reuptake inhibitors have been shown to be beneficial (Soni et al., 2007).

The symptoms of PWS can put significant stress on families. School professionals should work closely with families in educating, supporting treatment plans, and planning for the future. Given the behavioral challenges posed by children with PWS, teaching parents effective behavior management approaches, including identifying antecedents, teaching replacement behaviors, and adjusting contingencies, may help support behavior at home and school. School professionals should maintain regular communication with parents and may want to use a daily report card to communicate information to the parent. In addition, due to the low prevalence of PWS, it may be difficult for families to connect with other families of children with PWS; however, school professionals can also connect families with PWS organizations like those described in the Resources section.

CONCLUSION

PWS is a complex disorder marked by excessive appetite, obesity, behavioral problems, and intellectual disability. Management of PWS is optimized with a multidisciplinary approach that considers medical, cognitive, academic, behavior, mental health, and family needs.

RESOURCES

Butler, M. G., Lee, P. D. K., & Whitman, B. Y. (Eds.). (2006). *Management of Prader–Willi syndrome* (3rd ed.). Springer. https://doi.org/10.1007/978-0-387-33536-0
Prader–Willi Syndrome Association. https://www.pwsausa.org/
Foundation for Prader–Willi Research. https://www.fpwr.org

REFERENCES

Angulo, M. A., Butler, M. G., & Cataletto, M. E. (2015). Prader–Willi syndrome: A review of clinical, genetic, and endocrine findings. *Journal of Endocrinological Investigation, 38*(12), 1249–1263. https://doi.org/10.1007/s40618-015-0312-9

Bellicha, A., Coupaye, M., Mosbah, H., Tauber, M., Oppert, J. M., & Poitou, C. (2021). Physical activity in patients with Prader–Willi syndrome—A systematic review of observational and interventional studies. *Journal of Clinical Medicine, 10*(11), Article 2528. https://doi.org/10.3390/jcm10112528

Cassidy, S. B., & Driscoll, D. J. (2009). Prader–Willi syndrome. *European Journal of Human Genetics, 17*(1), 3–13. https://doi.org/10.1038/ejhg.2008.165

Cassidy, S. B., Schwartz, S., Miller, J. L., & Driscoll, D. J. (2012). Prader–Willi syndrome. *Genetics in Medicine, 14*(1), 10–26. https://doi.org/10.1038/gim.0b013e31822bead0

Chedd, N., Levine, K., & Wharton, R. H. (2006). Educational considerations for children with Prader–Willi syndrome. In M. Butler, P. D. K. Lee, & B. Y. Whitman (Eds.), *Management of Prader–Willi syndrome* (3rd ed., pp. 302–316). Springer. https://doi.org/10.1007/978-0-387-33536-0_11

Crinò, A., Fintini, D., Bocchini, S., & Grugni, G. (2018). Obesity management in Prader–Willi syndrome: Current perspectives. *Diabetes, Metabolic Syndrome and Obesity, 11*, 579–593. https://doi.org/10.2147/DMSO.S141352

Driscoll, D., Miller, J. L., Schwartz, S., & Cassidy, S. B. (2017). Pradar–Willi syndrome. In M. P. Adam, G. M. Mirzaa, R. A. Pagon, S. E. Wallace, L. J. H. Bean, K. W Gripp, & A. Amemiya (Eds.), *GeneReviews*. University of Washington. https://www.ncbi.nlm.nih.gov/books/NBK1116/

Eiholzer, U., Nordmann, Y., l'Allemand, D., Schlumpf, M., Schmid, S., & Kromeyer-Hauschild, K. (2003). Improving body composition and physical activity in Prader–Willi syndrome. *The Journal of Pediatrics, 142*(1), 73–78. https://doi.org/10.1067/mpd.2003.mpd0334

Goldstone, A. P., Holland, A. J., Hauffa, B. P., Hokken-Koelega, A. C., & Tauber, M.. (2008). Recommendations for the diagnosis and management of Prader–Willi syndrome. *The Journal of Clinical Endocrinology and Metabolism, 93*(11), 4183–4197. https://doi.org/10.1210/jc.2008-0649

Lambert, J. M., Parikh, N., Stankiewicz, K. C., Houchins-Juarez, N. J., Morales, V. A., Sweeney, E. M., & Milam, M. E. (2019). Decreasing food stealing of child with Prader–Willi syndrome through function-based differential reinforcement. *Journal of Autism and Developmental Disorders, 49*(2), 721–728. https://doi.org/10.1007/s10803-018-3747-y

Maglieri, K. A., DeLeon, I. G., Rodriguez-Catter, V., & Sevin, B. M. (2000). Treatment of covert food stealing in an individual with Prader–Willi syndrome. *Journal of Applied Behavior Analysis, 33*(4), 615–618. https://doi.org/10.1901/jaba.2000.33-615

McCandless, S. E., & Committee on Genetics. (2011). Health supervision for children with Prader–Willi syndrome. *Pediatrics, 127*(1), 195–204. https://doi.org/10.1542/peds.2010-2820

Page, T. J., Finney, J. W., Parrish, J. M., & Iwata, B. A. (1983). Assessment and reduction of food stealing in Prader–Willi children. *Applied Research in Mental Retardation, 4*(3), 219–228. https://doi.org/10.1016/S0270-3092(83)80003-4

Soni, S., Whittington, J., Holland, A. J., Webb, T., Maina, E., Boer, H., & Clarke, D. (2007). The course and outcome of psychiatric illness in people with Prader–Willi syndrome: Implications for management and treatment. *Journal of Intellectual Disability Research, 51*(1), 32–42. https://doi.org/10.1111/j.1365-2788.2006.00895.x

24

Rett Syndrome

Nicholas W. Gelbar

Rett syndrome is one of the leading known causes of intellectual disability in girls (Lyst & Bird, 2015). The disorder was first described by Andreas Rett in 1966 in a paper published in Austria. He reported on 31 girls with a history of a regression of intellectual and motor skills leading to intellectual disability and loss of purposeful hand movements coupled with the presence of a repetitive "hand-wringing behavior" (Rett, 1966). The first publication to comprehensively discuss Rett syndrome in English appeared in 1983 (Hagberg et al., 1983) and studied 35 cases, describing the syndrome as a "progressive syndrome of autism, dementia, ataxia, and loss of purposeful hand use in girls" (p. 234).

ETIOLOGY

Rett syndrome has been linked to mutations in the gene that encodes the methyl-CpG-binding protein 2 (*MECP2*; Amir et al., 1999). *MECP2* is an important

Nicholas W. Gelbar was supported in part by the Health Resources and Services Administration (HRSA) under the Leadership Education in Neurodevelopmental Disabilities Grant T73MC30115 and by the Administration on Intellectual and Developmental Disabilities under the University Center of Excellence in Developmental Disabilities Grant 90DDUC0071-01-00 of the U.S. Department of Health and Human Services (HHS). This information or content and conclusions are those of the author and should not be construed as the official position or policy of, nor should any endorsements be inferred by, HRSA, HHS, or the U.S. government.

https://doi.org/10.1037/0000349-024
Health-Related Disorders in Children and Adolescents: A Guidebook for Educators and Service Providers, Second Edition, M. M. Perfect, C. A. Riccio, and M. A. Bray (Editors)

contributor to "neuronal development and function, through its ability to bind to methylated DNA, and it interacts with coregulatory transcription protein partners in neuronal cells" (Gold et al., 2018, p. 168), although the exact processes by which it contributes to these functions are still unknown. These mutations in *MECP2* occur at or after conception (i.e., de novo mutations). Thus, the disorder generally does not have a hereditary component. Familial cases are incredibly rare (Neul et al., 2010) but were utilized to initially determine the impact of *MECP2* on the disorder (Amir et al., 1999).

Mutations in *MECP2* are linked to approximately 95% of cases of classic Rett syndrome (Neul et al., 2008) and 50% to 75% of atypical Rett syndrome (Neul et al., 2010). Different mutations are likely linked to clinical severity (Gold et al., 2018) as well as whether these mutations occur in all cells (i.e., mosaicism; Zhang et al., 2019). Similar to Down syndrome, it is likely that Rett syndrome may have a "mosaic" component depending on the timing of the mutation relative to conception (Zhang et al., 2019). Regardless, the presence of *MECP2* mutations is not sufficient to make a diagnosis of Rett syndrome, as *MECP2* mutations have also been linked to other disorders, such as learning disability in female individuals (Lombardi et al., 2015), male neonatal encephalopathy (Kankirawatana et al., 2006), autism spectrum disorder (Carney et al., 2003), Angelman syndrome (Watson et al., 2001), psychiatric disorders (Lombardi et al., 2015), and unspecified intellectual disabilities in male and female individuals (Lombardi et al., 2015). Further, Rett syndrome also has been linked to mutations in the *CDKL5* (Bahi-Buisson et al., 2008), *FOXG1* (Ariani et al., 2008), *MEF2C* (Armani et al., 2012), and *TCF4* genes (Armani et al., 2012). For these reasons, the clinical guidelines must be utilized in addition to information from genetic screening when diagnosing Rett syndrome.

PREVALENCE AND INCIDENCE

Rett syndrome affects approximately one in 10,000 female individuals (Lyst & Bird, 2015) and is the second leading known cause of intellectual disability among girls, with Down syndrome being the leading cause (Gold et al., 2018). The impacted protein is linked to the X chromosome, which is why the disorder is almost exclusively present in female individuals (Gold et al., 2018). In rare cases, boys are born with the disorder, and a systematic review indicated that 57 such cases have been reported in the research literature (Reichow et al., 2015).

SYMPTOMS

The latest clinical diagnostic guidelines for Rett syndrome were developed in 2010 and integrated the latest information regarding the interplay between genetics and behavioral manifestations of the disorder (Neul et al., 2010). Considerations include at least partial loss of purposeful hand movements and language, gait abnormalities (ranging from impaired walking to absence of walking), and the repetitive hand movements classically described as handwringing. Individuals with evidence of acquired brain injury either in utero or during the postnatal period or abnormal motor development during the first 6 months of life are not considered to have Rett syndrome. Instead, the individual with Rett syndrome must have a history of typical development followed by a regression; however, the regression can be followed by some level of recovery or at least a period where the skill loss plateaus. Additional symptoms include awake breathing abnormalities, teeth grinding while awake, scoliosis, inappropriate laughing, and intense use of the eyes to communicate (i.e., eye pointing; Neul et al., 2010). In the fifth edition of the *Diagnostic and Statistical Manual of Mental Disorders* (*DSM-5*; American Psychiatric Association, 2013), the diagnostic criteria for Rett syndrome were removed.

Three variants of atypical Rett syndrome have been specified. The first, known as the preserved speech or Zappella variant, involves individuals whose speech remains preserved and who have better outcomes than those with other forms of Rett syndrome (Renieri et al., 2009; Zappella, 1992). The second, known as the early seizure or Hanefield variant, involves the presence of seizures during the first 5 months of life (i.e., prior to the regression of skills). The third, known as the congenital or Rolando variant, is the only variant of Rett syndrome that allows for the presence of abnormal initial development. It also specifies that this period has to be followed by a regression of skills and notes that individuals with this variant have severe microcephaly during the first 4 months of life.

IMPACT ON THE STUDENT AND OUTCOMES

There is incredible variation in the presentation of Rett syndrome across domains, which ranges from the profound impairments characterized by the congenital variant to the relatively milder impairments characterized by the preserved speech variant. The classical and early seizure onset variants represent a moderate presentation of the disease. Further, it is important to note that there is incredible variation across individuals with Rett syndrome within each of these variants.

Medical

Approximately 60% to 80% of individuals with Rett syndrome will develop seizures (Tarquinio et al., 2015), and approximately 80% will experience reduced head growth (Tarquinio et al., 2012). Reduced physical growth among individuals with Rett syndrome is also relatively common (Gold et al., 2018). Other common comorbid conditions include "breathing disturbances with hyperventilation and/or apneas, gastrointestinal complications, gait disturbances, and scoliosis" (Gold et al., 2018, p. 168). Further, feeding difficulties leading to poor weight gain, osteoporosis, and the development of parkinsonian-like features are also common (Gold et al., 2018). Most individuals with Rett syndrome develop the ability to walk with an abnormal gait, but about a third lose this ability over time (Gold et al., 2018). Although a classic feature of the disorder is repetitive hand-wringing behavior, some individuals will develop the ability to engage in some form of purposeful hand movements (Cass et al., 2003).

Cognitive/Academic

All individuals with Rett syndrome meet the diagnostic criteria for intellectual disability, but the severity of their intellectual impairments ranges from moderate to profound (Smeets et al., 2011). This variation in the severity of intellectual impairment is linked to the level of communication difficulties present (Neul et al., 2010). Individuals with Rett syndrome vary from those who do not engage in purposeful communication to those who have some form of verbal communication (either using single words or sentences; Bartolotta et al., 2011). The use of eye gaze is the most frequently indicated form of communication (Bartolotta et al., 2011).

Social-Emotional and Behavioral

Behavior comorbidities include the presence of autism spectrum disorder, anxiety, mood disorders, and self-injury. Individuals with Rett syndrome display repetitive behaviors indicative of autism spectrum disorder and have significant difficulties engaging in social interactions, as their communication skills interfere with their ability to successfully do so. In addition, they engage in social withdrawal and avoid eye contact (Neul, 2012). Being highly agitated has also been reported (Vignoli et al., 2012). Other researchers have described individuals with Rett syndrome as showing signs of anxiety, especially in novel environments (Neul, 2012). Self-injury is reported to occur in 28% to 73% of clinical samples, and abrupt changes in mood were observed in 66% to 77% of clinical samples (Cianfaglione et al., 2016).

PSYCHOEDUCATIONAL IMPLICATIONS AND SCHOOL-BASED INTERVENTIONS

Given the ubiquity of the medical and behavioral comorbidities coupled with the presence of severe physical and intellectual limitations, individuals with Rett syndrome present with unique psychoeducational needs and require an interdisciplinary team and robust interventions across all domains. They will likely be qualified to receive special education services under the multiple disability or intellectual disability classifications.

Medical and Health Management

Individuals with Rett syndrome are medically complex and will be involved with a variety of medical disciplines, which will likely lead to greater involvement of the school nurse and may require specialized training for staff who are working with these individuals due to difficulties with physical mobility, feeding, and breathing. Individuals with Rett syndrome will likely require an individualized health plan developed by the school nurse in addition to their individualized education program. They will likely also be working with a team of outside providers across disciplines including, but not limited to, physical therapists, occupational therapists, speech/language pathologists, neurologists, and pulmonologists (Gold et al., 2018). The treatment plans developed by these disciplines should be aligned with the interventions utilized by school-based personnel.

Cognitive/Academic

Individuals with Rett syndrome will require individualized programming and intensive intervention similar to other individuals with severe intellectual disabilities; see Browder et al. (2014) for a comprehensive guide to developing programming for individuals with severe disabilities. Given the communication, gross motor, and fine motor difficulties experienced by these individuals, they will require intensive interventions from in-school and out-of-school service providers, such as speech/language, occupational, and physical therapists.

Academically, individuals with Rett syndrome will require a highly individualized curriculum that focuses on developing functional skills. The use of applied behavior analysis to provide instruction is highly recommended, as individuals with Rett syndrome will require highly structured and systematic forms of instruction. It will also likely be necessary to utilize strategies such as prompting hierarchies to develop skills. The presence of the hand-wringing behavior will affect how academic programming is provided, so it may be necessary to focus more on gross motor activities. Individuals with Rett syndrome will require assistance via both intensive speech/language therapy and the use of applied behavior analysis to develop and maintain skills for forms of communication. They will also require intensive therapies for their gross and fine motor difficulties, which will necessitate the involvement of both occupational and physical therapists.

Social-Emotional and Behavioral

As many individuals with Rett syndrome will have limited communication skills, they will often use their behavior to communicate their needs. Developing any form of purposeful communication will be an important part of managing their behavior. All individuals with Rett syndrome will require the use of comprehensive behavior intervention plans based on a functional assessment of their behaviors. This should be done in concert with developing highly structured academic programs for these individuals.

CONCLUSION

Individuals with Rett syndrome are incredibly complex medically, cognitively, and behaviorally. All will have some form of intellectual disability, and most will also meet the diagnostic criteria of autism spectrum disorder. The variation in the presentation of symptoms and functional abilities across individuals with Rett syndrome requires that their educational programs be highly individualized. Providing highly individualized, robust academic and behavioral programs in collaboration with school-based and community-based providers is the most efficacious approach for maximizing the outcomes of individuals with Rett syndrome.

RESOURCES

International Rett Syndrome Foundation. https://www.rettsyndrome.org

MedlinePlus. (2018). *Rett syndrome*. National Library of Medicine. https://medlineplus.gov/genetics/condition/rett-syndrome/

National Institute of Neurological Disorders and Stroke. (2022). *Rett syndrome fact sheet.* National Institutes of Health. https://www.ninds.nih.gov/Disorders/Patient-Caregiver-Education/Fact-Sheets/Rett-Syndrome-Fact-Sheet

Eunice Kennedy Shriver National Institute of Child Health and Development. (2022). *What are the treatments for Rett syndrome?* National Institutes of Health. https://www.nichd.nih.gov/health/topics/rett/conditioninfo/treatments

REFERENCES

American Psychiatric Association. (2013). *Diagnostic and statistical manual of mental disorders* (5th ed.). https://doi.org/10.1176/appi.books.9780890425596

Amir, R. E., Van den Veyver, I. B., Wan, M., Tran, C. Q., Francke, U., & Zoghbi, H. Y. (1999). Rett syndrome is caused by mutations in X-linked *MECP2*, encoding methyl-CpG-binding protein 2. *Nature Genetics, 23*(2), 185–188. https://doi.org/10.1038/13810

Ariani, F., Hayek, G., Rondinella, D., Artuso, R., Mencarelli, M. A., Spanhol-Rosseto, A., Pollazzon, M., Buoni, S., Spiga, O., Ricciardi, S., Meloni, I., Longo, I., Mari, F., Broccoli, V., Zappella, M., & Renieri, A. (2008). *FOXG1* is responsible for the congenital variant of Rett syndrome. *American Journal of Human Genetics, 83*(1), 89–93. https://doi.org/10.1016/j.ajhg.2008.05.015

Armani, R., Archer, H., Clarke, A., Vasudevan, P., Zweier, C., Ho, G., Williamson, S., Cloosterman, D., Yang, N., & Christodoulou, J. (2012). Transcription factor 4 and myocyte enhancer factor 2C mutations are not common causes of Rett syndrome. *American Journal of Medical Genetics: Part A, 158A*(4), 713–719. https://doi.org/10.1002/ajmg.a.34206

Bahi-Buisson, N., Nectoux, J., Rosas-Vargas, H., Milh, M., Boddaert, N., Girard, B., Cances, C., Ville, D., Afenjar, A., Rio, M., Héron, D., N'guyen Morel, M. A., Arzimanoglou, A., Philippe, C., Jonveaux, P., Chelly, J., & Bienvenu, T. (2008). Key clinical features to identify girls with *CDKL5* mutations. *Brain, 131*(10), 2647–2661. https://doi.org/10.1093/brain/awn197

Bartolotta, T., Zipp, G., Simpkins, S., & Glazewski, B. (2011). Communication skills in girls with Rett syndrome. *Focus on Autism and Other Developmental Disabilities, 26*(1), 15–24. https://doi.org/10.1177/1088357610380042

Browder, D. M., Wood, L., Thompson, J., & Ribuffo, C. (2014). *Evidence-based practices for students with severe disabilities* (Document No. IC-3). University of Florida, Collaboration for Effective Educator, Development, Accountability, and Reform Center. http://ceedar.education.ufl.edu/tools/innovation-configurations/

Carney, R. M., Wolpert, C. M., Ravan, S. A., Shahbazian, M., Ashley-Koch, A., Cuccaro, M. L., Vance, J. M., & Pericak-Vance, M. A. (2003). Identification of *MeCP2* mutations in a series of females with autistic disorder. *Pediatric Neurology, 28*(3), 205–211. https://doi.org/10.1016/S0887-8994(02)00624-0

Cass, H., Reilly, S., Owen, L., Wisbeach, A., Weekes, L., Slonims, V., Wigram, T., & Charman, T. (2003). Findings from a multidisciplinary clinical case series of females with Rett syndrome. *Developmental Medicine and Child Neurology, 45*(5), 325–337. https://doi.org/10.1111/j.1469-8749.2003.tb00404.x

Cianfaglione, R., Meek, A., Clarke, A., Kerr, M., Hastings, R. P., & Felce, D. (2016). Direct observation of the behaviour of females with Rett syndrome. *Journal of Developmental and Physical Disabilities, 28*(3), 425–441. https://doi.org/10.1007/s10882-016-9478-0

Gold, W. E., Krishnarajy, R., Ellawat, C., & Christodoulou, J. (2018). Rett syndrome: A genetic update and clinical review focusing on comorbidities. *ACS Chemical Neuroscience, 9*, 167–176. https://doi.org/10.1021/acschemneuro.7b00346

Hagberg, B., Aicardi, J., Dias, K., & Ramos, O. (1983). A progressive syndrome of autism, dementia, ataxia, and loss of purposeful hand use in girls: Rett's syndrome: Report of 35 cases. *Annals of Neurology, 14*(4), 471–479. https://doi.org/10.1002/ana.410140412

Kankirawatana, P., Leonard, H., Ellaway, C., Scurlock, J., Mansour, A., Makris, C. M., Dure, L. S., IV, Friez, M., Lane, J., Kiraly-Borri, C., Fabian, V., Davis, M., Jackson, J., Christodoulou, J., Kaufmann, W. E., Ravine, D., & Percy, A. K. (2006). Early progressive encephalopathy in boys and *MECP2* mutations. *Neurology, 67*(1), 164–166. https://doi.org/10.1212/01.wnl.0000223318.28938.45

Lombardi, L. M., Baker, S. A., & Zoghbi, H. Y. (2015). *MECP2* disorders: From the clinic to mice and back. *The Journal of Clinical Investigation, 125*(8), 2914–2923. https://doi.org/10.1172/JCI78167

Lyst, M. J., & Bird, A. (2015). Rett syndrome: A complex disorder with simple roots. *Nature Reviews Genetics, 16*(5), 261–275. https://doi.org/10.1038/nrg3897

Neul, J. L. (2012). The relationship of Rett syndrome and *MECP2* disorders to autism. *Dialogues in Clinical Neuroscience, 14*(3), 253–262. https://doi.org/10.31887/DCNS.2012.14.3/jneul

Neul, J. L., Fang, P., Barrish, J., Lane, J., Caeg, E. B., Smith, E. O., Zoghbi, H., Percy, A., & Glaze, D. G. (2008). Specific mutations in methyl-CpG-binding protein 2 confer different severity in Rett syndrome. *Neurology, 70*(16), 1313–1321. https://doi.org/10.1212/01.wnl.0000291011.54508.aa

Neul, J. L., Kaufmann, W. E., Glaze, D. G., Christodoulou, J., Clarke, A. J., Bahi-Buisson, N., Leonard, H., Bailey, M. E., Schanen, N. C., Zappella, M., Renieri, A., Huppke, P., & Percy, A. K. (2010). Rett syndrome: Revised diagnostic criteria and nomenclature. *Annals of Neurology, 68*(6), 944–950. https://doi.org/10.1002/ana.22124

Reichow, B., George-Puskar, A., Lutz, T., Smith, I. C., & Volkmar, F. R. (2015). Brief report: Systematic review of Rett syndrome in males. *Journal of Autism and Developmental Disorders, 45*(10), 3377–3383. https://doi.org/10.1007/s10803-015-2519-1

Renieri, A., Mari, F., Mencarelli, M. A., Scala, E., Ariani, F., Longo, I., Meloni, I., Cevenini, G., Pini, G., Hayek, G., & Zappella, M. (2009). Diagnostic criteria for the Zappella variant of Rett syndrome (the preserved speech variant). *Brain & Development, 31*(3), 208–216. https://doi.org/10.1016/j.braindev.2008.04.007

Rett, A. (1966). Über ein eigenartiges hirnatrophisches Syndrom bei Hyperammonämie im Kindersalter [On an unusual brain atrophy syndrome in hyperammonemia in childhood]. *Wiener Medizinische Wochenschrift, 116*(37), 723–726.

Smeets, E. E. J., Pelc, K., & Dan, B. (2011). Rett syndrome. *Molecular Syndromology, 2,* 113–127. https://doi.org/10.1159/000337637

Tarquinio, D. C., Hou, W., Neul, J. L., Kaufmann, W. E., Glaze, D. G., Motil, K. J., Skinner, S. A., Lee, H. S., & Percy, A. K. (2015). The changing face of survival in Rett syndrome and *MECP2*-related disorders. *Pediatric Neurology, 53*(5), 402–411. https://doi.org/10.1016/j.pediatrneurol.2015.06.003

Tarquinio, D. C., Motil, K. J., Hou, W., Lee, H. S., Glaze, D. G., Skinner, S. A., Neul, J. L., Annese, F., McNair, L., Barrish, J. O., Geerts, S. P., Lane, J. B., & Percy, A. K. (2012). Growth failure and outcome in Rett syndrome: Specific growth references. *Neurology, 79*(16), 1653–1661. https://doi.org/10.1212/WNL.0b013e31826e9a70

Vignoli, A., La Briola, F., Peron, A., Turner, K., Savini, M., Cogliati, F., Russo, S., & Canevini, M. P. (2012). Medical care of adolescents and women with Rett syndrome: An Italian study. *American Journal of Medical Genetics: Part A, 158A*(1), 13–18. https://doi.org/10.1002/ajmg.a.34367

Watson, P., Black, G., Ramsden, S., Barrow, M., Super, M., Kerr, B., & Clayton-Smith, J. (2001). Angelman syndrome phenotype associated with mutations in *MECP2,* a gene encoding a methyl CpG binding protein. *Journal of Medical Genetics, 38*(4), 224–228. https://doi.org/10.1136/jmg.38.4.224

Zappella, M. (1992). The Rett girls with preserved speech. *Brain and Development, 14*(2), 98–101. https://doi.org/10.1016/s0387-7604(12)80094-5

Zhang, Q., Yang, X., Wang, J., Li, J., Wu, Q., Wen, Y., Zhao, Y., Zhang, X., Yao, H., Wu, X., Yu, S., Wei, L., & Bao, X. (2019). Genomic mosaicism in the pathogenesis and inheritance of a Rett syndrome cohort. *Genetics in Medicine, 21*(6), 1330–1338. https://doi.org/10.1038/s41436-018-0348-2

25

Spina Bifida

Fay Roseman and Agnes Shine

Spina bifida (SB), one of the most common neural tube defects, occurs when the neural tube fails to close during the first 4 weeks of gestation. SB occulta occurs in about 5% of the population, where the defect is internal and may not be diagnosed (Sandler, 2010). If there is a swollen lesion outside of the body (most likely in the lumbar area) with an enclosed spinal cord, the term *meningocele* is used, and *meningomyelocele/myelomeningocele* (the most severe form) is used where the lesion is open and contains meninges and cerebrospinal fluid.

ETIOLOGY

Although the etiology is unclear, SB is linked to environmental factors such as low folic intake, obesity, maternal codeine use, and antiepileptic medication taken during the first trimester (Centers for Disease Control and Prevention, 2009; Fishman et al., 2019). Low levels of folic acid during pregnancy also have been indicated as a risk factor (Burro et al., 2018; Fishman et al., 2019; Sandler, 2010). As environmental factors do not contribute to all infants born with SB, research is also focusing on the possibility of a genetic component.

This chapter is dedicated to the memory of Darius McGinnis, who was born with spina bifida and always had a smile for everyone.

https://doi.org/10.1037/0000349-025
Health-Related Disorders in Children and Adolescents: A Guidebook for Educators and Service Providers, Second Edition, M. M. Perfect, C. A. Riccio, and M. A. Bray (Editors)

PREVALENCE AND INCIDENCE

Prior to 1998, neural tube defects occurred in about one in 1,000 live births. After 1998, when the Food and Drug Administration required that grain cereals include folic acid, the prevalence rate decreased and then stabilized at about two to three in 10,000 live births in the United States (Cooper et al., 2017; Joyeux et al., 2019; Sandler, 2010; Williams et al., 2015). Prevalence rates for SB are higher for Hispanic and White non-Hispanic women and for infant girls than boys (Williams et al., 2015). Women who have previously given birth to a child with SB are more likely to have another child with SB, and women with SB who had a child with SB are 5 to 10 times more likely to have another child with SB (Phillips et al., 2017).

SYMPTOMS

Most babies with SB (90%) are born with hydrocephalus, the accumulation of fluid in the brain due to infection or blockage (Patel et al., 2019). Surgical intrauterine procedures or surgical procedures done within 24 to 72 hours of birth have lessened the sequelae of SB and have improved the survival rate. Mortality rates are high during the 1st year of life especially for babies born with low birth weight and heart defects (Shin et al., 2012). Due to medical advances, individuals with SB are living longer, with about 75% to 80% living until adulthood (Hopson et al., 2018).

The severity of SB depends upon the site of the lesion, as nerves do not develop below that point. Individuals with SB have difficulty with sensation, ambulation, and bowel and bladder control (Lindsay et al., 2016; Patel et al., 2019). Individuals with SB have a wide variety of health challenges, such as hydrocephalus, surgeries for shunt and shunt revision, bladder control with urine and fecal incontinence, potential for urinary tract infections that could lead to kidney disease and failure, skin ulcers, neurological difficulties (e.g., seizures in children with shunts), and lower body paralysis (Cai et al., 2016). Some individuals with SB have abnormal breathing patterns and sleep apnea (Patel et al., 2019). Most infants with SB have Chiari malformation type II, a displacement of the cerebellum and medulla resulting in brain compression (Patel et al., 2019) and accompanying hydrocephalus, but only about 33% have accompanying symptoms (e.g., swallowing difficulties, airway obstructions). About 90% of individuals with Chiari malformation type II need a shunt to address the hydrocephalus (Sandler, 2010).

IMPACT ON THE STUDENT AND OUTCOMES

Depending on the severity of their condition, there are various impacts on a person with SB. Outcomes other than medical include social, cognitive, behavioral, and emotional. Some of these are lifetime outcomes, whereas interventions may mitigate others.

Medical

With medical advances, individuals with SB are living longer and thus need a lifetime of supports. As the severity of SB is mostly dependent upon the site of the lesion, children and adolescents with SB face many challenges to their quality of life. Children under the age of 2 with SB may be at a higher risk for maltreatment (e.g., medical neglect) than children without birth defects (Van Horne et al., 2015). Limited mobility leads to about 20% of those with SB being obese, and SB may present with small stature. In addition, female adolescents with SB attain puberty earlier than those without SB (Patel et al., 2019). As with any chronic medical condition, individuals with SB may have increased depression symptomatology, which could interfere with taking more responsibility for their medical care (Stern et al., 2018).

Cognitive/Academic

Intellectual functioning can range from normal to mild to severe deficits, with difficulties in attention, visual processing, short-term visual memory, visuomotor functioning, and processing time and space, along with problems in executive functioning (Burro et al., 2018; Dennis & Barnes, 2010; Sandler, 2010). Executive functioning as measured by the Behavior Rating Inventory of Executive Function found significantly higher scores in areas of metacognition (Initiate, Working Memory, and Plan/Organize subscales) and behavioral regulation, thus suggesting potential deficits in metacognition and behavioral regulation that could affect academic performance (Tarazi et al., 2008). Deficits in sustained attention (errors of omission and commission) are related to an inability to ignore irrelevant stimuli that overburden attentional processes (Dyhr Caspersen & Habekost, 2013). Children with SB may have similar attentional difficulties as children diagnosed with attention-deficit/hyperactivity disorder, inattentive type, but have more lapses (omission) in attention. Multiple shunt revisions are related to poorer attentional skills and more frequent lapses in attention (De la Torre et al., 2017).

As the number of deficits in functioning increases (e.g., mobility, cognitive executive functioning, memory, attention), some children with SB may struggle academically, which may lead to internalizing disorders such as anxiety and depression. Alternatively, others may excel and pursue higher education.

Social-Emotional and Behavioral

In addition to studying the physical and cognitive challenges faced by individuals with SB, research also has examined the impact of SB on social and emotional experiences across and within different age groups and severities of condition

(Devine et al., 2012; Holbein et al., 2017; Landry et al., 2013; Stiles-Shields et al., 2019). The consensus across studies suggests varying levels of challenges in social skills, social competence, and social acceptance across multiple age groups (Devine et al., 2012; Landry et al., 2013). Many children with SB have difficulty interpreting their own emotions and the emotions of others, and this may lead to a high rate of externalizing behavior (Kelly et al., 2012). Physical and medical challenges faced by those living with SB (e.g., surgeries, illness, limited mobility, bowel/bladder incontinence) are likely to be contributing factors to a sense of not belonging, along with being victims of bullying and teasing.

Children as young as preschool age face challenges with problem-solving skills and are sometimes uncomfortable when adding new people to an already established group of children (Landry et al., 2013), yet prosocial behavior and positive affect increases with age, as does the perception of the level of support received from friends (Stiles-Shields et al., 2019). The increase in the ability to acquire friends and to perform socially may be related to the child's ability to concentrate and engage in higher order thinking as they mature (Holbein et al., 2017). Although these results are initially promising in the classroom, they do not always apply to after-school contact and they are not often sustained into adulthood (Fletcher & Brei, 2010; Lindsay, 2014). Gender differences do not appear to play a role in friendship development (Devine et al., 2012; Stiles-Shields et al., 2019).

Another developmental area of importance in adolescents is the exploration of sexuality and romantic relationships. Akre et al. (2015) identified four main areas of concern in their sample of 13- to 28-year-old individuals with SB: romantic relationships, sexuality, fertility and parenthood, and the need for more discussion about these subjects with professionals in the field. Although some of the issues faced by those with SB are no different from the typical developmental angst that accompanies this stage (e.g., flirting, dating, self-confidence), the deterioration in physical health can present additional challenges, and Murray et al. (2015) noted that quality of life scores were lower among those with SB than in the nonclinical samples used in their study.

PSYCHOEDUCATIONAL IMPLICATIONS AND SCHOOL-BASED INTERVENTIONS

Understanding the challenges these children face provides an opportunity for appropriate planning and for the transition to the academic setting to be welcoming and safe. By using a multidisciplinary approach to psychoeducational and school-based interventions, schools can address their health, academics, and socioemotional needs more broadly.

Medical and Health Management

The lifelong challenges that people with SB may face necessitate high-quality medical care. Children with SB need frequent evaluation by medical professionals to identify their unique needs across development. Further, based on the findings of Akre and colleagues (2015), ensuring health education specific to sexuality is needed. In meeting the individual needs of students with SB, a multidisciplinary or coordinated care process that links the knowledge and needs from appropriate medical staff with those providing the educational program is optimal. In a school setting, classrooms should be user-friendly to students in wheelchairs, using a walker, or on crutches so that they can participate in everyday school activities. It is important that teachers help the students have as much independence as possible in their self-care and that age-appropriate chores are assigned to help increase self-esteem.

Cognitive/Academic

Determining cognitive, sensory, and physical limitations can help with designing appropriate interventions so that the individual can participate in school-related activities and manage their medical (e.g., participating in training for incontinence) and physical needs (e.g., putting on braces, complying with medical regimens). By meeting these challenges in the classroom, students can fully engage, opening the door to more effective cognitive and academic development. Although motor functioning may be impaired, individuals with SB have intact motor sequence learning (Vinck et al., 2012) and can improve their learning through motor tasks as do typically developing individuals. The use of repetition and explicit instruction can benefit individuals with SB. Vocabulary skills and speed in performing tasks influence success in reading and writing fluency (Cirino et al., 2019). Teachers and others should continue to challenge the individual with SB cognitively and academically rather than assuming that cognitive function is impaired and academic achievement will be low.

Social-Emotional/Behavioral

Teachers need to assist children with SB by creating an environment in which their social and emotional development can be fostered. The challenges these children face in this domain directly affect their functioning in a classroom setting (Paloma & Maricle, 2021). Opportunities for relationship development can occur by setting clear rules about acceptable classroom behavior and having open conversations about bullying and teasing. In addition, giving these children the opportunity to take on typical classroom tasks (e.g., assisting the teacher, passing out and collecting work) can provide them with the opportunity to feel safe and a part of the classroom experience (Holmbeck et al., 2003; Paloma & Maricle, 2021). In-service sessions for staff and students related to the differences to expect with a student or peer with SB can minimize unkind comments and bullying and help a child with SB feel more comfortable in school and the classroom (Porter et al., 2009). However, it must also be noted that the connection and bond these children experience within their family unit can be evidenced in the classroom setting. Papadakis et al. (2018) noted that "greater family cohesion fosters a more active and less passive youth interaction style" (p. 11), which may result in externalizing behaviors in the classroom.

In addition to the challenges of peer relationships in the classroom, adolescents with SB must also manage sexual and romantic relationships (Akre et al., 2015). Dating, romantic relationships, and sexual relationships are a developmental task for all adolescents, and this is exacerbated in adolescents with SB. As adolescents with SB tend to exhibit more loneliness, immaturity, and passivity (Kritikos et al., 2020), dating, romantic relationships, and sexual relationships are harder to manage. Questions about their condition relative to developing physical relationships and reproductive health need to be addressed not only by medical personnel but also by personnel who can help the adolescent/young adult explore their feelings (Akre et al., 2015).

CONCLUSION

The increase in understanding about the medical challenges faced by those with SB has provided the academic and mental health communities with a clearer picture of what may be necessary to support this population during their development in childhood. Proper support and guidance must be offered in the school setting to provide opportunities for them to meet both academic and socioemotional developmental milestones despite the physical challenges they may face. In addition, considerably more attention must be paid to including those with SB in conversations regarding their physical and emotional needs, most specifically as they relate to the developmental tasks of relationship development and sexuality in adolescence.

RESOURCES

National Easter Seal Society. 70 East Lake Street, Chicago, IL 60601; 312-726-6200. https://www.easterseals.com

Spina Bifida Association of America. 4590 MacArthur Boulevard, NW, Suite 250, Washington, DC 20007-4226; 800-621-3141, 202-944. http://www.sbaa.org

REFERENCES

Akre, C., Light, A., Sherman, L., Polvinen, J., & Rich, M. (2015). What young people with spina bifida want to know about sex and are not being told. *Child: Care, Health and Development, 41*(6), 963–969. https://doi.org/10.1111/cch.12282

Burro, F., Cama, A., Lertora, V., Veneselli, E., Rossetti, S., & Pezzuti, L. (2018). Intellectual efficiency in children and adolescents with spina bifida myelomeningocele and shunted hydrocephalus. *Developmental Neuropsychology, 43*(3), 198–206. https://doi.org/10.1080/87565641.2018.1439035

Cai, B., McDermott, S., Wang, Y., Royer, J. A., Mann, J. R., Hardin, J. W., Ozturk, O., & Ouyang, L. (2016). Skin ulcers and mortality among adolescents and young adults with spina bifida in South Carolina during 2000–2010. *Journal of Child Neurology, 31*(3), 370–377. https://doi.org/10.1177/0883073815596611

Centers for Disease Control and Prevention. (2009). Racial/ethnic differences in the birth prevalence of spina bifida—United States, 1995–2005. *Morbidity and Mortality Weekly Report, 57*(53), 1409–1413.

Cirino, P. T., Kulesz, P. A., Child, A. E., Ware, A. L., Barnes, M. A., Fletcher, J. M., & Dennis, M. (2019). Role of neurocognitive factors in academic fluency for children and adults with spina bifida myelomeningocele. *Journal of the International Neuropsychological Society, 25*(3), 249–265. https://doi.org/10.1017/S1355617718001200

Cooper, J., Chisolm, D., & McLeod, D. J. (2017). Sociodemographic characteristics, health literacy, and care compliance in families with spina bifida. *Global Pediatric Health, 4*, 1–7. https://doi.org/10.1177/2333794X17745765

De la Torre, G. G., Martin, A., Cervantes, E., Guil, R., & Mestre, J. M. (2017). Attention lapses in children with spina bifida and hydrocephalus and children with attention-deficit/hyperactivity disorder. *Journal of Clinical and Experimental Neuropsychology, 39*(6), 563–573. https://doi.org/10.1080/13803395.2016.1249828

Dennis, M., & Barnes, M. A. (2010). The cognitive phenotype of spina bifida meningomyelocele. *Developmental Disabilities Research Reviews, 16*(1), 31–39. https://doi.org/10.1002/ddrr.89

Devine, K. A., Holmbeck, G. N., Gayes, L., & Purnell, J. Q. (2012). Friendships of children and adolescents with spina bifida: Social adjustment, social performance, and social skills. *Journal of Pediatric Psychology, 37*(2), 220–231. https://doi.org/10.1093/jpepsy/jsr075

Dyhr Caspersen, I., & Habekost, T. (2013). Selective and sustained attention in children with spina bifida myelomeningocele. *Child Neuropsychology, 19*(1), 55–77. https://doi.org/10.1080/09297049.2011.639753

Fishman, B., Daniel, S., Koren, G., Lunenfeld, E., & Levy, A. (2019). Pregnancy outcome following opioid exposure: A cohort study. *PLOS ONE, 14*(7), Article e0219061. https://doi.org/10.1371/journal.pone.0219061

Fletcher, J. M., & Brei, T. J. (2010). Introduction: Spina bifida—A multidisciplinary perspective. *Developmental Disabilities Research Reviews, 16*(1), 1–5. https://doi.org/10.1002/ddrr.101

Holbein, C. E., Peugh, J. L., & Holmbeck, G. N. (2017). Social skills in youth with spina bifida: A longitudinal multimethod investigation comparing biopsychosocial predictors. *Journal of Pediatric Psychology, 42*(10), 1133–1143. https://doi.org/10.1093/jpepsy/jsx069

Holmbeck, G. N., Westhoven, V. C., Phillips, W. S., Bowers, R., Gruse, C., Nikolopoulos, T., Totura, C. M., & Davison, K. (2003). A multimethod, multi-informant, and multidimensional perspective on psychosocial adjustment in preadolescents with spina bifida. *Journal of Consulting and Clinical Psychology, 71*(4), 782–796. https://doi.org/10.1037/0022-006X.71.4.782

Hopson, B., Rocque, B. G., Joseph, D. B., Powell, D., McLain, A. B. J., Davis, R. D., Wilson, T. S., Conklin, M. J., & Blount, J. P. (2018). The development of a lifetime care model in comprehensive spina bifida care. *Journal of Pediatric Rehabilitation Medicine, 11*(4), 323–334. https://doi.org/10.3233/PRM-180548

Joyeux, L., Engels, A. C., Van Der Merwe, J., Aertsen, M., Patel, P. A., Deprez, M., Khatoun, A., Pranpanus, S., da Cunha, M. G. M. C. M., De Vleeschauwer, S., Parra, J., Apelt, K., Laughlin, M. M., Van Calenbergh, F., Radaelli, E., & Deprest, J. (2019). Validation of the fetal lamb model of spina bifida. *Scientific Reports, 9*(1), Article 9327. https://doi.org/10.1038/s41598-019-45819-3

Kelly, N. C., Ammerman, R. T., Rausch, J. R., Ris, M. D., Yeates, K. O., Oppenheimer, S. G., & Enrile, B. G. (2012). Executive functioning and psychological adjustment in children and youth with spina bifida. *Child Neuropsychology, 18*(5), 417–431. https://doi.org/10.1080/09297049.2011.613814

Kritikos, T. K., Smith, K., & Holmbeck, G. N. (2020). Mental health guidelines for the care of people with spina bifida. *Journal of Pediatric Rehabilitation Medicine, 13*(4), 525–534. https://doi.org/10.3233/PRM-200719

Landry, S. H., Taylor, H. B., Swank, P. R., Barnes, M., & Juranek, J. (2013). Longitudinal mediators of social problem solving in spina bifida and typical development. *Rehabilitation Psychology, 58*(2), 196–205. https://doi.org/10.1037/a0032500

Lindsay, S. (2014). A qualitative synthesis of adolescents' experiences of living with spina bifida. *Qualitative Health Research, 24*(9), 1298–1309. https://doi.org/10.1177/1049732314546558

Lindsay, S., Cruickshank, H., McPherson, A. C., & Maxwell, J. (2016). Implementation of an inter-agency transition model for youth with spina bifida. *Child: Care, Health and Development, 42*(2), 203–212. https://doi.org/10.1111/cch.12303

Murray, C. B., Holmbeck, G. N., Ros, A. M., Flores, D. M., Mir, S. A., & Varni, J. W. (2015). A longitudinal examination of health-related quality of life in children and adolescents with spina bifida. *Journal of Pediatric Psychology, 40*(4), 419–430. https://doi.org/10.1093/jpepsy/jsu098

Paloma, N. S., & Maricle, D. E. (2021). Spina bifida: What school psychologists should know. *Communique, 50*(2), 10–12.

Papadakis, J. L., Acevedo, L., Ramirez, S., Stern, A., Driscoll, C. F., & Holmbeck, G. N. (2018). Psychosocial and family functioning among Latino youth with spina bifida. *Journal of Pediatric Psychology, 43*(2), 105–119. https://doi.org/10.1093/jpepsy/jsx096

Patel, S. K., Staarmann, B., Heilman, A., Mains, A., Woodward, J., & Bierbrauer, K. S. (2019). Growing up with spina bifida: Bridging the gaps in the transition of care from childhood to adulthood. *Neurosurgical Focus, 47*(4), Article E16. https://doi.org/10.3171/2019.7.FOCUS19441

Phillips, L. A., Burton, J. M., & Evans, S. H. (2017). Spina bifida management. *Current Problems in Pediatric and Adolescent Health Care, 47*(7), 173–177. https://doi.org/10.1016/j.cppeds.2017.06.007

Porter, P., Obst, B., & Zabel, A. (2009). *A guide for school personnel working with students with spina bifida*. Maryland State Department of Education, Division of Special Education/Early Intervention Services.

Sandler, A. D. (2010). Children with spina bifida: Key clinical issues. *Pediatric Clinics of North America, 57*(4), 879–892. https://doi.org/10.1016/j.pcl.2010.07.009

Shin, M., Kucik, J. E., Siffel, C., Lu, C., Shaw, G. M., Canfield, M. A., & Correa, A. (2012). Improved survival among children with spina bifida in the United States. *The Journal of Pediatrics, 161*(6), 1132–1137.e3. https://doi.org/10.1016/j.jpeds.2012.05.040

Stern, A., Driscoll, C. F. B., Ohanian, D., & Holmbeck, G. N. (2018). A longitudinal study of depressive symptoms, neuropsychological functioning, and medical responsibility in youth with spina bifida: Examining direct and mediating pathways. *Journal of Pediatric Psychology, 43*(8), 895–905. https://doi.org/10.1093/jpepsy/jsy007

Stiles-Shields, C., Driscoll, C. F. B., Rausch, J. R., & Holmbeck, G. N. (2019). Friendship quality over time in youth with spina bifida compared to peers. *Journal of Pediatric Psychology, 44*(5), 601–610. https://doi.org/10.1093/jpepsy/jsy111

Tarazi, R. A., Zabel, T. A., & Mahone, E. M. (2008). Age-related differences in executive function among children with spina bifida/hydrocephalus based on parent behavior ratings. *The Clinical Neuropsychologist, 22*(4), 585–602. https://doi.org/10.1080/13854040701425940

Van Horne, B. S., Moffitt, K. B., Canfield, M. A., Case, A. P., Greeley, C. S., Morgan, R., & Mitchell, L. E. (2015). Maltreatment of children under age 2 with specific birth defects: A population study. *Pediatrics, 136*(6), e1504–e1512. https://doi.org/10.1542/peds.2015-1274

Vinck, A., Maassen, B. A. M., Hulstijn, W., Diender, M. G., Mullaart, R. A., Rotteveel, J. J., & Nijhuis-van der Sanden, M. W. G. (2012). Motor sequence learning in children with spina bifida. *Developmental Neuropsychology, 37*(7), 601–616. https://doi.org/10.1080/87565641.2012.697502

Williams, J., Mai, C. T., Mulinare, J., Isenburg, J., Flood, T. J., Ethen, M., Frohnert, B., Kirby, R. S., & the Centers for Disease Control and Prevention. (2015). Updated estimates of neural tube defects prevented by mandatory folic acid fortification—United States, 1995–2011. *Morbidity and Mortality Weekly Report, 64*(1), 1–5.

26

Williams Syndrome

Carly B. Gilson, Terry Monkaba, Maria Paula Mello, and Robin Pegg

Williams syndrome (WS) is a rare genetic disorder that affects many parts of the body. This condition is characterized by mild to moderate intellectual disability or learning problems, unique personality characteristics, distinctive facial features, and heart and blood vessel problems.

ETIOLOGY

Although there have been some cases of inherited WS, it generally occurs randomly (i.e., no family history of WS). WS is caused by the deletion of 26 to 28 genes from the long arm of chromosome 7. This deletion gives people with WS their facial, health, social, and cognitive characteristics. In particular, the deletion of the elastin gene may affect the tissues, joints, digestive system, and heart (e.g., supravalvular aortic stenosis, peripheral pulmonary stenosis). The elastin gene is often used to diagnose WS using FISH testing (fluorescent in situ hybridization) because most individuals with WS are missing the elastin gene (Martens et al., 2008). However, with recent developments, WS has been diagnosed using chromosomal microarray. This method of diagnosis provides more information about the level of deletion that can help one understand the impact of the deletion on the person with WS.

https://doi.org/10.1037/0000349-026
Health-Related Disorders in Children and Adolescents: A Guidebook for Educators and Service Providers, Second Edition, M. M. Perfect, C. A. Riccio, and M. A. Bray (Editors)

PREVALENCE AND INCIDENCE

WS impacts one in 10,000 people globally (approximately 20,000–30,000 people in the United States), affecting both female and male individuals of any racial/ethnic background equally at birth. Although the rate and prevalence of WS is similar across different countries and cultures, some slight variations on the phenotype depending on culture may be found. For example, although the social phenotype of individuals with WS remains consistent across cultures, some studies have found that the sociability of those with WS may vary in intensity depending on the culture of the individual (Zitzer-Comfort et al., 2007). Zitzer-Comfort et al. (2007) found stronger hypersociability characteristics in American children compared with Japanese children with WS.

SYMPTOMS

WS is characterized by cardiovascular anomalies, distinctive facies, connective tissue abnormalities, cognitive impairment, unique personality characteristics, growth abnormalities, and endocrine abnormalities (Mervis & Morris, 2007). Most people with WS have either a mild intellectual disability (i.e., impairment in intellectual functioning and adaptive behaviors) or learning disability. Even though people with WS may have an intellectual disability, they often exhibit abundant social skills and language abilities. In some cases, they are described as hypersociable, which can include such traits as being talkative, friendly, empathetic, polite, and happy (Martens et al., 2008). Emotionally and behaviorally, people with WS may be characterized by anxious behaviors, such as having specific fears or generalized anxiety at a higher rate than others with intellectual disabilities and typical peers (Royston et al., 2017). People with WS often have a strong affinity to music and exemplary musical abilities, though they may also have hyperacusis (Martens et al., 2008). Although people with WS might exhibit similar traits, the characteristics of WS cover a wide spectrum, and each person is different and unique.

IMPACT ON THE STUDENT AND OUTCOMES

Medical

WS is often characterized by distinct facial features, such as an upturned nose, long upper lip, broad brow, wide mouth, full lips, missing or small teeth, small chin, star-shaped irises, and flat nasal bridge (Martens et al., 2008). The appearance of certain facial features may differ across people with WS. In addition to facial characteristics, individuals with WS often have blocked tear ducts and a hoarse, deep voice. Individuals with WS may also experience reduced depth perception, which can cause difficulty in navigating uneven or sloped surfaces, such as stairs. It is critical to arrange an ophthalmologic exam within the 1st year of the child's life and annual vision screening thereafter.

Hyperacusis, or unusual sensitivity to sound, and early onset phonophobia (fear of noises) are common concerns for most children with WS. Several studies based on parental report and informal observation have pointed to the high prevalence of aversion responses to commonly encountered sounds (e.g., lawnmowers, vacuum cleaners, blenders, fire alarms, thunder, fireworks); as many as 95% of individuals with WS have been described as showing these behaviors (Gothelf et al., 2006; Levitin et al., 2005). In an observational study of sound sensitivity, Gallo et al. (2008) found that 90% of young children with WS showed overt behavioral reactivity to mild intensity sounds in comparison with 20% of children in a mixed etiology contrast group. This behavioral reactivity included covering ears, crying, verbalizing to stop the sound, backing away from the sound, seeking caregiver support, or obvious cringing. Children with WS often exhibit these behaviors in anticipation of the sound when they see the object or have reason to expect the sound. Though little research has been conducted on the effectiveness of approaches to manage this sound sensitivity, strategies to address these concerns include the provision of noise-canceling headphones, distraction, construction of social stories about situations in which there are likely to be aversive sounds to encourage more adaptive responses, and gradual exposure to the sounds with reinforcement of coping behaviors. There is ongoing research about the utility of play and humor-infused exposure approaches as described in the Replays approach (Levine & Chedd, 2007).

Noise tolerance tends to improve with age. In fact, it is common for the source of sound sensitivity to become a special interest over time. Specifically, individuals with WS often exhibit a strong affinity to music and a gift for musical sense and fluency. Even though they may experience global delays in early language development, young children with WS may learn best when learning through songs or rhythmic patterns. For example, preschool children with WS often memorize songs and storybooks and begin to follow along with the text long before they can actually read.

Cognitive/Academic

Although there is substantial variation, children with WS generally have intellectual abilities within the borderline to mild or moderate range of intellectual disability. Most children with WS have relative strengths in language and nonverbal reasoning and significant weakness in visuospatial construction. The typical cognitive profile for individuals with WS includes strengths in expressive vocabulary, retention of language, and short- and long-term auditory memory. Moreover, individuals with WS are often gregarious and exhibit exceptional articulation and language skills. Additionally, stories told by children with WS tend to be coherent and complex (Reilly et al., 1990). Young children with WS often experience developmental delays and may achieve developmental milestones, such as walking, talking, and toilet training, substantially later than do their peers. Individuals with WS tend to have poor achievement on performance tasks and exhibit weaknesses in visuospatial cognition, fine motor skills (e.g., buttoning, handwriting, drawing), abstract reasoning, concentration, and sequencing. Most individuals with WS test within the mild to moderate range of cognitive impairment and adaptive behavior, leading to a diagnosis of intellectual disability. Common behavioral issues include overfriendliness, excessive empathy, attention deficit, anxiety, and specific phobias.

After conducting developmental and neuropsychological evaluations to assist in early intervention, parents and caregivers should consult with medical and educational professionals to determine the best course of services in special education, occupational therapy, physical therapy, speech language therapy, and potentially behavioral therapy for anxiety and other related disorders.

Students with WS can generally learn to read well and develop extensive vocabularies when they have intensive phonics instruction. They are able to hear and distinguish a wide variety of sounds but struggle to create the "mental movie" when reading due to the visuospatial deficits that are an inherent part of the syndrome. Students with WS are generally able to complete the concrete phase of instructional tasks but can demonstrate struggles with the representational phase of math instruction. There is emerging anecdotal evidence that students with WS have the ability to make progress in more advanced math if educational staff help them work around the impact of their visuospatial challenges (Pegg et al., 2016).

Social-Emotional and Behavioral

Individuals with WS are often characterized as overly friendly, exuberant, empathetic, and abundantly social. They experience the normal desire to build relationships with others but may lack an in-depth understanding of social nuances and conventions. Moreover, as individuals with WS mature beyond the school years and structure of family activities, they often experience social isolation, which can lead to depression. To promote lasting friendships, social skills development should be an explicitly targeted intervention for children with WS. Peer supports and group activities in the classroom can help children with WS form relationships in school.

PSYCHOEDUCATIONAL IMPLICATIONS AND SCHOOL-BASED INTERVENTIONS

Medical and Health Management

There are no specific medical conditions exclusive to children with WS. The personality characteristics of children with WS often include enthusiastic mannerisms, strong sensitivity to the emotions of others, and excellent memory for people met infrequently or long ago. However, these strengths may mask the many challenges associated with WS. It is important to acknowledge the charismatic appeal of most children with WS as well as to capitalize on these strengths to help minimize and overcome the challenges to learning that confront each child with WS. In fact, the effective utilization of their personal strengths and their innate ability to access technology can help improve success in more challenging areas and allow access to age-appropriate curriculum with their same-age peers.

Cognitive/Academic

In general, students with WS learn best with consistency, structured instructional routines, clear and realistic expectations, social stories, scripts and visual schedules, and technology. In particular, students with WS are often very effective users of computers and tablets. They also benefit from "chunking" of material into manageable parts, sequential learning through task analyses, audio and dynamic visual supports, rhyme, rhythm and cadence, finding materials that they have an emotional connection with, and specific praise. Above all, it is critical to provide the material in a variety of ways. Adapting strategies to preteach, teach, and then reteach in order to enforce concepts can be very helpful (Pegg et al., 2016).

Language pragmatics is another area of need for students with WS. This difficulty is often most apparent in the social skills area. Another pragmatic difficulty for many children with WS is that they often do not realize that they misunderstood what their conversational partner or teacher has said to them. Even if they do realize that they did not understand what was said, they may not ask for clarification. Students with WS often have expressive and receptive language challenges that lead to delayed processing time and struggles with multistep directions.

Relational language concepts are generally very difficult for children with WS. These include spatial terms (e.g., behind, between), temporal terms (e.g., before, after), quantitative terms (e.g., most, least), and comparative adjectives (e.g., shortest, tallest), as well as more complex relational terms (e.g., neither, nor, unless).

Teachers and other educational providers should be aware that very weak visuospatial skills (especially visuospatial construction) do not only affect reading and math. This deficit can also affect school subjects that require fine and visual motor skills, such as art, geography, and physical education. Due to poor handwriting, individuals with WS often require the use of an alternate pencil or technology (e.g., computer, label maker). They often appear to understand more than they actually do, generally struggle with attention and focus (but are not necessarily hyperactive), and often have difficulty modulating emotion. Additionally, they may have mild to high anxiety and/or phobias, which can interfere with their ability to concentrate and focus on a task. In some cases, individuals with WS will take a prescribed antidepressant and anxiolytic medication to help with anxiety symptoms (Martens et al., 2012). However, some preliminary research suggests that mindfulness-based interventions may also help reduce stress and anxiety levels in individuals with WS (Miodrag et al., 2013).

Social-Emotional and Behavioral

Social support for students with WS is often overlooked due to their generally social and friendly nature, combined with their verbal skills. However, students genuinely need social skills support. They lack the skills to build legitimate friendships and have difficulty understanding social and linguistic nuances (e.g., sarcasm, metaphor, irony), and their desire to please others may lead them to follow poor examples from other students and be more susceptible to bullying and abuse.

Some adults with WS live independently in the community, whereas others succeed best in supported living environments, surrounded by family or professional support staff. Most adults with WS can advance to supportive postsecondary education programs designed for individuals with intellectual and developmental disabilities (Think College, 2019). They may also pursue competitive, integrated employment in settings that match their strengths and interests.

CONCLUSION

Proper assessment is a critical component for identifying supports for children with WS. Additionally, the right test will vary for students with WS at different ages, and the recommended tests for students with WS may be different from the tests that are typically given by school psychologists. In the very early years, the Mullen Scales of Early Learning (Mullen, 1995) is a good choice for children with WS. The Kaufman Brief Intelligence Test–2 (KBIT-2; Kaufman & Kaufman, 2004) is the most commonly used assessment in American research on WS. However, the KBIT is not normally used by school psychologists and is not recommended for formal assessments because it provides an IQ estimate that does not include visuospatial construction (the area of greatest weakness for most people with WS). The Wechsler Individual Achievement Test–III is generally a good test to use for those with WS as a predictor of academic achievement, and most children with WS perform much better on the reading than the math scales.

RESOURCES

Health Care Watch Table—Williams Syndrome. (2019). *Health care for adults with intellectual and developmental disabilities: Toolkit for primary care providers.* https://iddtoolkit.vkcsites.org/physical-health/health-watch-tables-2/williams-syndrome/

Williams Syndrome Association. https://williams-syndrome.org

REFERENCES

Gallo, F. J., Klein-Tasman, B. P., Gaffrey, M. S., & Curran, P. (2008). Expecting the worst: Observations of reactivity to sound in young children with Williams syndrome. *Research in Developmental Disabilities, 29*(6), 567–581. https://doi.org/10.1016/j.ridd.2007.09.003

Gothelf, D., Farber, N., Raveh, E., Apter, A., & Attias, J. (2006). Hyperacusis in Williams syndrome: Characteristics and associated neuroaudiologic abnormalities. *Neurology, 66*(3), 390–395. https://doi.org/10.1212/01.wnl.0000196643.35395.5f

Kaufman, A. S., & Kaufman, N. L. (2004). *Kaufman Brief Intelligence Test* (2nd ed.). Pearson.

Levine, K., & Chedd, N. (2007). *Replays: Using play to enhance emotional and behavioral development for children with autism spectrum disorders.* Jessica Kingsley Publishers.

Levitin, D. J., Cole, K., Lincoln, A., & Bellugi, U. (2005). Aversion, awareness, and attraction: Investigating claims of hyperacusis in the Williams syndrome phenotype. *Journal of Child Psychology and Psychiatry, 46*(5), 514–523. https://doi.org/10.1111/j.1469-7610.2004.00376.x

Martens, M. A., Seyfer, D. L., Andridge, R. R., Foster, J. E. A., Chowdhury, M., McClure, K. E., & Coury, D. L. (2012). Parent report of antidepressant, anxiolytic, and antipsychotic medication use in individuals with Williams syndrome: Effectiveness and adverse effects. *Research in Developmental Disabilities, 33*(6), 2106–2121. https://doi.org/10.1016/j.ridd.2012.06.006

Martens, M. A., Wilson, S. J., & Reutens, D. C. (2008). Research review: Williams syndrome: A critical review of the cognitive, behavioral, and neuroanatomical phenotype. *Journal of Child Psychology and Psychiatry, 49*(6), 576–608. https://doi.org/10.1111/j.1469-7610.2008.01887.x

Mervis, C. B., & Morris, C. A. (2007). Williams syndrome. In M. M. M. Mazzocco & J. L. Ross (Eds.), *Neurogenetic developmental disorders: Variation of manifestation in childhood* (pp. 199–262). Massachusetts Institute of Technology.

Miodrag, N., Lense, M. D., & Dykens, E. M. (2013). A pilot study of mindfulness intervention for individuals with Williams syndrome: Physiological outcomes. *Mindfulness, 4*(2), 137–147. https://doi.org/10.1007/s12671-012-0178-2

Mullen, E. M. (1995). *Mullen Scales of Early Learning.* American Guidance Service.

Pegg, R., Mervis, C. B., Klein-Tasman, B., Levine, K., & Martens, M. (2016). *The educational profile for Williams syndrome.* Williams Syndrome Association. https://williams-syndrome.org/resources/factinfo-sheet/ws-educational-profile-fact-sheet

Reilly, J., Klima, E. S., & Bellugi, U. (1990). Once more with feeling: Affect and language in atypical populations. *Development and Psychopathology, 2*(4), 367–391. https://doi.org/10.1017/S0954579400005782

Royston, R., Howlin, P., Waite, J., & Oliver, C. (2017). Anxiety disorders in Williams syndrome contrasted with intellectual disability and the general population: A systematic review and meta-analysis. *Journal of Autism and Developmental Disorders, 47*(12), 3765–3777. https://doi.org/10.1007/s10803-016-2909-z

Think College. (2019). *What is Think College?* https://thinkcollege.net/about/what-is-think-college

Zitzer-Comfort, C., Doyle, T., Masataka, N., Korenberg, J., & Bellugi, U. (2007). Nature and nurture: Williams syndrome across cultures. *Developmental Science, 10*(6), 755–762. https://doi.org/10.1111/j.1467-7687.2007.00626.x

IV

DIGESTIVE SYSTEM DISORDERS

27

Overview of Digestive System Disorders

Cheryl Maykel, Lauren Gammie, and Johanna deLeyer-Tiarks

The digestive system breaks down food and drinks that are ingested in order to absorb nutrients that power the body. Disorders associated with the digestive system often have a genetic cause and can be aggravated by specific foods. Digestive disorders vary in intensity, they can be acute or chronic, and whereas some can be treated at home, others require long-term medication or surgery to correct or manage symptoms.

BODY SYSTEM INVOLVEMENT AND FUNCTIONING

The human digestive system is complex and involves multiple organs with specific functions. It includes the gastrointestinal (GI) tract, which consists of the mouth, esophagus, stomach, small intestine, large intestine, and anus, as well as the liver, pancreas, and gallbladder. Various hormones, enzymes, and nerves also play a role in digestion (National Institute of Diabetes and Digestive and Kidney Diseases, 2017).

COMMON COMPLAINTS AND INDICATORS OF DYSFUNCTION

Several common childhood conditions list disrupted GI functioning as a symptom, including the stomach flu, constipation, and food allergies. In addition to the physical causes for stomach/GI upset, there are social and behavioral

https://doi.org/10.1037/0000349-027
Health-Related Disorders in Children and Adolescents: A Guidebook for Educators and Service Providers, Second Edition, M. M. Perfect, C. A. Riccio, and M. A. Bray (Editors)

components associated with various feeding problems. Further, stomachaches are a common physical manifestation of anxiety among children. Common characteristics of digestive disorders (e.g., fatigue, discomfort, flatulence, strict diets, hospitalization) can also limit an individual's ability to engage in various activities that promote socialization. Research suggests that youth with digestive disorders experience significant rates of depression, anxiety, school absenteeism, and missed leisure activities (Calsbeek et al., 2006; Nabors et al., 2008).

Another common condition, gastroesophageal reflux, is caused when stomach acid contacts the esophagus and results in the sensation known as heartburn (National Institute of Diabetes and Digestive and Kidney Diseases, 2020). This is generally not problematic unless it is persistent. Lactose intolerance results from the inability to digest lactose, the sugar found in milk (National Institute of Diabetes and Digestive and Kidney Diseases, 2018). Individuals with lactose intolerance typically experience some combination of GI symptoms that occur from 30 minutes to 2 hours after ingesting dairy products (MedlinePlus, 2020).

Functional gastrointestinal disorders involve various GI symptoms with no known biological cause and, thus, are often missed by traditional diagnostic methods. Some research suggests that these conditions may stem from some sort of miscommunication along the gut–brain axis, and there is an association with psychological disorders (Wu, 2012). Although functional gastrointestinal disorders are becoming more commonly diagnosed, further research is needed to fully understand the cause and course of these disorders.

PREVIEW OF MAJOR DIGESTIVE CONDITIONS IN PEDIATRICS

Four specific digestive disorders with serious implications and a low prevalence rate are covered in detail in this part of the book. These include celiac disease, Hirschsprung's disease, inflammatory bowel disease, and phenylketonuria. Next is a brief overview of each disorder; for more information, please refer to the corresponding chapter.

Celiac Disease

Celiac disease is a condition that causes an individual's immune system to react to gluten, a common ingredient in various foods, medications, and cosmetics. The immune system tackles healthy cells, causing damage to the small intestine and other areas of the body over time. It is therefore considered a food-induced autoimmune systemic disorder (Popp & Mäki, 2019). Prevalence varies somewhat around the world, though it is believed that many subclinical cases of celiac disease often go undetected for years (Popp & Mäki, 2019). As a result of intestinal damage, early signs in children may include malabsorption of nutrients and failure to thrive (Popp & Mäki, 2019). Although an individual does not always have significant symptoms, children often experience painful gas, diarrhea or constipation, weight loss, and fatigue (American Gastroenterological Association, 2017). For more information on celiac disease, see Chapter 28 by Maykel et al.

Hirschsprung's Disease

Hirschsprung's disease is a congenital disease often diagnosed within a few days of birth when an infant is unable to pass stool. However, in less severe cases, it may not be diagnosed until later in childhood. It is highly heritable, though more research is needed to fully understand what causes this disease. Hirschsprung's disease results in underdeveloped nerve cells in a child's large intestine, which prevent the body from being able to continue moving stool. It almost always requires surgery, which might entail removing the part of the intestine that does not have the necessary nerve cells. In some cases, more complicated procedures may be necessary. Following surgery, the prognosis is generally very good. Please see Chapter 29 by Jimenez et al. for additional information on Hirschsprung's disease.

Inflammatory Bowel Disease: Crohn's Disease and Ulcerative Colitis

Inflammatory bowel disease refers to disorders of chronic inflammation in the digestive tract, including both ulcerative colitis and Crohn's disease. These are typically diagnosed in adolescence and young adulthood, although the rate of diagnosis among children is rising. Common symptoms among children and adolescents include weight loss, abdominal pain, diarrhea, and rectal bleeding, although some children may only experience poor growth or anemia. Although there appears to be a genetic component to developing inflammatory bowel disease, environmental influences are implicated by significant evidence, such as a low concordance rate among twins, a drastic rise in rate that could not be explained by evolutionary changes in genetics, and the influence of exposure to a Western lifestyle (see Rosen et al., 2015). For more information on Crohn's disease, please refer to Chapter 30 by Puckett-Perez and Vaughan.

Phenylketonuria

Phenylketonuria, often referred to as PKU, is a genetic disorder that impairs the body's ability to break down phenylalanine. This leads to a buildup of this amino acid in the body, which can cause damage to the central nervous system, including various neurological and intellectual complications, that cannot be reversed. Phenylalanine is found in most foods that contain protein; therefore, the diet for someone with PKU is typically low in protein. PKU is usually identified in the United States as part of the standard newborn screening involving a blood test. The prognosis is generally good when individuals follow the diet. Medications are being developed to help increase an individual's tolerance to phenylalanine; however, the main treatment at this time is controlling diet

(Cleary & Skeath, 2019). For more information on PKU, please refer to Chapter 31 by Ogg and Strissel.

HEALTH CARE NEEDS AND MEDICAL SPECIALTIES

In addition to managing various symptoms and the disruption they cause, the child and family may be overwhelmed by health care needs. Primary health care providers serve as a vital resource in diagnosing and providing proper care but also in educating families on how to manage pediatric digestive disorders. Children who experience more severe digestive problems may also be referred to a pediatric gastroenterologist who can offer more specialized training and knowledge during treatment.

In addition to addressing the medical components of the digestive disorder, it is important to consider the effects on social–emotional/behavioral functioning. Many students with illness will be eligible for and could benefit from school accommodations. Thus, it is important that mental health and educational professionals (e.g., nurses, psychologists, counselors, social workers, teachers) also be involved in meeting the needs of these children and their families as part of a team-based approach.

CONCLUSION

A child with a digestive disorder may experience lifelong symptoms and impairments that can change, for better or worse, over time. Continuous communication and collaboration among parents, school staff, and health care providers is imperative to properly monitor and evaluate the current functioning and needs of a student. Proper diagnosis, treatment, and healthy lifestyle habits can help children with digestive disorders live active, fulfilling lives.

REFERENCES

American Gastroenterological Association. (2017). Celiac disease. *Clinical Gastroenterology and Hepatology, 15*(9), Article A25. https://doi.org/10.1016/j.cgh.2017.06.047

Calsbeek, H., Rijken, M., Bekkers, M. J. T. M., Dekker, J., & van Berge Henegouwen, G. P. (2006). School and leisure activities in adolescents and young adults with chronic digestive disorders: Impact of burden of disease. *International Journal of Behavioral Medicine, 13*(2), 121–130. https://doi.org/10.1207/s15327558ijbm1302_3

Cleary, M. A., & Skeath, R. (2019). Phenylketonuria. *Paediatrics and Child Health, 29*(3), 111–115. https://doi.org/10.1016/j.paed.2019.01.001

MedlinePlus. (2020). *Lactose intolerance*. National Library of Medicine. https://medlineplus.gov/genetics/condition/lactose-intolerance/

Nabors, L. A., Little, S. G., Akin-Little, A., & Iobst, E. A. (2008). Teacher knowledge of and confidence in meeting the need of children with chronic medical conditions: Pediatric psychology's contribution to education. *Psychology in the Schools, 45*(3), 217–226. https://doi.org/10.1002/pits.20292

National Institute of Diabetes and Digestive and Kidney Diseases. (2017, December). *Your digestive system and how it works*. U.S. Department of Health and Human Services. https://www.niddk.nih.gov/health-information/digestive-diseases/digestive-system-how-it-works

National Institute of Diabetes and Digestive and Kidney Diseases. (2018, February). *Symptoms and causes of lactose intolerance*. U.S. Department of Health and Human Services. https://www.niddk.nih.gov/health-information/digestive-diseases/lactose-intolerance/symptoms-causes

National Institute of Diabetes and Digestive and Kidney Diseases. (2020, November). *Definition and facts for GER and GERD in children*. https://www.niddk.nih.gov/health-information/digestive-diseases/digestive-system-how-it-works

Popp, A., & Mäki, M. (2019). Changing pattern of childhood celiac disease epidemiology: Contributing factors. *Frontiers in Pediatrics, 7*, Article 357. https://doi.org/10.3389/fped.2019.00357

Rosen, M. J., Dhawan, A., & Saeed, S. A. (2015). Inflammatory bowel disease in children and adolescents. *JAMA Pediatrics, 169*(11), 1053–1060. https://doi.org/10.1001/jamapediatrics.2015.1982

Wu, J. C. Y. (2012). Psychological comorbidity in functional gastrointestinal disorders: Epidemiology, mechanisms and management. *Journal of Neurogastroenterology and Motility, 18*(1), 13–18. https://doi.org/10.5056/jnm.2012.18.1.13

28

Celiac Disease (Coeliac Disease)

Emily M. Jimenez, Daphne J. Hill, and Anita Sohn McCormick

Celiac or coeliac disease (CD) is an autoimmune disorder of the small intestine. The disease is characterized by T cells attacking proteins found in wheat (gliadin), rye (secalin), and barley (hordein), which are collectively called *gluten* (Krupa-Kozak, 2014). When gluten is absorbed by villi, hairlike projections in the intestines, the villi atrophy, or break down, and the body is alerted. Autoantibodies then attack the wall of the intestines, causing the villi to become blunted and damaged and to eventually die (Lowth, 2014). The villi are an important element in the body's absorption of nutrients; therefore, when they are damaged, nutrient absorption declines. Because of this occurrence, some researchers say CD is a malabsorption disorder as well as an autoimmune disorder (Johns Hopkins Medicine, 2011). The only treatment for CD is a strict gluten-free diet (Wagner et al., 2008).

ETIOLOGY

CD can be diagnosed using a blood test to identify the presence of tissue transglutaminase IgA antibodies. The presence of these antibodies confirms a diagnosis of CD in approximately 95% of patients who suffer from the disease. However, there is a slightly higher risk of a false positive for CD when using blood tests on patients with other autoimmune disorders, such as Type 1 diabetes, rheumatoid arthritis, or heart disease. A genetic predisposition to developing CD has also been established, so genetic testing can provide some information

https://doi.org/10.1037/0000349-028
Health-Related Disorders in Children and Adolescents: A Guidebook for Educators and Service Providers, Second Edition, M. M. Perfect, C. A. Riccio, and M. A. Bray (Editors)

regarding the presence of CD. Currently, the most accurate method to diagnose CD is an intestinal biopsy; however, it is more common for children to undergo serological testing. Best practice is currently to have both types of testing administered for diagnosis (Cichewicz et al., 2019).

The etiology of CD is largely attributed to the human leukocyte antigen (HLA), particularly the HLA-DQ2 and HLA-DQ8 heterodimers. These HLAs, when gluten is present, are antigens to the body's T cells, which then attack the gluten protein, damaging the villi of the child's intestines (Howell et al., 1986; Kaur et al., 2017). Approximately 95% of patients with CD have the DQ2 heterodimer, and the other 5% have the DQ8 heterodimer (Howell et al., 1986). However, some research suggests that HLA-DQ2/8 likely are not solely responsible for the development of CD, as approximately 40% of the White population has the HLA-DQ2 and/or the -DQ8, yet only approximately 1% of the world's population develops CD (Laass et al., 2015).

PREVALENCE AND INCIDENCE

In the past 2 decades, the rate of diagnosis for CD has more than doubled (Kang et al., 2013) in the United States. Population-based studies indicate that the current CD prevalence ranges from 0.31% to 0.9% for children and adolescents (Krupa-Kozak, 2014). In other words, one out of 150 people are estimated to have CD. Seventy percent of CD cases occur in female individuals, and 10% of patients have a close relative diagnosed with CD. CD is most common in Whites and people of European descent (Johns Hopkins Medicine, 2011). One explanation for the low prevalence of CD is the low rate of appropriate diagnostic techniques. For example, in the United States an estimated 83% of CD cases go undiagnosed (Rubio-Tapia et al., 2012). It is common for patients with CD to remain undiagnosed due to a prior diagnosis with a different disease, not showing evident symptoms of CD, or being financially unable to afford CD diagnostic screenings (Cascella et al., 2011). In more rare situations, CD can also go undetected if the patient is not consuming much gluten in their diet (Rubio-Tapia et al., 2012).

SYMPTOMS

Clinical presentation of CD can vary based on age, severity of disease, duration of symptoms, and manifestation of disease (Chand & Mihas, 2006). More than 200 symptoms can be associated with CD, categorized as both intestinal or extraintestinal, and these vary from person to person (Celiac Disease Foundation, n.d.-c). Common intestinal symptoms in children and adolescents are chronic diarrhea, weight loss (Tonutti & Bizzaro, 2014), nausea or vomiting, cramping, abdominal pain (Lowth, 2014; Tonutti & Bizzaro, 2014), and bloating (Johns Hopkins Medicine, 2011). Extraintestinal symptoms often present in the form of neurological complications (e.g., ataxia, epilepsy, migraines; Briani et al., 2008), dermatitis herpetiformis, fatigue, mouth ulcers, dental enamel defects, angular stomatitis, irritability, and malabsorption (Cruz et al., 2018; Lowth, 2014).

IMPACT ON THE STUDENT AND OUTCOMES

Medical

A childhood diagnosis of CD has been shown to significantly affect health-related quality of life, academic outcomes, and the overall functioning of the family (Bacigalupe & Plocha, 2015; Skjerning et al., 2014). The malabsorption of important vitamins and nutrients (e.g., vitamins E, D, K, and calcium) in patients with CD has also been linked to the presence of comorbidities such as anemia and osteoporosis (Krupa-Kozak, 2014; Larussa et al., 2012). Weight and body mass index (BMI) have been shown to fluctuate, with 75% of patients exhibiting an elevated BMI at the time of their CD diagnosis. Many patients end up decreasing their BMI significantly after adherence to a gluten-free diet, normalizing it in 44% of cases. However, in some patients with a normal BMI at diagnosis, weight increases significantly after adherence to a gluten-free diet, with 13% becoming overweight (Reilly et al., 2011). Other long-term medical outcomes of CD can be growth failure (Tonutti & Bizzaro, 2014), delayed puberty, and dental problems (Cruz et al., 2018). CD diagnosis in children has also been associated with internalizing and externalizing disorders, most prominently anxiety, depression, and aggression problems (Smith et al., 2017). Additionally, CD symptoms may mimic behaviors associated with attention-deficit/hyperactivity disorder (Niederhofer & Pittschieler, 2006).

Cognitive/Academic

The symptoms of CD can vary in their severity of impact on the child's education and academic success. The adjustment to lifestyle changes necessary for someone with CD, as well as the doctor's appointments for diagnosis, and the chronic pain that can be caused by CD can reduce time spent in school and social contact with peers. After a CD diagnosis is made, which can take months, school personnel should monitor the student to ensure healthy social functioning and continuity of school work that may have been missed during the diagnosis process.

Social-Emotional and Behavioral

Aside from the potential loss of school-based social interactions that children with CD experience due to illness, the entire family may also experience a decrease in socialization. Children with CD reported feeling socially stigmatized and isolated by their peers for their dietary restrictions (Bacigalupe & Plocha, 2015). Sarkhy et al. (2016) suggested that a gluten-free diet can lead to a decline in a family's participation in social activities and social outings. Over half the population of families surveyed (n = 113) reported a decrease in their desire to attend social gatherings, eat in restaurants, and travel. This was attributed to the challenges of eating differently (Bacigalupe & Plocha, 2015).

Another less researched area that has been shown to be affected by a childhood CD diagnosis is the socioeconomic stability of the family. Due to the additional expenses associated with the substitution or modification of foods in order to maintain a gluten-free diet, families can also experience financial hardships (Sarkhy et al., 2016). The limited availability and generally greater expense of gluten-free foods have both been cited as some of the leading contributors to poor compliance to a gluten-free diet, leading to poorer overall health outcomes (Barratt et al., 2011; Singh & Whelan, 2011).

PSYCHOEDUCATIONAL IMPLICATIONS AND SCHOOL-BASED INTERVENTIONS

As with many chronic illnesses, the inclusion of psychoeducational interventions along with disease management has significant implications for the academic outcomes of students with CD. Increased knowledge about the condition, its consequences, and how to manage it are associated with better diet adherence and better overall outcomes (Werbrouck et al., 2018).

Medical and Health Management

The health benefits of gluten-free diet adherence are favorable to the intestinal and extraintestinal symptom presentation in CD children, but the diet can negatively affect other areas of the child's health (Reilly et al., 2011). Many patients' intestines never fully heal after diagnosis, even with gluten-free diet adherence, usually due to the accidental ingestion of gluten and cross-contamination. Cross-contamination concerns can be severe, with many patients needing to request glove changes and separate stoves or cabinets and even having to avoid publicly prepared foods altogether. Medical trials are hoping to develop medications that can help reduce the burden of the gluten-free diet, the fears associated with cross-contamination, and consequently the effects of CD, in order to improve long-term health outcomes (Celiac Disease Foundation, n.d.-b). Compliance with a strict gluten-free diet is the leading choice of treatment for individuals with CD, making fidelity a key factor in physical and emotional outcomes of children with CD. In adolescents, gluten-free diet compliance has been reported to be somewhere between 52% and 81%, with female and younger adolescents being the most compliant (Stockman, 2010). For children with a CD diagnosis, the greatest fidelity in gluten-free diet compliance was found among patients who were diagnosed as young children (before age 6), and the most transgressions were found among patients diagnosed as adolescents (Wagner et al., 2008).

Cognitive/Academic

Although there are no specific cognitive impairments associated with CD, students with this disease may face challenges when attending school. Students with CD are more prone to miss classes due to stomachaches and to suffer long school absences that affect their continued access to education. A 504 plan or an individualized education program to address the student's needs associated with this disease may be necessary in order to aid in their dietary requirements and to assist with the missed school work (Celiac Disease Foundation, n.d.-a). The recommendations offered in the individualized plan may include modifications to attendance policies, extra time to turn in assignments, the ability to pause and later resume exams, and extended time for work completion due to absence or feeling ill.

Social-Emotional and Behavioral

School psychologists and other school-based professionals can be important advocates for students with CD by helping create awareness of the consequences of living with a chronic illness in schools as well as in the community. Additionally, more targeted interventions to address the social, emotional, and psychological effects of the disease are critical. As in most chronic illnesses, the use of cognitive behavioral and mindful therapeutic interventions has been found to be effective to address patients' emotional and psychological issues, such as self-efficacy, self-management of disease, psychosocial well-being, anxiety, and isolation (Howarth et al., 2016). Additionally, school mental health professionals can help foster understanding among students about the consequences of CD to facilitate the social integration of students with this disease. Using a small group approach for psychoeducational purposes can be an effective way of fostering an inclusive attitude among students.

CONCLUSION

Considering the day-to-day challenges faced by families of children with CD, particularly associated with social isolation, health professionals as well as school psychologists are in an excellent position to help support parents and facilitate the integration of students into the school fabric. They can provide families with an accepting environment and put in place strategies that support the student's social, emotional, and academic development. Even more importantly, school psychologists should foster an inclusive atmosphere that focuses on cultural/ethnic issues but also on the acceptance and inclusion of students with chronic illness such as CD.

RESOURCES

General Information About Celiac Disease

Celiac Disease Foundation. https://celiac.org/

Celiac Disease Foundation. (n.d.). *What is celiac disease?* https://celiac.org/about-celiac-disease/what-is-celiac-disease/

Beyond Celiac. (n.d.). *What is celiac disease?* https://www.beyondceliac.org/celiac-disease/

National Celiac Association. https://nationalceliac.org/

Celiac Disease in Children

KidsHealth. (2021). *Celiac disease*. https://kidshealth.org/en/parents/celiac-disease.html

Children's Hospital of Philadelphia. *Celiac disease resources*. https://www.chop.edu/conditions-diseases/celiac-disease/health-resources

Celiac Disease Foundation. *Back-to-school and 504 plan guide*. https://celiac.org/about-celiac-disease/celiac-disease-in-children/504-plan/

National Celiac Association. *Back to school resources for parents and students*. https://nationalceliac.org/resources/school-resources/

REFERENCES

Bacigalupe, G., & Plocha, A. (2015). Celiac is a social disease: Family challenges and strategies. *Families, Systems, & Health, 33*(1), 46–54. https://doi.org/10.1037/fsh0000099

Barratt, S. M., Leeds, J. S., & Sanders, D. S. (2011). Quality of life in coeliac disease is determined by perceived degree of difficulty adhering to a gluten-free diet, not the level of dietary adherence ultimately achieved. *Journal of Gastrointestinal and Liver Diseases, 20*(3), 241–245.

Briani, C., Zara, G., Alaedini, A., Grassivaro, F., Ruggero, S., Toffanin, E., Albergoni, M. P., Luca, M., Giometto, B., Ermani, M., De Lazzari, F., D'Odorico, A., & Battistin, L. (2008). Neurological complications of celiac disease and autoimmune mechanisms: A prospective study. *Journal of Neuroimmunology, 195*(1–2), 171–175. https://doi.org/10.1016/j.jneuroim.2008.01.008

Cascella, N. G., Kryszak, D., Bhatti, B., Gregory, P., Kelly, D. L., Mc Evoy, J. P., Fasano, A., & Eaton, W. W. (2011). Prevalence of celiac disease and gluten sensitivity in the United States clinical antipsychotic trials of intervention effectiveness study population. *Schizophrenia Bulletin, 37*(1), 94–100. https://doi.org/10.1093/schbul/sbp055

Celiac Disease Foundation. (n.d.-a). *Back to school and 504 plan guide*. https://celiac.org/about-celiac-disease/celiac-disease-in-children/504-plan/

Celiac Disease Foundation. (n.d.-b). *Future therapies*. https://celiac.org/about-celiac-disease/future-therapies-for-celiac-disease/

Celiac Disease Foundation. (n.d.-c). *Symptoms of celiac disease*. https://celiac.org/about-celiac-disease/symptoms-of-celiac-disease/

Chand, N., & Mihas, A. A. (2006). Celiac disease: Current concepts in diagnosis and treatment. *Journal of Clinical Gastroenterology, 40*(1), 3–14. https://doi.org/10.1097/01.mcg.0000190644.01661.2b

Cichewicz, A. B., Mearns, E. S., Taylor, A., Boulanger, T., Gerber, M., Leffler, D. A., Drahos, J., Sanders, D. S., Thomas Craig, K. J., & Lebwohl, B. (2019). Diagnosis and treatment patterns in celiac disease. *Digestive Diseases and Sciences, 64*(8), 2095–2106. https://doi.org/10.1007/s10620-019-05528-3

Cruz, I. T. S. A., Fraiz, F. C., Celli, A., Amenabar J.-M., & Assunção, L. R. D. S. (2018). Dental and oral manifestations of celiac disease. *Medicina Oral, Patología Oral y Cirugia Bucal, 23*(6), e639–e645. https://doi.org/10.4317/medoral.22506

Howarth, A., Perkins-Porras, L.. Copland, C., & Ussher, M. (2016). Views on a brief mindfulness intervention among patients with long-term illness. *BMC Psychology, 4*(1), Article 56. https://doi.org/10.1186/s40359-016-0163-y

Howell, M. D., Austin, R. K., Kelleher, D., Nepom, G. T., & Kagnoff, M. F. (1986). An HLA-D region restriction fragment length polymorphism associated with celiac disease. *Journal of Experimental Medicine, 164*(1), 333–338. https://doi.org/10.1084/jem.164.1.333

Johns Hopkins Medicine. (2011). *Celiac disease*. https://www.hopkinsmedicine.org/health/conditions-and-diseases/celiac-disease

Kang, J. Y., Kang, A. H. Y., Green, A., Gwee, K. A., & Ho, K. Y. (2013). Systematic review: Worldwide variation in the frequency of coeliac disease and changes over time. *Alimentary Pharmacology & Therapeutics, 38*(3), 226–245. https://doi.org/10.1111/apt.12373

Kaur, A., Shimoni, O., & Wallach, M. (2017). Celiac disease: From etiological factors to evolving diagnostic approaches. *Journal of Gastroenterology, 52*(9), 1001–1012. https://doi.org/10.1007/s00535-017-1357-7

Krupa-Kozak, U. (2014). Pathologic bone alterations in celiac disease: Etiology, epidemiology, and treatment. *Nutrition, 30*(1), 16–24. https://doi.org/10.1016/j.nut.2013.05.027

Laass, M. W., Schmitz, R., Uhlig, H. H., Zimmer, K. P., Thamm, M., & Koletzko, S. (2015). The prevalence of celiac disease in children and adolescents in Germany: Results from the KiGGS study. *Deutsches Ärzteblatt International, 112*(33–34), 553–560. https://doi.org/10.3238/arztebl.2015.0553

Larussa, T., Suraci, E., Nazionale, I., Abenavoli, L., Imeneo, M., & Luzza, F. (2012). Bone mineralization in celiac disease. *Gastroenterology Research and Practice, 2012*, Article 198025. https://doi.org/10.1155/2012/198025

Lowth, M. (2014). Coeliac disease: Clinical features, diagnosis and management. *Practice Nursing, 44*, 36–40.

Niederhofer, H., & Pittschieler, K. (2006). A preliminary investigation of ADHD symptoms in persons with celiac disease. *Journal of Attention Disorders, 10*(2), 200–204. https://doi.org/10.1177/1087054706292109

Reilly, N. R., Aguilar, K., Hassid, B. G., Cheng, J., DeFelice, A. R., Kazlow, P., Bhagat, G., & Green, P. H. (2011). Celiac disease in normal-weight and overweight children: Clinical features and growth outcomes following a gluten-free diet. *Journal of Pediatric Gastroenterology and Nutrition, 53*(5), 528–531. https://doi.org/10.1097/MPG.0b013e3182276d5e

Rubio-Tapia, A., Ludvigsson, J. F., Brantner, T. L., Murray, J. A., & Everhart, J. E. (2012). The prevalence of celiac disease in the United States. *The American Journal of Gastroenterology, 107*(10), 1538–1544. https://doi.org/10.1038/ajg.2012.219

Sarkhy, A., El Mouzan, M. I., Saeed, E., Alanazi, A., Alghamdi, S., Anil, S., & Assiri, A. (2016). Socioeconomic impacts of gluten-free diet among Saudi children with celiac disease. *Pediatric Gastroenterology, Hepatology & Nutrition, 19*(3), 162–167. https://doi.org/10.5223/pghn.2016.19.3.162

Singh, J., & Whelan, K. (2011). Limited availability and higher cost of gluten-free foods. *Journal of Human Nutrition and Dietetics, 24*(5), 479–486. https://doi.org/10.1111/j.1365-277X.2011.01160.x

Skjerning, H., Mahony, R. O., Husby, S., & DunnGalvin, A. (2014). Health-related quality of life in children and adolescents with celiac disease: Patient-driven data from focus group interviews. *Quality of Life Research, 23*(6), 1883–1894. https://doi.org/10.1007/s11136-014-0623-x

Smith, L. B., Lynch, K. F., Kurppa, K., Koletzko, S., Krischer, J., Liu, E., Johnson, S. B., Agardh, D., & the TEDDY study group. (2017). Psychological manifestations of celiac disease autoimmunity in young children. *Pediatrics, 139*(3), Article e20162848. https://doi.org/10.1542/peds.2016-2848

Stockman, J. A., III. (2010). Quality of life in adolescents with treated coeliac disease: Influence of compliance and age at diagnosis. In *Year book of pediatrics* (pp. 141–143). https://doi.org/10.1016/S0084-3954(09)79423-0

Tonutti, E., & Bizzaro, N. (2014). Diagnosis and classification of celiac disease and gluten sensitivity. *Autoimmunity Reviews, 13*(4–5), 472–476. https://doi.org/10.1016/j.autrev.2014.01.043

Wagner, G., Berger, G., Sinnreich, U., Grylli, V., Schober, E., Huber, W. D., & Karwautz, A. (2008). Quality of life in adolescents with treated coeliac disease: Influence of compliance and age at diagnosis. *Journal of Pediatric Gastroenterology and Nutrition, 47*(5), 555–561. https://doi.org/10.1097/MPG.0b013e31817fcb56

Werbrouck, A., Swinnen, E., Kerckhofs, E., Buyl, R., Beckwée, D., & De Wit, L. (2018). How to empower patients? A systematic review and meta-analysis. *Translational Behavioral Medicine, 8*(5), 660–674. https://doi.org/10.1093/tbm/iby064

29

Hirschsprung's Disease

Craig L. Frisby

Hirschsprung's disease (HD) is a congenital disorder characterized by a lack of nerve cells (i.e., ganglion cells) in a portion of the colon of variable length (Kenny et al., 2010). During normal development, nerve cells start growing at the beginning of the bowel and grow toward the end of the bowel. Prior to birth, however, nerve cells may stop growing. In HD, the nerve cells do not reach the end of the baby's bowel. As a result, stool elimination fails to work properly after birth.

ETIOLOGY

This condition of the lack of ganglion cells is called *aganglionosis* (Kenny et al., 2010). Most often, the areas missing the nerve cells are the rectum and the sigmoid (S-shaped) colon. In short-segment HD, nerve cells are missing from the last part of the large intestine. In long-segment HD, nerve cells are missing from most or all of the large intestine and sometimes the last part of the small intestine. In rarer cases, nerve cells are missing in the entire large and small intestine (National Institute of Diabetes and Digestive and Kidney Diseases [NIDDKD], 2015).

https://doi.org/10.1037/0000349-029
Health-Related Disorders in Children and Adolescents: A Guidebook for Educators and Service Providers, Second Edition, M. M. Perfect, C. A. Riccio, and M. A. Bray (Editors)

PREVALENCE AND INCIDENCE

HD occurs in approximately one in 5,000 newborns (Kenny et al., 2010). Notably, one recent survey of HD prevalence rates in California between 1995 and 2013 found significant racial/ethnic differences in prevalence rates, with the highest rates among African Americans and Asian/Pacific Islanders (Anderson et al., 2018). HD also has a skewed gender distribution, with a female-to-male ratio of 1:4 (Granéli et al., 2017). Having one child with HD increases the chances of having more children with HD. In addition, a parent who has HD has a greater chance of having a child with HD compared with a parent without HD (Kenny et al., 2010).

SYMPTOMS

In a child with HD, the stool moves through the small and large intestines until it reaches the part of the intestine that lacks nerve cells. At that point, the movement of the stool slows significantly or stops altogether. Symptoms of HD are first noted as bowel obstruction in the days after birth, and the condition is fatal if left untreated. With HD, the intestine becomes blocked with stool, and the child will be constipated and will fail to have a first bowel movement within 48 hours after birth (NIDDKD, 2015). Other infant symptoms may include brown or green vomit, explosive stools after a doctor inserts a finger into the newborn's rectum, swelling of the abdomen, diarrhea with blood, growth failure, and/or unexplained fevers (NIDDKD, 2015). Symptoms of HD that may occur in toddlers and older children include a failure to pass stools without enemas or suppositories.

IMPACT ON THE STUDENT AND OUTCOMES

There are no known cognitive or academic impacts of HD. The following section covers medical and social–emotional impacts affecting children.

Medical

A general practitioner who suspects HD may refer the child to a pediatric gastroenterologist (i.e., a doctor who specializes in digestive diseases in children). The gastroenterologist diagnoses HD from a physical exam; a medical and family history; and test results from a rectal biopsy, an abdominal X-ray, an anorectal manometry (i.e., a test that measures how well a child's rectum is working), and an X-ray of the lower gastrointestinal series (NIDDKD, 2015).

Children with HD typically do not respond to constipation medicines taken orally. Because HD is life threatening, it requires surgery. The most common medical procedure for treating patients with HD is called the *pull-through procedure* (Boston Children's Hospital, 2019). The goal is to remove the diseased section of the child's intestine and then pull the healthy portion of the intestine down to the anus. In a majority of cases, the pull-through procedure can be performed in a single operation with minimally invasive techniques. Although a pull-through procedure can be performed by entering the patient through the abdomen or the anus, over time the latter has become more popular and has shown better follow-up results (Gosemann et al., 2013).

A smaller percentage of children with HD have symptoms that are sufficiently severe to warrant a colostomy (i.e., a surgical operation in which a piece of the colon is diverted to an artificial opening in the abdominal wall so as to bypass a damaged part of the colon). In the event that a colostomy is performed, the intestines will work as they did before the operation; however, the colon and rectum (normal storage area for the stool) may be disconnected or removed (American Cancer Society, 2019). A removable external collection pouch, called an ostomy pouch or ostomy appliance, is attached to the opening in the abdomen and worn outside the body to collect the stool.

The ostomy procedure may be temporary or permanent. The temporary ostomy procedure may be performed as a prelude to a pull-through procedure, and the child will undergo a second surgery to close the ostomy and reattach the intestine. When a long segment of the bowel is missing nerve cells or when the child has repeated episodes of bowel inflammation, then a permanent ostomy procedure is required (NIDDKD, 2015).

Even though surgery for HD may be successful, incontinence (i.e., loss of ability to control liquid or solid stools) may still occur due to sphincter damage at the time of the surgery, loss of sensation, or overflow due to long-lasting constipation (Norton, 2008).

Medical concerns are not limited to elimination issues. Because factors that are involved in the migration of cells during the development of HD also may affect the migration of cells associated with other anomalies, HD has been known to co-occur in 4% to 35% of cases of sensorineural deafness, cardiovascular skeletal and limb anomalies, cleft palate, mental retardation, undescended testes, and microcephaly (Kenny et al., 2010).

Part of the job of the large intestine is to absorb water. Some nutritional and dietary changes are designed to counteract the effects of HD surgery. Infants may require a feeding tube (passed through the nose), which serves as a passageway to receive formula or liquid food directly into the stomach or small intestine, and the doctor may recommend a more permanent feeding tube that is surgically placed in the child's abdomen. If a child has an ostomy and part of the child's colon is removed, then they will need to drink more liquids to make up for water loss and prevent dehydration. In addition, these children require twice as much salt intake as a healthy child does (NIDDK, 2015).

Social-Emotional and Behavioral

If a child with HD undergoes a pull-through surgical procedure or a temporary/permanent ostomy, they will need sufficient time to adjust to the new structure of their intestine. Infants will be able to pass gas and stool more easily. Most children feel significantly better after surgery, although some may experience complications (e.g., narrowing of the anus, constipation, diarrhea, leaking of stool from the anus, delayed toilet training, inflammation of the colon). When the colon becomes inflamed (called enterocolitis), doctors can prescribe a special antibiotic to be taken orally. In other cases, the doctor must insert a small amount of salt water into the child's rectum and allow it to come back out (called rectal irrigation).

Older children who have undergone an ostomy must learn to properly take care of the surgical opening in the abdomen, as well as how to change the ostomy pouch. These children can lead a relatively normal life with minimal lifestyle changes; however, some may experience natural anxieties around feeling different from their friends. Daily functional issues related to HD can lead to impaired social acceptance, social relations, and psychosocial development. Observable soiling evokes revulsion from peers, parents, and caregivers, which in turn can lead to frequent shaming, blaming, and punishment for a condition that is largely beyond the child's control (see the review by Friman et al., 2006).

PSYCHOEDUCATIONAL IMPLICATIONS AND SCHOOL-BASED INTERVENTIONS

Medical and Health Management

As noted previously, HD has been known to occur in 4% to 35% of cases of sensorineural deafness, cardiovascular skeletal and limb anomalies, cleft palate, mental retardation, undescended testes, and microcephaly (Kenny et al., 2010).

The primary physician for a child with HD is the most important medical professional with whom school professionals should consult about school-based interventions or accommodations. Physicians are intimately familiar with the physical effects of postoperative procedures, the care and management of ostomy pouches, the use of stool softeners and laxatives, and dietary issues.

School professionals can enlist the help of the child's physician by asking them to write a letter to the school (Norton, 2008). The letter would explain that the student has a gastrointestinal disorder that may require them to use the bathroom more frequently and often suddenly, with little warning. The school professional can then work with the classroom teacher to work out a system where the student can go to the bathroom without asking or drawing attention to themselves. Alternatively, school professionals can work out times when the student can use a bathroom when other students are unlikely to be there in order to reduce the potential for embarrassment. Having a plan in place can make strides in reducing the child's anxiety about their condition within the school context.

Social-Emotional and Behavioral

Suggestions from the research literature on how to address psychoeducational conditions related to HD are framed within the context of the more general issue of how to respond to involuntary *functional encopresis* (FE; Friman et al., 2006; also sometimes called *functional defecation*; Beaudry-Bellefeuille et al., 2017). According to the fifth edition of the *Diagnostic and Statistical Manual of Mental Disorders* (American Psychiatric Association, 2013), FE is defined as the repeated (and usually involuntary) passage of feces into inappropriate places (e.g., into clothing or on the floor) by a child who is at least 4 years of age (or at an equivalent level of development). The diagnosis would be made if this occurs at least once a month for 3 months.

In schools, the elements of successful intervention for soiling problems include a proper assessment, which includes a review of the child's medical history, toileting habits, eating habits, and bowel movements with the parent or other significant caregiver, with particular attention to symptoms of constipation.

Friman et al. (2006) recommended a demystifying of the elimination process, where the teacher, school psychologist, school counselor, or other school professional should meet jointly with both the parent/caregiver and child. In this joint meeting, the school professional communicates optimism about intervention outcomes, employs a diagram of abnormal bowel functioning when discussing bodily functions, reinforces clearly that these problems are not the child's fault, and discourages any punitive responses to the child from the parent/caregiver. Most toileting interventions prescribed for FE require constant adult monitoring and prescribed regular defecation attempts, regardless of whether the child feels an urge to defecate, particularly after surgery to correct HD problems. Sometimes this can only happen through enrollment in an outpatient or inpatient behavioral treatment program where treatment can be monitored by nurse practitioners and/or behavioral psychologists (e.g., see Hankinson et al., 2018).

As a result, Friman et al. (2006) urged caution in recommending intensive toileting-related interventions that need to occur during school hours. Sometimes, a knowledgeable and sensitive school professional, who is familiar with postoperative HD conditions, can assist parents and caregivers with home-based interventions. Specifically, school professionals can assist parents/caregivers with (a) setting up a consistent home schedule for frequent monitoring of bowel movements; (b) helping the child feel maximally comfortable, relaxed, pleasant, and private when defecating at home; (c) helping caregivers give positive feedback for bowel movements and nonjudgmental instructions for cleaning oneself after accidents; and (d) how to ensure that (per physician instructions) the child's diet is rich in fiber.

There may be situations where families affected by HD need to access articles and research studies that discuss specific behaviors related to defecation problems. These can include, but are not limited to, manifestations of pain or fear when defecating or experiencing the urge to defecate, refusing to use the school toilet and only preferring the home toilet, not being upset by soiling behaviors, or hiding soiled underwear from adults. Readers are encouraged to consult Beaudry-Bellefeuille et al. (2017) for a thorough inventory of such specific behaviors and a directory of research studies tailored to each.

CONCLUSION

HD is an unfortunate congenital malady involving the inability to properly pass stool. HD can be diagnosed early and treated effectively with surgery, although postoperative outcomes can vary due to any number of associated factors. With close consultation between the child's primary physician and school personnel, the school experience of a child with HD can be relatively normal.

RESOURCES

National Organization for Rare Disorders. (2017). *Hirschsprung disease.* https://rarediseases.org/rare-diseases/hirschsprungs-disease/

Pediatric Colorectal and Pelvic Learning Consortium. (n.d.). *Resources for patients and families.* https://www.pcplc.org/newpage16c7f0d4

REFERENCES

American Cancer Society. (2019, October). *What is a colostomy?* https://www.cancer.org/treatment/treatments-and-side-effects/physical-side-effects/ostomies/colostomy/what-is-colostomy.html

American Psychiatric Association. (2013). *Diagnostic and statistical manual of mental disorders* (5th ed.). https://doi.org/10.1176/appi.books.9780890425596

Anderson, J. E., Vanover, M. A., Saadai, P., Stark, R. A., Stephenson, J. T., & Hirose, S. (2018). Epidemiology of Hirschsprung disease in California from 1995 to 2013. *Pediatric Surgery International, 34*(12), 1299–1303. https://doi.org/10.1007/s00383-018-4363-9

Beaudry-Bellefeuille, I., Booth, D., & Lane, S. J. (2017). Defecation-specific behavior in children with functional defecation issues: A systematic review. *The Permanente Journal, 21*(4), Article 17-047. https://doi.org/10.7812/TPP/17-047

Boston Children's Hospital. (2019). *Pull-through procedure for Hirschsprung's disease.* http://www.childrenshospital.org/conditions-and-treatments/treatments/pull-through-procedure

Friman, P. C., Hofstadter, K. L., & Jones, K. M. (2006). A biobehavioral approach to the treatment of functional encopresis in children. *Journal of Early and Intensive Behavior Intervention, 3*(3), 263–272. https://doi.org/10.1037/h0100340

Gosemann, J. H., Friedmacher, F., Ure, B., & Lacher, M. (2013). Open versus transanal pull-through for Hirschsprung disease: A systematic review of long-term outcome. *European Journal of Pediatric Surgery, 23*(2), 94–102. https://doi.org/10.1055/s-0033-1343085

Granéli, C., Dahlin, E., Börjesson, A., Arnbjörnsson, E., & Stenström, P. (2017). Diagnosis, symptoms, and outcomes of Hirschsprung's disease from the perspective of gender. *Surgery Research and Practice, 2017,* Article 9274940. https://doi.org/10.1155/2017/9274940

Hankinson, J. C., Borden, L., Allen, T., Santo Domingo, L., Oliva-Hemker, M., Mathews, T., Brock, K., Perry-Parrish, C., Reynolds, E. K., Specht, M., & Ostrander, R. (2018). Outcomes of combined medical and behavioral treatments for constipation within a specialty outpatient clinic. *Clinical Practice in Pediatric Psychology, 6*(1), 31–41. https://doi.org/10.1037/cpp0000202

Kenny, S. E., Tam, P. K., & Garcia-Barcelo, M. (2010). Hirschsprung's disease. *Seminars in Pediatric Surgery, 19*(3), 194–200. https://doi.org/10.1053/j.sempedsurg.2010.03.004

National Institute of Diabetes and Digestive and Kidney Diseases. (2015, September). *Hirschsprung disease.* U.S. Department of Health and Human Services. https://www.niddk.nih.gov/health-information/digestive-diseases/hirschsprung-disease

Norton, W. F. (2008). An overview of bowel incontinence: What can go wrong? *Exceptional Parent, 38*(9), 67–69. https://eric.ed.gov/?id=EJ810570

30

Inflammatory Bowel Disease: Crohn's Disease and Ulcerative Colitis

Stevie Puckett-Perez and Chelsea Vaughan

Inflammatory bowel disease (IBD) is a term for conditions characterized by symptoms of chronic inflammation and ulceration of the gastrointestinal tract, diarrhea, intestinal bleeding, vomiting, malabsorption of nutrients, and abdominal pain. Although gastrointestinal symptoms compose the primary presentation of the disease, individuals with IBD may also experience chronic fatigue, joint pains, weight loss, fever, skin changes, and delayed physical and sexual development. IBD is a chronic disease requiring lifelong treatment, with implications across all areas of functioning. The two most common types of IBD are Crohn's disease and ulcerative colitis, which are differentiated based on the location and depth of affected tissue. IBD should not be confused with or compared with irritable bowel syndrome, which is a very common functional gastrointestinal disorder involving bowel changes and discomfort and does not have the same severe disease correlates and sequelae.

ETIOLOGY

The etiology of IBD is not yet fully understood, but it is thought to be multifactorial and polygenic, in that the interaction between genetic susceptibility, gut microbiome, immune responses, and environmental triggers affects disease onset and outcomes. More than 160 genes are implicated in IBD, and researchers have identified numerous gene variants associated with reduced immunity, increased permeability of mucosal barriers, and abnormal autophagy (destruction and

https://doi.org/10.1037/0000349-030
Health-Related Disorders in Children and Adolescents: A Guidebook for Educators and Service Providers, Second Edition, M. M. Perfect, C. A. Riccio, and M. A. Bray (Editors)

renewal of cells). IBD is most often characterized as an overactive immune response that ultimately leads to chronic inflammation in the gut. Resultant changes in gut microbiota can subsequently increase host vulnerability to environmental triggers, which may include environmental toxins, viral illnesses, or food sensitivities (Knights et al., 2013).

PREVALENCE AND INCIDENCE

According to the most recent data reported by the Centers for Disease Control and Prevention (CDC) as part of the 2015 National Health Interview Survey, IBD affects an estimated 3.1 million Americans, which is approximately 1.3% of the population (Dahlhamer et al., 2016). Approximately one in four individuals with IBD are diagnosed before the age of 18 (Benchimol et al., 2011). The incidence of pediatric IBD is increasing worldwide, with high-population, developing countries being especially affected, possibly due to population exposure to environmental toxins that are not well regulated (Hanauer, 2006).

SYMPTOMS

The path to diagnosis of IBD may begin with patient complaints of disruptive or painful gastrointestinal symptoms that require further medical workup involving the use of endoscopic procedures and imaging studies to confirm diagnosis. In very young children, chronic diarrhea, frequent crying and distress, failure to thrive, and perianal disease may indicate the need for further testing for IBD. Although Crohn's disease and ulcerative colitis tend to share symptoms of inflammation, diarrhea, abdominal pain, and weight loss, individuals with Crohn's are more likely to present with systemic symptoms such as joint pain, eye inflammation, and skin lesions, whereas symptoms of ulcerative colitis tend to be isolated to the gastrointestinal tract (Waugh et al., 2013).

IMPACT ON THE STUDENT AND OUTCOMES

Medical

In most cases, IBD is chronic and incurable. Most patients with IBD experience lifelong episodic exacerbations of disease activity (flares) followed by periods of remission. The aims of IBD treatment are symptom management, prevention of complications, and prolonged periods of remission. Treatment recommendations may include pharmacotherapy, lifestyle interventions such as dietary changes and stress management, and surgery. Pharmacotherapy is effective for symptom reduction in most individuals; however, side effects, which can include fatigue, weight gain, facial swelling, joint pain, and reduced immunity, can be extreme. Surgical intervention to remove affected tissues in the digestive tract (resections) may be part of treatment for some individuals, whereas others may require placement of an ostomy pouching system, which involves surgical diversion of waste into an external pouch. Ostomies may be temporary or permanent.

Cognitive/Academic

There is no evidence that IBD directly affects cognitive functioning; however, students with IBD are more likely to have difficulties in school functioning due to increased absences secondary to illness exacerbations and frequent medical visits. In addition, when in class, students with IBD may experience fatigue, pain, and frequent urge to stool, which can have practical implications for their ability to focus and learn. To this end, students often report that they have difficulty attending to and retaining information learned in class due to exhaustion, internal physical sensations competing for their attention, and stress or worry related to feeling that they are lagging behind their peers.

Social-Emotional and Behavioral

Children with IBD are at increased risk for psychopathology, reduced health-related quality of life (HRQOL), and poorer family and social functioning in comparison to healthy peers (Mackner et al., 2013). Later age of diagnosis is associated with increased risk for mood disorders. This may be due to the fact that, when diagnosed in earlier childhood, IBD becomes an accepted part of the child's life, whereas a later diagnosis creates more disruption, leading to potential anxiety or depression.

Pediatric IBD patients are significantly more likely to experience reduced HRQOL as compared with healthy children. Youth with active and/or severe disease endorse lower scores on HRQOL domains relative to healthy peers (Kunz et al., 2010). Notably, scores in the domain of "school functioning" on HRQOL measures are generally lower for children with IBD relative to youth with other chronic illnesses.

Youth with IBD also report greater social difficulties relative to same-age peers. Mackner et al. (2006) reported that 22% of children with IBD had difficulties with social competence, as compared with 6% of healthy children. In this vein, children and adolescents with IBD report more difficulties with peer interaction, which may occur secondary to social isolation during flares and less frequent involvement in sports or other extracurricular activities that promote social development.

Body image issues are another frequently cited area of concern for individuals with IBD. Female patients are more likely than male patients to report body image dissatisfaction in the wake of an IBD diagnosis. Higher rates of body image dissatisfaction are reported for youth with older median age, older age of diagnosis, higher rates of active disease, higher steroid use, and higher rates of depression and anxiety (Claytor et al., 2018). Additionally, IBD can impact physical and sexual development, and pharmacotherapy can cause weight gain and observable facial swelling.

PSYCHOEDUCATIONAL IMPLICATIONS AND SCHOOL-BASED INTERVENTIONS

Medical and Health Management

It is particularly helpful for educators working with students with IBD to have an understanding of the illness and its chronic, relapsing and remitting nature. School personnel, including administrators, should be aware of the numerous limitations faced by students with IBD. These students are likely to need support for managing special medical needs, including medication administration, toileting needs, dietary accommodations, and fatigue or discomfort.

One accommodation that proves to be particularly helpful is the provision of an unlimited pass to the nurse's office. Students may frequently need the services of the school nurse for daily or as-needed medications or assessment of fatigue, pain, or other discomforts that might mandate a rest break or additional medical care. Additionally, students with IBD will almost certainly need more frequent restroom visits than their peers due to bowel urgency or ostomy care; thus, an unlimited bathroom pass is recommended as well. Some students may have special materials to use to support toileting (e.g., wipes, skin creams, ostomy care supplies, spare clothing as needed) and may feel more comfortable using a private restroom. When available, use of a single-stall restroom is preferred so that students may have the comfort of privacy and the ability to store supplies as needed. If a younger student has an ostomy, they may need support from a nurse or aide to help with emptying or changing their bag, caring for their stoma, or dealing with complications such as leaks. Students with IBD may also have special dietary requirements that require accommodation, such as restricting certain food types or being allowed opportunities to eat more frequently. Allowing students to bring safe snacks that they can access as needed can be helpful, as is having a readily available record of their food restrictions so that alternatives can be provided as necessary.

Students with IBD can usually participate in the same activities as other children; however, students with IBD may get fatigued more easily and may require activity modifications such as frequent rest breaks or, in some cases, exemption from physical education requirements altogether. Each student's needs vary greatly, and it is recommended that parents, physicians, and the students themselves advocate for appropriate educational planning according to their disease and symptom severity.

Cognitive/Academic

Although students with IBD typically have normal cognitive profiles and intact academic ability, frequent absences for medical appointments and disease flares have a notable effect on school life. Additionally, children with IBD are likely to struggle with fatigue and discomfort, which can affect their ability to focus and learn. The Crohn's and Colitis Foundation recommends that youth with IBD have education plans in place that highlight academic accommodations, such as stop-the-clock testing, options to make up missed class time without penalty, additional time on assignments, tutoring after absences, and full participation in extracurricular activities despite absence rates. During periods of worsened disease, students may require hospitalization or extended absences from school, in which case homebound services should be given strong consideration. Disease flares can happen on multiple occasions throughout the school year; thus, having a plan in place to initiate services quickly so as to not lose valuable learning time is particularly important (Carreon et al., 2018).

Social-Emotional and Behavioral

School faculty can play a vital role in helping students with IBD adjust to the demands of school, navigate social difficulties, and receive support for mood or adjustment challenges. Due to frequent absences and symptoms, students are at risk of feeling behind or different from their peers, and they may have a reduced sense of belonging in their school environment. This sense of otherness can worsen psychosocial outcomes (Muse et al., 2021). One way of combating this problem is to establish a trusted adult who can act as a mentor or student liaison on campus. The CDC's (2017) research brief for supporting students with chronic illness in the school setting recommends identifying faculty in the school to be the point person for the child and family; these mentors may be responsible for checking in with the student frequently, getting updates from the family when the student is out, supporting the student in problem solving challenges as they arise, and facilitating communication between the school and family as needed to make for a smoother school experience.

Students with IBD may have a range of preferences concerning how much or how little information about their diagnosis should be shared with peers. It is recommended that educators and faculty follow students' lead and take care not to inadvertently share private information or force students to share information by asking questions or making illness-related comments in front of peers. However, many students *do* want peers to know about their illness and may struggle with how to share this information. With the permission of students with IBD and their parents, teachers or counselors may wish to provide disease-specific education to the students' peers, with the aim of facilitating open discussion about IBD in order to normalize disease symptoms and to decrease students' sense of social isolation (e.g., assuring peers that IBD is not a contagious illness).

Although most students with IBD are able to continue to thrive in the school setting after diagnosis, up to 60% may experience mood or adjustment challenges related to their illness, including anxiety, depression, and body image issues. Having a counselor or school psychologist available to periodically monitor these students can help facilitate timely support and treatment. Therapeutic interventions, such as cognitive behavior therapy, acceptance and commitment therapy, and general supportive and reflective listening in the spirit of unconditional positive regard, can be helpful (Levy et al., 2016; Parmar et al., 2021). If these resources are not available in the school setting, faculty may provide the families referrals for further treatment. Faculty may also help students and their families to identify other supportive resources such as local support groups, local chapters of the Crohn's and Colitis Foundation, and IBD-themed camps (e.g., Camp Oasis in the United States) or facilitate communication among peers with IBD who are open to sharing information.

CONCLUSION

Overall, children and adolescents with IBD are more likely to have compromised psychosocial functioning in areas of mood, HRQOL, school functioning, social functioning, and body image relative to their same-age peers. Educators are well positioned to partner with students, families, and medical providers in maximizing the school experience for children with IBD.

RESOURCES

Crohn's and Colitis Foundation. https://www.crohnscolitisfoundation.org/

Crohn's and Colitis Foundation. (n.d.). *Information about IBD.* https://www.crohnscolitisfoundation.org/justlikeme

Crohn's and Colitis Foundation. (2022). *504 accommodation plan.* https://www.crohnscolitisfoundation.org/504-accommodation-plan

Crohn's and Colitis Foundation IBD Help Center. 888-MY-GUT-PAIN (888-694-8872)

Crohn's and Colitis Foundation. (n.d.). *Camp Oasis: A summer camp for youth with IBD.* https://www.crohnscolitisfoundation.org/get-involved/camp-oasis

REFERENCES

Benchimol, E. I., Fortinsky, K. J., Gozdyra, P., Van den Heuvel, M., Van Limbergen, J., & Griffiths, A. M. (2011). Epidemiology of pediatric inflammatory bowel disease: A systematic review of international trends. *Inflammatory Bowel Diseases, 17*(1), 423–439. https://doi.org/10.1002/ibd.21349

Carreon, S. A., Bugno, L. T., Wojtowicz, A. A., & Greenley, R. N. (2018). School functioning in adolescents with inflammatory bowel diseases: An examination of disease and demographic correlates. *Inflammatory Bowel Diseases, 24*(8), 1624–1631. https://doi.org/10.1093/ibd/izy026

Centers for Disease Control and Prevention. (2017). *Research brief: Addressing the needs of students with chronic health conditions: Strategies for schools.* https://www.cdc.gov/healthyschools/chronic_conditions/pdfs/2017_02_15-How-Schools-Can-Students-with-CHC_Final_508.pdf

Claytor, J., Kochar, B., Kappelman, M., Martin, C. F., Robb, A., & Long, M. D. (2018). Body image dissatisfaction in pediatric patients with inflammatory bowel diseases. *Gastroenterology, 154*(1 Suppl.), S8–S9. https://doi.org/10.1053/j.gastro.2017.11.047

Dahlhamer, J. M., Zammitti, E. P., Ward, B. W., Wheaton, A. G., & Croft, J. B. (2016). Prevalence of inflammatory bowel disease among adults aged ≥18 years—United States, 2015. *Morbidity and Mortality Weekly Report, 65*(42), 1166–1169. https://doi.org/10.15585/mmwr.mm6542a3

Hanauer, S. B. (2006). Inflammatory bowel disease: Epidemiology, pathogenesis, and therapeutic opportunities. *Inflammatory Bowel Diseases, 12*(Suppl. 1), S3–S9. https://doi.org/10.1097/01.MIB.0000195385.19268.68

Knights, D., Lassen, K. G., & Xavier, R. J. (2013). Advances in inflammatory bowel disease pathogenesis: Linking host genetics and the microbiome. *Gut, 62*(10), 1505–1510. https://doi.org/10.1136/gutjnl-2012-303954

Kunz, J. H., Hommel, K. A., & Greenley, R. N. (2010). Health-related quality of life of youth with inflammatory bowel disease: A comparison with published data using the PedsQL 4.0 generic core scales. *Inflammatory Bowel Diseases, 16*(6), 939–946. https://doi.org/10.1002/ibd.21128

Levy, R. L., van Tilburg, M. A. L., Langer, S. L., Romano, J. M., Walker, L. S., Mancl, L. A., Murphy, T. B., Claar, R. L., Feld, S. I., Christie, D. L., Abdullah, B., DuPen, M. M., Swanson, K. S., Baker, M. D., Stoner, S. A., & Whitehead, W. E. (2016). Effects of a cognitive behavioral therapy intervention trial to improve disease outcomes in children with inflammatory bowel disease. *Inflammatory Bowel Diseases, 22*(9), 2134–2148. https://doi.org/10.1097/MIB.0000000000000881

Mackner, L. M., Crandall, W. V., & Szigethy, E. M. (2006). Psychosocial functioning in pediatric inflammatory bowel disease. *Inflammatory Bowel Diseases, 12*(3), 239–244. https://doi.org/10.1097/01.MIB.0000217769.83142.c6

Mackner, L. M., Greenley, R. N., Szigethy, E., Herzer, M., Deer, K., & Hommel, K. A. (2013). Psychosocial issues in pediatric inflammatory bowel disease: Report of the North American Society for Pediatric Gastroenterology, Hepatology, and Nutrition. *Journal of Pediatric Gastroenterology and Nutrition, 56*(4), 449–458. https://doi.org/10.1097/MPG.0b013e3182841263

Muse, K., Johnson, E., & David, A. L. (2021). A feeling of otherness: A qualitative research synthesis exploring the lived experiences of stigma in individuals with inflammatory bowel disease. *International Journal of Environmental Research and Public Health, 18*(15), Article 8038. https://doi.org/10.3390/ijerph18158038

Parmar, A., Esser, K., Barreira, L., Miller, D., Morinis, L., Chong, Y.-Y., Smith, W., Major, N., Church, P., Cohen, E., & Orkin, J. (2021). Acceptance and commitment therapy for children with special health care needs and their parents: A systematic review and meta-analysis. *International Journal of Environmental Research and Public Health, 18*(15), Article 8205. https://doi.org/10.3390/ijerph18158205

Waugh, N., Cummins, E., Royle, P., Kandala, N. B., Shyangdan, D., Arasaradnam, R., Clar, C., & Johnston, R. (2013). Faecal calprotectin testing for differentiating amongst inflammatory and noninflammatory bowel diseases: Systematic review and economic evaluation. *Health Technology Assessment, 17*(55), 1–211. https://doi.org/10.3310/hta17550

31

Phenylketonuria

Julia Ogg and Dan Strissel

Phenylketonuria (PKU) is the most common of the generally rare disorders caused by inborn errors of metabolism (Blau et al., 2010). With PKU, individuals are limited in their capacity to produce the enzyme phenylalanine hydroxylase (PAH), resulting in dangerous concentrations of the essential amino acid phenylalanine (Phe) in the blood and brain (Blau et al., 2010). Without early intervention, the resulting neurotoxicity can lead to developmental delay, intellectual disability, and adverse psychosocial outcomes (MacDonald et al., 2010).

ETIOLOGY

Recent changes in the nomenclature of PKU recognized that there is a continuum of PAH deficiencies. These range from individuals with *classical PKU,* which refers to the most severe form of PAH deficiency, resulting in impaired Phe levels when left untreated, to those individuals with higher blood Phe levels than normal (but not as severe as PKU), which is referred to as *hyperphenylalaninemia* (National Institutes of Health Consensus Development Panel, 2001). Thus, PKU is considered a severe form of PAH deficiency. PKU is caused by an inborn error of metabolism (Blau et al., 2010). Inborn errors of metabolism are genetic disorders in which enzymes in the body fail to metabolize food (i.e., convert food into energy). In the case of PKU, mutations of the *PAH* gene limit its ability to produce PAH, an enzyme that is

https://doi.org/10.1037/0000349-031
Health-Related Disorders in Children and Adolescents: A Guidebook for Educators and Service Providers, Second Edition, M. M. Perfect, C. A. Riccio, and M. A. Bray (Editors)

required to metabolize Phe to tyrosine, an amino acid necessary for the production of dopamine and serotonin (de Sonneville et al., 2011). When PAH cannot convert Phe, dangerous concentrations are left to accumulate in the blood and brain (Blau et al., 2010).

In addition to the deficient production of neurotransmitters like dopamine and serotonin, hypomyelination and demyelination are common neuropathological markers among treated and untreated PKU patients (Dyer, 1999). Myelin is a lipid-rich substance that insulates and sheathes nerve fibers to increase impulse transmission and protect them from damage (Miller et al., 2012). The connectivity that myelination establishes is critical in the developing brain, facilitating the rapid synchronization of information transfer across neural systems, a crucial process for higher order cognition (Miller et al., 2012). Evidence supports that Phe exerts its neurotoxic effects via direct inhibition of the cholesterol metabolism in the oligodendrocyte, a neuroglial cell responsible for myelin production (Dyer, 1999). PKU follows an autosomal recessive inheritance pattern (National Institutes of Health Consensus Development Panel, 2001). For a child to inherit PKU, both parents must pass on a mutated copy of the PAH gene. Thus, for two parents who are carriers of the PAH gene, there is a one in four chance that the child will develop PKU. There is also a 50% chance that one of the parents will pass on a defective PAH gene to their child; that child will be a nonaffected carrier of PKU.

PREVALENCE AND INCIDENCE

Overall, the worldwide incidence of PKU is approximately one in 10,000 (Gundorova et al., 2018). However, frequencies of monogenic diseases like PKU can differ greatly across regions and among various ethnic groups (Gundorova et al., 2018). For example, in the Karachay-Cherkess Republic of Russia, the estimated incidence of PKU is one in 850, the highest in the world (Gundorova et al., 2018), whereas in Japan, the incidence is far lower at one in 125,000. The prevalence rate of PKU in the United States closely approximates the worldwide incidence rate. Between 1991 and 2001 in the United States, the overall birth prevalence of classical PKU and significant hyperphenylalaninemia was one in 11,400 (Hertzberg et al., 2011).

SYMPTOMS

The severity of symptoms of PKU is linked with the levels of Phe in the blood and brain (Blau et al., 2010), such that higher concentrations of Phe are typically related to worse symptoms. Absent intervention, the resulting neurotoxicity can lead to developmental delay, intellectual disability, and adverse psychosocial outcomes (MacDonald et al., 2010). These include elevated levels of psychiatric symptoms, especially anxiety and depression, as well as attention problems. Additional symptoms may include autism, seizures, and motor deficits (Blau et al., 2010).

IMPACT ON THE STUDENT AND OUTCOMES

Although the symptoms and outcomes are much less severe for individuals who are treated early, a pattern of cognitive, social, and emotional outcomes may emerge to a lesser extent for individuals who maintain treatment and to a greater extent for those individuals who lose dietary control as they get older.

Medical

PKU may result in microcephaly (i.e., abnormally small head), speech delays or absent speech, skin rashes, lightly pigmented skin, a musty odor, and seizures (de Baulny et al., 2007; Kaye & Committee on Genetics, 2006).

Cognitive/Academic

PKU's neurotoxicity can lead to developmental delay and subsequent intellectual disability without early intervention. At the same time, research has suggested significant variation in cognitive ability among individuals with PKU. For instance, levels of intellectual functioning have been shown to correlate with levels and stability of Phe, which vary widely across individuals with PKU (Anastasoaie et al., 2008; Romani et al., 2017). One study found that almost 98% of the early-diagnosed patients had average IQs, whereas almost half of the late-diagnosed patients had significant cognitive impairments (González et al., 2011). Visual and verbal learning has also been found to be mildly impaired in children with early-treated PKU. White et al. (2001) found that children with early-treated PKU showed poorer learning and were less likely to employ an effective verbal memory strategy (e.g., semantic clustering) than controls. Anderson et al. (2007) showed that in addition to overall lower levels of IQ, attention, and information processing, children with early-treated PKU were less efficient than controls in their learning of visual designs.

Youth with PKU may experience neurocognitive impairments even with early intervention. One primary area of impairment is executive functioning (Christ et al., 2010). Although prior research has demonstrated that working memory is affected in some adults, these results are not as strong in youth with early-treated PKU, suggesting that this impairment may emerge through aging. In contrast, on measures of inhibitory control, individuals with PKU, including children with early-treated PKU, are likely to display a deficit (Christ et al., 2010). In addition to laboratory-based executive function tasks, studies using rating scales of executive functioning have suggested that youth with PKU experience difficulties with executive functioning in their daily life (Christ et al., 2010).

Social-Emotional and Behavioral

Behavioral challenges are also seen with PKU, such as hyperactivity and signs of autism or schizophrenia (de Baulny et al., 2007). Since adopting early dietary treatment, the social, emotional, and psychological impairments associated with PKU have lessened. Among youth with PKU, findings suggest an increased likelihood of attention problems, depression, anxiety, and low self-esteem (Vockley et al., 2014). Some research suggests that the behavioral profile is similar to attention-deficit/hyperactivity disorder, including a short attention span, low frustration tolerance, difficulty concentrating, hyperactivity, and fidgeting (Vockley et al., 2014). Youth with PKU have shown lower quality social skills, with the level of impairment tied to Phe levels (Jahja et al., 2016). Generally, research has supported a connection between higher Phe levels and more detrimental social and emotional outcomes, with higher Phe levels during childhood and early adolescence predicting later functioning (Jahja et al., 2016).

Adolescence can be particularly challenging for youth with PKU. Loss of dietary control can occur, as adherence to a specialized diet at this time may be difficult due to adolescents striving for autonomy and seeking peer approval, as well as natural increases in rebellious behavior (Vockley et al., 2014). The loss of dietary control can result in changes in cognitive and developmental functioning (Vockley et al., 2014). Some complicating factors include emerging behaviors that occur with loss of dietary control, such as increasing challenges with executive functioning, which can make it increasingly difficult to monitor dietary consumption.

Beyond the maintenance of healthy Phe levels as adolescents transition to adulthood, another related and critical component of health for women is pregnancy. Elevated Phe levels can create teratogenic effects on the developing fetus, termed *maternal PKU syndrome*, and can result in fetal growth issues, heart defects, and intellectual disability (Vockley et al., 2014). Prevention of maternal PKU depends on control of Phe levels in utero, with higher Phe being related to more adverse effects (National Institutes of Health Consensus Development Panel, 2001).

PSYCHOEDUCATIONAL IMPLICATIONS AND SCHOOL-BASED INTERVENTIONS

Medical and Health Management

Newborn screening for PKU, implemented in the 1960s, has resulted in most individuals with PKU being identified at birth (Christ et al., 2010) and has allowed individuals to be placed on a low-Phe diet to prevent the levels of Phe from becoming toxic. High levels of Phe are found in protein-rich foods, including meat, fish, poultry, eggs, nuts, beans, dairy, and some artificial sweeteners. The low-Phe diet is mainly vegetarian and is aimed at providing sources of protein that are low in Phe. The low-Phe diet is also accompanied by supplementation with reduced or Phe-free amino acid mixtures, which are often referred to as formulas, to buffer the loss of protein and nutrients from the low-Phe diet. The goal is to maintain a Phe level below 2 to 6 mg/dL (Vockley et al., 2014). The levels of Phe and other essential nutrients are monitored through frequent blood testing (National Institutes of Health Consensus Development Panel, 2001). The restrictive nature of the diet and the expense associated with allowable foods and medical formulas can result in variable levels of adherence (Romani et al., 2017). Several recently developed medications are now available that also help regulate levels of Phe. However, the only medication currently approved by the U.S. Food and Drug Administration for PKU is sapropterin dihydrochloride, which can help the body break down Phe (Vockley et al., 2014). Unfortunately, fewer than half of patients with PAH deficiencies are responsive to this medication (Vockley et al., 2014).

In order to support youth with PKU, school professionals need to know the basics of PKU. Specifically, understanding the PKU diet and products high in Phe can help the child maintain dietary compliance in the school setting, which is critical to avoid the adverse effects of Phe. Implementing a 504 plan or individualized education program can facilitate communication regarding the needs of the students. Specific elements of an intervention plan will likely need to include coordination and supervision about the formula, coordination to ensure adequate storage (refrigerated if necessary), and supervision to ensure that the student consumes the formula in its entirety while at school. Communication is vital to track what has been eaten at school so daily protein can be calculated. In addition, communication about the food available through the lunch program at the school (e.g., menus sent home early, information about ingredients provided) can be given. Planning for special events at school where food will be served (e.g., parties, field trips) should also be considered. It is helpful for school professionals to be aware that until children are 12, it is recommended that Phe levels are monitored twice per month and then monthly after 12 years (National Institutes of Health Consensus Development Panel, 2001). In addition, it is recommended that dietary monitoring and blood testing be increasingly managed by the child (National Institutes of Health Consensus Development Panel, 2001), and school professionals could support parents in encouraging independence in these endeavors.

Cognitive/Academic

Concerns with executive functioning, primarily inhibitory control and working memory, and mild reductions in mental processing speed have been noted in individuals with PKU, even for early- and well-treated students (Gentile et al., 2010). Often, these subtle deficits in cognition contribute to difficulties in reading comprehension, work completion, and overall school performance (Gentile et al., 2010). School-based information, including classroom observational data from teachers, could provide important insights into how these deficits are contributing uniquely to students with PKU (Christ et al., 2010). In addition, for youth who have executive function difficulties, school professionals can implement intervention strategies (e.g., behavior management and academic interventions) to support learning. For example, teachers could help support visual or verbal learning deficits with graphic organizers, cognitive organizers, cognitive and concept maps, structured overviews, and tree diagrams. Reducing or eliminating time constraints on assessments and assignments would also likely be indicated, given this population's pattern of reduced processing speed (Anderson et al., 2007). Implementing a 504 plan or individualized education program, wherein professionals could document these and other student-specific strategies, is likely necessary to support cognitive and academic outcomes for youth who experience difficulties.

Social–Emotional and Behavioral

Given the increased incidence of behavioral and mental health concerns among youth with PKU, helping parents and teachers recognize the early warning signs is essential. Current guidelines recommend frequent monitoring of mental health concerns, including monitoring of executive functioning, internalizing and externalizing behaviors, and adaptive skills every 2 to 3 years or as needed (Vockley et al., 2014). School-based supports to intervene with these concerns may be warranted. Ongoing dietary management has been linked with more positive social–emotional and behavioral outcomes (Ashe et al., 2019), highlighting the importance of providing support at school to help youth maintain their dietary treatment as outlined previously. In addition, school professionals can provide interventions matched to the particular concerns (e.g., behavior management for externalizing challenges, cognitive and behavioral approaches to address internalizing concerns, skills training to support adaptive skill development).

Finally, families of children with PKU are likely to encounter elevated stress levels due to the supervisory demands of their child's nutritional needs and frequent medical appointments. The stress may be more impactful on parents of younger children with PKU (Bosch et al., 2015). School professionals can support parents by implementing the diet in the school setting, helping train school staff on the child's needs, and connecting the parents with resources on PKU.

CONCLUSION

PKU is a progressive disease that may result in developmental delay, intellectual disability, and adverse psychosocial outcomes. However, with dietary control, many of the adverse outcomes can be avoided. School professionals should work closely with families to support positive outcomes for youth with PKU.

RESOURCES

New England Consortium of Metabolic Programs. (n.d.). *Phenylketonuria (PKU)*. https://www.newenglandconsortium.org/phenylketonuria

Logue, J. C. (n.d.). *An educator's guide to PKU*. Boston Children's Hospital. https://www.newenglandconsortium.org/educators-pku

National PKU Alliance. https://www.npkua.org/

REFERENCES

Anastasoaie, V., Kurzius, L., Forbes, P., & Waisbren, S. (2008). Stability of blood phenylalanine levels and IQ in children with phenylketonuria. *Molecular Genetics and Metabolism, 95*(1–2), 17–20. https://doi.org/10.1016/j.ymgme.2008.06.014

Anderson, P. J., Wood, S. J., Francis, D. E., Coleman, L., Anderson, V., & Boneh, A. (2007). Are neuropsychological impairments in children with early-treated phenylketonuria (PKU) related to white matter abnormalities or elevated phenylalanine levels? *Developmental Neuropsychology, 32*(2), 645–668. https://doi.org/10.1080/87565640701375963

Ashe, K., Kelso, W., Farrand, S., Panetta, J., Fazio, T., De Jong, G., & Walterfang, M. (2019). Psychiatric and cognitive aspects of phenylketonuria: The limitations of diet and promise of new treatments. *Frontiers in Psychiatry, 10*, Article 561. https://doi.org/10.3389/fpsyt.2019.00561

Blau, N., van Spronsen, F. J., & Levy, H. L. (2010). Phenylketonuria. *The Lancet, 376*(9750), 1417–1427. https://doi.org/10.1016/S0140-6736(10)60961-0

Bosch, A. M., Burlina, A., Cunningham, A., Bettiol, E., Moreau-Stucker, F., Koledova, E., Benmedjahed, K., & Regnault, A. (2015). Assessment of the impact of phenylketonuria and its treatment on quality of life of patients and parents from seven European countries. *Orphanet Journal of Rare Diseases, 10*(1), Article 80. https://doi.org/10.1186/s13023-015-0294-x

Christ, S. E., Huijbregts, S. C. J., de Sonneville, L. M. J., & White, D. A. (2010). Executive function in early-treated phenylketonuria: Profile and underlying mechanisms. *Molecular Genetics and Metabolism, 99*(Suppl.), S22–S32. https://doi.org/10.1016/j.ymgme.2009.10.007

de Baulny, H. O., Abadie, V., Feillet, F., & de Parscau, L. (2007). Management of phenylketonuria and hyperphenylalaninemia. *The Journal of Nutrition, 137*(6, Suppl. 1), 1561S–1563S. https://doi.org/10.1093/jn/137.6.1561S

de Sonneville, L. M., Huijbregts, S. C., Licht, R., Sergeant, J. A., & van Spronsen, F. J. (2011). Pre-attentive processing in children with early and continuously-treated PKU: Effects of concurrent Phe level and lifetime dietary control. *Journal of Inherited Metabolic Disease, 34*(4), 953–962. https://doi.org/10.1007/s10545-011-9321-9

Dyer, C. A. (1999). Pathophysiology of phenylketonuria. *Mental Retardation and Developmental Disabilities Research Reviews, 5*(2), 104–112. https://doi.org/10.1002/(SICI)1098-2779(1999)5:2<104::AID-MRDD2>3.0.CO;2-7

Gentile, J. K., Ten Hoedt, A. E., & Bosch, A. M. (2010). Psychosocial aspects of PKU: Hidden disabilities—A review. *Molecular Genetics and Metabolism, 99*(Suppl.), S64–S67. https://doi.org/10.1016/j.ymgme.2009.10.183

González, M. J., Gutiérrez, A. P., Gassió, R., Fusté, M. E., Vilaseca, M. A., & Campistol, J. (2011). Neurological complications and behavioral problems in patients with phenylketonuria in a follow-up unit. *Molecular Genetics and Metabolism, 104*(Suppl.), S73–S79. https://doi.org/10.1016/j.ymgme.2011.07.015

Gundorova, P., Zinchenko, R. A., Kuznetsova, I. A., Bliznetz, E. A., Stepanova, A. A., & Polyakov, A. V. (2018). Molecular-genetic causes for the high frequency of phenylketonuria in the population from the North Caucasus. *PLOS ONE, 13*(8), Article e0201489. https://doi.org/10.1371/journal.pone.0201489

Hertzberg, V. S., Hinton, C. F., Therrell, B. L., & Shapira, S. K. (2011). Birth prevalence rates of newborn screening disorders in relation to screening practices in the United States. *The Journal of Pediatrics, 159*(4), 555–560. https://doi.org/10.1016/j.jpeds.2011.04.011

Jahja, R., van Spronsen, F. J., de Sonneville, L. M. J., van der Meere, J. J., Bosch, A. M., Hollak, C. E. M., Rubio-Gozalbo, M. E., Brouwers, M. C. G. J., Hofstede, F. C., de Vries, M. C., Janssen, M. C. H., van der Ploeg, A. T., Langendonk, J. G., & Huijbregts, S. C. J. (2016). Social-cognitive functioning and social skills in patients with early treated phenylketonuria: A PKU-COBESO study. *Journal of Inherited Metabolic Disease, 39*(3), 355–362. https://doi.org/10.1007/s10545-016-9918-0

Kaye, C. I., & Committee on Genetics. (2006). Introduction to the newborn screening fact sheets. *Pediatrics, 118*(3), 1304–1312. https://doi.org/10.1542/peds.2006-1782

MacDonald, A., Gokmen-Ozel, H., van Rijn, M., & Burgard, P. (2010). The reality of dietary compliance in the management of phenylketonuria. *Journal of Inherited Metabolic Disease, 33*(6), 665–670. https://doi.org/10.1007/s10545-010-9073-y

Miller, D. J., Duka, T., Stimpson, C. D., Schapiro, S. J., Baze, W. B., McArthur, M. J., Fobbs, A. J., Sousa, A. M., Sestan, N., Wildman, D. E., Lipovich, L., Kuzawa, C. W., Hof, P. R., & Sherwood, C. C. (2012). Prolonged myelination in human neocortical evolution. *Proceedings of the National Academy of Sciences of the United States of America, 109*(41), 16480–16485. https://doi.org/10.1073/pnas.1117943109

National Institutes of Health Consensus Development Panel. (2001). National Institutes of Health Consensus Development Conference Statement: Phenylketonuria: Screening and management, October 16–18, 2000. *Pediatrics, 108*(4), 972–982. https://doi.org/10.1542/peds.108.4.972

Romani, C., Palermo, L., MacDonald, A., Limback, E., Hall, S. K., & Geberhiwot, T. (2017). The impact of phenylalanine levels on cognitive outcomes in adults with phenylketonuria: Effects across tasks and developmental stages. *Neuropsychology, 31*(3), 242–254. https://doi.org/10.1037/neu0000336

Vockley, J., Andersson, H. C., Antshel, K. M., Braverman, N. E., Burton, B. K., Frazier, D. M., Mitchell, J., Smith, W. E., Thompson, B. H., Berry, S. A., & the American College of Medical Genetics and Genomics Therapeutics Committee. (2014). Phenylalanine hydroxylase deficiency: Diagnosis and management guideline. *Genetics in Medicine, 16*(2), 188–200. https://doi.org/10.1038/gim.2013.157

White, D. A., Nortz, M. J., Mandernach, T., Huntington, K., & Steiner, R. D. (2001). Deficits in memory strategy use related to prefrontal dysfunction during early development: Evidence from children with phenylketonuria. *Neuropsychology, 15*(2), 221–229. https://doi.org/10.1037/0894-4105.15.2.221

V

ENDOCRINE AND REPRODUCTIVE SYSTEM DISORDERS

32

Overview of Endocrine and Reproductive System Disorders

Cindy Chin, Graciela E. Silva, and Mark Wheeler

The conditions described in this part involve endocrinopathies and genetic disorders, the latter of which can affect the reproductive system (i.e., Klinefelter and Turner syndromes). *Endocrinology* refers to the study of hormones, which are regulatory chemical messengers that control essential bodily functions involved in metabolism, stress response, water balance, growth, and sexual development. Reproductive system disorders manifest as abnormal pubertal development in the pediatric age group.

BODY SYSTEM INVOLVEMENT AND FUNCTIONING

Given the wide range of action, the endocrine system involves many organs. Endocrine glands include the hypothalamus, pituitary, parathyroid, thyroid, adrenal, and gonads (ovaries and testes). In addition to endocrine glands, individual cells within organs can produce endocrine hormones (e.g., the brain, heart, lungs, kidneys, liver, thymus, skin, pancreas, gastrointestinal tract, fat tissue).

The endocrine system involves endocrine glands and their targets (i.e., the tissues on which hormones act). The targets of hormone action may be (a) distant to the endocrine gland from which it is produced (endocrine), (b) cells adjacent to the endocrine gland (paracrine), (c) cells within the endocrine gland itself (autocrine), or (d) within the cell from which the hormone is produced (intracrine; Geffner, 2009). Endocrine function is often controlled with a negative feedback loop, such that excess hormone production from endocrine

https://doi.org/10.1037/0000349-032
Health-Related Disorders in Children and Adolescents: A Guidebook for Educators and Service Providers, Second Edition, M. M. Perfect, C. A. Riccio, and M. A. Bray (Editors)

glands (e.g., excess thyroid hormone) results in down-regulation of regulatory hormones (e.g., thyroid-stimulating hormone). Conversely, deficiency of hormone production results in the up-regulation of regulatory hormones.

Aneuploidy refers to an abnormal number of chromosomes (e.g., trisomy 21, also known as Down syndrome; see Chapter 18 by Gelbar). When the abnormal copy number is in the sex chromosomes, the condition is categorized as a sex chromosome aneuploidy syndrome, such as Klinefelter syndrome (Chapter 35 by Suorsa-Johnson and Sandberg) and Turner syndrome (Chapter 37 by Suorsa-Johnson and Sandberg). The medical conditions associated with Klinefelter and Turner syndromes are not limited to the reproductive consequences of these genetic disorders. Their phenotypes can be seen throughout the body, as is further discussed in their respective chapters.

COMMON COMPLAINTS AND INDICATORS OF DYSFUNCTION

Endocrinopathies may be isolated to a specific hormone system (e.g., abnormal thyroid function laboratory tests) but may manifest diffusely. Regular evaluation of growth parameters (i.e., height and weight) by a health care provider can greatly aid endocrine dysfunction identification. Poor linear growth accompanied by preserved weight gain increases suspicion for an endocrine hormone deficiency. In contrast, the opposite circumstance (i.e., poor weight gain with preserved linear growth) may signal nutritional deficits. Deviations from the standard growth curve offer clues to evaluate for an endocrinopathy. Children with endocrine disorders may also have vague symptoms (e.g., fatigue, joint pain, abdominal complaints, learning difficulties), posing a diagnostic challenge. The conditions included in this part are often a result of single hormone derangements. However, disorders involving endocrine regulation (i.e., hypothalamus and pituitary) may affect more than one endocrine system. Children with endocrinopathies may present in a relatively benign fashion (e.g., history of polyuria elicited during a routine well-child visit) or present with critical illness (e.g., diabetic ketoacidosis) as in the case of Type 1 diabetes mellitus. For classification of endocrinopathies, please see Table 32.1.

TABLE 32.1. Endocrinopathy Classification by Etiology

Problem with	Classification	Example
Endocrine gland	Primary	Acquired autoimmune thyroiditis • Deficiency: hypothyroidism • Excess: hyperthyroidism
Hormone regulation in		
• Pituitary	Secondary	Secondary hypothyroidism due to tumor involving the pituitary
• Hypothalamus	Tertiary	
Target tissue	Resistance	Resistance to thyroid hormone

PREVIEW OF MAJOR ENDOCRINE SYSTEM CONDITIONS IN PEDIATRICS

Conditions Associated With Growth Failure and Short Stature

Concern about linear growth is a common reason parents seek medical advice and children see an endocrinologist. As discussed in Chapter 33 by Sandberg and Suorsa-Johnson, *growth failure* with accompanying short stature may be a symptom of other medical processes warranting evaluation and possible treatment. Medical, educational, and psychosocial impacts of growth failure, as well as resources to aid in understanding when short stature should be considered problematic, are provided in the chapter.

Congenital Adrenal Hyperplasia

Congenital adrenal hyperplasia (CAH; Chapter 34, Fairchild & Preece) refers to several autosomal recessive disorders that affect cortisol production. In this condition, an enzyme required for cortisol synthesis is deficient. Newborns in the United States are routinely screened for the most common form of classical CAH (i.e., 21-α-hydroxylase deficiency), which can be life threatening if untreated. Classical CAH in female infants may be suspected in the setting of ambiguous genitalia; affected male infants are often indistinguishable from their nonaffected peers. Less severe enzyme deficiencies (i.e., late-onset CAH) may manifest in school-aged children with signs of early puberty (e.g., increased body odor or pubic hair from excess androgens). Given the potential life-threatening consequences of inadequate treatment, educational professionals should be aware of the condition.

Klinefelter Syndrome

As noted by Suorsa-Johnson and Sandberg (Chapter 35), *Klinefelter syndrome*, the most common chromosomal abnormality in male individuals, is characterized by an extra X chromosome or, more rarely, several X chromosomes. In some cases, the presence of the extra X chromosome may not be identified until after puberty. In other cases, identification may occur earlier due to delayed or stalled puberty and treated with medical intervention (i.e., testosterone). The complexity and variability in the presentation and its associated medical, cognitive, and psychosocial features require careful consideration by health care specialists and educational professionals.

Thyroid Disorders

Thyroid disorders account for a large portion of endocrine disorders in pediatric populations, most commonly hypothyroidism and hyperthyroidism. In Chapter 36, Coyle and Stettler discuss these two conditions in more detail. The primary goal of medical treatment for both hypothyroidism and hyperthyroidism is to normalize thyroid hormone levels. In addition to pharmacological therapy, educational and psychosocial issues should be addressed. With proper medication management and continued monitoring of the thyroid hormones, outcomes for individuals with thyroid disorders are generally positive.

Turner Syndrome

Turner syndrome is one of the more common sex chromosome anomalies. Unlike Klinefelter syndrome (see Chapter 35, Suorsa-Johnson and Sandberg), Turner syndrome (Chapter 37, Suorsa-Johnson & Sandberg) is restricted to phenotypic female individuals with only one intact X chromosome; the second X chromosome is partial or missing. The syndrome may be diagnosed prenatally, at birth, in childhood due to growth concerns, in adolescence after delayed puberty, or in adulthood. Diagnosis at birth or during childhood provides a range of potential benefits, including early treatment for growth failure with recombinant human growth hormone, screening and treatment of medical comorbidities, and assessment for educational concerns in a timely manner. The variability of features associated with Turner syndrome often requires these patients to be followed by multiple medical specialists across the lifespan.

Type 1 Diabetes Mellitus

Type 1 diabetes mellitus (T1DM) is an endocrine disorder caused by the destruction of insulin-producing beta cells in the pancreas and eventual absence of insulin production. It is the second most prevalent chronic illness among youth (Rawshani et al., 2018) and is considered an autoimmune disorder, a clear distinction from Type 2 diabetes. Medical intervention is lifelong, requiring constant monitoring of T1DM as well as associated problems in dealing with different environments and social situations. Larez and Perfect (Chapter 38) emphasize the need to take into consideration the individual's ability to self-manage and to be mindful of the potential risks if T1DM is not well managed.

Type 2 Diabetes Mellitus

Like T1DM, *Type 2 diabetes mellitus* (T2DM) results from insufficient insulin production to meet a body's demands. Unlike those with T1DM, individuals with T2DM experience a period of insulin resistance with elevated insulin levels (compared with reference norms) to maintain normal glucose readings before symptomatic disease. Obesity increases the risk for T2DM. Although previously diagnosed primarily in adults, the number of pediatric patients with T2DM is increasing. Medical therapy may range from lifestyle changes to oral medication to intensive insulin therapy. T2DM has implications for academic performance and school attendance, as discussed by Chamberlain and Bello (Chapter 39).

HEALTH CARE NEEDS AND MEDICAL SPECIALTIES

When disorders arise in the endocrine system, the child is seen by specialists in this field. In addition, a child's medical care team may involve other health care specialists to address associated issues and monitor outcomes of medical interventions as appropriate across the lifespan. These may include cardiologists, developmental pediatricians, geneticists, nephrologists, neurologists, and urologists. For associated educational issues, educational professionals may be involved in ensuring appropriate support. Finally, as many of these disorders include potential psychosocial or adjustment issues, involvement of mental health professionals may be appropriate.

CONCLUSION

Children diagnosed with endocrine disorders are cared for by primary care providers and specialists throughout their childhood and into adulthood. Screening and observation of developmental deviations can identify the wide-ranging conditions included in this part as well as potential treatments and supports needed. Given the variability and involvement of the endocrine system across life tasks, an integrated approach to care and outcome monitoring is recommended.

REFERENCES

Geffner, M. (2009). Hormone-resistant states. In N. Lavin (Ed.), *Manual of endocrinology and metabolism* (4th ed., pp. 11–30). Lippincott Williams & Wilkins.

Rawshani, A., Sattar, N., Franzén, S., Rawshani, A., Hattersley, A. T., Svensson, A. M., Eliasson, B., & Gudbjörnsdottir, S. (2018). Excess mortality and cardiovascular disease in young adults with Type 1 diabetes in relation to age at onset: A nationwide, register-based cohort study. *The Lancet, 392*(10146), 477–486. https://doi.org/10.1016/S0140-6736(18)31506-X

33

Conditions Associated With Growth Failure and Short Stature

David E. Sandberg and Kristina I. Suorsa-Johnson

Abnormal growth is an important indicator of general health. Children grow an average of 10 inches in the 1st year, 4 inches per year between ages 1 and 4 years, and 2 inches per year until the onset of puberty. The onset of puberty is typically preceded by a deceleration of growth, followed by marked acceleration over the course of puberty. The pubertal growth spurt begins, on average, at around 9 years in girls and around 11 years in boys. Pubertal growth accounts for approximately 17% of adult height: around 12 inches in boys and around 11 inches in girls (Abbassi, 1998). Growth velocity (i.e., height gain over time) that falls below norms for the healthy population of developing children and adolescents is referred to as *growth failure*. *Short stature* is defined statistically as a measured height two standard deviations or more below the mean for age- and gender-specific norms (Cooke et al., 2020).

ETIOLOGY

Growth failure and abnormal growth can be due to numerous pathological processes. Conditions resulting in *proportionate short stature* (i.e., exhibiting typical body proportions) include growth hormone deficiency, chronic renal insufficiency, Turner syndrome, Prader–Willi syndrome, children born small for gestational age, Noonan syndrome, and malnutrition (Cooke et al., 2020). In contrast, *disproportionate short stature* (or dwarfism) refers to either short limbs or a short torso and results from genetic conditions causing disorders of skeletal

https://doi.org/10.1037/0000349-033
Health-Related Disorders in Children and Adolescents: A Guidebook for Educators and Service Providers, Second Edition, M. M. Perfect, C. A. Riccio, and M. A. Bray (Editors)

development, that is, skeletal dysplasia. The most common skeletal dysplasia is achondroplasia, associated with an average adult height of 4 feet, 4 inches and 4 feet, 1 inch in men and women, respectively.

Short stature, as an isolated physical characteristic, is not necessarily an indicator of an underlying medical condition. For example, *idiopathic short stature* is a condition in which the individual's height is two standard deviations or more below the corresponding mean height for a given age and sex without evidence of systemic, endocrine, nutritional, or chromosomal abnormalities (Cohen et al., 2008).

PREVALENCE AND INCIDENCE

Although the specific medical causes responsible for growth failure may be individually rare, the frequency of short stature is not; by definition, approximately 2.5% of the population have short stature. An equal number of boys and girls display this characteristic. As mentioned, those categorized as having idiopathic short stature are healthy youth, a portion of whom are exhibiting constitutional delay of growth and puberty (i.e., "late bloomers") or familial short stature (i.e., healthy short stature that "runs in the family"). It is important to distinguish between short stature that is largely explained by healthy family genetics versus short stature that develops as a consequence of poor growth linked to an underlying medical condition (Cooke et al., 2020). Despite the common belief that population genetics contribute to significant variability in growth rates in different regions of the world, the World Health Organization (WHO) determined that uniform growth standards for young children aged birth to 5 years are appropriate. This standard describes the growth of healthy children living in well-supported environments in six countries (Brazil, Ghana, India, Norway, Oman, and the United States; WHO Multicentre Growth Reference Study Group, 2006).

IMPACT ON THE STUDENT AND OUTCOMES

Medical

As noted in the Etiology section, growth failure with associated short stature can be a consequence of many discrete and complex medical conditions. For all of these, poor growth can signal the health care provider to investigate the cause and provide condition-specific treatments, as indicated (Cooke et al., 2020). Each of these conditions—Turner syndrome, Prader–Willi syndrome, Noonan syndrome, among others—has syndrome-specific features requiring a combination of surveillance and treatment. The reader is referred to the specific chapters in this volume focusing on those conditions for details (see Chapter 9 by Margiano on Noonan syndrome, Chapter 23 by Wendel and Ogg on Prader–Willi syndrome, and Chapter 37 by Suorsa-Johnson and Sandberg on Turner syndrome). One group not mentioned elsewhere are those children or adolescents who have grown poorly as a consequence of pregnancy risk factors. A large body of animal experimental and human clinical research, conducted under the umbrella of the *fetal origins of adult disease hypothesis*, has shown the lasting consequences of inimical prenatal environments on physical health and cognitive development (Gentner & Leppert, 2019). For example, malnutrition and smoking during pregnancy are predictors of intrauterine growth retardation, low birth weight, and lack of catch-up growth for a significant minority. These same conditions are causally responsible for cognitive disabilities and the development of chronic disease in middle age (Gentner & Leppert, 2019).

Cognitive/Academic

Syndromes sharing short stature as a feature may also be associated with characteristic neurocognitive profiles (e.g., Turner syndrome). The reader is advised to refer to sources focusing on those specific conditions for details. Studies suggest an association between short stature and poorer academic functioning (e.g., Stabler et al., 1994), although others attribute these differences to social class and IQ rather than height (e.g., Downie et al., 1997). This observation notwithstanding, the relatively large group of children born low birth weight (< 2,500 grams) are at risk for continued poor growth, general health, and both developmental and learning disabilities (Boulet et al., 2011). Approximately 314,000 children were born low birth weight in 2018 (or 8.28% of all U.S. births), implying that this population warrants early and sustained health surveillance because of risks to physical health, cognitive function, and general well-being.

Social-Emotional and Behavioral

Short stature is predictably associated with psychosocial stressors, in particular, teasing about height and juvenilization (i.e., being treated as younger than the person's chronological age; Sandberg & Gardner, 2015). Studies of patients (some with normal growth pattern variants, others with pathologic growth) who were consecutively referred to pediatric endocrinologists showed slightly more than half were regularly teased about being short; roughly the same proportion experienced juvenilization (Sandberg & Michael, 1998; Voss & Mulligan, 2000). These studies corroborate anecdotal reports that short stature is associated with psychosocial stress. At the same time, not all children of small stature in these studies shared these experiences; furthermore, stressors were not related to the degree of short stature, nor was it predictive of impairment in the child's psychosocial or educational adaptation (Sandberg & Michael, 1998).

The majority of studies on the psychosocial impact of short stature have recruited participants in medical clinics where growth evaluations are performed. Because only a subset of children and adolescents with short stature are referred to specialists for evaluation, the possibility exists that selection biases produce study samples unrepresentative of youth with comparable short stature who have not been referred for medical evaluation. To address this issue, a school-based study conducted in the United States (n = 956, 11–18 years old) assessed the influence of height on students' peer status (i.e., popularity, friendships, and reputation) using peer nomination techniques (Sandberg et al., 2004). Height was unrelated to popularity, total number of friends, or whether friendships were reciprocated. In terms of reputation among peers, short youths were distinguished from classmates on only one item ("looking younger"), but even here, being judged as younger was unrelated to social acceptance among peers. Short students were not more likely to have the reputation of being someone who "gets picked on," "is often left out," or "is a class clown." Findings did not vary by gender, peer report, or self-report (Sandberg et al., 2004).

PSYCHOEDUCATIONAL IMPLICATIONS AND SCHOOL-BASED INTERVENTIONS

The medical conditions identified in this chapter, which share short stature as a feature, put patients at increased risk of educational and behavioral deficits that call for early intervention based on detailed cognitive assessment and followed by tailored educational and social interventions.

Medical and Health Management

Persistent growth failure can reflect a wide range of underlying pathological processes (Cooke et al., 2020). Accordingly, a precise diagnosis is essential to establishing a roadmap for optimal care. A corollary of this proposition is the importance of differentiating the causes of growth failure from short stature. Short stature is not a disease, but it can serve as a marker of health problems.

At present, recombinant human growth hormone (rhGH) is approved for the treatment of short stature in growth hormone deficiency, chronic renal insufficiency, Turner syndrome, Prader–Willi syndrome, children born small for gestational age, SHOX deficiency, Noonan syndrome, and idiopathic short stature. Predicting the response to rhGH is far from a perfect science for any of these conditions but is particularly challenging in the case of idiopathic short stature. In these short but otherwise physically healthy youth, it can be difficult to differentiate spontaneous catch-up growth during puberty from any additional growth stemming from treatment with rhGH (Richmond & Rogol, 2017).

Shared decision making is recommended before starting rhGH treatment (Grimberg et al., 2016). The process of prescribing rhGH should include an assessment of physical and psychological traits and a discussion of risks and benefits with the child and family. The discussion should contain information on rhGH treatment efficacy to ensure the child and family have appropriate expectations of treatment, in addition to outlining potential adverse side effects (Laventhal et al., 2013; Sandberg & Gardner, 2015). Children and parents should be informed of the treatment regimen for rhGH, including daily injections, the potential use of puberty blockers to prolong the growth-potential window, and the need for regular (typically quarterly) return visits to the medical clinic, which may be experienced by some as a significant burden.

Cognitive/Academic

The particular origin of poor growth and short stature informs the health care provider, educator, and the family regarding the cognitive and social challenges the child is likely to experience. Cases in point include Turner syndrome (Gravholt et al., 2017; Hutaff-Lee et al., 2019), Prader–Willi syndrome (Whittington & Holland, 2017), and being born small for gestational age (Walker & Marlow, 2008).

Social-Emotional and Behavioral

A psychosocial and educational screening assessment should be completed with all children and adolescents with growth failure and marked short stature (Sandberg & Gardner, 2015), followed by any necessary referrals for treatment. Given the likelihood that problems observed among these youths are easily misattributed to the negative social experiences related to short stature, caution must be exercised to ensure that root causes of the child's difficulties are identified and appropriately managed. For those youths experiencing growth problems that are a consequence of an underlying medical condition, meeting with a pediatric psychologist to provide psychoeducational counseling specific to the condition and support in its clinical management can be helpful. This specialist can recommend referrals for additional assessment, as indicated, and assist the family and patient in integrating this component of care in the overall treatment plan.

Anticipation of predictable social experiences related to short stature can be helpful. In the case of juvenilization, a number of recommendations have been made, but their efficacy has not been established in a clinical trial. These include psychoeducational counseling regarding the tendency for the short child to be perceived as chronologically younger than their age. Parents and teachers should be sensitized to this bias and look for opportunities to reinforce the child's independence and self-help skills. Younger children who are relatively short sometimes adopt the role of teacher's pet; this tendency should be countered. Anticipation of and practice with preparing for situations that evoke juvenilization can be quite helpful. For example, having a restaurant server provide the short and pubertally delayed 13-year-old a child's menu can be experienced very negatively. With encouragement from the family, the youth in this situation can develop confidence in immediately asking the restaurant host for an adult menu. Variations on this theme can be applied to comparable situations.

Teasing is a prevalent phenomenon in childhood and adolescence, and its expression changes developmentally (Warm, 1997). However, being teased about an objective physical characteristic might be experienced as particularly hurtful because the provocation is factually based, unlike less personalized taunts. In the case of boys, research has shown that physical weakness and parental overprotection are potent predictors of victimization (Olweus, 1993). A child's anxiety over such experiences can further exacerbate the situation. A study of a cognitive behavioral intervention for adolescents experiencing anxiety and facing bullying demonstrated that the intervention was effective in significantly reducing victimization experiences, as well as anxiety and depressive symptoms (Berry & Hunt, 2009). Growth hormone treatment has not been convincingly demonstrated to enhance adaptive psychosocial coping, and given that appreciable increases in height are only very gradual, this treatment should never be considered a standalone remedy for psychosocial difficulties.

CONCLUSION

Growth failure with accompanying short stature is most often a symptom of other medical processes warranting evaluation and possible treatment. Although the advent of rhGH and its unlimited supply have led to the view that short stature itself is a problem to be treated, evidence is lacking that this physical characteristic, in otherwise healthy youth, is a risk factor for poor psychosocial adaptation. Instead, marked short stature accompanied by growth failure can be a symptom of an underlying medical condition and should be addressed for that reason. Educators and health care providers can counter common stereotypes about the negative aspects of short stature by becoming more familiar with and sharing empirical evidence with parents and the affected youth.

RESOURCES

Human Growth Foundation. http://hgfound.org/

Little People of America. https://www.lpaonline.org. This organization focuses on support of individuals with disproportionate short stature (i.e., dwarfism).

The MAGIC Foundation. https://www.magicfoundation.org/

REFERENCES

Abbassi, V. (1998). Growth and normal puberty. *Pediatrics, 102*(Suppl. 3), 507–511. https://doi.org/10.1542/peds.102.S3.507

Berry, K., & Hunt, C. J. (2009). Evaluation of an intervention program for anxious adolescent boys who are bullied at school. *Journal of Adolescent Health, 45*(4), 376–382. https://doi.org/10.1016/j.jadohealth.2009.04.023

Boulet, S. L., Schieve, L. A., & Boyle, C. A. (2011). Birth weight and health and developmental outcomes in U.S. children, 1997–2005. *Maternal and Child Health Journal, 15*(7), 836–844. https://doi.org/10.1007/s10995-009-0538-2

Cohen, P., Rogol, A. D., Deal, C. L., Saenger, P., Reiter, E. O., Ross, J. L., Chernausek, S. D., Savage, M. O., & Wit, J. M. (2008). Consensus statement on the diagnosis and treatment of children with idiopathic short stature: A summary of the Growth Hormone Research Society, the Lawson Wilkins Pediatric Endocrine Society, and the European Society for Paediatric Endocrinology Workshop. *The Journal of Clinical Endocrinology and Metabolism, 93*(11), 4210–4217. https://doi.org/10.1210/jc.2008-0509

Cooke, D. W., DiVall, S. A., & Radovick, S. (2020). Normal and aberrant growth in children. In S. Melmed, R. J. Auchus, A. B. Goldfine, R. J. Koenig, & C. J. Rosen (Eds.), *Williams textbook of endocrinology* (14th ed., pp. 937–1022). Elsevier.

Downie, A. B., Mulligan, J., Stratford, R. J., Betts, P. R., & Voss, L. D. (1997). Are short normal children at a disadvantage? The Wessex growth study. *BMJ, 314*(7074), 97–100. https://doi.org/10.1136/bmj.314.7074.97

Gentner, M. B., & Leppert, M. L. O. (2019). Environmental influences on health and development: Nutrition, substance exposure, and adverse childhood experiences. *Developmental Medicine and Child Neurology, 61*(9), 1008–1014. https://doi.org/10.1111/dmcn.14149

Gravholt, C. H., Andersen, N. H., Conway, G. S., Dekkers, O. M., Geffner, M. E., Klein, K. O., Lin, A. E., Mauras, N., Quigley, C. A., Rubin, K., Sandberg, D. E., Sas, T. C. J., Silberbach, M., Söderström-Anttila, V., Stochholm, K., van Alfen-van derVelden, J. A., Woelfle, J., & Backeljauw, P. F. (2017). Clinical practice guidelines for the care of girls and women with Turner syndrome: Proceedings from the 2016 Cincinnati International Turner Syndrome Meeting. *European Journal of Endocrinology, 177*(3), G1–G70. https://doi.org/10.1530/EJE-17-0430

Grimberg, A., DiVall, S. A., Polychronakos, C., Allen, D. B., Cohen, L. E., Quintos, J. B., Rossi, W. C., Feudtner, C., & Murad, M. H. (2016). Guidelines for growth hormone and insulin-like growth factor-I treatment in children and adolescents: Growth hormone deficiency, idiopathic short stature, and primary insulin-like growth factor-I deficiency. *Hormone Research in Paediatrics, 86*(6), 361–397. https://doi.org/10.1159/000452150

Hutaff-Lee, C., Bennett, E., Howell, S., & Tartaglia, N. (2019). Clinical developmental, neuropsychological, and social–emotional features of Turner syndrome. *American Journal of Medical Genetics: Part C, Seminars in Medical Genetics, 181*(1), 42–50. https://doi.org/10.1002/ajmg.c.31687

Laventhal, N. T., Shuchman, M., & Sandberg, D. E. (2013). Warning about warnings: Weighing risk and benefit when information is in a state of flux. *Hormone Research in Paediatrics, 79*(1), 4–8. https://doi.org/10.1159/000346381

Olweus, D. (1993). Victimization by peers: Antecedents and long-term outcomes. In K. H. Rubin & J. B. Asendorpf (Eds.), *Social withdrawal, inhibition, and shyness in childhood* (pp. 315–341). Lawrence Erlbaum Associates.

Richmond, E. J., & Rogol, A. D. (2022). Growth hormone treatment for idiopathic short stature. *UpToDate*. Retrieved December 7, 2022, from https://www.uptodate.com/contents/growth-hormone-treatment-for-idiopathic-short-stature

Sandberg, D. E., Bukowski, W. M., Fung, C. M., & Noll, R. B. (2004). Height and social adjustment: Are extremes a cause for concern and action? *Pediatrics, 114*(3), 744–750. https://doi.org/10.1542/peds.2003-1169-L

Sandberg, D. E., & Gardner, M. (2015, August). Short stature: Is it a psychosocial problem and does changing height matter? *Pediatric Clinics of North America, 62*(4), 963–982. https://doi.org/10.1016/j.pcl.2015.04.009

Sandberg, D. E., & Michael, P. (1998). Psychosocial stresses related to short stature: does their presence imply psychiatric dysfunction? In D. Drotar (Ed.), *Assessing pediatric health-related quality of life and functional status: Implications for research* (pp. 287–312). Lawrence Erlbaum Associates.

Stabler, B., Clopper, R. R., Siegel, P. T., Stoppani, C., Compton, P. G., & Underwood, L. E. (1994). Academic achievement and psychological adjustment in short children.

Journal of Developmental and Behavioral Pediatrics, 15(1), 1–6. https://doi.org/10.1097/00004703-199402000-00001

Voss, L. D., & Mulligan, J. (2000). Bullying in school: Are short pupils at risk? Questionnaire study in a cohort. *BMJ, 320*(7235), 612–613. https://doi.org/10.1136/bmj.320.7235.612

Walker, D. M., & Marlow, N. (2008). Neurocognitive outcome following fetal growth restriction. *Archives of Disease in Childhood: Fetal and Neonatal Edition, 93*(4), F322–F325. https://doi.org/10.1136/adc.2007.120485

Warm, T. R. (1997). The role of teasing in development and vice versa. *Journal of Developmental and Behavioral Pediatrics, 18*(2), 97–101. https://doi.org/10.1097/00004703-199704000-00004

Whittington, J., & Holland, A. (2017). Cognition in people with Prader–Willi syndrome: Insights into genetic influences on cognitive and social development. *Neuroscience and Biobehavioral Reviews, 72,* 153–167. https://doi.org/10.1016/j.neubiorev.2016.09.013

World Health Organization Multicentre Growth Reference Study Group. (2006). Assessment of differences in linear growth among populations in the WHO Multicentre Growth Reference Study. *Acta Paediatrica, S450,* 56–65. https://doi.org/10.1111/j.1651-2227.2006.tb02376.x

34

Congenital Adrenal Hyperplasia

Allison Fairchild and Madison Preece

Congenital adrenal hyperplasia (CAH) was first documented in 1865 by an Italian anatomist, Luigi DeCrecchio, who noted enlarged adrenal glands, male-appearing genitals, and an internal female reproductive system in a patient (Texas Department of State Health Services, 2021). Commonly referred to as an invisible illness because many of its symptoms are unnoticeable to the naked eye, CAH is now known to be a collection of inherited disorders that affect the adrenal glands. Although some forms of CAH can be life-threatening if left untreated, lifelong treatments have been developed to address many of the symptoms and allow affected individuals to lead generally healthy and independent lives (Carroll et al., 2020).

ETIOLOGY

CAH refers to a group of autosomal recessive genetic conditions that affect hormone production in the adrenal glands (Gidlöf et al., 2013). The adrenal glands are responsible for producing corticosteroids, which gauge the body's response to illness or injury; mineralocorticoids, which regulate salt and water levels; and androgens, which are male sex hormones. The most common form of CAH occurs because of mutations in the gene encoding the 21-hydroxylase enzyme. This mutation causes an impairment in the production of cortisol and aldosterone and an excess of androgen (El-Maouche et al., 2017). This type of CAH accounts for 95% of all CAH cases and is subcategorized into classic CAH and

https://doi.org/10.1037/0000349-034
Health-Related Disorders in Children and Adolescents: A Guidebook for Educators and Service Providers, Second Edition, M. M. Perfect, C. A. Riccio, and M. A. Bray (Editors)

nonclassic CAH (El-Maouche et al., 2017). An analysis of fetal DNA can detect a 21-hydroxylase deficiency, and standard newborn screening procedures can find an imbalance in cortisol and aldosterone (Nimkarn & New, 2009). These procedures are able to identify most male and female babies who have inherited classic CAH. However, nonclassic CAH can be more difficult to detect and often goes undiagnosed until the onset of symptoms, typically between childhood and early adulthood (Witchel & Azziz, 2011).

PREVALENCE AND INCIDENCE

Classic CAH affects approximately one in 15,000 children. Nonclassic CAH is one of the most common autosomal recessive genetic disorders, affecting approximately one in 150 individuals (Therrell et al., 1998). Those from specific ethnic backgrounds, such as individuals with Ashkenazi Jewish or Italian heritage, are more likely to inherit the nonclassic form of the disorder (Vogiatz & Poppas, n.d.). Khalid et al. (2012) found that CAH is present in approximately an equal number of girls and boys during the first year of life. However, boys tend to present with more severe cases of the disorder. Most female infants with CAH will be diagnosed within the first day of life or after newborn screening has been completed, around day 14 of life; approximately only 6% of girls and 50% of boys will go undiagnosed (Khalid et al., 2012).

SYMPTOMS

The symptoms of CAH may vary greatly depending on the underlying gene mutation and level of deficiency (Gidlöf et al., 2013). A deficiency in the enzyme 21-hydroxylase causes 95% of all CAH cases, which can be classified as classic or nonclassic CAH (El-Maouche et al., 2017). The remaining diagnoses of CAH are a result of five other enzyme deficiencies and are considered rare forms of CAH (rare diseases).

Classic CAH is further subdivided into simple virilizing CAH and salt-wasting CAH. *Simple virilizing CAH* is caused by too little cortisol and too much androgen. Female individuals with simple virilizing CAH most often present with ambiguous or atypical genitalia (e.g., fused labia, enlarged clitoris) while having normal internal reproductive organs (Carroll et al., 2020). Both sexes can also experience other symptoms, such as premature pubarche (i.e., early onset of puberty occurring before age 8 for girls and 9 for boys, including the development of pubic hair and body odor), fast body growth, and premature completion of growth leading to short stature (Witchel & Azziz, 2011).

Known as the most severe form of classic CAH, *salt-wasting CAH* may lead to death if undiagnosed and untreated. This type of CAH is a result of aldosterone deficiency, resulting in the body not being able to retain enough salt (i.e., too much sodium is lost in urine). Symptoms include dehydration, poor feeding, diarrhea, vomiting, heart rhythm problems, low blood pressure, very low sodium levels, low glucose, weight loss, and shock (National Institutes of Health [NIH], 2021). Individuals with salt-wasting CAH can also have simple virilizing CAH symptoms and are also at risk for adrenal crisis, especially when ill or physically stressed (NIH, 2021). Adrenal crisis occurs when the body does not produce enough cortisol, causing lightheadedness or dizziness, weakness, sweating, abdominal pain, nausea, vomiting, and even loss of consciousness (NIH, 2021).

Nonclassic CAH is a common genetic disorder that is non-life-threatening and often goes undiagnosed until symptoms appear between childhood and early adulthood. The most common symptom is hirsutism, the development of excessive facial or body hair, occurring in 59% of diagnosed female adolescents and adults (Witchel & Azziz, 2011). Other symptoms include oligomenorrhea (i.e., infrequent menstruations), acne, alopecia, decreased fertility, male-pattern baldness, enlarged penis, and small testicles (Witchel & Azziz, 2011). Because the symptoms of nonclassic CAH can be very mild, some individuals remain undiagnosed (Genetic and Rare Diseases Information Center [GRDIC], n.d.). Individuals with a rare form of CAH have also presented with various combinations of classic and nonclassic CAH symptoms. One of these disorders with combined symptoms, congenital lipoid adrenal hyperplasia, is the most fatal form of CAH due to risk of susceptibility to an adrenal crisis (Kim, 2014).

IMPACT ON THE STUDENT AND OUTCOMES

Children with CAH and their caregivers reported good overall health-related quality of life regarding physical well-being, emotional well-being, self-esteem, family, friends, everyday functioning, and school, with self-reports of self-esteem and school having the lowest quality scores (Carroll et al., 2021).

Medical

Classic CAH can be treated with steroids, such as hydrocortisone, to replace the low cortisol levels (NIH, 2021). Cortisol is a hormone produced by the adrenal gland to regulate various functions in the body, such as the stress response, metabolism, blood pressure, blood sugar, and the sleep–wake cycle. Lower than normal levels of cortisol can be harmful to health, due to dysregulation of these bodily functions, and can lead to fatigue, unintentional weight loss, poor appetite, and low blood pressure. Cortisol replacement treatment should begin soon after birth and requires daily medication with multiple doses for the rest of an individual's life to remain symptom free (NIH, 2021). Medication levels require close monitoring by health care providers because cortisol levels naturally fluctuate throughout the lifespan and increase during times of physical stress (GRDIC, n.d.). Those with classic CAH are at risk of Cushing's syndrome if medication dose is too high or too low. When individuals with classic CAH undergo physical stress (e.g., illness, surgery, major injury), they will require additional medication.

CAH is the most common cause of female intersex disorder of sexual development. Therefore, for individuals with CAH, the presence of various sexual characteristics (e.g., chromosomes, primary and secondary sex characteristics) are all important considerations for development. The decision and timing of gender assignment in the individual's development require a multidisciplinary decision that includes the individual and family members (Kumar et al., 2010). Nonclassic CAH requires treatment if the individual experiences early puberty, excess body hair, irregular menstrual periods, or infertility. If necessary, individuals with nonclassic CAH are given a low-dose steroid to replace their low cortisol levels (NIH, 2021).

Cognitive/Academic

Research on cognitive abilities of individuals with CAH has yielded mixed results. Some studies have found that individuals with CAH have impaired cognitive functioning, including deficits in memory, spatial abilities, and quantitative reasoning when compared with the general population. However, studies have also shown that women with CAH display superior spatial abilities. These mixed results may be due to the synthetic glucocorticoid (GC) replacement therapy individuals with CAH receive throughout the lifespan. As the receptors for GC are highly expressed within the hippocampus, amygdala, and prefrontal cortex, high doses of GC may have various impacts on skills related to these areas of the brain, including executive functioning, emotional regulation, and memory (Messina et al., 2020). A recent study by Messina et al. (2020) found that when children with CAH are diagnosed and treated early, they score within the average range of general intelligence and executive functioning.

Even though early detection and appropriate treatment methods can lessen the impact of CAH on cognitive functioning, children with CAH still face challenges at school. In interviews, children with CAH reported having to miss class to take medication, having to handle the negative or misperceptions of school personnel regarding CAH, and coping with stigma when peers become aware of their diagnosis (Carroll et al., 2020). According to Carroll et al. (2021), a large majority of educators and school nurses report lacking general knowledge and training around the needs of students with CAH. School personnel's attitudes, biases, and fears regarding liability (e.g., concerns about a medical emergency occurring while a child is engaging in activities) can lead to teachers prohibiting participation in certain activities, which contributes to the negative experience of school for children with CAH. Perceived stigma is an important aspect of the disorder that affects psychological well-being and overall health. By gaining an accurate understanding of which activities are safe for these students to participate in, educators can promote inclusion with peers, reduce stigma, and support the health of students with CAH (Carroll et al., 2021).

Social-Emotional and Behavioral

Psychological functioning and well-being of children with CAH can be affected by anticipated and real stigma and feelings of shame for taking medication and/or for having a sex disorder (Carroll et al., 2021). In a qualitative study, Carroll et al. (2020) found that, among girls, young children shared feelings of embarrassment and shame, whereas older children tended to describe feelings of fear. All of these children expressed feeling stigmatized due to their invisible illness and how they believed others perceived them.

Research focusing on the behavior of children with CAH has found that girls affected by CAH displayed more aggression and higher levels of activity in comparison with those unaffected by the disorder. However, these differences were not noted in boys with CAH in comparison with those without the disorder (Pasterski et al., 2007). Additionally, other studies have found that girls with CAH show greater preferences for toys and activities typically preferred by boys and for boys as playmates (Hines & Kaufman, 1994; Pasterski et al., 2005).

PSYCHOEDUCATIONAL IMPLICATIONS AND SCHOOL-BASED INTERVENTIONS

Medical and Health Management

While CAH cannot be cured, it can be effectively treated. Treatment of classic CAH typically starts immediately after birth and should continue throughout an individual's lifespan. Treatment of this disorder requires great variation depending on the type of CAH (e.g., classic) and the severity. Research suggests that treatment by a multidisciplinary team typically yields the best results, due to improved communication between practitioners during times of transition. However, for many patients, this option is not available. The clinical management of CAH involves suppression of adrenal androgen production and treatment of the adrenal insufficiency these individuals experience. If the adrenal androgen is not adequately suppressed, children may experience early onset of puberty, infertility, and psychological effects. In addition, excess levels of the medication needed to suppress the adrenal androgen may result in obesity, growth suppression, decreased bone density, and, again, psychological impacts. Because the levels of excess androgen production need to be closely monitored and symptoms vary in levels of severity, this disorder requires clinicians to provide individualized therapy (Messina et al., 2020).

Cognitive/Academic

In order to ensure students with CAH do not miss more classroom instruction than necessary and to ensure their physical safety, it is important for all school personnel to be trained on the signs and symptoms of an adrenal crisis. In addition to staff training, measures can be put in place in the classroom to accommodate physical health needs, such as incorporating rest breaks, providing snacks, and allowing students to carry electrolyte replacement drinks, and allowing check-ins with the school nurse between class periods. It may be beneficial for students to bring symptom cards to school, which can help staff and other students understand when an adrenal emergency may be occurring. As students may still experience disruptions to their classroom environment due to physical health issues, academic interventions should also be put in place, including extended time for assignments, assistance in note taking, and specialized seating near a teacher or classroom aide (Adrenal Insufficiency United, 2022). These accommodations allow students to function within the classroom setting, even when time is needed to resolve disorder-related health issues, by allowing for immediate support from adults when necessary and eliminating the need for schoolwork-related tasks to be completed in a limited amount of time.

Social-Emotional and Behavioral

Due to hormone changes during puberty and psychological issues that may arise during adolescence, treatment side effects and adherence to medication need to be closely monitored during this time. As sexual maturation occurs during adolescence, this is a time during which clinicians can play a major role in supporting development of a healthy body image. Additionally, girls with CAH are at risk for developing an anxiety disorder (Kyritsi et al., 2017). An important aspect of social–emotional management for those with CAH is disclosure of sex development-related information to the child, in order to prepare for changes during puberty and ways in which they may appear differently from other children and adolescents. Coupled with therapy, best mental health outcomes occur when clinicians assist parents in developing a strategy to gradually educate children on these topics. For example, some young girls and adolescents may develop an enlarged clitoris later in life, if they did not have a clitoral surgery as an infant, due to medication noncompliance. These children may need social–emotional support, as they might present with "clitoral erections" that may be noticeable in a bathing suit or tight clothing (Fleming et al., 2017).

CONCLUSION

Often referred to as an invisible illness, CAH affects adrenal hormone production, resulting in a variety of symptoms. Depending on the underlying mutations and level of deficiency, symptoms can vary in levels of severity and may require specialized and closely monitored medical treatment. With proper medical treatment and support from parents, school staff, and mental health practitioners, children and adolescents with CAH can function and succeed within the school setting.

RESOURCES

CARESFoundation. 2414 Morris Avenue, Ste 110, Union, NJ 07083. https://caresfoundation.org

Hsu, C. Y., & Rivkees, S. A. (2005). *Congenital adrenal hyperplasia: A parent's guide.* AuthorHouse.

National Adrenal Diseases Foundation. PO Box 95149, Newton, MA 02495. https://www.nadf.us

REFERENCES

Adrenal Insufficiency United. (2022). *School resources.* https://united4rare.org/school-resources/

Carroll, L., Graff, C., Wicks, M., & Diaz Thomas, A. (2020). Living with an invisible illness: A qualitative study exploring the lived experiences of female children with congenital adrenal hyperplasia. *Quality of Life Research, 29*(3), 673–681. https://doi.org/10.1007/s11136-019-02350-2

Carroll, L., Graff, C., Wicks, M., Jones, T., & Diaz Thomas, A. (2021). Health-related quality of life of children with congenital adrenal hyperplasia: A mixed methods study. *Journal of Pediatric Nursing, 58,* 88–94. https://doi.org/10.1016/j.pedn.2021.01.008

El-Maouche, D., Arlt, W., & Merke, D. P. (2017). Congenital adrenal hyperplasia. *The Lancet, 390*(10108), 2194–2210. https://doi.org/10.1016/S0140-6736(17)31431-9

Fleming, L., Van Riper, M., & Knafl, K. (2017). Management of childhood congenital adrenal hyperplasia—An integrative review of the literature. *Journal of Pediatric Health Care, 31*(5), 560–577. https://doi.org/10.1016/j.pedhc.2017.02.004

Genetic and Rare Diseases Information Center. (n.d.). *Congenital adrenal hyperplasia.* National Institutes of Health. https://rarediseases.info.nih.gov/diseases/1467/congenital-adrenal-hyperplasia

Gidlöf, S., Falhammar, H., Thilén, A., von Döbeln, U., Ritzén, M., Wedell, A., & Nordenström, A. (2013). One hundred years of congenital adrenal hyperplasia in Sweden: A retrospective, population-based cohort study. *The Lancet Diabetes & Endocrinology, 1*(1), 35–42. https://doi.org/10.1016/S2213-8587(13)70007-X

Hines, M., & Kaufman, F. R. (1994). Androgen and the development of human sex-typical behavior: Rough-and-tumble play and sex of preferred playmates in children with congenital adrenal hyperplasia (CAH). *Child Development, 65*(4), 1042–1053. https://doi.org/10.2307/1131303

Khalid, J. M., Oerton, J. M., Dezateux, C., Hindmarsh, P. C., Kelnar, C. J., & Knowles, R. L. (2012). Incidence and clinical features of congenital adrenal hyperplasia in Great Britain. *Archives of Disease in Childhood, 97*(2), 101–106. https://doi.org/10.1136/archdischild-2011-300234

Kim, C. J. (2014). Congenital lipoid adrenal hyperplasia. *Annals of Pediatric Endocrinology & Metabolism, 19*(4), 179–183. https://doi.org/10.6065/apem.2014.19.4.179

Kumar, A., Mohanty, N. K., Jain, M., Prakash, S., & Arora, R. P. (2010). Gender identity in a female with intersex disorder of sexual development due to congenital adrenal hyperplasia: A management dilemma. *UroToday International Journal, 3*(2). Advance online publication. https://doi.org/10.3834/uij.1944-5784.2010.04.06

Kyritsi, E. M., Koltsida, G., Farakla, I., Papanikolaou, A., Critselis, E., Mantzou, E., Zoumakis, E., Kolaitis, G., Chrousos, G. P., & Charmandari, E. (2017). Psychological vulnerability to stress in carriers of congenital adrenal hyperplasia due to 21-hydroxylase deficiency. *Hormones, 16*(1), 42–53. https://doi.org/10.14310/horm.2002.1718

Messina, V., Karlsson, L., Hirvikoski, T., Nordenström, A., & Lajic, S. (2020). Cognitive function of children and adolescents with congenital adrenal hyperplasia: Importance of early diagnosis. *The Journal of Clinical Endocrinology and Metabolism, 105*(3), e683–e691. https://doi.org/10.1210/clinem/dgaa016

National Institutes of Health. (2021, May 17). *What are the symptoms of congenital adrenal hyperplasia (CAH)?* Eunice Kennedy Shriver National Institute of Child Health and Human Development. https://www.nichd.nih.gov/health/topics/cah/conditioninfo/symptoms

Nimkarn, S., & New, M. I. (2009). Prenatal diagnosis and treatment of congenital adrenal hyperplasia due to 21-hydroxylase deficiency. *Molecular and Cellular Endocrinology, 300*(1–2), 192–196. https://doi.org/10.1016/j.mce.2008.11.027

Pasterski, V. L., Geffner, M. E., Brain, C., Hindmarsh, P., Brook, C., & Hines, M. (2005). Prenatal hormones and postnatal socialization by parents as determinants of male-typical toy play in girls with congenital adrenal hyperplasia. *Child Development, 76*(1), 264–278. https://doi.org/10.1111/j.1467-8624.2005.00843.x

Pasterski, V., Hindmarsh, P., Geffner, M., Brook, C., Brain, C., & Hines, M. (2007). Increased aggression and activity level in 3- to 11-year-old girls with congenital adrenal hyperplasia (CAH). *Hormones and Behavior, 52*(3), 368–374. https://doi.org/10.1016/j.yhbeh.2007.05.015

Texas Department of State Health Services. (2021, March 8). *History of congenital adrenal hyperplasia*. Texas Health and Human Services. https://dshs.texas.gov/newborn/histor~1.shtm

Therrell, B. L., Jr., Berenbaum, S. A., Manter-Kapanke, V., Simmank, J., Korman, K., Prentice, L., Gonzalez, J., & Gunn, S. (1998). Results of screening 1.9 million Texas newborns for 21-hydroxylase-deficient congenital adrenal hyperplasia. *Pediatrics, 101*(4), 583–590. https://doi.org/10.1542/peds.101.4.583

Vogiatz, M., & Poppas, D. (n.d.). *Non-classical congenital adrenal hyperplasia (NC-CAH): Adolescents and adults*. The Comprehensive Center for Congenital Adrenal Hyperplasia. https://www.nyp.org/pdf/komansky/NC-CAH_Adolescents_and_Adults.pdf

Witchel, S. F., & Azziz, R. (2011). Congenital adrenal hyperplasia. *Journal of Pediatric and Adolescent Gynecology, 24*(3), 116–126. https://doi.org/10.1016/j.jpag.2010.10.001

35

Klinefelter Syndrome

Kristina I. Suorsa-Johnson and David E. Sandberg

Klinefelter syndrome (KS), the most common chromosomal abnormality in male individuals, is characterized by an extra X chromosome (47,XXY) or, more rarely, several X chromosomes (Davis et al., 2016).

ETIOLOGY

KS is caused by meiotic nondisjunction of the sex chromosomes during gametogenesis. Nondisjunction occurs in cell division when chromosomes do not divide properly (Gottlieb et al., 2022).

PREVALENCE AND INCIDENCE

Approximately 250,000 male individuals in the United States have KS (Paduch et al., 2009). The annual birth rate is approximately one in 500 to 650 live male births (Groth et al., 2013). There have not been any reports of ethnic differences in KS prevalence.

This work was supported in part by grants from the Eunice Kennedy Shriver National Institute of Child Health and Human Development (R01 HD093450 and R01 HD086583).

https://doi.org/10.1037/0000349-035
Health-Related Disorders in Children and Adolescents: A Guidebook for Educators and Service Providers, Second Edition, M. M. Perfect, C. A. Riccio, and M. A. Bray (Editors)

SYMPTOMS

The medical features of KS have significant variability. The most common features include small testes, tall stature, hypergonadotropic hypogonadism (i.e., impaired response of the gonads to gonadal stimulating factors—gonadotropins—secreted from the pituitary gland), gynecomastia (breast development in a male individual), learning disabilities, increased incidence of psychiatric symptoms, and infertility (Groth et al., 2013). There are also a range of less common characteristics, including osteopenia, Type 2 diabetes, cryptorchidism, decreased penis size, congenital malformations, mitral valve prolapse, and breast or mediastinal cancer (Groth et al., 2013). Due to the broad range of presentation and subtle characteristics of KS, making an early diagnosis can be difficult (Bojesen et al., 2003): An estimated 75% of men with KS remain undiagnosed (Bojesen et al., 2003; Davis et al., 2016; Swerdlow et al., 2005), and only 10% are identified before puberty (Wosnitzer & Paduch, 2013). This finding suggests that detection may be more likely for those more severely affected (Groth et al., 2013), representing a case ascertainment bias.

IMPACT ON THE STUDENT AND OUTCOMES

Medical

Although the additional X chromosome in boys with KS is associated with progressive gonadal failure, germ cell depletion, and reduced testosterone production by the testes, boys with KS tend to start puberty at the same time as their peers and tend to progress through early puberty at about the same speed (Davis et al., 2016). However, as boys continue to age, puberty may stall due to decreasing testosterone levels. Medical features of particular relevance in the school setting are those related to physical appearance, including tall stature, gynecomastia, and small penis size. Although some features will not be directly observable in an academic setting, they may negatively impact body image and social relationships with peers. This is of particular significance due to the increased social difficulties already experienced by boys with KS (discussed further later). KS is also associated with a range of medical comorbidities, including diabetes, lung diseases, epilepsy, cerebrovascular disease, and vascular insufficiency of the intestine (Belling et al., 2017).

Cognitive/Academic

As with the medical characteristics of KS, the cognitive features are equally variable. The most common cognitive deficits impact verbal functioning (Gravholt et al., 2018). Verbal functioning deficits cause downstream impairment in early language development; language-based learning problems; and difficulty in syntax production, word retrieval, and nonsemantic cues in spoken language (Davis et al., 2016). Additional cognitive deficits can include verbal and nonverbal memory impairment, poor motor skills, executive functioning deficits, and arithmetic abilities in the mildly impaired range (Boone et al., 2001; Davis et al., 2016; DeLisi et al., 2005; Fales et al., 2003; N. R. Lee et al., 2011). Problems with motor functioning have been linked to involvement in fewer extracurricular activities for boys with KS (Bender et al., 1995). The overall cognitive profile of boys with KS results in lower educational attainment (Bojesen et al., 2011). In addition to the cognitive profile, for some boys with KS, increased rates of inattention, hyperactivity, and impulsivity likely contribute to academic problems. Rates of attention-deficit/hyperactivity disorder (ADHD) in boys with KS range from 41% to 63% (Bruining et al., 2009; N. R. Lee et al., 2011; Ross et al., 2012).

Social-Emotional and Behavioral

Boys with KS are at risk for increased behavior problems, low frustration tolerance, social and emotional immaturity, low self-esteem, and emotional sensitivity (Davis et al., 2016). KS is generally associated with lower health-related quality of life among children and adolescents (Close et al., 2015). Psychiatric symptoms are also elevated among boys with KS. For example, Bruining and colleagues (2009) reported that 24% of boys (6–19 years old) with KS met criteria for a past or current episode of a depressive disorder, 18% had experienced generalized anxiety, and 14% had experienced separation anxiety disorder. In a study of boys with KS (8–19 years old) who had never received testosterone replacement therapy, lower endogenous testosterone was associated with increased social anxiety (van Rijn, 2018).

The presence of autistic traits affects an estimated 11% to 27% of boys with KS (Bishop et al., 2011; Bruining et al., 2009). Specific deficit areas include difficulty with expression, understanding complex language, social reciprocity, and abnormalities in communication (Bishop et al., 2011; Bruining et al., 2009). Symptoms of gender dysphoria have been reported to be higher among adults with KS, although this relationship appears to be mediated by the presence of autistic features (Fisher et al., 2016). The possible association between KS and gender dysphoria has not been studied in boys with KS.

PSYCHOEDUCATIONAL IMPLICATIONS AND SCHOOL-BASED INTERVENTIONS

Individuals with KS would benefit if basic information about the process of sex development of the body was covered in the core educational curriculum. Sensitive discussion of sex chromosomes in disorders of sex development (P. A. Lee et al., 2016) in the context of health and/or biology classes would not only reflect a more accurate story about the diversity of our biology but would also hopefully reduce the taboo sometimes associated with these conditions and the perceived need for secrecy.

Medical and Health Management

Early diagnosis and intervention for boys with KS lead to the most promising outcomes across the lifespan. Due to the benefits of early detection, parents of children with KS and primary care providers support the use of newborn screening to promote early detection of KS (Gies et al., 2016). For detection in children and adults, Close and colleagues (2015) developed a KS screening tool, which considers the common physical traits of this diagnosis (e.g., tall stature, eunuchoid body proportion, wide arm span, large waist circumference, high body mass index, gynecomastia). A factor contributing to low rates of early diagnosis in KS is health care provider unfamiliarity with the features and associated sequelae (Turriff et al., 2017).

Testosterone replacement therapy should occur at the beginning of puberty to promote progression through this developmental milestone at a similar time as peers (Gravholt et al., 2018; Groth et al., 2013). Given that endogenous production of testosterone wanes with increasing age, lifelong testosterone treatment is indicated to prevent osteoporosis, obesity, metabolic syndrome, and diabetes (Gravholt et al., 2018; Groth et al., 2013). Contrary to popular belief, testosterone replacement therapy is helpful in reducing behavior problems (Annell et al., 1970; Nielsen & Pelsen, 1987) and in increasing energy levels (Nielsen & Pelsen, 1987).

The importance of providers educating boys and their families about KS and associated medical and psychosocial features cannot be overstated. As with all diagnoses, information should be repeatedly provided in a developmentally sensitive manner (Dennis et al., 2015; Metcalfe et al., 2008). Gaining the knowledge to understand their—or for parents, their child's—diagnosis promotes positive coping and the ability to correctly share information about KS with others (e.g., school), as appropriate to circumstance.

Cognitive/Educational

Recommended interventions for cognitive and educational deficits experienced by children and adolescents with KS are broadly based on supporting the deficit area, rather than on providing a specific intervention for all boys with KS. This is particularly relevant due to the variability of presentations in KS. Therefore, neuropsychological evaluation is recommended if a child has a KS diagnosis, even if particular areas of concern have not been identified. Davis and colleagues (2016) suggested providers take a preventative stance and advocate that boys with KS receive services as early as possible through either an individualized education program or 504 plan, as unremedied concerns can quickly devolve into significant delays.

Early identification of KS is beneficial due to the ability to evaluate and provide any indicated supports for children exhibiting cognitive or developmental deficits. In those identified prenatally, evaluations of cognitive functioning, speech-language and motor development, social engagement, and adaptive functioning are recommended at regular intervals (e.g., 9–15 months, 18–24 months, and 30–36 months; Davis et al., 2016). Based on findings from testing, early intervention for developmental, speech, occupational, physical, or behavioral therapies may be warranted. Finally, some research supports that testosterone therapy, initiated prior to puberty, has beneficial effects on cognitive performance and behavior (Ross et al., 2017; Samango-Sprouse et al., 2013). However, current recommendations are to initiate treatment at the beginning of puberty, corresponding with an atypical elevation of the gonadotropins luteinizing hormone and follicle stimulating hormone (Groth et al., 2013).

Given the known verbal deficits in boys with KS, evaluation by a pediatric speech and language pathologist is recommended annually before the age of 4 years old and every 2 to 3 years after that, as warranted, due to symptom persistence (Davis et al., 2016). Verbal/language difficulties can have a presentation similar to autism spectrum disorder. Therefore, evaluations need to consider the co-occurrence of these features in KS. Interventions for reading disorders include Lindamood-Bell, which focuses on developing phonemic skills (https://lindamoodbell.com/), and Orton-Gillingham, a multisensory phonics-based approach to reading (Davis et al., 2016; Ritchey & Goeke, 2006). If problems with handwriting, play activities, extracurricular activities, dressing, eating, or general self-care skills are detected, these can be addressed through physical or occupational therapy (Davis et al., 2016).

A student's ADHD diagnosis should be incorporated into any preexisting individualized education program in order to provide additional supports in the academic setting. Empirically supported behavioral therapy strategies, such as behavior parent training, can be useful in helping parents and children gain mastery of ADHD management strategies within a positive framework (Chronis et al., 2004). Psychopharmacologic treatment for ADHD has been shown to be effective in the majority of boys with KS (Ross et al., 2012).

Social-Emotional and Behavioral

Concerns over behavioral, emotional, or social adaptation should trigger a referral for psychological services (Davis et al., 2016; Gravholt et al., 2018). Due to the variability in the presentation of KS, no sweeping recommendations for treatment are warranted. A comprehensive evaluation, guided by knowledge of the cognitive, psychosocial, and psychosexual aspects of KS, will generate strong recommendations for indicated services. Psychoeducational counseling for the individual with KS and their family is an essential element of optimal care. Accordingly, misunderstandings regarding the implications of atypical sex chromosomes for the person's health, sense of self, and worries regarding potential stigmatization need to be addressed early and repeatedly. Strong adherence to medical recommendation for lifelong health surveillance and testosterone replacement therapy, in particular, is predicated on an accurate understanding of KS and emotional acceptance of its personal meaning in order to avert any tendency to cope through avoidance. Peer support can also be helpful and occur through referral to a national or international support network or through one-to-one engagement with another affected person arranged through the specialty clinic where care is being received.

The combination of verbal difficulties, autism spectrum features, and ADHD likely contribute to the social skills deficits experienced by boys and men with KS. Social skills training or individual therapy may be helpful in alleviating some symptoms. Participation in groups or clubs with peers who share similar interests can also be beneficial. If features of autism spectrum disorder are present, applied behavior analysis therapies, such as the Early Start Denver Model (Ryberg, 2015) are recommended (Davis et al., 2016). The Program for the Education and Enrichment of Relational Skills (Laugeson et al., 2012) is an evidence-based approach that potentially could translate well to the KS population.

Psychologists can help in the development of a script that can be used to share information about the diagnosis with relatives and friends. This method can be critical in reducing the occurrence of internalized stigma. Among people with a medical or psychological condition, privacy can be confused with secrecy in an effort to protect the individual and prevent bias. Secrecy can result in adverse psychosocial outcomes (Newheiser & Barreto, 2014). With respect to the school setting, some parents and affected youth may be wary of sharing medical information (in particular, karyotype) with schools due to concerns about misunderstandings, the perceived risk of unwanted disclosures, and associated stigma. This approach can be counterproductive, as sharing such information might accelerate the provision of child's reception of appropriate accommodations to ensure academic success.

CONCLUSION

The complexity and variability in presentation of KS and its associated medical, cognitive, and psychosocial features require careful surveillance by health care specialists and educators. Early detection of KS is made difficult by its varied and subtle presentation, yet early diagnosis and intervention are associated with the most positive outcomes.

RESOURCES

Association for X and Y Chromosome Variations. https://genetic.org/

MedlinePlus. (2019). *Klinefelter syndrome*. National Library of Medicine. https://medlineplus.gov/genetics/condition/klinefelter-syndrome/

National Organization for Rare Diseases. (2020). *47,XXY (Klinefelter syndrome)*. https://rarediseases.org/rare-diseases/xyy-syndrome/

American Association for Klinefelter Syndrome Information and Support. http://www.aaksis.org/

REFERENCES

Annell, A.-L., Gustavson, K. H., & Tenstam, J. (1970). Symptomatology in schoolboys with positive sex chromatin (the Klinefelter syndrome). *Acta Psychiatrica Scandinavica, 46*(1), 71–80. https://doi.org/10.1111/j.1600-0447.1970.tb02102.x

Belling, K., Russo, F., Jensen, A. B., Dalgaard, M. D., Westergaard, D., Rajpert-De Meyts, E., Skakkebæk, N. E., Juul, A., & Brunak, S. (2017). Klinefelter syndrome comorbidities linked to increased X chromosome gene dosage and altered protein interactome activity. *Human Molecular Genetics, 26*(7), 1219–1229. https://doi.org/10.1093/hmg/ddx014

Bender, B. G., Harmon, R. J., Linden, M. G., & Robinson, A. (1995). Psychosocial adaptation of 39 adolescents with sex chromosome abnormalities. *Pediatrics, 96*(2), 302–308. https://doi.org/10.1542/peds.96.2.302

Bishop, D. V., Jacobs, P. A., Lachlan, K., Wellesley, D., Barnicoat, A., Boyd, P. A., Fryer, A., Middlemiss, P., Smithson, S., Metcalfe, K., Shears, D., Leggett, V., Nation, K., & Scerif, G. (2011). Autism, language and communication in children with sex chromosome trisomies. *Archives of Disease in Childhood, 96*(10), 954–959. https://doi.org/10.1136/adc.2009.179747

Bojesen, A., Juul, S., & Gravholt, C. H. (2003). Prenatal and postnatal prevalence of Klinefelter syndrome: A national registry study. *The Journal of Clinical Endocrinology and Metabolism, 88*(2), 622–626. https://doi.org/10.1210/jc.2002-021491

Bojesen, A., Stochholm, K., Juul, S., & Gravholt, C. H. (2011). Socioeconomic trajectories affect mortality in Klinefelter syndrome. *The Journal of Clinical Endocrinology and Metabolism, 96*(7), 2098–2104. https://doi.org/10.1210/jc.2011-0367

Boone, K. B., Swerdloff, R. S., Miller, B. L., Geschwind, D. H., Razani, J., Lee, A., Gonzalo, I. G., Haddal, A., Rankin, K., Lu, P., & Paul, L. (2001). Neuropsychological profiles of adults with Klinefelter syndrome. *Journal of the International Neuropsychological Society, 7*(4), 446–456. https://doi.org/10.1017/S1355617701744013

Bruining, H., Swaab, H., Kas, M., & van Engeland, H. (2009). Psychiatric characteristics in a self-selected sample of boys with Klinefelter syndrome. *Pediatrics, 123*(5), e865–e870. https://doi.org/10.1542/peds.2008-1954

Chronis, A. M., Chacko, A., Fabiano, G. A., Wymbs, B. T., & Pelham, W. E., Jr. (2004). Enhancements to the behavioral parent training paradigm for families of children with ADHD: Review and future directions. *Clinical Child and Family Psychology Review, 7*(1), 1–27. https://doi.org/10.1023/B:CCFP.0000020190.60808.a4

Close, S., Fennoy, I., Smaldone, A., & Reame, N. (2015). Phenotype and adverse quality of life in boys with Klinefelter syndrome. *The Journal of Pediatrics, 167*(3), 650–657. https://doi.org/10.1016/j.jpeds.2015.06.037

Davis, S., Howell, S., Wilson, R., Tanda, T., Ross, J., Zeitler, P., & Tartaglia, N. (2016). Advances in the interdisciplinary care of children with Klinefelter syndrome. *Advances in Pediatrics, 63*(1), 15–46. https://doi.org/10.1016/j.yapd.2016.04.020

DeLisi, L. E., Maurizio, A. M., Svetina, C., Ardekani, B., Szulc, K., Nierenberg, J., Leonard, J., & Harvey, P. D. (2005). Klinefelter's syndrome (XXY) as a genetic model for psychotic disorders. *American Journal of Medical Genetics: Part B, Neuropsychiatric Genetics, 135B*(1), 15–23. https://doi.org/10.1002/ajmg.b.30163

Dennis, A., Howell, S., Cordeiro, L., & Tartaglia, N. (2015). "How should I tell my child?": Disclosing the diagnosis of sex chromosome aneuploidies. *Journal of Genetic Counseling, 24*(1), 88–103. https://doi.org/10.1007/s10897-014-9741-4

Fales, C. L., Knowlton, B. J., Holyoak, K. J., Geschwind, D. H., Swerdloff, R. S., & Gonzalo, I. G. (2003). Working memory and relational reasoning in Klinefelter syndrome. *Journal of the International Neuropsychological Society, 9*(6), 839–846. https://doi.org/10.1017/S1355617703960036

Fisher, A. D., Ristori, J., Fanni, E., Castellini, G., Forti, G., & Maggi, M. (2016). Gender identity, gender assignment and reassignment in individuals with disorders of sex development: A major of dilemma. *Journal of Endocrinological Investigation, 39*(11), 1207–1224. https://doi.org/10.1007/s40618-016-0482-0

Gies, I., Tournaye, H., & De Schepper, J. (2016). Attitudes of parents of Klinefelter boys and pediatricians towards neonatal screening and fertility preservation techniques in Klinefelter syndrome. *European Journal of Pediatrics, 175*(3), 399–404. https://doi.org/10.1007/s00431-015-2657-7

Gottlieb, S. F., Tupper, C., Kerndt, C. C., & Tegay, D. H. (2022). *Genetics, nondisjunction*. StatPearls Publishing. https://www.ncbi.nlm.nih.gov/books/NBK482240/

Gravholt, C. H., Chang, S., Wallentin, M., Fedder, J., Moore, P., & Skakkebæk, A. (2018). Klinefelter syndrome: Integrating genetics, neuropsychology, and endocrinology. *Endocrine Reviews, 39*(4), 389–423. https://doi.org/10.1210/er.2017-00212

Groth, K. A., Skakkebæk, A., Høst, C., Gravholt, C. H., & Bojesen, A. (2013). Klinefelter syndrome—A clinical update. *The Journal of Clinical Endocrinology and Metabolism, 98*(1), 20–30. https://doi.org/10.1210/jc.2012-2382

Laugeson, E. A., Frankel, F., Gantman, A., Dillon, A. R., & Mogil, C. (2012). Evidence-based social skills training for adolescents with autism spectrum disorders: The UCLA PEERS program. *Journal of Autism and Developmental Disorders, 42*(6), 1025–1036. https://doi.org/10.1007/s10803-011-1339-1

Lee, N. R., Wallace, G. L., Clasen, L. S., Lenroot, R. K., Blumenthal, J. D., White, S. L., Celano, M. J., & Giedd, J. N. (2011). Executive function in young males with Klinefelter (XXY) syndrome with and without comorbid attention-deficit/hyperactivity disorder. *Journal of the International Neuropsychological Society, 17*(3), 522–530. https://doi.org/10.1017/S1355617711000312

Lee, P. A., Nordenström, A., Houk, C. P., Ahmed, S. F., Auchus, R., Baratz, A., Baratz Dalke, K., Liao, L. M., Lin-Su, K., Looijenga, L. H., III, Mazur, T., Meyer-Bahlburg, H. F., Mouriquand, P., Quigley, C. A., Sandberg, D. E., Vilain, E., Witchel, S., & the Global DSD Update Consortium. (2016). Global disorders of sex development update since 2006: Perceptions, approach and care. *Hormone Research in Paediatrics, 85*(3), 158–180. https://doi.org/10.1159/000442975

Metcalfe, A., Coad, J., Plumridge, G. M., Gill, P., & Farndon, P. (2008). Family communication between children and their parents about inherited genetic conditions: A meta-synthesis of the research. *European Journal of Human Genetics, 16*(10), 1193–1200. https://doi.org/10.1038/ejhg.2008.84

Newheiser, A. K., & Barreto, M. (2014). Hidden costs of hiding stigma: Ironic interpersonal consequences of concealing a stigmatized identity in social interactions. *Journal of Experimental Social Psychology, 52*, 58–70. https://doi.org/10.1016/j.jesp.2014.01.002

Nielsen, J., & Pelsen, B. (1987). Follow-up 20 years later of 34 Klinefelter males with karyotype 47,XXY and 16 hypogonadal males with karyotype 46,XY. *Human Genetics, 77*(2), 188–192. https://doi.org/10.1007/BF00272390

Paduch, D. A., Bolyakov, A., Cohen, P., & Travis, A. (2009). Reproduction in men with Klinefelter syndrome: The past, the present, and the future. *Seminars in Reproductive Medicine, 27*(2), 137–148. https://doi.org/10.1055/s-0029-1202302

Ritchey, K. D., & Goeke, J. L. (2006). Orton-Gillingham and Orton-Gillingham-based reading instruction. *The Journal of Special Education, 40*(3), 171–183. https://doi.org/10.1177/00224669060400030501

Ross, J. L., Kushner, H., Kowal, K., Bardsley, M., Davis, S., Reiss, A. L., Tartaglia, N., & Roeltgen, D. (2017). Androgen treatment effects on motor function, cognition, and behavior in boys with Klinefelter syndrome. *The Journal of Pediatrics, 185*, 193–199.e4. https://doi.org/10.1016/j.jpeds.2017.02.036

Ross, J. L., Roeltgen, D. P., Kushner, H., Zinn, A. R., Reiss, A., Bardsley, M. Z., McCauley, E., & Tartaglia, N. (2012). Behavioral and social phenotypes in boys with 47,XYY syndrome or 47,XXY Klinefelter syndrome. *Pediatrics, 129*(4), 769–778. https://doi.org/10.1542/peds.2011-0719

Ryberg, K. H. (2015). Evidence for the implementation of the Early Start Denver Model for young children with autism spectrum disorder. *Journal of the American Psychiatric Nurses Association, 21*(5), 327–337. https://doi.org/10.1177/1078390315608165

Samango-Sprouse, C. A., Sadeghin, T., Mitchell, F. L., Dixon, T., Stapleton, E., Kingery, M., & Gropman, A. L. (2013). Positive effects of short course androgen therapy on the neurodevelopmental outcome in boys with 47,XXY syndrome at 36 and 72 months of age. *American Journal of Medical Genetics: Part A, 161*(3), 501–508. https://doi.org/10.1002/ajmg.a.35769

Swerdlow, A. J., Higgins, C. D., Schoemaker, M. J., Wright, A. F., Jacobs, P. A. (2005). Mortality in patients with Klinefelter syndrome in Britain: A cohort study. *The Journal of Clinical Endocrinology and Metabolism, 90*(12), 6516–6522. https://doi.org/10.1210/jc.2005-1077

Turriff, A., Macnamara, E., Levy, H. P., & Biesecker, B. (2017). The impact of living with Klinefelter syndrome: A qualitative exploration of adolescents and adults. *Journal of Genetic Counseling, 26*(4), 728–737. https://doi.org/10.1007/s10897-016-0041-z

van Rijn, S. (2018). Salivary testosterone in relation to social cognition and social anxiety in children and adolescents with 47,XXY (Klinefelter syndrome). *PLOS ONE, 13*(7), Article e0200882. https://doi.org/10.1371/journal.pone.0200882

Wosnitzer, M. S., & Paduch, D. A. (2013). Endocrinological issues and hormonal manipulation in children and men with Klinefelter syndrome. *American Journal of Medical Genetics: Part C, Seminars in Medical Genetics, 163*(1), 16–26. https://doi.org/10.1002/ajmg.c.31350

36

Thyroid Disorders

Samantha Coyle and Brooke R. Stettler

Thyroid disease is a common endocrine disorder characterized by structural abnormalities or disruptions in thyroid gland functioning and includes multiple conditions such as hypothyroidism, hyperthyroidism, autoimmune thyroiditis, thyroid nodules and goiters, and thyroid cancer (Golden et al., 2009; Hanley et al., 2016). Thyroid disease accounts for the majority of endocrine disorders in pediatric populations (Donaldson & Jones, 2013). Given the scope and variety of thyroid disorders, the current chapter focuses on hypothyroidism and hyperthyroidism in youth.

ETIOLOGY

Hypothyroidism is the more common of the two conditions. Worldwide, the most common cause is iodine deficiency; however, in iodine-replete countries such as the United States, hypothyroidism is oftentimes the result of autoimmune or structural abnormalities (Hanley et al., 2016). Hypothyroidism can be present at birth (congenital) or be acquired later in development (Hanley et al., 2016). *Congenital hypothyroidism* (CH) is most commonly caused by thyroid dysgenesis, or abnormal/incomplete development of the thyroid gland during prenatal development, which explains approximately 80% to 85% of all cases (Hanley et al., 2016). *Acquired hypothyroidism,* or autoimmune hypothyroidism, is most often caused by autoimmune thyroiditis, or Hashimoto's disease (Garber et al., 2012). Other preexisting medical conditions, including Down syndrome and

https://doi.org/10.1037/0000349-036
Health-Related Disorders in Children and Adolescents: A Guidebook for Educators and Service Providers, Second Edition, M. M. Perfect, C. A. Riccio, and M. A. Bray (Editors)

Turner syndrome, may predispose youth to autoimmune hypothyroidism (Hanley et al., 2016). *Hyperthyroidism* is another thyroid condition, which accounts for approximately 15% of pediatric thyroid disorders; about 95% of hyperthyroid cases in children are the result of autoimmune hyperthyroidism, or Graves' disease (Bettendorf, 2002; Hanley et al., 2016).

PREVALENCE AND INCIDENCE

Researchers believe that CH occurs in about one in 1,500 to 3,000 births (Hanley et al., 2016). Estimates of CH incidence have increased over the years, likely due to the inclusion of thyroid disorders as part of newborn screening routines (Wassner, 2017). Rates of CH in the United States appear to be about equal among boys and girls (Nandi-Munshi & Taplin, 2015). Autoimmune hypothyroidism occurs in approximately 1% to 2% of the population, although some studies report rates as high as approximately 5% (Golden et al., 2009; Hanley et al., 2016). Acquired hypothyroidism is more common among female than male individuals, with a 4:1 predominance ratio (Golden et al., 2009; Hanley et al., 2016).

Hyperthyroidism is rare in children and adolescents, with only about 1% to 5% of cases beginning before the age of 16 (Bettendorf, 2002). The prevalence is around 1.2%, with common rates between 0.5% and 2% (Golden et al., 2009). Incidence of hyperthyroid Graves' disease are variable and range from one case in 10,000 in the United States to one in 100,000 in other countries, including the United Kingdom and Ireland (Hanley et al., 2016). As with acquired hypothyroidism, hyperthyroidism is more common in female than male individuals, with ratios ranging from 3:1 to 5:1 (Bettendorf, 2002).

SYMPTOMS

Symptoms of hypothyroidism depend on age of onset and include jaundice, lethargy, constipation, and feeding difficulties in early infancy. Symptoms later in development include delays in meeting developmental milestones, decreased linear growth (i.e., height), weakness, fatigue, weight gain, puffy face, cold intolerance, constipation, dry skin, joint and muscle pain, and menstrual irregularities (Bettendorf, 2002; Garber et al., 2012; Hanley et al., 2016). An enlarged thyroid (goiter) is also common, although this symptom is nonspecific and found in cases of both hypo- and hyperthyroidism (Hanley et al., 2016).

Symptoms of hyperthyroidism are more overt and observable than those of hypothyroidism and include restlessness or fidgetiness, warm moist skin, palpitations and tremors, difficulties sleeping, increased sweating, proximal muscle weakness, growth acceleration, advanced bone age, and delayed puberty (Hanley et al., 2016). Children with hyperthyroidism may present as anxious, irritable, and overactive, often leading to misdiagnoses for behavioral and attentional disorders (Hanley et al., 2016).

IMPACT ON THE STUDENT AND OUTCOMES

Thyroid disorders are important for school professionals to understand, as thyroid disorders may place youth at risk for other medical problems. They may also be associated with students' academic, social, and emotional well-being.

Medical

Problems with thyroid functioning result in a disruption of essential hormone production within the body. The endocrine system regulates the thyroid gland and the secretion of the thyroid hormone, thyroxine (T4), in the bloodstream. The hypothalamic–pituitary–thyroid axis monitors thyroxine levels, secreting thyroid-stimulating hormone (TSH) when increased levels of thyroxine are needed and suppressing thyroxine secretion when levels rise to a specific set point, creating a feedback loop that maintains homeostasis of the thyroid hormones in the body (Wassner, 2017). *Hypothyroidism* refers to an underactive thyroid gland resulting in low production of the thyroid hormone and an excess of TSH (Wassner, 2017). *Hyperthyroidism* refers to an excessively active thyroid gland resulting in the overproduction of the thyroid hormones, with low or unmeasurable levels of TSH (Hanley et al., 2016). Thyroid dysfunction can be caused by defects in the thyroid gland itself (referred to as primary) or can result from dysfunction within the hypothalamic–pituitary–thyroid axis or another medical condition (Donaldson & Jones, 2013).

There is an increased frequency of other autoimmune disorders in individuals with hypothyroidism, most commonly Type 1 diabetes, myasthenia gravis, celiac disease, and pernicious anemia (Garber et al., 2012). In addition to co-occurring medical conditions, it is possible that the treatments used to manage hypothyroidism might cause a variety of complications, such as cardiovascular, skeletal, and potentially affective disturbances when overtreated as well as lower cognitive functioning when overtreated early in life (Bongers-Schokking et al., 2013; Garber et al., 2012). Furthermore, the overtreatment of hypothyroidism by use of hormone replacement therapy can in turn cause symptoms of hyperthyroidism (Hanley et al., 2016).

Some individuals with hyperthyroidism due to Graves' disease experience a co-occurring eye disease (ophthalmopathy), which occurs in about one third of pediatric cases but is often milder than in adults (Hanley et al., 2016). Dermopathy is another complication that develops in a small minority of individuals with hyperthyroidism and presents as firm lesions on the skin (Little, 2006). Additional features of hyperthyroidism include weight loss in the presence of an increased appetite, rashes, polyarthritis, agranulocytosis, arthralgias, and hepatic abnormalities (Reid & Wheeler, 2005). Similar to hypothyroidism, overtreatment for hyperthyroidism can cause symptoms of the reverse (Reid & Wheeler, 2005). Hyperthyroidism has also been associated with muscular and motor deficits, including abnormal muscle tone, ataxia, and difficulties in motor coordination, correlating with severity of disease (Nandi-Munshi & Taplin, 2015). These sequelae may interfere with school functioning, particularly in regard to writing activities and physical education classes.

Cognitive/Academic

Failing to identify CH early can cause significant cognitive deficits, including intellectual disabilities. Left untreated, CH can cause significant cognitive impairments, placing hypothyroidism among the most common preventable causes of intellectual disabilities (Nandi-Munshi & Taplin, 2015; Rovet & Alvarez, 1996). Some studies have suggested that youth with CH have similar global IQ scores compared with those with normal thyroid functioning (Nandi-Munshi & Taplin, 2015) and no differences in academic performance and grade promotion at sixth grade (Léger et al., 2001). However, school delay was linked with low adherence to treatment, highlighting the importance of carefully following a medical treatment plan in order to reduce any disruptions in learning and academic growth (Léger et al., 2001).

Social-Emotional and Behavioral

Although cognitive and motor correlates of the disorder are well studied, less is known about the social and emotional correlates of hypo- and hyperthyroidism. Limited research has investigated quality of life and self-esteem in youth treated for CH and discovered that adolescents with CH self-reported more difficulty in areas including depressed mood, cognitive functioning, social development, and self-esteem (van der Sluijs Veer et al., 2008). In addition, research has suggested that youth with endocrine disorders, including thyroid disorders, may be at greater risk for negative outcomes in the face of peer victimization and may be at greater risk of experiencing continued victimization over time (Devine et al., 2008; Storch et al., 2004). Because psychosocial problems are linked with decreased adherence to medical treatment plans (Storch et al., 2004), it is important that educators look out for potential factors, such as victimization, that might place students with chronic medical conditions at risk for these problems and implement appropriate interventions to address these concerns.

PSYCHOEDUCATIONAL IMPLICATIONS AND SCHOOL-BASED INTERVENTIONS

Although thyroid disorders are detected only by a licensed medical professional, several school-based interventions and accommodations may help to improve outcomes for students with an identified thyroid disorder.

Medical and Health Management

Advancements in the identification and treatment of thyroid disorders have led to significant improvements in outcomes overall. Specifically, testing for CH has become routine in the newborn screening process, and hypothyroidism is typically treated with medication (Hanley et al., 2016). As a result, some children may take their medications during the school day, and if a child is taking medication at school, it is important that educators are aware of the drug interactions and diet of the child, as levothyroxine tablets, the drug approved by the U.S. Food and Drug Administration to treat hypothyroidism, are typically administered once daily before food consumption and cannot be taken with foods or supplements containing calcium, iron, or soy (Hanley et al., 2016). One additional drug-related consideration involving thyroid disorders is that as medical advances continue, children and adolescents with significant behavioral and mood disorders are being prescribed psychotropic medications to address their symptoms (Correll & Carlson, 2006). One of the commonly associated side effects of these medications includes thyroid dysfunction, with elevated levels of TSH.

Cognitive/Academic

Adherence to treatment is critical in ensuring continued positive outcomes related to cognitive and academic performance (Sandberg & Barrick, 1995). Youth with hypothyroidism may suffer from fatigue and "brain fog," which can be extreme at times, making it difficult to concentrate and learn in the classroom (Rovet & Alvarez, 1996). Providing youth with frequent breaks and movement throughout the day to help increase alertness may be an effective support for children with hypothyroidism. On the other hand, hyperactivity is a side effect of hyperthyroidism and a side effect of overtreatment of hypothyroidism (Hanley et al., 2016). Educators and school staff should monitor and report any changes in attention, concentration, and energy levels noticed throughout the school day to parents. In addition, the use of behavioral strategies such as self-monitoring techniques and consistent and clear prompts to redirect students may be effective in improving attention and concentration within the school setting. Students may also benefit from extended time on tests and testing in a distraction-free or alternative environment, as well as shortened assignments/extended deadlines to address both chronic fatigue and symptoms of hyperactivity. Motor deficits associated with the disorder can also be addressed by reducing the amount of note-taking, providing written notes or an outline, or using computer technology in the classroom. In addition, students with thyroid disorders may display increased sensitivity to the physical environment (e.g., temperature) and may benefit from access to layered clothing or the use of a fan to adapt appropriately to the climate. Students with thyroid disorders may also benefit from additional instructional support and explicit and direct instruction to support their learning. Tutoring sessions and extra classroom support may be helpful to catch students up on any material missed due to absences resulting from their condition.

Social-Emotional and Behavioral

Importantly, it is essential that educational professionals working with children presenting as irritable, anxious, or hyperactive rule out the possibility of a thyroid condition before labeling the child with an emotional and/or behavioral disorder, as these behaviors are often misinterpreted and not commonly attributed to possible thyroid dysfunction, despite their connection. In addition, adults working with children who have a chronic disease should also be aware of the impact that living with a chronic condition may have on the social and emotional well-being of youth and should provide these students with additional supports and guidance. Checking in with students regularly and providing them with emotional support when needed may be effective in promoting positive outcomes for youth with thyroid disorders. Fortunately, with proper treatment and adherence to a closely monitored medical treatment plan, children and adolescents with a thyroid disorder typically maintain normal lives and development.

CONCLUSION

The primary goal of treatment for hypo- and hyperthyroidism is to stabilize thyroid hormone production and ensure that youth are growing and meeting their developmental milestones appropriately (Hanley et al., 2016). Patients who do not respond to antithyroid drugs or experience negative side effects as a result of this method of treatment may consider a more definitive option: permanently inhibiting the thyroid and placing the client into a permanent state of hypothyroidism, which is considered to be more stable and easier to treat (Hanley et al., 2016). Treatment of hypothyroidism involves thyroid hormone replacement therapy to stabilize thyroxine levels (Wassner, 2017). With proper medication management and continued monitoring of the thyroid hormones, outcomes for individuals with thyroid disorders are generally positive.

RESOURCES

American Thyroid Association. 6066 Leesburg Pike, #550, Falls Church, VA 22041. https://www.thyroid.org

Endocrine Society. 2055 L St NW, Suite 600, Washington, DC 20036. https://www.endocrine.org/topics/thyroid-disorders-and-cancer

REFERENCES

Bettendorf, M. (2002). Thyroid disorders in children from birth to adolescence. *European Journal of Nuclear Medicine and Molecular Imaging, 29*(2), S439–S446.

Bongers-Schokking, J. J., Resing, W. C., de Rijke, Y. B., de Ridder, M. A., & de Muinck Keizer-Schrama, S. M. (2013). Cognitive development in congenital hypothyroidism: Is overtreatment a greater threat than undertreatment? *The Journal of Clinical Endocrinology and Metabolism, 98*(11), 4499–4506. https://doi.org/10.1210/jc.2013-2175

Correll, C. U., & Carlson, H. E. (2006). Endocrine and metabolic adverse effects of psychotropic medications in children and adolescents. *Journal of the American Academy of Child & Adolescent Psychiatry, 45*(7), 771–791. https://doi.org/10.1097/01.chi.0000220851.94392.30

Devine, K. A., Storch, E. A., Geffken, G. R., Freddo, M., Humphrey, J. L., & Silverstein, J. H. (2008). Prospective study of peer victimization and social-psychological adjustment in children with endocrine disorders. *Journal of Child Health Care, 12*(1), 76–86. https://doi.org/10.1177/1367493507085620

Donaldson, M., & Jones, J. (2013). Optimising outcome in congenital hypothyroidism; current opinions on best practice in initial assessment and subsequent management. *Journal of Clinical Research in Pediatric Endocrinology, 5*(Suppl. 1), 13–22.

Garber, J. R., Cobin, R. H., Gharib, H., Hennessey, J. V., Klein, I., Mechanick, J. I., Pessah-Pollack, R., Singer, P. A., & Woeber, K. A.. (2012). Clinical practice guidelines for hypothyroidism in adults: Cosponsored by the American Association of Clinical Endocrinologists and the American Thyroid Association. *Thyroid, 22*(12), 1200–1235. https://doi.org/10.1089/thy.2012.0205

Golden, S. H., Robinson, K. A., Saldanha, I., Anton, B., & Ladenson, P. W. (2009). Clinical review: Prevalence and incidence of endocrine and metabolic disorders in the United States: A comprehensive review. *The Journal of Clinical Endocrinology and Metabolism, 94*(6), 1853–1878. https://doi.org/10.1210/jc.2008-2291

Hanley, P., Lord, K., & Bauer, A. J. (2016). Thyroid disorders in children and adolescents: A review. *JAMA Pediatrics, 170*(10), 1008–1019. https://doi.org/10.1001/jamapediatrics.2016.0486

Léger, J., Larroque, B., Norton, J., & the Association Française pour le Dépistage et la Prévetion des Handicaps de l'Enfant. (2001). Influence of severity of congenital hypothyroidism and adequacy of treatment on school achievement in young adolescents: A population-based cohort study. *Acta Paediatrica, 90*(11), 1249–1256. https://doi.org/10.1111/j.1651-2227.2001.tb01570.x

Little, J. W. (2006). Thyroid disorders. Part I: Hyperthyroidism. *Oral Surgery, Oral Medicine, Oral Pathology, Oral Radiology, and Endodontics, 101*(3), 276–284. https://doi.org/10.1016/j.tripleo.2005.05.069

Nandi-Munshi, D., & Taplin, C. E. (2015). Thyroid-related neurological disorders and complications in children. *Pediatric Neurology, 52*(4), 373–382. https://doi.org/10.1016/j.pediatrneurol.2014.12.005

Reid, J. R., & Wheeler, S. F. (2005). Hyperthyroidism: Diagnosis and treatment. *American Family Physician, 72*(4), 623–630.

Rovet, J., & Alvarez, M. (1996). Thyroid hormone and attention in school-age children with congenital hypothyroidism. *Journal of Child Psychology and Psychiatry, 37*(5), 579–585. https://doi.org/10.1111/j.1469-7610.1996.tb01444.x

Sandberg, D. E., & Barrick, C. (1995). Endocrine disorders in childhood: A selective survey of intellectual and educational sequelae. *School Psychology Review, 24*(2), 146–170. https://doi.org/10.1080/02796015.1995.12085759

Storch, E. A., Lewin, A. B., Silverstein, J. H., Heidgerken, A. D., Strawser, M. S., Baumeister, A., & Geffken, G. R. (2004). Social-psychological correlates of peer victimization in children with endocrine disorders. *The Journal of Pediatrics, 145*(6), 784–789. https://doi.org/10.1016/j.jpeds.2004.08.025

van der Sluijs Veer, L., Kempers, M. J. E., Last, B. F., Vulsma, T., & Grootenhuis, M. A. (2008). Quality of life, developmental milestones, and self-esteem of young adults with congenital hypothyroidism diagnosed by neonatal screening. *The Journal of Clinical Endocrinology and Metabolism, 93*(7), 2654–2661. https://doi.org/10.1210/jc.2007-1560

Wassner, A. J. (2017). Pediatric hypothyroidism: Diagnosis and treatment. *Pediatric Drugs, 19*(4), 291–301. https://doi.org/10.1007/s40272-017-0238-0

37

Turner Syndrome

Kristina I. Suorsa-Johnson and David E. Sandberg

Turner syndrome (TS) is one of the more common sex chromosome anomalies. The definition of TS is restricted to individuals with a predominantly female genital phenotype.

ETIOLOGY

TS is characterized as a sex chromosome aneuploidy (an abnormal number of chromosomes in a cell) affecting phenotypic female individuals with one X chromosome and complete or partial absence of the second sex chromosome. The most common karyotype in TS is 45,X (40%–50% of cases), but TS is also observed in girls/women with genetic mosaicism, that is, the presence of two different cell lines in the body. The most common TS variants are 45,X/46,XX (15%–20%) and 45,X/46,XY (10%–12%; Gravholt et al., 2017).

PREVALENCE AND INCIDENCE

TS affects approximately one in 2,000 to one in 2,500 live female births (Gravholt et al., 2017). Although a range of traits are characteristic of TS, the

This work was supported in part by grants from the Eunice Kennedy Shriver National Institute of Child Health and Human Development (R01 HD093450 and R01 HD086583).

https://doi.org/10.1037/0000349-037
Health-Related Disorders in Children and Adolescents: A Guidebook for Educators and Service Providers, Second Edition, M. M. Perfect, C. A. Riccio, and M. A. Bray (Editors)

most prominent features present in virtually all girls and women with TS are linear growth failure and gonadal dysgenesis, which is associated with infertility and lack of spontaneous puberty.

SYMPTOMS

Beyond these characteristics, there are a range of other presenting features (see Gravholt et al., 2017). Due to the broad range of presentations, diagnosis can occur prenatally, at birth, in childhood due to poor growth, in adolescence after delayed puberty, or in adulthood following fertility problems. Diagnosis of TS at birth or during childhood provides a range of potential benefits, including early treatment for growth failure with recombinant human growth hormone, aggressive treatment of middle ear infections, and educational supports. The broad range of features associated with TS often requires these patients to be followed by multiple medical specialists across the lifespan (Gravholt et al., 2017).

IMPACTS ON THE STUDENT AND OUTCOMES

Medical

TS is associated with characteristic medical features and health problems (Gravholt et al., 2017) leading to increased rates of morbidity and mortality (Stochholm et al., 2012), including cardiac and kidney anomalies, diabetes, thyroid dysfunction, and celiac disease. The majority of girls with TS will not experience spontaneous puberty, a consequence of gonadal dysgenesis without medical intervention. In addition to hormone-related issues, hearing impairment in TS is a common feature that may require intervention (Gravholt et al., 2017).

Cognitive/Academic

As in other genetic syndromes, there is a high degree of individual variability in the physical, cognitive, and psychosocial presentations of girls and women with TS. Only a subset of individuals with TS, approximately 10%, meet criteria for an intellectual disability (Sybert & McCauley, 2004). Nonetheless, many female individuals with TS experience neurocognitive deficits compared with the general population, including difficulty with nonverbal and perceptual motor skills and visuospatial awareness. For these individuals, performance on verbal and visuospatial working memory tends to be one to two standard deviations below the mean (Hart et al., 2006; Zinn et al., 2007), with additional impaired performance on tasks requiring visuospatial and perceptual motor skills (Downey et al., 1991; Romans et al., 1998). Broader memory deficits also may manifest among some individuals with TS. Areas of impairment can include object, location, and facial memory. Furthermore, girls with TS are at an increased risk for motor delays, including difficulty with perceptual motor tasks (El-Mansoury et al., 2009; Wahlberg et al., 2013).

Despite neurocognitive weaknesses, the educational attainment of women with TS is on par or above expectation when compared with their peers (Næss et al., 2010); however, deficits in perceptual motor and visuospatial skills can manifest as mathematics or reading disorders in the academic setting. Thus, 50% to 75% of girls with TS experience poor mathematics performance and numerical processing deficits (Mazzocco & Hanich, 2010; Murphy et al., 2006). Further, TS is often associated with weaknesses in phonological word processing, word reading, and reading comprehension (Rae et al., 2004). In contrast, these also can be areas of strength, and girls with TS have been reported as outperforming their peers in oral and written communication (Temple & Carney, 1996).

Social-Emotional and Behavioral

Girls and women with TS face multiple burdens, placing them at risk for emotional distress and problems in their social and romantic relationships. Distress may be a reaction to medical complications, as well as the delayed growth and puberty and knowledge of infertility. These condition-specific issues affect psychological well-being, with many women reporting experiences of teasing due to their short stature and general appearance and feeling they would be rejected by potential partners due to their short stature and infertility. Further, there is a tendency to treat children according to their height age rather than their chronological age. This effect is compounded for children with delayed puberty (Sandberg & Gardner, 2015). Reduced social demands may be placed on the child or adolescent who is perceived as younger. A lack of age-appropriate social experiences may lead to distancing from peers and a preference for younger children or adults. All of these factors can contribute to emergence of clinically significant mental health problems, social isolation, and low self-concept (Hong et al., 2011; Lagrou et al., 2006; Suzigan et al., 2011).

Attention-deficit/hyperactivity disorder (ADHD) is reported at higher rates among individuals with TS compared with their peers (Green et al., 2015; McCauley et al., 2001). Specific areas of concern include difficulty with attentional control, problems orienting attention, and some evidence for deficits in sustained attention (Green et al., 2015). Executive functioning skills may also be affected, including problems with planning, response inhibition, and mental flexibility. Symptoms of ADHD for individuals with TS can manifest as distractibility, poor organization, and inability to sit still. Problems specific to executive function deficits include difficulty planning, rigid and black-and-white thinking, and inability to inhibit thoughts and behaviors (Green et al., 2015; Russell et al., 2006).

Girls and women with TS have consistently been shown to experience difficulty with social cognition. These deficits are linked to difficulty with facial processing and affect recognition in children with TS (Adams et al., 2011; Hong et al., 2014). Parents report their daughters experience greater overall impairments in social functioning compared with their unaffected peers and siblings (Hong et al., 2011; McCauley et al., 2001; Suzigan et al., 2011); girls with TS also perceive themselves as less socially competent (Lagrou et al., 2006).

Among children and adolescents with TS, across studies, symptoms of depression were consistently within the nonclinical range (Green et al., 2015; Hong et al., 2011). Among adults with TS, however, the extant literature continues to be inconsistent, with some studies showing higher rates of depression (Cardoso et al., 2004) and others indicating symptoms in the nonclinical range.

PSYCHOEDUCATIONAL IMPLICATIONS AND SUCCESSFUL INTERVENTIONS

Medical and Health Management

Due to the numerous medical complications associated with TS, regular follow-up with a multidisciplinary team is recommended (Gravholt et al., 2017; Turner Syndrome Society of the United States [TSS], 2017). As primary care providers and specialists often act as gatekeepers for additional specialized health care and mental health resources, awareness of the physical and psychological challenges these individuals face can help greatly improve quality of life (Green et al., 2015). Decisions regarding estrogen replacement will need to take into consideration the trade-off between the perceived psychosexual benefits of an on-time puberty versus taller adult stature, with input from the teen and her family (Sandberg & Gardner, 2015). Special care should be given to sharing information with girls over time. From an early age, girls with TS should be provided with accurate information about ways to achieve parenthood, as well as the risks of pregnancy due to the high prevalence of cardiac anomalies among patients with TS (TSS, 2017).

Providers should consider the psychoeducational implications of missed school due to medical visits. Some medical facilities have worked to overcome this barrier by providing care through multidisciplinary teams, such that patients are able to attend one comprehensive clinic visit where they meet with multiple providers. Additionally, 504 plans can help ensure schools are understanding of any missed school days (for additional information on 504 plans, see U.S. Department of Education, 2018).

Cognitive/Academic

Annual developmental and behavioral screenings are recommended for children and adolescents with TS to help identify and remediate noted deficiencies as early as possible (TSS, 2017). As a result of the potential for motor delays, referrals to occupational and physical therapy services are recommended in early childhood. These services can promote learning of specific motor skills and facilitate the implementation of appropriate academic accommodations (Gravholt et al., 2017).

Problems in cognitive and academic areas should be monitored with early intervention. Problems with working memory may present as difficulty multitasking, problems with mental calculations, and struggling to hold information "in mind." To address these difficulties, classroom modifications, such as shortening the length of assignments/activities, presenting new information within the context of familiar content, allowing repetition of tasks to promote familiarity, repeating instructions or providing written instructions, using memory aids, and coaching the child to use their strengths to help compensate for deficit areas, may prove beneficial. Given the potential visuospatial deficits, utilizing verbal strengths and providing verbal information in conjunction with visuals (e.g., verbal descriptions, mnemonics) as well as other interventions may be appropriate (Gravholt et al., 2017).

Difficulties with visuospatial issues and memory also can impact math. Mathematics mastery can be addressed with empirically supported remediation methods aimed at underlying mathematics disorders (e.g., numerical magnitude representation, linking exact numbers with number symbols). In addition, neuropsychological evaluations are recommended to tailor intervention (Gravholt et al., 2017; TSS, 2017) and also may serve as an opportunity for career counseling due to the tendency for underemployment (Robitschek & Woodson, 2006).

Social-Emotional and Behavior

As noted, girls and women with TS may exhibit a number of social–emotional and behavioral problems. Depending on the presenting problem, behavioral therapy and behavioral parent training may be beneficial, particularly if the child also has ADHD (Chronis et al., 2004). As a general principle, a referral for psychological or psychiatric services is warranted in TS if significant behavioral or social–emotional symptomatology is suspected (Gravholt et al., 2017). Meaningful recommendations are predicated on completion of a comprehensive evaluation from a behavioral health perspective due to the overlapping medical and psychosocial factors. In girls, therapy may be helpful in developing scripts for sharing details of their condition with select others in ways more likely to promote sympathetic understanding rather than confusion. It is also important to make a distinction between privacy and secrecy, as the latter is known to be predictive of negative psychological and social consequences (Newheiser & Barreto, 2014). Pediatric psychologists can also provide resources for peer support for girls and women with TS in order to facilitate networking with other similarly affected persons.

Social deficits may manifest as difficulty identifying emotions through facial expressions, impaired recognition of nonverbal cues, and problems initiating or retaining friendships, possibly diagnosed as social communication disorder or autism spectrum disorder. Social skills group therapy can be beneficial in the school or community setting. Further, girls with TS may benefit from strategies for how to manage teasing by peers, in or outside of school, and how to be assertive in responding to negative comments (Rickert et al., 1996). Counseling and educational intervention should include education about sex chromosomes and the process of sexual differentiation of the body. Educators need to be able to round out the story of sex development of the human body by providing details that are inclusive of boys/men and girls/women born with atypical sex chromosomes.

CONCLUSION

TS is a complex condition requiring support from numerous health care providers, including for mental health, across the lifespan. Early detection of TS is beneficial but complicated by the range in presentations. It is essential that providers view comprehensive care as encompassing the medical/physical as well as the cognitive, academic, and psychosocial aspects of TS and their implications across the lifespan.

RESOURCES

Turner Syndrome Society of the United States. https://www.turnersyndrome.org/

Turner Syndrome Society of Canada. http://www.turnersyndrome.ca/

Turner Syndrome Global Alliance. http://tsgalliance.org/

National Institute of Child Health and Human Development. (2021). *More information on Turner syndrome*. U.S. Department of Health and Human Services. https://www.nichd.nih.gov/health/topics/turner/resources/default

REFERENCES

Adams, R. E., Santo, J. B., & Bukowski, W. M. (2011). The presence of a best friend buffers the effects of negative experiences. *Developmental Psychology, 47*(6), 1786–1791. https://doi.org/10.1037/a0025401

Cardoso, G., Daly, R., Haq, N. A., Hanton, L., Rubinow, D. R., Bondy, C. A., & Schmidt, P. (2004). Current and lifetime psychiatric illness in women with Turner syndrome. *Gynecological Endocrinology, 19*(6), 313–319. https://doi.org/10.1080/09513590400021227

Chronis, A. M., Chacko, A., Fabiano, G. A., Wymbs, B. T., & Pelham, W. E., Jr. (2004). Enhancements to the behavioral parent training paradigm for families of children with ADHD: Review and future directions. *Clinical Child and Family Psychology Review, 7*(1), 1–27. https://doi.org/10.1023/B:CCFP.0000020190.60808.a4

Downey, J., Elkin, E. J., Ehrhardt, A. A., Meyer-Bahlburg, H. F., Bell, J. J., & Morishima, A. (1991). Cognitive ability and everyday functioning in women with Turner syndrome. *Journal of Learning Disabilities, 24*(1), 32–39. https://doi.org/10.1177/002221949102400107

El-Mansoury, M., Barrenäs, M.-L., Bryman, I., Hanson, C., & Landin-Wilhelmsen, K. (2009). Impaired body balance, fine motor function and hearing in women with

Turner syndrome. *Clinical Endocrinology, 71*(2), 273–278. https://doi.org/10.1111/j.1365-2265.2008.03473.x

Gravholt, C. H., Andersen, N. H., Conway, G. S., Dekkers, O. M., Geffner, M. E., Klein, K. O., Lin, A. E., Mauras, N., Quigley, C. A., Rubin, K., Sandberg, D. E., Sas, T. C. J., Silberbach, M., Söderström-Anttila, V., Stochholm, K., van Alfen-van derVelden, J. A., Woelfle, J., Backeljauw, P. F., & the International Turner Syndrome Consensus Group. (2017). Clinical practice guidelines for the care of girls and women with Turner syndrome: Proceedings from the 2016 Cincinnati International Turner Syndrome Meeting. *European Journal of Endocrinology, 177*(3), G1–G70.

Green, T., Bade Shrestha, S., Chromik, L. C., Rutledge, K., Pennington, B. F., Hong, D. S., & Reiss, A. L. (2015). Elucidating X chromosome influences on attention deficit hyperactivity disorder and executive function. *Journal of Psychiatric Research, 68*, 217–225. https://doi.org/10.1016/j.jpsychires.2015.06.021

Hart, S. J., Davenport, M. L., Hooper, S. R., & Belger, A. (2006). Visuospatial executive function in Turner syndrome: Functional MRI and neurocognitive findings. *Brain, 129*(5), 1125–1136. https://doi.org/10.1093/brain/awl046

Hong, D. S., Bray, S., Haas, B. W., Hoeft, F., & Reiss, A. L. (2014). Aberrant neurocognitive processing of fear in young girls with Turner syndrome. *Social Cognitive and Affective Neuroscience, 9*(3), 255–264. https://doi.org/10.1093/scan/nss133

Hong, D. S., Dunkin, B., & Reiss, A. L. (2011). Psychosocial functioning and social cognitive processing in girls with Turner syndrome. *Journal of Developmental and Behavioral Pediatrics, 32*(7), 512–520. https://doi.org/10.1097/DBP.0b013e3182255301

Lagrou, K., Froidecoeur, C., Verlinde, F., Craen, M., De Schepper, J., François, I., & Massa, G. (2006). Psychosocial functioning, self-perception and body image and their auxologic correlates in growth hormone and oestrogen-treated young adult women with Turner syndrome. *Hormone Research, 66*(6), 277–284. https://doi.org/10.1159/000095547

Mazzocco, M. M. M., & Hanich. L. B. (2010). Math achievement, numerical processing, and executive functions in girls with Turner syndrome: Do girls with Turner syndrome have math learning disability? *Learning and Individual Differences, 20*(2), 70–81. https://doi.org/10.1016/j.lindif.2009.10.011

McCauley, E., Feuillan, P., Kushner, H., & Ross, J. L. (2001). Psychosocial development in adolescents with Turner syndrome. *Journal of Developmental and Behavioral Pediatrics, 22*(6), 360–365. https://doi.org/10.1097/00004703-200112000-00003

Murphy, M. M., Mazzocco, M. M., Gerner, G., & Henry, A. E. (2006). Mathematics learning disability in girls with Turner syndrome or fragile X syndrome. *Brain and Cognition, 61*(2), 195–210. https://doi.org/10.1016/j.bandc.2005.12.014

Næss, E. E., Bahr, D., & Gravholt, C. H. (2010). Health status in women with Turner syndrome: A questionnaire study on health status, education, work participation and aspects of sexual functioning. *Clinical Endocrinology, 72*(5), 678–684. https://doi.org/10.1111/j.1365-2265.2009.03715.x

Newheiser, A.-K., & Barreto, M. (2014). Hidden costs of hiding stigma: Ironic interpersonal consequences of concealing a stigmatized identity in social interactions. *Journal of Experimental Social Psychology, 52*, 58–70. https://doi.org/10.1016/j.jesp.2014.01.002

Rae, C., Joy, P., Harasty, J., Kemp, A., Kuan, S., Christodoulou, J., Cowell, C. T., & Coltheart, M. (2004). Enlarged temporal lobes in Turner syndrome: An X-chromosome effect? *Cerebral Cortex, 14*(2), 156–164. https://doi.org/10.1093/cercor/bhg114

Rickert, V. I., Hassed, S. J., Hendon, A. E., & Cunniff, C. (1996). The effects of peer ridicule on depression and self-image among adolescent females with Turner syndrome. *The Journal of Adolescent Health, 19*(1), 34–38. https://doi.org/10.1016/1054-139X(95)00225-H

Robitschek, C., & Woodson, S. J. (2006). Vocational psychology: Using one of counseling psychology's strengths to foster human strength. *The Counseling Psychologist, 34*(2), 260–275. https://doi.org/10.1177/0011000005281321

Romans, S. M., Stefanatos, G., Roeltgen, D. P., Kushner, H., & Ross, J. L. (1998). Transition to young adulthood in Ullrich–Turner syndrome: Neurodevelopmental changes. *American Journal of Medical Genetics, 79*(2), 140–147. https://doi.org/10.1002/(SICI)1096-8628(19980901)79:2<140::AID-AJMG10>3.0.CO;2-J

Russell, H. F., Wallis, D., Mazzocco, M. M., Moshang, T., Zackai, E., Zinn, A. R., Ross, J. L., & Muenke, M. (2006). Increased prevalence of ADHD in Turner syndrome with no evidence of imprinting effects. *Journal of Pediatric Psychology, 31*(9), 945–955. https://doi.org/10.1093/jpepsy/jsj106

Sandberg, D. E., & Gardner, M. (2015). Short stature: Is it a psychosocial problem and does changing height matter? *Pediatric Clinics of North America, 62*(4), 963–982. https://doi.org/10.1016/j.pcl.2015.04.009

Stochholm, K., Hjerrild, B., Mortensen, K. H., Juul, S., Frydenberg, M., & Gravholt, C. H. (2012). Socioeconomic parameters and mortality in Turner syndrome. *European Journal of Endocrinology, 166*(6), 1013–1019.

Suzigan, L. Z., de Paiva e Silva, R. B., Guerra-Júnior, G., Marini, S. H., & Maciel-Guerra, A. T. (2011). Social skills in women with Turner syndrome. *Scandinavian Journal of Psychology,.52*(5), 440–447. https://doi.org/10.1111/j.1467-9450.2011.00887.x

Sybert, V. P., & McCauley, E. (2004). Turner's syndrome. *The New England Journal of Medicine, 351*(12), 1227–1238. https://doi.org/10.1056/NEJMra030360

Temple, C. M., & Carney, R. (1996). Reading skills in children with Turner's syndrome: An analysis of hyperlexia. *Cortex, 32*(2), 335–345. https://doi.org/10.1016/S0010-9452(96)80055-4

Turner Syndrome Society of the United States. (2017). *Clinical practice guidelines for the care of girls and women with Turner syndrome: Brief synopsis for Turner syndrome girls and women and for their parents/caregivers/families.* https://www.turnersyndrome.org/_files/ugd/8fb9de_96c65fef38194ab59df4841d7d744ed6.pdf

U.S. Department of Education. (2018). *Protecting students with disabilities.* https://www2.ed.gov/about/offices/list/ocr/504faq.html

Wahlberg, J., Sydsjö, G., Ledin, T., Bågesund, M., & Ekman, B. (2013). Impaired postural balance in Turner syndrome. *Hormone and Metabolic Research, 45*(7), 537–540. https://doi.org/10.1055/s-0033-1333718

Zinn, A. R., Roeltgen, D., Stefanatos, G., Ramos, P., Elder, F. F., Kushner, H., Kowal, K., & Ross, J. L. (2007). A Turner syndrome neurocognitive phenotype maps to Xp22.3. *Behavioral and Brain Functions, 3*(1), Article 24. https://doi.org/10.1186/1744-9081-3-24

38

Type 1 Diabetes Mellitus

Natalie A. Lárez and Michelle M. Perfect

Type 1 diabetes mellitus (T1DM) is an endocrine disorder caused by the destruction of insulin-producing beta cells in the pancreas, resulting in the body not producing insulin (Butalia et al., 2016). In the 1980s, Eisenbarth proposed that everyone is born with varying degrees of genetic susceptibility to T1DM. The subsequent events of the development of T1DM are due to environmental factors that activate the genetic predisposition (Butalia et al., 2016).

ETIOLOGY

T1DM is the second most prevalent chronic illness among youth (Rawshani et al., 2018). Due to the self-destructive nature of the disease, T1DM is an autoimmune disorder, a clear distinction from Type 2 diabetes, which is a metabolic dysfunction of the pancreas. Currently, there are two main factors when considering the susceptibility of the development of T1DM: genetic predisposition that leaves certain individuals more vulnerable and environmental factors that may initiate autoimmunity or beta-cell destruction (Acharjee et al., 2013). Researchers have been trying to isolate environmental conditions implicated in disease onset; risk factors have included pollutants, viruses, and toxins (Butalia et al., 2016). Antibodies that underlie the autoimmunity against the beta cells that characterize the disease include glutamic acid decarboxylase, tyrosine

Support for work on this chapter was provided in part from the National Institutes of Health, Diversity Supplement (#3RO1DK110528-03S1).

https://doi.org/10.1037/0000349-038
Health-Related Disorders in Children and Adolescents: A Guidebook for Educators and Service Providers, Second Edition, M. M. Perfect, C. A. Riccio, and M. A. Bray (Editors)

phosphates IA-2 and IA-2β, and zinc transporter 8. Researchers have identified at least one of these antibodies in more than 85% of youth who eventually develop T1DM (Kahanovitz et al., 2017). Additionally, having the human leukocyte antigen genotypes DQA and DQB increases the risk of developing T1DM (Kahanovitz et al., 2017; Xia et al., 2019).

PREVALENCE AND INCIDENCE

T1DM has been on the rise in recent decades worldwide. There has been an overall 21% increase in the United States alone since 2001 (Xia et al., 2019). When considering younger children, 15% to 20% of all new diagnoses are among children under 5 years old (Streisand & Monaghan, 2014). About 50% of diagnoses of T1DM occur preadolescence (Rawshani et al., 2018). In summarizing the SEARCH for Diabetes in Youth study, Spanakis and Golden (2013) reported the following rates per 1,000 for youth under 10 years old: 1.03 in non-Hispanic Whites, 0.57 in African Americans, and 0.44 in Latinxs. Between the ages of 10 and 19 years, the prevalence per 1,000 was 2.89 in non-Hispanic White youth, 2.04 in African American youth, and 1.59 in Latinx youth. Worldwide, Finland and Canada have the highest incidence rates of T1DM in youth (Xia et al., 2019).

SYMPTOMS

Symptoms for T1DM often do not present until enough insulin-producing cells have been destroyed. Many youths and families are unaware of their illness until months and maybe years after the (as yet unidentified) causal insult. Signs and symptoms of T1DM include excessive thirst, appetite, weight loss, and urination (Kahanovitz et al., 2017). Treatment of T1DM can result in hyper- and hypoglycemia. *Hyperglycemia* is when blood sugar rises above target range. *Hypoglycemia* is when blood sugar levels have fallen below the recommended range for a specific age. Although target ranges are individualized, a general consensus for characterizing hypo- and hyperglycemia is glucose levels below 70 mg/dL and above 180 mg/dL, respectively (Agiostratidou et al., 2017).

IMPACT ON THE STUDENT AND OUTCOMES

Medical

The gold standard metric for diabetes control is hemoglobin A1c, which is a measure of blood glucose levels over 90 days (Agiostratidou et al., 2017). Hypoglycemic levels below 54 mg/dL or multiple repeated or prolonged episodes have been linked with neurophysiological changes in the prefrontal cortex and medial temporal lobes. Severe hypoglycemia may lead to light-headedness, visual disturbances, or seizures (Agiostratidou et al., 2017). If sugar levels rise too high, fat breakdown products that accumulate in the bloodstream can lead to ketoacidosis. Hyperglycemia also has long-term complications, including nerve damage, blindness, kidney disease, and cardiovascular repercussions (Agiostratidou et al., 2017). Individuals with T1DM are at an increased risk for other autoimmune conditions, such as celiac disease and thyroid dysfunction (American Diabetes Association [ADA], 2022). Researchers have found that 36% of children under the age of 6 do not meet the ADA goals for a hemoglobin A1c level of less than 8.5% (Streisand & Monaghan, 2014). A recent case-controlled study of thousands of young adults with T1DM found that diagnoses before the age of 10 had 5 to 90 times increased risk for various cardiovascular comorbidities (Rawshani et al., 2018).

Cognitive/Academic

Individuals with T1DM have a higher risk of adverse outcomes in reading, writing, attention, executive functioning, psychomotor functioning, and visuospatial processing (Agiostratidou et al., 2017; Naguib et al., 2009). Using repeated home-based assessments, researchers found that performance on brief mental math and choice reaction tasks was poorer when children were concurrently experiencing hypo- or hyperglycemia (Gonder-Frederick et al., 2009). Notably, a longitudinal study found that deteriorating glycemic control preceded a decline in academic performance (Winnick et al., 2017). In a study examining concurrent glucose levels during the administration of standardized achievement tests, youth with T1DM who had glucose levels in the suboptimal or hyperglycemic ranges performed worse on writing and reading fluency tasks than those with glucose levels in the target range. Additionally, more frequent and longer hypoglycemic episodes during the 12 hours preceding testing predicted lower scores on reading fluency, math calculation, and spelling tests (Knight & Perfect, 2019). Conversely, Perfect and Jaramillo (2012) found that adolescents who reported fewer diabetes-related stressors and more resilient characteristics also reported higher grades.

Social–Emotional and Behavioral

T1DM often means additional stressors associated with continuous management of the disease while still navigating the complexities of development. Researchers have found that fluctuations in glucose levels lead to symptoms that may affect the individual's concentration, alertness, and irritability (Winnick et al., 2017). Moreover, these associated symptoms may make it difficult for youth with T1DM to invest in their social relationships. Among younger children, fear of being away from caregivers is common due to their greater dependence for diabetes management. Due to the constant vigilance required from parents, managing diabetes may also lead to psychosocial repercussions among caregivers. Consequently, parents who reported higher levels of diabetes-related stress also reported a higher occurrence of behavioral problems among young children (Streisand & Monaghan, 2014). Both adolescents (Perfect & Jaramillo, 2012) and young children (Streisand & Monaghan, 2014) have increased incidence of internalizing disorders, such as depression and anxiety. Although lifestyle factors are not primary contributors to T1DM progression, factors such as poor diet, lack of physical activity, and poor sleep hygiene make these youth more vulnerable to poor psychosocial outcomes and difficulties at school (Åman et al., 2009; Perfect, 2014). Conversely, resilient characteristics combat diabetes-related risk factors, demonstrating that self-efficacy, family support, and a positive attitude are associated with good diabetes management (Hillard et al., 2017).

PSYCHOEDUCATIONAL IMPLICATIONS AND SCHOOL-BASED INTERVENTIONS

The findings discussed thus far have led to insights into how professionals in schools can better serve students who may have fluctuating glucose levels throughout the day. They underscore the risks associated with T1DM and demonstrate the importance of fostering a strength-based approach to support youth diabetes management.

Medical and Health Management

Exogenous insulin is typically administered to patients to stabilize glucose levels and avoid severe hyper- and hypoglycemia and ketoacidosis. Typically, youth with T1DM require a dose of basal insulin once daily. In some cases, patients with T1DM will have an insulin pump, which is a small, computerized device that delivers small amounts of insulin over time through a subcutaneous catheter in place of the basal insulin injection. Additionally, youth need rapid-acting insulin (referred to as bolus) several times a day based on glucose values above a certain threshold and the anticipated carbohydrate intake for an upcoming meal or snack (ADA Professional Practice Committee, 2022). Youth can use either a glucometer or a continuous glucose monitor to check glucose levels in real time (Knight & Perfect, 2019).

Due to the continuous monitoring required in T1DM, a diabetes management plan should be in place for each student. Younger children may need assistance with administering their insulin and checking blood glucose levels, which requires staff and family to be knowledgeable in diabetes care (Streisand & Monaghan, 2014). Middle and high school students may be completely self-sufficient in their diabetes care, but staff should still be aware of the extra time they may need between classes and other activities (ADA, 2014). To manage hypoglycemia, students should have easy access to fast-acting carbohydrates and, in severe cases, glucagon to increase glucose levels. In the chronic health plan, the student and educators should be clear about requirements for glucose testing frequency (e.g., 15 minutes before each meal), testing location (e.g., classroom vs. nurse's office), and flexibility to self-administer insulin when needed.

Cognitive/Academic

Although academic interventions are lacking, several accommodations, modifications, and interventions have been proposed to best support the needs of youth with T1DM. Due to the known areas that are affected, Knight and Perfect (2019) suggested that students with T1DM be allotted extra time for reading and writing assignments, have access to a spell checker, and be provided with larger print passages to support students who experience frequent and out-of-range glucose levels. Considerations must be taken to allow for extended or delayed testing and accommodate recurring intermittent absences. The most recent ADA standards recommended screening for cognitive function in youth and for those who experience hypoglycemia, making referral for formal testing as warranted (ADA Professional Practice Committee, 2022). Planning for after high school is an autonomous task in which adolescents will participate; moreover, transitioning to a new diabetes care team is essential to prepare for the future (ADA, 2014). School professionals can be intentional in creating cohesive plans with medical professionals across settings. Additionally, school counselors or psychologists can work with adolescents to develop self-advocacy and self-efficacy skills, such as helping them create a plan for treatment while managing other obligations (e.g., college course work, industry schedules) and involving youth as key stakeholders in decision making (Perfect et al., 2017).

Social-Emotional and Behavioral

Due to the high comorbidity of psychological disorders among youth with T1DM, universal screening of psychological functioning has been recommended (ADA Professional Practice Committee, 2022; Cameron et al., 2007). Allowing for flexibility in the schedule of youth with T1DM can allow space for peer interaction (ADA, 2014). When children adhere to their management plan, positive reinforcement is vital for continued optimal care and fostering independence (Silverstein et al., 2005). Given the self-care nature of T1DM, caregivers and patients should identify effective coping mechanisms to alleviate stress associated with managing their condition (Perfect & Jaramillo, 2012). Moreover, current interventions include parent and child support groups to devise stress management strategies (Streisand & Monaghan, 2014). Positive affect promotes positive outcomes for youth with T1DM (Hillard et al., 2017; Lord et al., 2015). Consequently, interventions focused on fostering positive affect among youth, such as practicing gratitude and self-affirmations, may lead to promising improvements for optimal health outcomes (Lord et al., 2015). Schools should implement interventions that target increasing school personnel knowledge of diabetes or those that focus on improving student self-management to increase self-efficacy and quality of life (Pansier & Schulz, 2015). Research has shown that particularly intermittent reinforcement may increase self-care behaviors and improve glycemic control (Lasecki et al., 2008). Consultation models, such as behavioral consultation and conjoint behavioral consultation, may allow a provider to support school personnel in working with students to manage their diabetes better (Lasecki et al., 2008).

CONCLUSION

The constant vigilance of T1DM and the associated health outcomes may lead to multiple repercussions in youths' ever-changing environments and development. Even so, patients have demonstrated a resilient ability to perform well in school while managing their condition. When working with students with T1DM, it is crucial to take into consideration their ability to self-manage and be mindful of the potential risks.

RESOURCES

Centers for Disease Control and Prevention. (2022). *Managing diabetes at school.* https://www.cdc.gov/diabetes/library/features/managing-diabetes-at-school.html

Juvenile Diabetes Research Foundation. (n.d.). *Type 1 diabetes resources and support.* https://www.jdrf.org/t1d-resources/

American Diabetes Association. (n.d.). *Help for schools.* https://diabetes.org/tools-support/know-your-rights/safe-at-school-state-laws/help-for-schools

Applications for monitoring glucose: MySugr (free, available for iPhone and Android), BG Monitor Diabetes (free, available for Android), Glucose Buddy (free, available for iPhone and Android).

REFERENCES

Acharjee, S., Ghosh, B., Al-Dhubiab, B. E., & Nair, A. B. (2013). Understanding Type 1 diabetes: Etiology and models. *Canadian Journal of Diabetes, 37*(4), 269–276. https://doi.org/10.1016/j.jcjd.2013.05.001

Agiostratidou, G., Anhalt, H., Ball, D., Blonde, L., Gourgari, E., Harriman, K. N., Kowalski, A. J., Madden, P., McAuliffe-Fogarty, A. H., McElwee-Malloy, M., Peters, A., Raman, S., Reifschneider, K., Rubin, K., & Weinzimer, S. A. (2017). Standardizing clinically meaningful outcome measures beyond HbA1c for Type 1 diabetes: A consensus report of the American Association of Clinical Endocrinologists, the American Association of Diabetes Educators, the American Diabetes Association, the Endocrine Society, JDRF International, the Leona M. and Harry B. Helmsley Charitable Trust, the Pediatric Endocrine Society, and the T1D Exchange. *Diabetes Care, 40*(12), 1622–1630. https://doi.org/10.2337/dc17-1624

Åman, J., Skinner, T. C., de Beaufort, C. E., Swift, P. G. F., Aanstoot, H. J., Cameron, F., & the Hvidoere Study Group on Childhood Diabetes. (2009). Associations between physical activity, sedentary behavior, and glycemic control in a large cohort of adolescents with Type 1 diabetes: The Hvidoere Study Group on Childhood

Diabetes. *Pediatric Diabetes, 10*(4), 234–239. https://doi.org/10.1111/j.1399-5448.2008.00495.x

American Diabetes Association. (2014). Diabetes care in school and day care setting. *Diabetes Care, 37*(Suppl. 1), S91–S96. https://doi.org/10.2337/dc14-S091

American Diabetes Association Professional Practice Committee. (2022). Facilitating behavior change and well-being to improve health outcomes: *Standards of Medical Care in Diabetes—2022. Diabetes Care, 45*(Suppl. 1), S60–S82. https://doi.org/10.2337/dc22-S005

Butalia, S., Kaplan, G. G., Khokhar, B., & Rabi, D. M. (2016). Environmental risk factors and Type 1 diabetes: Past, present, and future. *Canadian Journal of Diabetes, 40*(6), 586–593. https://doi.org/10.1016/j.jcjd.2016.05.002

Cameron, F. J., Northam, E. A., Ambler, G. R., & Daneman, D. (2007). Routine psychological screening in youth with Type 1 diabetes and their parents: A notion whose time has come? *Diabetes Care, 30*(10), 2716–2724. https://doi.org/10.2337/dc07-0603

Gonder-Frederick, L. A., Zrebiec, J. F., Bauchowitz, A. U., Ritterband, L. M., Magee, J. C., Cox, D. J., & Clarke, W. L. (2009). Cognitive function is disrupted by both hypo- and hyperglycemia in school-aged children with Type 1 diabetes: A field study. *Diabetes Care, 32*(6), 1001–1006. https://doi.org/10.2337/dc08-1722

Hillard, M. E., Hagger, V., Hendrieckx, C., Anderson, B. J., Trawley, S., Jack, M. M., Pouwer, F., Skinner, T., & Speight, J. (2017). Strengths, risk factors, and resilience outcomes in adolescents with Type 1 diabetes: Results from Diabetes MILES youth–Australia. *Diabetes Care, 40*(7), 849–855. https://doi.org/10.2337/dc16-2688

Kahanovitz, L., Sluss, P. M., & Russell, S. J. (2017). Type 1 diabetes—A clinical perspective. *Point of Care, 16*(1), 37–40. https://doi.org/10.1097/POC.0000000000000125

Knight, M. F., & Perfect, M. M. (2019). Glycemic control influences on academic performance in youth with Type 1 diabetes. *School Psychology, 34*(6), 646–655. https://doi.org/10.1037/spq0000320

Lasecki, K., Olympia, D., Clark, E., Jenson, W., & Heathfield, L. T. (2008). Using behavioral interventions to assist children with Type 1 diabetes manage blood glucose levels. *School Psychology Quarterly, 23*(3), 389–406. https://doi.org/10.1037/1045-3830.23.3.389

Lord, J. H., Rumburg, T. M., & Jaser, S. S. (2015). Staying positive: Positive affect as a predictor of resilience in adolescents with Type 1 diabetes. *Journal of Pediatric Psychology, 40*(9), 968–977. https://doi.org/10.1093/jpepsy/jsv042

Naguib, J. M., Kulinskaya, E., Lomax, C. L., & Garralda, M. E. (2009). Neuro-cognitive performance in children with Type 1 diabetes—A meta-analysis. *Journal of Pediatric Psychology, 34*(3), 271–282. https://doi.org/10.1093/jpepsy/jsn074

Pansier, B., & Schulz, P. J. (2015). School-based diabetes interventions and their outcomes: A systematic literature review. *Journal of Public Health Research, 4*(1), Article 467. https://doi.org/10.4081/jphr.2015.467

Perfect, M. M. (2014). The relations of sleep and quality of life to school performance in youth with Type 1 diabetes. *Journal of Applied School Psychology, 30*(1), 7–28. https://doi.org/10.1080/15377903.2013.853718

Perfect, M. M., Frye, S., Bauman, S., Kroeger, S., Chou, C. C., & Shaw, L. (2017). A model for facilitating an inclusive experience for college students with health-related conditions: Application for students with diabetes. *The School Psychologist, 71*(3), 45–57. https://www.researchgate.net/publication/321487460_A_Model_for_Facilitating_an_Inclusive_Experience_for_College_Students_with_Health-Related_Conditions_Application_for_Students_with_Diabetes

Perfect, M. M., & Jaramillo, E. (2012). Relations between resiliency, diabetes-related quality of life, and disease markers to school-related outcomes in adolescents with diabetes. *School Psychology Quarterly, 27*(1), 29–40. https://doi.org/10.1037/a0027984

Rawshani, A., Sattar, N., Franzén, S., Rawshani, A., Hattersley, A. T., Svensson, A. M., Eliasson, B., & Gudbjörnsdottir, S. (2018). Excess mortality and cardiovascular disease in young adults with Type 1 diabetes in relation to age at onset: A nation-wide, register-based cohort study. *The Lancet, 392*(10146), 477–486. https://doi.org/10.1016/S0140-6736(18)31506-X

Silverstein, J., Klingensmith, G., Copeland, K., Plotnick, L., Kaufman, F., Laffel, L., Deeb, L., Grey, M., Anderson, B., Holzmeister, L. A., Clark, N., & American Diabetes Association. (2005). Care of children and adolescents with Type 1 diabetes. *Diabetes Care, 28*(1), 186–212. https://doi.org/10.2337/diacare.28.1.186

Spanakis, E. K., & Golden, S. H. (2013). Race/ethnic difference in diabetes and diabetic complications. *Current Diabetes Reports, 13*(6), 814–823. https://doi.org/10.1007/s11892-013-0421-9

Streisand, R., & Monaghan, M. (2014). Young children with Type 1 diabetes: Challenges, research, and future directions. *Current Diabetes Reports, 14*(9), Article 520. https://doi.org/10.1007/s11892-014-0520-2

Winnick, J. B., Berg, C. A., Wiebe, D. J., Schaefer, B. A., Lei, P. W., & Butner, J. E. (2017). Metabolic control and academic achievement over time among adolescents with Type 1 diabetes. *School Psychology Quarterly, 32*(1), 105–117. https://doi.org/10.1037/spq0000190

Xia, Y., Xie, Z., Huang, G., & Zhou, Z. (2019). Incidence and trend of Type 1 diabetes and the underlying environmental determinants. *Diabetes/Metabolism Research and Reviews, 35*(1), Article e3075. https://doi.org/10.1002/dmrr.3075

39

Type 2 Diabetes Mellitus

Stihlyn Chamberlain and Savina Maria Bello

Karamanou et al. (2016) reported that an ancient Greek physician, Araetus of Cappadocia, first coined the term "diabetes." Flash forward to the year 1675, and "mellitus," meaning honey sweet, was added to the term "diabetes." The Ancient Indians first noticed an excess of sugar in individuals' urine; however, a British physician, Thomas Willis, rediscovered this and confirmed the presence of excess sugar in the urine of individuals presenting with diabetes. Later in 1857, a French physiologist, Claude Bernard, discovered the role of the liver in glycogenesis, or the formation of glycogen from sugar. In 1889, Mering and Minkowski discovered the role of the pancreas in diabetes. These discoveries were significant turning points in experimental medicine. Diabetes and its effects on the body were slowly being understood, thus shaping accurate diagnosis and treatment. Furthermore, these discoveries led to the identification of two types of diabetes: Type 1 and Type 2 (Karamanou et al., 2016).

ETIOLOGY

The two hallmark features of Type 2 diabetes mellitus (T2DM) are insulin resistance and dysfunction in the beta cells in the pancreas (American Diabetes Association [ADA], 2019). Insulin resistance is when the body is unable to suppress the liver's glucose output and disposal of glucose. Dysfunction in the beta cells occurs when pancreatic insulin release is not meeting the same degree of insulin resistance. Insulin resistance and reduced sensitivity in skeletal muscle

https://doi.org/10.1037/0000349-039
Health-Related Disorders in Children and Adolescents: A Guidebook for Educators and Service Providers, Second Edition, M. M. Perfect, C. A. Riccio, and M. A. Bray (Editors)

are two of the first detectable signs of T2DM (Taylor, 2013). An excess of fat accumulation in the liver can occur before the onset of T2DM as well (Taylor, 2013).

Obesity increases the risk substantially for T2DM (Cefalu et al., 2019; Hannon & Arslanian, 2015; McGarry, 2002; Pettitt et al., 2014; Xu & Verre, 2018). Historically, T2DM has been diagnosed later in life, but an increase in younger onset is being seen (ADA, 2017; Cefalu et al., 2019; Mayo Clinic, 2019; Xu & Verre, 2018). However, T2DM precursors can occur at different time points.

PREVALENCE AND INCIDENCE

T2DM has been increasing worldwide for the past 3 decades and is one of the fastest growing public health problems (Alonso-Magdalena et al., 2011; Xu & Verre, 2018). This continual increase has occurred concomitantly with the obesity epidemic in the United States. Pettitt et al. (2014) found 0.24 cases of T2DM per 1,000 American youth under 20 years old in a sample of around 3.5 million individuals with physician-diagnosed diabetes (Type 1, Type 2, and other). The prevalence of T2DM increased with age and was higher in female and non-Hispanic White populations. Notably, T2DM was most prevalent in Native American and African American youth (Pettitt et al., 2014). In 2001, the overall prevalence in the United States was 0.34 per 1,000 and increased to 0.46 per 1,000 in 2009 (Dabelea et al., 2014). This is a prevalence increase of 35% between the years 2001 and 2009 for T2DM in youths under the age of 20. These increases were found in both sexes, as well as for White, Black, and Latinx youth (Dabelea et al., 2014). Although there was a statistically significant increase for both sexes in the age range of 10 to 14 years, the prevalence of T2DM was found to be higher for female individuals ages 15 to 19 than for male individuals (Dabelea et al., 2014). With the increase of T2DM among youth, children who are around the age of 10 years, at the beginning of puberty, or obese should be screened for T2DM (Cefalu et al., 2019; Reinehr, 2013).

SYMPTOMS

Type 1 and Type 2 diabetes share features during symptomatic disease. T2DM is distinguished by hyperglycemia with insulin resistance and impaired insulin production (Xu & Verre, 2018). T2DM is typically diagnosed by urine and blood tests in individuals who are asymptomatic, meaning they display no physical symptoms of hyperglycemia (Sperry, 2006). Hyperglycemia symptoms can include increased appetite and thirst, blurred vision, weight loss, fatigue, frequent urination, slow-healing sores, tingling pain, or numbness in hands and feet (ADA, 2019; Mayo Clinic, 2019). Patches of darkened skin, typically in the armpit or neck (i.e., acanthosis nigricans), are consistent with insulin resistance. Distinguishing between Type 1 and Type 2 diabetes in obese pediatric patients can be challenging. Pediatric patients with features indicative of T2DM can present with diabetes-associated autoantibodies and ketosis (Cefalu et al., 2019).

Diabetes mellitus is diagnosed when any two of the following are found: a fasting plasma glucose level greater than or equal to 126 mg/dL, a 2-hour plasma glucose level greater than or equal to 200 mg/dL during an oral glucose tolerance test, or a laboratory-tested hemoglobin A1c level greater than or equal to 6.5%. If only one criterion is met, that abnormal result should be retested. A single random plasma glucose level greater than or equal to 200 mg/dL with classic hyperglycemia symptoms (e.g., polydipsia, polyuria, unintentional weight loss) also meets the diagnostic criteria (Xu & Verre, 2018).

IMPACT ON THE STUDENT AND OUTCOMES

Medical

T2DM is a serious disease with poorer outcomes the younger the onset. Comparing Type 1 and Type 2 participants, the Type 2 cohort had a significant excess in mortality at 11% versus 6.8% in Type 1 (Constantino et al., 2013). Mortality occurred significantly faster and at a younger age (with a shorter diabetes duration) for T2DM at 26.9 years versus 36.5 years (Constantino et al., 2013). Those with T2DM also had more cardiovascular deaths (50% vs. 30%; Constantino et al., 2013). Additionally, complications associated with T2DM include skin, eye (cataracts, glaucoma), and foot complications (poor circulation and amputation in severe cases); neuropathy; kidney disease; high blood pressure; and stroke (ADA, 2019). Due to common severe comorbidities with T2DM, individuals should have a lipid panel and a liver function test annually, as well as an evaluation for microalbuminuria, retinopathy, and sleep apnea (Xu & Verre, 2018).

The hemoglobin A1c test should be conducted approximately every 3 months to assess glycemic control (Cefalu et al., 2019; Wyckoff et al., 2015). The hemoglobin A1c level goal for those with diabetes is less than 7%; the higher the level, the higher blood sugar levels were in the past 3 months, which puts the individual at a higher risk for complications (ADA, 2019).

Diabetic ketoacidosis (DKA) is a life-threatening condition associated with diabetes. DKA occurs when the individual's body does not have enough insulin to use glucose and begins to break down fats too fast because of the lack of glucose, pushing the liver to make the fat into ketones, which then causes the individual's blood to become acidic (ADA, 2019). DKA can lead to a diabetic coma and is a sign that the individual's disease management is suboptimal. Approximately 25% of children and adolescents who present with DKA have T2DM (ADA, 2019).

Cognitive/Academic

Individuals with T2DM have been found to perform more poorly in learning and memory domains, especially reading and spelling (McCrimmon et al.,

2012; Ryan et al., 2016). They also have been found to have lower scores on intelligence and academic achievement measurements, as well as on tasks of attention, psychomotor speed, and executive functions (Ryan et al., 2016). Unlike Type 1, individuals with T2DM often manifest mild learning and memory deficits (Ryan et al., 2016). Additionally, the longer the individual suffers from T2DM, the more reduction in mental efficiency and brain volume they experience, which is worsened by poor metabolic control and accelerates the rate of cognitive decline (Ryan et al., 2016). Chronic hyperglycemia and microvascular disease contribute to the cognitive dysfunction seen in T2DM (McCrimmon et al., 2012). These more severe consequences are typically seen between the ages of 40 and 64 (Ryan et al., 2016). Yau et al. (2010) studied 18 obese T2DM adolescents and found all the participants performed poorly in all cognitive domains assessed. The most significant areas of poor performance were found in intellectual functioning, verbal memory, and psychomotor efficiency (Yau et al., 2010). An adolescent's intellectual capacity and verbal memory impairments were found to be consistent with middle-aged individuals with T2DM. Yau et al. proposed that impairments in vascular reactivity found with insulin resistance or T2DM may play a part in the reductions seen with cognitive performance.

Variability in blood sugar levels can affect cognitive functioning. There is a medical link between individuals with T2DM and academic achievement, such that suboptimal glycemic control is a risk factor for student academic underperformance and increased absenteeism (ADA, 2017). Yau et al. (2010) found adolescents who were diagnosed with T2DM and were obese performed poorly on an academic achievement measure. If an individual's cognition is not functioning properly, they tend to fall behind academically. Thus, it is crucial for school providers to have the resources and procedures to ensure the safety and well-being of the student. Academically, younger patients with T2DM tend to need more resources than the average student to keep up with their health. Dysglycemia, including in school settings, can result from inadequate carbohydrate intake and inaccurate insulin doses due to delayed meals or overeating (ADA, 2006). Recommendations for students with T2DM are discussed later in the chapter.

Social-Emotional and Behavioral

Diabetes mellitus is one of the most prevalent chronic health conditions identified among school-age children (Wyckoff et al., 2015). Students with T2DM are suffering not only from a chronic disease but also from possible social stigma or isolation. Depending on the age of onset, the understanding of their disease plays a major factor in their ability to plan for their meals/snacks with injections. Misusing insulin for weight management can become an issue for students (Wyckoff et al., 2015). Psychosocial issues found with T2DM youth can include caregiver overprotection, lack of independence, perceived helplessness, and student authority control issues (Butler et al., 2013, as cited in Wyckoff et al., 2015). Students do not want to appear different from their peers, and this can greatly affect their ability or willingness to adhere to their treatment regimen. Treatment adherence and other challenges extend past the school or peer setting. Family dynamics, socioeconomic status, concerns for privacy, weight and body image concerns, coordination of meals, school activities, sports management, skill level, and knowledge especially regarding self-management of their diabetes can all affect the individuals' adherence to their diabetes management, which can have serious consequences in the moment and long term (Halvorson et al., 2005, as cited in Wyckoff et al., 2015). The family dynamic and support should not be overlooked, as they can have a major impact on the child's management and understanding of their disease (Fritsch & Olshan, 2011, as cited in Wyckoff et al., 2015).

Financial strain is a significant stressor for those living with any chronic disease, especially those with T2DM. To mediate financial stress, it is recommended that T2DM individuals discuss alternative methods and plans with their health care providers to gather information on how to afford the equipment and appointments needed to properly manage their T2DM (Daly et al., 2009). The child's caregiver should facilitate these discussions with their health care provider or endocrinologist. These discussions provide the opportunity to mediate the child's feeling of stigma, as there are options for inconspicuous devices.

PSYCHOEDUCATIONAL IMPLICATIONS AND SCHOOL-BASED INTERVENTIONS

Medical and Health Management

Management of T2DM includes self-management, exercising, nutrition therapy, and educating the individual about living with diabetes (Sperry, 2006). The goal is to provide and maintain a healthy diet and exercise regimen that can be modified to fit their lifestyle, ethnicity, and culture. Unfortunately, only about 10% of individuals living with T2DM are able to control their diabetes by dieting and exercising alone; the remaining 90% utilize insulin injections to maintain their blood glucose levels (Sperry, 2006). Health care professionals recommend that children should limit sedentary activities, partake in physical activity, and be conscious of what they eat to mitigate the health risks associated with T2DM, especially obesity (ADA, 2000). T2DM is highly comorbid with obesity, insulin resistance, and high cholesterol and triglyceride levels (Ryan et al., 2016). Obesity is a greater health risk and concern especially in young children and adolescents, as this puts the individual at risk for other complications. Additionally, chronic hyperglycemia and microvascular disease have been found to contribute to cognitive dysfunction, changes in white matter tracts, mental and motor slowing in measures of attention and executive functioning, and neural slowing (McCrimmon et al., 2012; Ryan et al., 2016).

Due to the risks found with T2DM, common recommendations include the need for daily physical activity, proper nutrition, and adherence to their diabetes management plan. Physical activity for all students is important but especially for those with diabetes. It is highly recommended that these individuals participate in at least 30 to 60 minutes of moderate to vigorous exercise at least 5 days a week, including strength training on at least 3 of the days (Cefalu et al., 2019; Wyckoff et al., 2015). Nutrition and a healthy diet also play a major role in the effects and management of T2DM. The ADA recommends a diet of nutrient-dense, high-quality foods with reduced consumption of calorie-dense, nutrient-lacking, or sugary meals and beverages (Cefalu et al., 2019; Wyckoff et al., 2015). The child or adolescent's A1c should be measured every 3 months (Cefalu et al., 2019; Wyckoff et al., 2015).

School staff members need to be trained in understanding T2DM as well as in recognizing signs of danger and the correct responses (Wyckoff et al., 2015). These trained individuals should be available during school hours, and at least one should be present during extracurricular activities to ensure student safety. A student who is frequently absent, not succeeding, or presenting behavioral issues should be monitored for possible glycemic control issues and referred for further glycemic control (Wyckoff et al., 2015). An individualized health plan explaining how to treat symptoms of hypo- and hyperglycemia for the student should be created by the school nurse (Wyckoff et al., 2015). A diabetes medical management plan should be obtained from the student's care provider (Wyckoff et al., 2015). The school nurse should help with the implementation of the individualized health plan and diabetes medical management plan and communication with the student, their caregivers, and their health care provider (Wyckoff et al., 2015). A private area should be assigned for the student to use for their injections and care. Further information and explanation should be provided to both the student and their family as needed about proper nutrition at school and how to plan accordingly for their meals and snacks as well as for exercise.

Cognitive/Academic

Communication between medical personnel, family, and school personnel is crucial, as with other chronic illnesses. As with all other children, prompt identification of cognitive and academic deficits is critical for successful outcomes. The earlier the intervention, the less that student has to struggle and the less they fall behind. As was stated earlier in the chapter, cognitive performance and academic performance are highly correlated. T2DM affects memory and learning domains, especially in reading and spelling (McCrimmon et al., 2012; Ryan et al., 2016) as well as poor performance on academic achievement measures. Compounded by the effects of neural slowing, which includes slow information processing, the effects of these impacts are certain to be seen in the school setting (McCrimmon et al., 2012; Ryan et al., 2016). However, support can mediate these effects. Students suffering from any chronic illness, including T2DM, should have a 504 plan with their school. Because of the cognitive impacts seen with T2DM, it is recommended that students should have a comprehensive evaluation in order to determine the areas of support needed. This will provide an opportunity for an individualized education program.

Social-Emotional and Behavioral

Social factors, such as social support, are directly linked with glycemic control (Walker et al., 2014). These social factors allow the individual to become more aware of how to care for themselves. Lower distress about their T2DM was related to increased levels of social support from their loved ones and lower perceived stress, which is all correlated with moderating one's glycemic control (Walker et al., 2014). Typically, the more support an individual receives socially, the better their overall health becomes. Browne et al. (2013) analyzed how social stigma surrounding this chronic disease affected the students' lives and thoughts. Often, people associate T2DM with laziness and assume it is the individual's fault for not taking better care of themselves, thus leading individuals with T2DM to "blame and shame" themselves and feel inferior or excluded on certain occasions (Browne et al., 2013). Browne et al. recommended that more coping mechanisms be incorporated into the treatment plan for individuals to feel more at ease after being diagnosed and living with T2DM.

CONCLUSION

The prevalence of T2DM is increasing, especially in the United States among minority groups such as African Americans and Native American youth (Pettitt et al., 2014). Cognitive and academic impacts can occur in T2DM individuals, especially with poor health management. Individuals with T2DM have been found to perform lower in learning and memory domains, especially reading and spelling (McCrimmon et al., 2012; Ryan et al., 2016). Overall, individuals with T2DM should have daily physical activity and proper nutrition and should adhere to their diabetes management plan to decrease negative consequences.

RESOURCES

American Diabetes Association. (n.d.). *Tools and support*. https://www.diabetes.org/tools-support

American Diabetes Association. (n.d.). *Know your rights: Safe at school*. https://diabetes.org/tools-support/know-your-rights/safe-at-school-state-laws

Centers for Disease Control and Prevention. (2021). *Type 2 diabetes*. https://www.cdc.gov/diabetes/basics/type2.html

Association of Diabetes Care and Education Specialists. (n.d.). *Resources for people living with diabetes*. https://www.diabeteseducator.org/living-with-diabetes

National Institute of Diabetes and Digestive and Kidney Diseases. https://www.niddk.nih.gov/

Diabetes Research Institute Foundation. https://www.diabetesresearch.org/

International Diabetes Federation. https://www.idf.org/

American Association of Clinical Endocrinologists. https://www.aace.com/
Defeat Diabetes Foundation. https://defeatdiabetes.org/
CR3 Diabetes Association. https://www.cr3diabetes.org/
Huggins Salomon, S. (2021). What are the signs and symptoms of Type 2 diabetes? *Everyday Health*. https://www.everydayhealth.com/type-2-diabetes/guide/symptoms/
Lawler, M., & Bucklin, S. (2022). Type 2 diabetes treatment: Types, benefits, and side effects. *Everyday Health*. https://www.everydayhealth.com/type-2-diabetes/guide/treatment/

REFERENCES

Alonso-Magdalena, P., Quesada, I., & Nadal, A. (2011). Endocrine disruptors in the etiology of Type 2 diabetes mellitus. *Nature Reviews Endocrinology, 7*(6), 346–353. https://doi.org/10.1038/nrendo.2011.56

American Diabetes Association. (2000). Type 2 diabetes in children and adolescents. *Pediatrics, 105*(3), 671–680. https://doi.org/10.1542/peds.105.3.671

American Diabetes Association. (2006). Diabetes care in the school and day care setting. *Diabetes Care, 29*(Suppl. 1), S49–S55. https://doi.org/10.2337/diacare.29.s1.06.s49

American Diabetes Association. (2017). Children and adolescents. *Diabetes Care, 40*(Suppl. 1), S105–S113. https://doi.org/10.2337/dc17-S015

American Diabetes Association. (2019). *DKA (ketoacidosis) and ketones.*

Browne, J. L., Ventura, A., Mosely, K., & Speight, J. (2013). "I call it the blame and shame disease": A qualitative study about perceptions of social stigma surrounding Type 2 diabetes. *BMJ Open, 3*(11), Article e003384. https://doi.org/10.1136/bmjopen-2013-003384

Cefalu, W. T., Berg, E. G., Saraco, M., Petersen, M. P., Uelmen, S., Robinson, S., & the American Diabetes Association. (2019). Children and adolescents: *Standards of Medical Care in Diabetes—2019. Diabetes Care, 42*(Suppl. 1), S148–S164. https://doi.org/10.2337/dc19-S013

Constantino, M. I., Molyneaux, L., Limacher-Gisler, F., Al-Saeed, A., Luo, C., Wu, T., Twigg, S. M., Yue, D. K., & Wong, J. (2013). Long-term complications and mortality in young-onset diabetes: Type 2 diabetes is more hazardous and lethal than Type 1 diabetes. *Diabetes Care, 36*(12), 3863–3869. https://doi.org/10.2337/dc12-2455

Dabelea, D., Mayer-Davis, E. J., Saydah, S., Imperatore, G., Linder, B., Divers, J., Bell, R., Badaru, A., Talton, J. W., Crume, T., Liese, A. D., Merchant, A. T., Lawrence, J. M., Reynolds, K., Dolan, L., Liu, L. L., & Hamman, R. F. (2014). Prevalence of Type 1 and Type 2 diabetes among children and adolescents from 2001 to 2009. *JAMA, 311*(17), 1778–1786. https://doi.org/10.1001/jama.2014.3201

Daly, J. M., Hartz, A. J., Xu, Y., Levy, B. T., James, P. A., Merchant, M. L., & Garrett, R. E. (2009). An assessment of attitudes, behaviors, and outcomes of patients with Type 2 diabetes. *The Journal of the American Board of Family Medicine, 22*(3), 280–290. https://doi.org/10.3122/jabfm.2009.03.080114

Halvorson, M., Yasuda, P., Carpenter, S., & Kaiserman, K. (2005). Unique challenges for pediatric patients with diabetes. *Diabetes Spectrum, 18*(3), 167–173. https://doi.org/10.2337/diaspect.18.3.167

Hannon, T. S., & Arslanian, S. A. (2015). The changing face of diabetes in youth: Lessons learned from studies of Type 2 diabetes. *Annals of the New York Academy of Sciences, 1353*(1), 113–137. http://doi.org/10.1111/nyas.12939

Karamanou, M., Protogerou, A., Tsoucalas, G., Androutsos, G., & Poulakou-Rebelakou, E. (2016). Milestones in the history of diabetes mellitus: The main contributors. *World Journal of Diabetes, 7*(1), 1–7. https://doi.org/10.4239/wjd.v7.i1.1

Mayo Clinic. (2019). *Type 2 diabetes*. https://www.mayoclinic.org/diseases-conditions/type-2-diabetes/diagnosis-treatment/drc-20351199

McCrimmon, R. J., Ryan, C. M., & Frier, B. M. (2012). Diabetes and cognitive dysfunction. *The Lancet, 379*(9833), 2291–2299. https://doi.org/10.1016/S0140-6736(12)60360-2

McGarry, J. D. (2002). Banting lecture 2001: Dysregulation of fatty acid metabolism in the etiology of Type 2 diabetes. *Diabetes, 51*(1), 7–18. https://doi.org/10.2337/diabetes.51.1.7

Pettitt, D. J., Talton, J., Dabelea, D., Divers, J., Imperatore, G., Lawrence, J. M., Liese, A. D., Linder, B., Mayer-Davis, E. J., Pihoker, C., Saydah, S. H., Standiford, D. A., Hamman, R. F., & the SEARCH for Diabetes in Youth Study Group. (2014). Prevalence of diabetes in U.S. youth in 2009: The SEARCH for Diabetes in Youth Study. *Diabetes Care, 37*(2), 402–408. https://doi.org/10.2337/dc13-1838

Reinehr, T. (2013). Type 2 diabetes mellitus in children and adolescents. *World Journal of Diabetes, 4*(6), 270–281. https://doi.org/10.4239/wjd.v4.i6.270

Ryan, C. M., van Duinkerken, E., & Rosano, C. (2016). Neurocognitive consequences of diabetes. *American Psychologist, 71*(7), 563–576. https://doi.org/10.1037/a0040455

Sperry, L. (2006). *Psychological treatment of chronic illness: The biopsychosocial therapy approach*. American Psychological Association.

Taylor, R. (2013). Type 2 diabetes: Etiology and reversibility. *Diabetes Care, 36*(4), 1047–1055. https://doi.org/10.2337/dc12-1805

Walker, R. J., Gebregziabher, M., Martin-Harris, B., & Egede, L. E. (2014). Relationship between social determinants of health and processes and outcomes in adults with Type 2 diabetes: Validation of a conceptual framework. *BMC Endocrine Disorders, 14*(1), Article 82. https://doi.org/10.1186/1472-6823-14-82

Wyckoff, L., Hanchon, T., & Gregg, S. R. (2015). Psychological, behavioral, and educational considerations for children with classified disabilities and diabetes within the school setting. *Psychology in the Schools, 52*(7), 672–682. https://doi.org/10.1002/pits.21848

Xu, H., & Verre, M. C. (2018). Type 2 diabetes mellitus in children. *American Family Physician, 98*(9), 590–594.

Yau, P. L., Javier, D. C., Ryan, C. M., Tsui, W. H., Ardekani, B. A., Ten, S., & Convit, A. (2010). Preliminary evidence for brain complications in obese adolescents with Type 2 diabetes mellitus. *Diabetologia, 53*(11), 2298–2306. https://doi.org/10.1007/s00125-010-1857-y

VI

RESPIRATORY SYSTEM DISORDERS

40

Overview of Respiratory System Disorders

Melissa A. Bray, Cheryl Maykel, Lea A. Theodore, and Justina Petrullo

The primary function of the respiratory system is inhalation, or the intake of air that brings oxygen to the blood, and subsequent exhalation of carbon dioxide that occurs as the transfer from the blood to the lungs takes place. Respiratory illnesses can be acute or chronic in nature and can occur anywhere along the respiratory tract. Some of these are more prevalent in children and adolescents (World Health Organization [WHO], 2013).

BODY SYSTEM INVOLVEMENT AND FUNCTIONING

The respiratory system consists of the upper (nasal cavity, pharynx, larynx) and lower respiratory tracts (trachea, lungs). These anatomical structures are connected and acted upon by the neurological, lymphatic, immune, and circulatory systems (WHO, 2013). They work together to promote optimal respiration, primarily delivering oxygen and removing bodily waste.

COMMON COMPLAINTS AND INDICATORS OF DYSFUNCTION

Generally, the most common causes and risk factors for respiratory illnesses are air pollutants, environmental exposure to toxins, and genetics (London, 2007). Common indications of respiratory distress include apnea (the absence of breathing), rapid or shallow breathing, wheezing, and coughing (Johns Hopkins

https://doi.org/10.1037/0000349-040
Health-Related Disorders in Children and Adolescents: A Guidebook for Educators and Service Providers, Second Edition, M. M. Perfect, C. A. Riccio, and M. A. Bray (Editors)

Medicine, 2021). Acute illnesses can come on very suddenly but generally resolve within 3 months (WHO, 2013). Common examples of acute respiratory illnesses in children include influenza (flu), whooping cough (pertussis), croup, common cold, sinusitis, bronchitis, and pneumonia (WHO, 2013). Respiratory illnesses chronic in nature, such as asthma and cystic fibrosis, are more likely to develop over time and will continue beyond 3 months (Story, 2022).

PREVIEW OF MAJOR RESPIRATORY SYSTEM CONDITIONS IN PEDIATRICS

Asthma

Asthma, the most common chronic condition for children in the United States, is characterized by the experience of breathing difficulties due to a lack of airflow throughout the respiratory system. Asthma has various known causes and triggers, including both genetic and environmental factors. Children and adolescents with asthma may experience difficulty in certain circumstances, such as when they are outside during allergy season or engaging in physical activity and breathing more rapidly. People with asthma often utilize control medications, taken regularly, to maintain respiratory functioning and avoid experiencing severe asthmatic symptoms. Some also have what is considered a rescue medication on hand in the event of an asthma attack. Please see Chapter 41 by Maykel et al. for more information on asthma.

Cystic Fibrosis

Cystic fibrosis, a genetic disease, is usually diagnosed in childhood. It affects both respiratory and digestive systems, getting progressively worse over time, and is often life threatening. However, it is no longer considered a terminal illness of childhood, and many more individuals with cystic fibrosis are living into adulthood. Children and adolescents with cystic fibrosis have a buildup of sticky mucus in their lungs, which can mean that they are at a greater risk of respiratory infections and therefore should take additional precautions to avoid people who are sick. Newborn screening programs have led to earlier diagnosis, and advancements in treatment have helped to reduce symptoms and complications of the disease. Treatments often include medication and procedures to remove mucus (David, 2015). Please see Chapter 42 by Smith and Aoyagi for more information.

Cytomegalovirus

Cytomegalovirus falls under the Herpesvirales order. The effects are wide and varied, including pneumonia and other negative respiratory outcomes, some similar to those found in the common cold. This condition affects children and adolescents and is a concern in pregnancy. The typical diagnosis is done via blood testing, with follow-up treatment with antiviral antibiotics when needed. Often it settles on its own without intervention. Please see Chapter 43 by Santos for more information.

Sarcoidosis

Sarcoidosis appears to be an autoimmune disease that leads to inflammation in the lungs. These inflammatory responses create noncaseating granulomas to arise in the respiratory system. Diagnosis is typically arrived at using diffusion capacity, chest radiography, biopsies, and assessment of serum angiotensin-converting enzymes. Outcomes are relevant to physical, emotional, and cognitive domains. In terms of treatment, medication, school-based interventions, and mind–body health treatments have been used to increase quality of life (Dioverti & Razonable, 2016). Please see Chapter 44 by Bray et al. for more information.

HEALTH CARE NEEDS AND MEDICAL SPECIALTIES

When a child experiences symptoms of a respiratory disorder, they should consult with their pediatrician first. The primary care provider would likely then refer them on to a specialist, such as a pediatric pulmonologist, a doctor who has special training in diagnosing and treating diseases of the lungs (National Cancer Institute, n.d.). Common assessment procedures may include spirometry (a measure of the amount of air inhaled and exhaled and the speed of exhalation), plethysmography (a measure of organ volume), bronchoscopy (use of an endoscope camera to view airways), magnetic resonance imaging, and chest X-ray. Traditional treatment includes various medications, oxygen therapy, and the use of a ventilator.

CONCLUSION

Living with a chronic illness that affects daily living can be difficult to accept and manage, especially for a child. Further, these children and adolescents may be concerned about experiencing severe symptoms, which not only may threaten physical health but also can be perceived as embarrassing. Further, students who miss class frequently or cannot fully participate in school activities may also experience difficulties with peer relationships. These difficulties may make the child feel socially and academically isolated.

REFERENCES

David, T. J. (2015). Cystic fibrosis in children and adults: Supplement to *Paediatric Respiratory Reviews*. *Paediatric Respiratory Reviews, 16*(Suppl. 1), 1. https://doi.org/10.1016/j.prrv.2015.07.005

Dioverti, M. V., & Razonable, R. R. (2016). Cytomegalovirus. *Microbiology Spectrum, 4*(4). https://doi.org/10.1128/microbiolspec.DMIH2-0022-2015

Johns Hopkins Medicine. (2021, November 10). *Signs of respiratory distress.* https://www.hopkinsmedicine.org/health/conditions-and-diseases/signs-of-respiratory-distress

London, S. J. (2007). Gene–air pollution interactions in asthma. *Proceedings of the American Thoracic Society, 4*(3), 217–220. https://doi.org/10.1513/pats.200701-031AW

National Cancer Institute. (n.d.). Pulmonologist. In *NCI dictionary of cancer terms.* Retrieved November 5, 2021, from https://www.cancer.gov/publications/dictionaries/cancer-terms/def/pulmonologist

Story, C. M. (2022, March 11). Chronic lung diseases: Causes and risk factors. *Healthline.* https://www.healthline.com/health/understanding-idiopathic-pulmonary-fibrosis/chronic-lung-diseases-causes-and-risk-factors

World Health Organization. (2013). Cough or difficulty in breathing. In *Pocket book of hospital care for children: Guidelines for the management of common childhood illnesses* (2nd ed., pp. 75–124).

41

Asthma

Cheryl Maykel, Melissa A. Bray, Meghan Long, and Lauren Gammie

Asthma is a condition that affects people of all ages and often progresses with age. It impairs breathing to varying degrees, ranging from a minor inconvenience to life-threatening attacks that require hospitalization. Careful management of this disorder is likely to lead to reduced impairment in functioning, increased quality of life, and an overall improved prognosis for the individual.

ETIOLOGY

The expression of asthmatic symptoms occurs as a result of both genetic and environmental factors. In addition to genetic heritability, airborne allergen exposure and sensitivity and respiratory infections early in life are thought to be the two main contributing factors to the development, persistence, and severity of asthma. This disease is characterized by chronic inflammation of the airways, resulting in reduced airflow and respiratory symptoms such as coughing and wheezing (National Heart, Lung, and Blood Institute, 2014).

PREVALENCE AND INCIDENCE

Prevalence rates for asthma have been increasing, and it is now considered the most common chronic condition among children in the United States (Akinbami et al., 2016). The national prevalence among children under 18 in the

https://doi.org/10.1037/0000349-041
Health-Related Disorders in Children and Adolescents: A Guidebook for Educators and Service Providers, Second Edition, M. M. Perfect, C. A. Riccio, and M. A. Bray (Editors)

United States is 7.5%. The rates are higher among older groups of children and boys (although rates are higher among women than men over 18), as well as among those in lower socioeconomic groups. Black youth have the highest rates of all racial groups (Centers for Disease Control and Prevention [CDC], 2020).

SYMPTOMS

The most typical symptoms people with asthma experience include wheezing, coughing, feelings of chest tightness, and labored breathing. Various factors contribute to the severity of symptoms, including overall health and exposure to respiratory viruses; a number of environmental irritants and allergens; and the ability of the individual to manage their symptoms through medication, the avoidance of known triggers, and remaining calm when experiencing symptoms.

IMPACT ON THE STUDENT AND OUTCOMES

Students with asthma may experience issues in multiple areas of functioning, including, but not limited to, their physical health. Student cognitive and academic functioning, behavior, and social relationships can also be impacted, either directly or indirectly, as a result of this condition.

Medical

Various types of asthma medications are given for different purposes, such as long-term control medications and fast-acting rescue medications (Sobieraj & Baker, 2018). Controller medications, such as inhaled corticosteroids and medications in pill form, are often utilized routinely. In addition, knowing one's triggers can help an individual with asthma avoid exposure or prevent the worsening of symptoms after exposure. Common triggers include environmental allergens (e.g., pollen, mold, pet dander) and irritants (e.g., smoke, strong scents/fumes), cold air, exercise, respiratory illness, and even strong emotions (e.g., anxiety).

Cognitive/Academic

Students with asthma may need to routinely leave class to take medication, and they may even be absent from school for days at a time in the event of a severe asthma attack. These students may need extra help or the ability to make up work that was missed. As a result of asthmatic symptoms, some students may also experience trouble sleeping, which can further affect overall health and functioning. For instance, adequate sleep has been associated with successful academic performance, including homework completion and attendance at school, as well as social functioning (Mitchell, 2015).

Social-Emotional and Behavioral

Asthma has been associated with psychological and behavioral disorders. For instance, if asthma increases in severity or persists beyond early childhood, the individual is at an increased risk of developing various mental health problems, including anxiety, depression, and disorders related to defiant behavior (Goodwin et al., 2013). In particular, asthma is highly comorbid with anxiety, with estimates of up to one third of children and adolescents with asthma also meeting criteria for an anxiety disorder (Katon et al., 2004).

Certainly, the experience of both asthmatic symptoms and anxiety can be frightening to anyone, let alone a child who is grappling with both. It is known that symptoms of asthma can understandably lead to the individual feeling anxious, which can then worsen symptoms, just as anxious thoughts can lead to worsening asthmatic symptoms (Chen & Miller, 2007). As is true for all youth, but particularly for those who experience chronic illnesses, it is important for parents and educators to nurture confidence and independence as the child learns how to manage their illness as well as their response to experiences of the illness.

Families of children with asthma often experience the impact and effects of the illness as well. Asthma can be a scary and unpredictable disease, causing family members of a child with asthma to experience stress and fear. Family member involvement, specifically parents/adult guardians, is imperative in the maintenance and care of young patients. Parents must be able to understand different asthma treatment options and methods, know how to monitor symptoms, and be able to quickly respond to changes in illness conditions. Experts encourage families of patients to take part in family empowerment programs, such as the National Asthma Education and Prevention Program, to help them obtain skills and learn about asthma control, use of inhalers and respiratory assist devices, and activity and nutrition of children with asthma (McCarty & Rogers, 2012). Improving asthma management requires family and child education regarding management responsibility (Brown et al., 2010). The active role of families is imperative for young asthma patients and can significantly affect the progression and management of symptoms and care.

PSYCHOEDUCATIONAL IMPLICATIONS AND SCHOOL-BASED INTERVENTIONS

Educators can effectively help students with asthma in a number of ways. Research has found that providing appropriate education for students, principals, custodians, and appropriate school staff can reduce asthma-related illnesses, improve asthma management, and decrease the number of school absences (Clark et al., 2004). First, having a point person, such as the school psychologist, serve as a case manager for the student's needs can set the foundation for a student's asthma management while in school. Designating an appropriate school staff member can help to alleviate confusion and ensure that the student stays on track, for instance, in the event that the student is absent or experiences anxiety as related to asthma symptoms.

Medical and Health Management

It is recommended that children undergo pulmonary function tests (PFTs) to properly measure lung function and determine necessary treatment and medication procedures (American Thoracic Society, 2014). The most common PFT is a spirometry test, which can be conducted as early as 6 years old. Spirometry testing measures how much air is moved in and out of the lungs and how fast the air moves. For younger children, a shorter test of lung function, called force oscillometry, is another method to measure lung function, specifically how easily air flows in the lungs (American Thoracic Society, 2014). Lung function tests help providers determine the level of treatment and possible medication a child with asthma may need. Based on the severity level of asthma, a child may require various quick-relief medications during the school day. Inhalers, oral beta agonists, short-course oral corticosteroids, and ipratropium (Atrovent) are common medications that should be kept in the school nurse's office and be available when symptoms warrant use (Kemp & Kemp, 2001).

The CDC has developed an asthma-specific, six-item list of strategies to promote healthy asthma management, based on the coordinated school health model. The strategies emphasize the importance of establishing management and support for asthma-friendly schools; providing appropriate mental health and school health services for students with asthma; providing asthma education and awareness programs for students and staff; ensuring the existence of safe and healthy school environments to reduce asthma triggers; implementing safe physical education and activities for students with asthma; and coordinating school, family, and community efforts to improve asthma symptom management and reduce school absences among students with asthma (CDC, 2015).

It is important to maintain communications between school personnel and parents, as well as with other providers who work with the student, so that everyone can have a clear understanding about triggers, medications, and what to do in the event of an asthma attack. Students with asthma can benefit most from school staff and family members participating in asthma education and professional development activities (National Asthma Education and Prevention Program, 2007).

Cognitive/Academic

Students with asthma may need to be excused from some activities, such as those involving strenuous physical exertion or strong odors, and they may need to stay inside during cold weather or when allergens are high. Educators should remain flexible for students who need to leave class to take medication, and if a student needs to be absent for a prolonged period of time, an educated school staff member can help to coordinate the delivery of lessons and schoolwork. This can help ensure that the child will not fall too far behind academically, but it can also help them to stay motivated and ease their transition back into the school setting when they are well. Further, it is beneficial for the student to remain connected to the school, their teachers, and their peers.

Social-Emotional and Behavioral

School counselors and school psychologists can work with students with asthma who also experience anxiety, depression, or other social or psychological issues. For instance, students with asthma and anxiety would likely benefit from talking through their concerns; identifying people within the school building whom they can go to in the event of an asthma attack or when experiencing feelings of anxiety; and learning strategies to manage anxiety in the moment, such as various relaxation techniques.

Understanding the symptoms and knowing what to do in various situations will likely help the child to cope and could prevent additional negative outcomes. For instance, children who experience asthma and anxiety are prone to overusing their quick-relief inhalers. It is believed that they misconstrue their psychological symptoms as having a physical basis (Goodwin et al., 2013). Therefore, therapy can be targeted to help the student with asthma distinguish between psychological and physical symptoms (Goodwin et al., 2013).

An effective cognitive behavior treatment, Creating Opportunities for Personal Empowerment (COPE), has been successful in reducing symptoms of asthma, depression, and related anxiety (McGovern et al., 2019). The intervention helps the students with asthma correctly identify symptoms that are psychological versus physical. COPE is a manualized small-group treatment program that runs for 7 weeks and targets students with asthma, depression, and anxiety. The program includes traditional cognitive behavior therapy components in addition to identifying asthma triggers, differentiating between controller and quick-relief medications, and practicing proper diaphragmatic breathing (McGovern et al., 2019). The program is feasible for implementation in the schools and has been well-received by students and teachers.

The physiological and psychological effects and symptoms of asthma have been found to be effectively managed through the use of mind–body interventions, such as meditation and relaxation. Mind–body methods offer alternative ways to manage asthma symptoms beyond the realm of medication. Practices such as prayer, relaxation, guided imagery, meditation, yoga, massage, herbs, vitamins, rubs, and diet modifications have all been reported to effectively help improve the management of the physical and mental discomforts of having asthma (Cotton et al., 2012).

CONCLUSION

Asthma is an increasingly common disease that educators will undoubtedly encounter through their work with youth in schools. Thus, they ought to be aware of the symptoms, common triggers, and protocols for students who have this diagnosis, as well as the increased likelihood that these students will also experience comorbid psychological issues, such as anxiety. Although asthma is common and manageable, accommodations and time away from class may at times be required for these students. Educators need also recognize that symptoms can be severe and students may require immediate medical attention beyond what the school nurse can provide in the school setting. School staff should be knowledgeable and remain flexible in order to best accommodate students' needs.

RESOURCES

American Lung Association. (n.d.). *Asthma*. https://www.lung.org/lung-health-and-diseases/lung-disease-lookup/asthma/

Centers for Disease Control and Prevention. (2022). *Agencies working on asthma*. https://www.cdc.gov/asthma/links.htm

Asthma and Allergy Foundation of America. https://www.aafa.org/

REFERENCES

Akinbami, L. J., Simon, A. E., & Rossen, L. M. (2016). Changing trends in asthma prevalence among children. *Pediatrics, 137*(1), Article e20152354. https://doi.org/10.1542/peds.2015-2354

Brown, N., Gallagher, R., Fowler, C., & Wales, S. (2010). The role of parents in managing asthma in middle childhood: An important consideration in chronic care. *Collegian, 17*(2), 71–76. https://doi.org/10.1016/j.colegn.2010.04.006

Centers for Disease Control and Prevention. (2015). *Strategies for addressing asthma within a coordinated school health program*. https://www.cdc.gov/healthyschools/asthma/strategies/asthmacsh.htm

Centers for Disease Control and Prevention. (2020, March 24). *Most recent national asthma data*. https://www.cdc.gov/asthma/most_recent_national_asthma_data.htm

Chen, E., & Miller, G. E. (2007). Stress and inflammation in exacerbations of asthma. *Brain, Behavior, and Immunity, 21*(8), 993–999. https://doi.org/10.1016/j.bbi.2007.03.009

Clark, N. M., Brown, R., Joseph, C. L., Anderson, E. W., Liu, M., & Valerio, M. A. (2004). Effects of a comprehensive school-based asthma program on symptoms, parent management, grades, and absenteeism. *Chest, 125*(5), 1674–1679. https://doi.org/10.1378/chest.125.5.1674

Cotton, S., Weekes, J. C., McGrady, M. E., Rosenthal, S. L., Yi, M. S., Pargament, K., Succop, P., Roberts, Y. H., & Tsevat, J. (2012). Spirituality and religiosity in urban adolescents with asthma. *Journal of Religion and Health, 51*(1), 118–131. https://doi.org/10.1007/s10943-010-9408-x

Goodwin, R. D., Robinson, M., Sly, P. D., McKeague, I. W., Susser, E. S., Zubrick, S. R., Stanley, F. J., & Mattes, E. (2013). Severity and persistence of asthma and mental health: A birth cohort study. *Psychological Medicine, 43*(6), 1313–1322. https://doi.org/10.1017/S0033291712001754

Katon, W. J., Richardson, L., Lozano, P., & McCauley, E. (2004). The relationship of asthma and anxiety disorders. *Psychosomatic Medicine, 66*(3), 349–355. https://doi.org/10.1097/01.psy.0000126202.89941.ea

Kemp, J. P., & Kemp, J. A. (2001). Management of asthma in children. *American Family Physician, 63*(7), 1341–1348, 1353–1354.

McCarty, K., & Rogers, J. (2012). Inpatient asthma education program. *Pediatric Nursing, 38*(5), 257–262.

McGovern, C. M., Arcoleo, K., & Melnyk, B. (2019). COPE for asthma: Outcomes of a cognitive behavioral intervention for children with asthma and anxiety. *School Psychology, 34*(6), 665–676. https://doi.org/10.1037/spq0000310

Mitchell, D. K. (2015). Asthma and school functioning in children: Still more work to do. *The Brown University Child and Adolescent Behavior Letter, 31*(9), 1–6. https://doi.org/10.1002/cbl.30064

National Asthma Education and Prevention Program. (2007). *Expert panel report 3: Guidelines for the diagnosis and management of asthma*. National Library of Medicine. https://www.ncbi.nlm.nih.gov/books/NBK7223/

National Heart, Lung, and Blood Institute (2014). *Managing asthma: A guide for schools*. U.S. Department of Health and Human Services. https://www.nhlbi.nih.gov/files/docs/resources/lung/NACI_ManagingAsthma-508%20FINAL.pdf

Sobieraj, D. M., & Baker, W. L. (2018). Medications for asthma. *JAMA, 319*(14), Article 1520. https://doi.org/10.1001/jama.2018.3808

42

Cystic Fibrosis

Jeanette Smith and Keiko Aoyagi

Cystic fibrosis (CF) is a genetic disorder marked by progressive and chronic deterioration of the respiratory and/or gastrointestinal systems that may affect the quality and length of one's life (Sanders & Fink, 2016). Recent medications that improve function of the CF transmembrane conductance regulator (*CFTR*) protein have given great hope of a different trajectory for many of those with CF. Candidacy for these medications is determined by each person's CF genetic mutations. Unfortunately, a small percentage of individuals with CF have mutations that are not responsive to the current *CFTR* modulators. Even with new medications, children with CF and their caregivers still must cope with a unique set of medical and psychosocial challenges, which can best be managed by well-coordinated multidisciplinary care.

ETIOLOGY

CF is an autosomal recessive disorder that is chronic, progressive, and can be life limiting (Mitchell & Cohn, 2006). In White people, CF is the most common autosomal recessive cause of early mortality worldwide (Sanders & Fink, 2016). It is an inherited disease that requires both parents to be carriers of the pathogenic mutation of the *CFTR* gene. The pathogenic mutation of the *CFTR* gene is carried in about one in 25 to 30 White persons (Sanders & Fink, 2016). Regulatory approval has recently occurred for highly effective *CFTR* modulator therapy (HEMT) that helps improve function of the *CFTR* protein for the majority

https://doi.org/10.1037/0000349-042
Health-Related Disorders in Children and Adolescents: A Guidebook for Educators and Service Providers, Second Edition, M. M. Perfect, C. A. Riccio, and M. A. Bray (Editors)

of those with CF. These medications are expected to greatly extend the current median survival age of 53 for those born between 2017 and 2021. That median age is expected to increase with HEMT being approved for younger age groups and as more treatments are developed for all of those with CF. Even before the recent advances in medications, treatment improvements led to adults with CF outnumbering children with CF for the first time in the United States in 2014 (Sanders & Fink, 2016). Although CF is not contagious, it can be life-threatening to the affected individual.

PREVALENCE AND INCIDENCE

Approximately 1,000 individuals in the United States are diagnosed with CF each year, and CF is more common among White people than other races and ethnicities (Sanders & Fink, 2016). CF occurs in about one in 3,000 to 4,000 live White births. For Latin Americans, CF occurs in one in 4,000 to 10,000, and in African Americans, CF occurs in one in 15,000 to 20,000. It is even less common in Asian Americans (Sanders & Fink, 2016). CF affects more than 70,000 individuals across the world, approximately 30,000 of whom reside in the United States. CF affects male and female individuals equally. With advances in technology and medicine, the majority of new cases are identified early through newborn screening, which now occurs in every state in the United States (Sanders & Fink, 2016). The diagnosis of CF involves both clinical observations and laboratory data (Mitchell & Cohn, 2006). Technological and medical advancements have allowed for early identification, diagnosis, and treatment of CF among the population, which in turn has enabled individuals with CF to enjoy longer and healthier lives. These adults with CF increasingly pursue tertiary education and/or move into the workforce (Burker et al., 2004). Although the dramatically longer life expectancy compared with a few decades ago is promising in terms of offering individuals with CF hope and opportunities they did not have before, it also presents the individuals with new challenges associated with life and career planning (e.g., Mahdavi, 2015; Storlie & Baltrinic, 2015).

SYMPTOMS

CF is a multisystem disease marked by a range of symptoms. The defective genes cause the production of unusually thick, sticky mucus, which can affect several organs, including the lungs, sinuses, intestines, pancreas, and the liver (Mitchell & Cohn, 2006). In the lungs, the mucus can plug the airway, making breathing harder for individuals with CF. The thick, sticky mucus also can provide a favorable environment for bacteria to stay and grow, causing lung infections. Furthermore, the mucus can hinder the lung's recovery from such infections. Thus, individuals with CF often suffer from chronic and reoccurring lung infections that gradually diminish their lung function. Experience and severity of symptoms depend on types of CF-causing genetic mutations, quality of received medical care, treatment adherence, and psychosocial support/resources (Mahdavi, 2015).

IMPACT ON THE STUDENT AND OUTCOMES

Medical

Some individuals with CF have recurrent sinus infections. Male individuals may have infertility. Individuals with CF also may have bowel obstructions or abnormal stools and pancreatic insufficiency. Additionally, failure to thrive affects about 50% of individuals with CF in infancy and childhood due to pancreatic insufficiency and increased caloric demands with CF. Pancreatic insufficiency also is linked to the high comorbidity rate of CF-related diabetes, which adds complexity to the medical and health routine of the affected individual with CF.

Cognitive/Academic

CF poses challenges to the affected individuals in terms of attaining healthy physical and cognitive growth and regular attendance in school. Comparing performances on cognitive and academic tests, researchers have found that students with CF did not significantly differ from their peers without CF in terms of their standardized test scores (Grieve et al., 2011). At the same time, absences were significantly associated with their grade-point average, which has important implications for educational attainment of children with CF (Grieve et al., 2011).

Social–Emotional and Behavioral

In the classroom, CF symptoms can be embarrassing for the student with CF. Persistent coughing occurs as their body's response to remove thick mucus from their lungs. Individuals with CF may have stress incontinence due to coughing attacks. They often require extra snacks in class to maintain their weight, which can also feel embarrassing to some students with CF. They may experience bloating, cramping, and abdominal distention, with more malodorous flatulence than the average person. Although exercise is generally encouraged with physician approval, some may experience shortness of breath with exertion activities (Cystic Fibrosis Foundation [CFF], 2019b).

Depression and anxiety are commonly reported symptoms among both adolescent and adult CF patients, as well as their parents, and these conditions have important implications for treatment outcomes and students' quality of life (Duff, 2015; Duff et al., 2014; Snell et al., 2014). Duff (2015) reported the results from the International Depression/Anxiety Epidemiological Study that examined depression and anxiety symptoms among CF patients who were ages 12 and older, as well as among their caregivers, from the United States and eight other Western countries. The international study confirmed that the rates of depression were significantly elevated among CF patients and their caregivers. Besides the increased risks of depression and anxiety, individuals with CF over the course of development are vulnerable to experience concerns over mortality, treatment adherence issues, identity crisis, difficulty developing/maintaining peer relations, and difficulty achieving independence (Mahdavi, 2015). Developing long-term life plans, including higher education, employment, marriage, and so on, as well as balancing medical and psychosocial responsibilities independently, are emerging challenges for many individuals with CF as they enjoy longer and healthier lives (Gathercole, 2019). In this regard, educators and mental health professionals play an important role in contributing to multidisciplinary CF care. By assisting individuals with CF and their families to address psychological issues inherent to living with CF (Mahdavi, 2015), they are facilitating development of a resilient mindset.

PSYCHOEDUCATIONAL IMPLICATIONS AND SCHOOL-BASED INTERVENTIONS

Medical and Health Management

CF care involves a multitude of treatments that are personalized to target chief symptoms experienced by each individual with CF. All students with CF have significant daily treatment demands from the time they are diagnosed with CF until the end of their life. A typical treatment regimen for a healthy student with CF includes up to an hour of breathing treatments every morning and evening, consisting of using a vest or other forms of airway clearance and using a nebulizer for inhaled medicines. Many individuals with CF have pancreatic insufficiency and require enzyme supplements with meals and snacks. Most also require a much higher caloric intake to reach and maintain an average weight, which is strongly associated with better health outcomes (Konstan et al., 2003). Medical visits also require time. In addition to their regular quarterly CF clinic appointments, which typically last a few hours when an individual is healthy, there are also CF clinic visits and/or hospitalizations when they are ill. If the lung function of an individual with CF becomes severely impaired to the extent that the breathing treatments and/or medications become insufficient, a lung transplant would be considered (CFF, 2019a). Managing these individual-specific treatments each day, as well as frequent clinic/hospital visits, often causes individuals with CF and their families difficulty juggling multiple responsibilities and obligations, including school and/or work (Gathercole, 2019).

Successful CF care and success in the classroom rely on cooperation and support from multiple parties, including the child with CF, parents, school nurses, teachers, and psychologists (Mahdavi, 2015). Maximizing a child's attendance in school is the goal, and this often necessitates school accommodations to decrease exposure to germs and to maintain medical treatment adherence. The following accommodations may assist with these goals (CFF, 2019a):

- Implement daily wiping of desks as well as handwashing for all.
- Assist the child in moving to a desk away from a sick peer to decrease the risk of the child with CF becoming ill.
- Allow the child with CF to have their own crayons, pencils, and other supplies to decrease the sharing of germs.
- Enable the child to keep their nebulizer machine and medication in the school nurse's office so extra treatments are available when needed to encourage school attendance.
- Encourage teachers to keep the child's pancreatic enzymes in a cabinet in the back of the class so the child can quickly take them before snacks and lunch and is thus able to walk to lunch with the rest of the children.
- Allow the child to have snacks throughout the school day and an extra 15 minutes at lunchtime to address the need for a high-calorie, high-fat diet that is true for most students with CF.
- Train teachers to not draw attention to the child's cough in the classroom, as coughing helps clear mucus from the lungs.
- Have tissues to cough/blow their nose as well as a trashcan near the child's desk.
- Allow water at the child's desk, as dehydration is a real concern for individuals with CF, especially with exercise.
- Encourage the child to participate in physical education/exercise as long as they feel able to. For most students with CF, physical education/exercise is recommended to the extent they feel comfortable with. Check with the student's parent or physician for their recommendations.
- Seat the child near the door that is closest to the bathroom, and allow breaks when needed, as children with CF may still experience abdominal pain, diarrhea, and foul-smelling gas, even when taking their enzymes.
- Take extra caution if there are other students in the school with CF. They must keep at least a safe 6-foot distance from each other at all times and never share common items.

Teachers, school nurses, and other school personnel will benefit from the information at https://CFF.org, and they can reach out to the student's local CF clinic with any questions or concerns.

Cognitive/Academic

Securing reasonable accommodations early in the educational process can effectively ensure the quality of the learning experience among students with CF. Individualized education programs and 504 plans can help students in Grades K–12 access accommodations (CFF, 2019b). In addition to the prior recommendations, accommodations for school absences due to appointments or illness may include minimizing the homework expectation while still assisting the student in learning the material needed.

Social-Emotional and Behavioral

Given the increased risks of depression and anxiety among individuals with CF (e.g., Duff et al., 2014), routine psychological screening and access to mental health services are highly recommended. Mental health professionals, including counselors, social workers, and psychologists, who work with individuals with CF need to be knowledgeable about CF as well as its treatments. They need to be skillful in addressing various concerns among these individuals that include, but are not limited to, coping with the diagnosis, managing the complexity of treatments, coping with declining health, developing a healthy and independent sense of self, and setting up long-term goals (Mahdavi, 2015). Along with everyone else, individuals with CF can experience a wide range of life challenges (e.g., childhood trauma, relationship issues, loss and grief, substance abuse) in addition to CF-specific challenges. Thus, students can greatly benefit from working with mental health professionals who are able to assist the student in developing the resiliency needed throughout their life. Promoting self-efficacy, or belief in one's own ability to accomplish a certain task (e.g., mastering math skills), can go a long way in terms of promoting academic achievement among students with CF (Grieve et al., 2011). To help promote self-efficacy or a sense of agency and capability, creating a supportive and caring school environment is crucial (Rehm, 2002). By doing so, the school is facilitating the student's development of resilience.

CONCLUSION

CF is a complex disease that significantly impacts one's life experience. An overview of the medical complexity of CF, some of the medical and psychosocial challenges, potential interventions, and the significant role of the school in the lives of students with CF was provided in this chapter. Given that the average lifespan of an individual with CF has dramatically increased due to medical developments (Sanders & Fink, 2016), it is crucial that individuals with CF are assisted in developing the resiliency they need to live a full life. The support needed for individuals with CF to thrive can be achieved through cooperation between themselves, their families, and interdisciplinary teams of professionals, including physicians, nurses, teachers, principals, social workers, and psychologists.

RESOURCES

Cystic Fibrosis Foundation. https://www.cff.org/

Cystic Fibrosis Foundation YouTube Channel. https://www.youtube.com/user/CysticFibrosisUSA

Cystic Fibrosis Research Institute. (2017–present). *CF Community Voices Podcast* [Video postcast]. https://www.cfri.org/education-support/cf-community-voices-podcast-series/

REFERENCES

Burker, E. J., Sedway, J., & Carone, S. (2004). Psychological and educational factors: Better predictors of work status than FEV_1 in adults with cystic fibrosis. *Pediatric Pulmonology, 38*(5), 413–418. https://doi.org/10.1002/ppul.20090

Cystic Fibrosis Foundation. (2019a). *Managing CF: Treatments and therapies.* https://www.cff.org/managing-cf#treatments-and-therapies

Cystic Fibrosis Foundation. (2019b). *Working with your child's school.* https://www.cff.org/Life-With-CF/Daily-Life/CF-and-School/

Duff, A. J. A. (2015). Depression in cystic fibrosis: Implications of the International Depression/Anxiety Epidemiological Study (TIDES) in cystic fibrosis. *Pediatric Respiratory Reviews, 16*(Suppl. 1), 2–5. https://doi.org/10.1016/j.prrv.2015.07.006

Duff, A. J. A., Abbott, J., Cowperthwaite, C., Sumner, C., Hurley, M. A., Quittner, A., & the TIDES-UK Group. (2014). Depression and anxiety in adolescents and adults with cystic fibrosis in the U.K.: A cross-sectional study. *Journal of Cystic Fibrosis, 13*(6), 745–753. https://doi.org/10.1016/j.jcf.2014.02.010

Gathercole, K. (2019). Managing cystic fibrosis alongside children's schooling: Family, nurse and teacher perspectives. *Journal of Child Health Care, 23*(3), 425–436. https://doi.org/10.1177/1367493518814930

Grieve, A. J., Tluczek, A., Racine-Gilles, C. N., Laxova, A., Albers, C. A., & Farrell, P. M. (2011). Associations between academic achievement and psychosocial variables in adolescents with cystic fibrosis. *Journal of School Health, 81*(11), 713–720. https://doi.org/10.1111/j.1746-1561.2011.00648.x

Konstan, M. W., Butler, S. M., Wohl, M. E., Stoddard, M., Matousek, R., Wagener, J. S., Johnson, C. A., Morgan, W. J., & the Investigators and Coordinators of the Epidemiologic Study of Cystic Fibrosis. (2003). Growth and nutritional indexes in early life predict pulmonary function in cystic fibrosis. *The Journal of Pediatrics, 142*(6), 624–630. https://doi.org/10.1067/mpd.2003.152

Mahdavi, S. (2015). Children with cystic fibrosis: A primer for school psychologists. *Communiqué, 44*(3), 4–7. https://www.nasponline.org/publications/periodicals/communique/issues/volume-44-issue-3

Mitchell, R. M., & Cohn, J. A. (2006). Cystic fibrosis: The science behind the disease. In A. McKenna & H. Goldsweig (Eds.), *Beyond lungs: Meeting the needs of adults with cystic fibrosis* (pp. 4–11). Felenstein CCCP.

Rehm, R. S. (2002). Creating a context of safety and achievement at school for children who are medically fragile/technology dependent. *Advances in Nursing Science, 24*(3), 71–84. https://doi.org/10.1097/00012272-200203000-00008

Sanders, D. B., & Fink, A. K. (2016). Background and epidemiology. *Pediatric Clinics of North America, 63*(4), 567–584. https://doi.org/10.1016/j.pcl.2016.04.001

Snell, C., Fernandes, S., Bujoreanu, I. S., & Garcia, G. (2014). Depression, illness severity, and healthcare utilization in cystic fibrosis. *Pediatric Pulmonology, 49*(12), 1177–1181. https://doi.org/10.1002/ppul.22990

Storlie, C., & Baltrinic, E. R. (2015). Counseling children with cystic fibrosis: Recommendations for practice and counselor self-care. *The Professional Counselor, 5*(2), 293–303. https://doi.org/10.15241/cas.5.2.293

43

Cytomegalovirus

Maryann Santos

Cytomegalovirus (CMV) is a common herpes virus that is part of the same group that contains viruses that cause infectious mononucleosis (Epstein–Barr virus), chickenpox, and shingles (Centers for Disease Control and Prevention [CDC], 2020; Kaye, 2021). Three forms of CMV are recognized: (a) CMV inclusion disease of the newborn, also known as congenital CMV; (b) acute acquired CMV infection; and (c) CMV in immune-compromised persons (National Organization of Rare Disorders, 2019).

ETIOLOGY

For the most part, the virus remains asymptomatic with no long-term health implications (Schleiss, 2018; Sommers & Fannin, 2014). CMV infection can have adverse outcomes, however, for individuals with impaired immune systems or for unborn children whose mothers become infected for the first time during pregnancy (Adler et al., 2007). CMV is transmitted through direct contact with small amounts of the virus shed in body fluids, including tears, saliva, urine, stools, semen, blood, and breast milk (Kaye, 2021; Sommers & Fannin, 2014); transmission also may occur through organ transplants, vaginal delivery, and sexual intercourse (CDC, 2020; Kaye, 2021). An important risk factor for primary infection is prolonged exposure to young children; the virus is particularly common among infants and toddlers in group day care, as contact with various bodily excretions (e.g., feces, tears, urine, saliva) is relatively

https://doi.org/10.1037/0000349-043
Health-Related Disorders in Children and Adolescents: A Guidebook for Educators and Service Providers, Second Edition, M. M. Perfect, C. A. Riccio, and M. A. Bray (Editors)

common in such settings. As a result, there is a high risk of exposure for nurses, day care workers, and preschool teachers (National CMV Foundation, 2019).

PREVALENCE AND INCIDENCE

CMV infects nearly one in three children by age 5 and over half of adults by age 40 (CDC, 2020). Although congenital CMV occurs in less than 1% of pregnancies (Anderholm et al., 2016), more than 25,000 children are affected each year in the United States (Schleiss, 2018); of these, one in every five children will have birth defects (CDC, 2020) or develop permanent health problems, and up to 400 infant fatalities will occur annually (National CMV Foundation, 2019). Of all congenital CMV-related deaths, 71% occur in the first year of life (Bristow et al., 2011). Poverty status has been associated with higher levels of CMV antibodies in children (Dowd et al., 2012).

SYMPTOMS

Congenital CMV infections are symptomatic in about 10% of newborns. Additionally, children who were asymptomatic at birth may develop symptoms later (Nigro et al., 2005). Clinical manifestations of congenital CMV include hearing loss, vision loss, microcephaly, low birth weight, jaundice, enlarged liver and spleen, seizures, retinitis, cerebral palsy, skin rashes, and mental retardation (Manicklal et al., 2013; Schleiss, 2018).

Although cases of pneumonia, hepatitis, and rash have been reported in CMV infections acquired after the newborn period, it is more common to have no or only mild symptoms, such as fever, sore throat, swollen glands, joint and muscle pain, and tiredness (Nordqvist, 2018). Individuals with weakened immune systems may experience symptoms affecting the eyes, lungs, liver, stomach, intestines, and/or brain (Bristow et al., 2011).

IMPACT ON THE STUDENT AND OUTCOMES

Medical

CMV is the most common cause of nongenetic childhood hearing loss and a significant cause of neurodevelopmental delay (Manicklal et al., 2013). There is some evidence of a direct relationship between the time in gestational development at which CMV infection occurs and the severity of damage (Adler et al., 2007; Nigro et al., 2005; Pass et al., 2006). In addition, it has been suggested that CMV may be an etiological agent in autism (Gentile et al., 2017). Although the CMV in women infected before pregnancy can be reactivated and transmitted to the fetus, it appears that their newborns receive protection from maternal antibodies and consequently rarely are seriously affected (CDC, 2020). At the same time, though these children are asymptomatic at birth, they may develop hearing, vision, coordination, or other medical problems later in life (National CMV Foundation, 2019). Healthy children and adolescents who contract CMV after birth generally have no long-term problems associated with the virus, although some may experience short-term illness that involves fever, sore throat, fatigue, joint stiffness, and swollen glands (Nordqvist, 2018).

Individuals who have impaired or suppressed immune systems are at risk for serious complications from either primary or reactivated CMV infections (Kaye, 2021). Indeed, CMV is a major cause of disease and death in these individuals. It may cause illness in a number of ways, including CMV retinitis, which gradually destroys light-sensitive tissue in the eye and is the most common form of blindness in individuals with autoimmune deficiencies (Turbert, 2022). CMV also may cause pneumonia; colitis; neuropathy (tingling in the hands or feet); and problems in the intestines, throat, brain, kidneys, gall bladder, liver, and other organs.

Cognitive/Academic

Children with visible symptoms of CMV at birth may experience neurological damage that becomes more evident in the early years of life in the form of hearing or vision impairment as well as attention, cognitive, speech, and/or developmental delays; as a result, parents of children with long-term impairment report school performance issues and an overall poorer quality of life (Korndewal et al., 2017). Children who contract CMV in utero but are asymptomatic at birth may develop cognitive problems later in life (National CMV Foundation, 2019).

Social–Emotional and Behavioral

Although specific social–emotional or behavioral issues do not appear directly related to the presence of CMV infection, it is possible that CMV-infected children may experience difficulties in social interactions or exhibit behavioral problems based on the specific manifestations of their impairments.

PSYCHOEDUCATIONAL IMPLICATIONS AND SCHOOL-BASED INTERVENTIONS

Medical and Health Management

No treatment regimen is recommended for healthy individuals with CMV, and currently there are no approved treatments for fetal CMV (Pass & Arav-Boger, 2018). No cure is available for CMV. Due to the many ways in which CMV may affect children, available treatment options will depend on the age of the individual as well as the number, type, and severity of symptoms, and a coordinated team-based approach has been recommended to address the child's specialized needs (Schleiss, 2018). Newborns and those with autoimmune difficulties often are treated with antiviral medications such as ganciclovir (Zirgan) and foscarnet (Foscavir) to slow the disease, although these drugs may result in toxic side effects that include neutropenia (a low white blood cell count) and renal toxicity (Kaye, 2021). Isolating individuals is not necessary, and excluding individuals with CMV infection from school, day care, or other group settings is not recommended. Because of the potential for risk to a fetus, female caregivers, educators, and HIV-infected individuals who work in these settings, as well as parents of childbearing age, should be informed of their increased risk of exposure to CMV, and those who may have future pregnancies may choose to be tested to determine the presence of CMV antibodies (National CMV Foundation, 2019; Siberry et al., 2013). To minimize the risk of infection, child care workers and educators are encouraged to practice standard hygiene procedures, including frequent handwashing after changing diapers, feeding a child, wiping a child's nose or mouth, and handling toys (National CMV Foundation, 2019). Other hygiene practices include wearing disposable gloves when in contact with body fluids, avoiding the shared use of eating utensils, substituting hugs for kisses, and sanitizing toys and surface areas regularly (Aronson, 1988).

Although universal screening for CMV infection in infants and toddlers previously was felt to be impractical, several states (Connecticut, Iowa, New York, and Utah) now require newborns to be tested for congenital CMV if they fail the newborn hearing screening. Numerous other states have proposed including targeted newborn screening and/or parent or professional education (National CMV Foundation, 2019).

Cognitive/Academic

Infants' growth and developmental patterns should be monitored closely throughout development with referral as needed to special education, physical therapy, and social services (Sommers & Fannin, 2014). Because of the potential for progressive decline, children who are known to have either symptomatic or asymptomatic forms of CMV should be closely monitored both medically and academically to quickly identify and begin treatment for emerging problems. Regular hearing and vision checks should be conducted to detect deteriorating acuity in these areas (CDC, 2020), with appropriate accommodations implemented. For example, children with hearing impairments may require hearing amplification, classroom seating modifications, and speech and language services, whereas those with fine and gross motor difficulties may require physical and occupational therapy and the use of adaptive devices. Children identified with cognitive developmental delays or learning disabilities may require additional academic support in the classroom through individualized instruction or with the use of assistive technology to facilitate learning in the specific areas of deficit. Such support may range from mild to intensive services.

Social-Emotional and Behavioral

Social–emotional difficulties should be addressed on a case-by-case basis and include coordination between parents, classroom teacher, and school psychologists and/or school counselors to enable the child to receive the best possible care. Given the high occurrence of CMV in the general population, children and other individuals with CMV should not be isolated from others or excluded from school unless they are too ill to attend. Instead, behavioral guidance should be provided to school personnel to regularly practice and encourage all students to exercise universal hygiene practices. Individuals with impaired immune systems should be informed of their increased risk and take appropriate preventive steps (Siberry, 2013).

CONCLUSION

CMV is a common virus found in a large percentage of children and adolescents. In most cases, CMV will not cause problems; however, it is a leading cause of congenital infections and a common cause of numerous types of birth defects, many with the potential for long-term impairment. Although only a small percentage of congenitally affected infants are symptomatic at birth, others may develop symptoms later. With no vaccine currently available, prevention efforts should focus on the use of universal hygiene practices. As there are many ways in which CMV can cause impairments, medical treatment and school-based interventions and accommodations should focus on how the virus manifests in each individual. Children who have received transplants or have impaired immune systems must be carefully monitored to prevent further severe medical issues.

RESOURCES

Centers for Disease Control and Prevention. (2020). *Cytomegalovirus (CMV) and congenital CMV infection*. U.S. Department of Health and Human Services. https://www.cdc.gov/cmv/

National CMV Foundation. https://www.nationalcmv.org/

Anthony, T. (2011). *Fact sheet: Spotlight on cytomegalovirus (CMV)*. Colorado Department of Education. https://www.cde.state.co.us/sites/default/files/documents/cdesped/download/pdf/dbcmv.pdf

Baylor College of Medicine. (n.d.). *Get involved: Parent to parent support network*. https://www.bcm.edu/departments/pediatrics/sections-divisions-centers/cmvregistry/get-involved

National PTA. (n.d.). *Special education toolkit*. https://www.pta.org/home/family-resources/Special-Education-Toolkit

Center for Parent Information and Resources. https://www.parentcenterhub.org/

REFERENCES

Adler, S. P., Nigro, G., & Pereira, L. (2007). Recent advances in the prevention and treatment of congenital cytomegalovirus infections. *Seminars in Perinatology, 31*(1), 10–18. https://doi.org/10.1053/j.semperi.2007.01.002

Anderholm, K. M., Bierle, C. J., & Schleiss, M. R. (2016). Cytomegalovirus vaccines: Current status and future prospects. *Drugs, 76*(17), 1625–1645. https://doi.org/10.1007/s40265-016-0653-5

Aronson, S. S. (1988). Health update: CMC and child care programs. *Child Care Information Exchange, 59*, 25–28.

Bristow, B. N., O'Keefe, K. A., Shafir, S. C., & Sorvillo, F. J. (2011). Congenital cytomegalovirus mortality in the United States, 1990–2006. *PLOS Neglected Tropical Diseases, 5*(4), Article e1140. https://doi.org/10.1371/journal.pntd.0001140

Centers for Disease Control and Prevention. (2020). *Cytomegalovirus (CMV) and congenital CMV infection*. U.S. Department of Health and Human Services. https://www.cdc.gov/cmv/

Dowd, J. B., Palermo, T. M., & Aiello, A. E. (2012). Family poverty is associated with cytomegalovirus antibody titers in U.S. children. *Health Psychology, 31*(1), 5–10. https://doi.org/10.1037/a0025337

Gentile, I., Zappulo, E., Riccio, M. P., Binda, S., Bubba, L., Pellegrinelli, L., Scognamiglio, D., Operto, F., Margari, L., Borgia, G., & Bravaccio, C. (2017). Prevalence of congenital cytomegalovirus infection assessed through viral genome detection in dried blood spots in children with autism spectrum disorders. *In Vivo, 31*(3), 467–473. https://doi.org/10.21873/invivo.11085

Kaye, K. M. (2021). Cytomegalovirus (CMV) infection. *Merck Manuals Professional Version*. https://www.merckmanuals.com/professional/infectious-diseases/herpesviruses/cytomegalovirus-cmv-infection

Korndewal, M. J., Oudesluys-Murphy, A. M., Kroes, A. C. M., Vossen, A. C. T. M., & de Melker, H. E. (2017). Congenital cytomegalovirus infection: Child development, quality of life and impact on daily life. *The Pediatric Infectious Disease Journal, 36*(12), 1141–1147. https://doi.org/10.1097/INF.0000000000001663

Manicklal, S., Emery, V. C., Lazzarotto, T., Boppana, S. B., & Gupta, R. K. (2013). The "silent" global burden of congenital cytomegalovirus. *Clinical Microbiology Reviews, 26*(1), 86–102. https://doi.org/10.1128/CMR.00062-12

National CMV Foundation. (2019). *Newborn screening*. https://www.nationalcmv.org/overview/newborn-screening

Nigro, G., Adler, S. P., La Torre, R., & Best, A. M. (2005). Passive immunization during pregnancy for congenital cytomegalovirus infection. *The New England Journal of Medicine, 353*(13), 1350–1362. https://doi.org/10.1056/NEJMoa043337

Nordqvist, C. (2018). Everything you need to know about cytomegalovirus. *Medical News Today*. https://www.medicalnewstoday.com/articles/173811

Pass, R. F., & Arav-Boger, R. (2018). Maternal and fetal cytomegalovirus infection: Diagnosis, management, and prevention. *F1000 Research, 7*, Article 255. https://doi.org/10.12688/f1000research.12517.1

Pass, R. F., Fowler, K. B., Boppana, S. B., Britt, W. J., & Stagno, S. (2006). Congenital cytomegalovirus infection following first trimester maternal infection: Symptoms at birth and outcome. *Journal of Clinical Virology, 35*(2), 216–220. https://doi.org/10.1016/j.jcv.2005.09.015

Schleiss, M. R. (2018). Congenital cytomegalovirus: Impact on child health. *Contemporary Pediatrics, 35*(7), 16–24.

Siberry, G. K., Abzug, M. J., & Nachman, S. (2013). Executive summary: Guidelines for the prevention and treatment of opportunistic infections in HIV-exposed and HIV-infected children: Recommendations from the National Institutes of Health, the

Centers for Disease Control and Prevention, the HIV Medicine Association of the Infectious Diseases Society of America, the Pediatric Infectious Diseases Society, and the American Academy of Pediatrics. *Journal of the Pediatric Infectious Diseases Society, 2*(4), 293–308. https://doi.org/10.1093/jpids/pit074

Sommers, M., & Fannin, E. (2014). *Diseases and disorders: A nursing therapeutics manual* (5th ed.). F. A. Davis.

Turbert, D. (2022). *What is cytomegalovirus retinitis?* American Academy of Ophthalmology. https://www.aao.org/eye-health/diseases/what-is-cytomegalovirus-retinitis

44

Sarcoidosis

Adeline M. Bray, Sai Sudha Aravala, and Craig Schramm

Sarcoidosis is classified as an autoimmune disease that results in inflammation in various sites in the body, such as the lungs, lymph nodes, and the skin (Autoimmune Association, 2018). Current findings suggest there is no one definitive cause for this condition. As an inflammatory response, noncaseating granulomas form in different sites of the body (Jadotte et al., 2018). A unique aspect of this condition is that many individuals have no symptoms that can be classified as sarcoidosis. Most commonly, the diagnosis is made using tests of lung function, including diffusion capacity, in addition to chest radiography (e.g., X-rays, high-resolution CT scans) and biopsies of any involved tissue (Autoimmune Association, 2018). Serum angiotensin-converting enzyme is often assessed, as levels are elevated in 60% to 80% of adult patients, but the test has poor diagnostic sensitivity and specificity.

ETIOLOGY

Sarcoidosis appears in individuals who are genetically predisposed and who are exposed to a currently unidentified antigen. The inflammatory response can potentially be triggered by self-antigens, indicative of an autoimmune contribution (Grunewald et al., 2019), and/or environmental antigens, in light of regional differences in prevalence. Genetic factors play a role in both the risk of disease development as well as the variability in the disease course (Grunewald et al., 2019). Current models suggest the involvement of oligoclonal T cell

https://doi.org/10.1037/0000349-044
Health-Related Disorders in Children and Adolescents: A Guidebook for Educators and Service Providers, Second Edition, M. M. Perfect, C. A. Riccio, and M. A. Bray (Editors)

expansion and T helper 1 cytokine polarization result in the granulomatous response (Chen & Moller, 2008).

PREVALENCE AND INCIDENCE

Sarcoidosis predominantly affects individuals from ages 20 to 40 years, among whom the prevalence has been reported to span from approximately one to as many as 40 cases per population of 100,000 people (Baculard et al., 2001; Baughman et al., 2016). The prevalence of childhood sarcoidosis is estimated to be lower than that of sarcoidosis in adults and is approximately 0.27 per population of 100,000 children per year (Baculard et al., 2001). The peak age of children diagnosed with sarcoidosis is 13 to 15 years old, with the majority of children being diagnosed at an age greater than 10 years (Baculard et al., 2001). Very few children younger than 5 years have sarcoidosis (Shetty & Gedalia, 2008). Overall, the lifetime prevalence across the lifespan is estimated to be 2.4% for Black people and 0.85% for White people, with slightly differing rates in northern countries (Iannuzzi et al., 2007).

Sarcoidosis can vary by geographic region as well as race. Nordic countries have shown higher prevalence and incidence. Black individuals, in comparison with Whites, Asians, and Latinxs, have at least a 10-fold higher incidence and prevalence (Arkema & Cozier, 2018; Kamangar et al., 2022). Prevalence is higher for individuals who are Black, estimated at approximately 34 in 100,000, compared with 11 in 100,000 for individuals who are White when adjusted for age. Sarcoidosis is twice as likely to occur in women, with Black women having the highest prevalence (Baughman et al., 2016).

SYMPTOMS

Sarcoidosis is a disorder that is diverse in both its clinical manifestations and disease severity (Ungprasert et al., 2019). The organ most commonly affected is the lungs. Other organs commonly involved include the lymph nodes, eyes, skin, and liver; less commonly implicated are the central nervous system, heart, joints, bone, spleen, and kidneys. In youth 10 years of age and older, the disease presents in the same manner as adults, primarily causing mediastinal/hilar lymph node enlargement and lung tissue inflammation. Pulmonary involvement results in symptoms such as dry hacking cough and, at times, chest pain and possible mild to moderate dyspnea (shortness of breath; Shetty & Gedalia, 2008) and rarely hemoptysis (coughing up blood; Kamangar et al., 2022). Peripheral lymph node hypertrophy occurs in 40% to 70% of children (Shetty & Gedalia, 2008).

Childhood sarcoidosis also affects the skin, with an erythematous rash occurring in 75% of young children and 24% to 40% of older children (Shetty & Gedalia, 2008). Eye involvement with iritis or uveitis (inflammation inside the eye) is present in 24% to 58% of affected children, often presenting with blurriness, red eyes, photophobia, and blurry vision (Shetty & Gedalia, 2008). Arthritis has been reported in 15% to 58% of children with sarcoidosis. Nonspecific constitutional symptoms are also common, including fever, fatigue, malaise, and weight loss (Shetty & Gedalia, 2008). Some patients will present with Löfgren syndrome, a triad of hilar lymphadenopathy, acute arthritis, and erythema nodosum (Kamangar et al., 2022). This syndrome is rare in Japanese and African American individuals and is less common in children than adults.

Across the age span, sarcoidosis can present in a multitude of ways and can be subacute, acute, or chronic (Bargagli & Prasse, 2018; Kamangar et al., 2022). About 5% of the chronic cases are asymptomatic and are recognized by chest imaging. In 45% of cases, patients present with systemic complaints. In the remaining 50% of cases, patients exhibit pulmonary issues. About 20% of the chronic severe patients are at risk for developing lung fibrosis (Bargagli & Prasse, 2018).

No treatment is indicated for asymptomatic children or for children with mild radiographic lung disease and normal to mildly abnormal lung function, as many of these patients will experience spontaneous remission of their disease (Prasse, 2016). The mainstay of treatment for more severely affected patients is systemic corticosteroids, usually a form of prednisone. Indications for treatment include severe, progressive disease in any organ system; deteriorating pulmonary status or development of pulmonary hypertension; any cardiac, neurologic, ocular, or renal lesions; or hypercalcemia, which can cause fatal cardiac dysrhythmias and renal failure. Other immunosuppressive or cytotoxic therapies are sometimes added, particularly in refractory or relapsing cases. For the most severe cases, procedures such as lung transplantation may be the best option (Egan, 2003).

IMPACT ON THE STUDENT AND OUTCOMES

Medical

On average, 40% of adults diagnosed with sarcoidosis experience a chronic severe condition, whereas less than 60% have reported the disease disappears over a span of 2 to 5 years without specific therapy (Baughman et al., 2018). Although this may present a sign of hope for those who see the condition's disappearance over time, quality of life is still affected (Baughman et al., 2018). Conversely, in more persistent cases, progression of lung inflammation to pulmonary fibrosis or uveitis to blindness may cause significant morbidity.

Cognitive/Academic

Sarcoidosis has been shown to negatively affect the quality of educational functioning. Cognitive impairment, characterized by cognitive processing dysfunction due to concentration problems and memory loss, has been found in 35% of adults with sarcoidosis and has been attributed to inflammation-induced changes in central neurotransmitter metabolism (Elfferich et al., 2010). Low cognitive performance is also associated with fatigue and depressive symptoms (Elfferich et al., 2010). Medications can induce cognitive impairments, such as impaired auditory processing and memory, as well as word-finding difficulties (Kenna et al., 2011). Further, individuals with this systemic inflammatory condition tend to experience alexithymia (Trombini & Trombini, 2012). Alexithymia is described as a cognitive processing deficiency in which the individual is unable to express their state of being, which includes aspects such as one's emotions and bodily sensations (Haviland, 2016). These deficits affect academic performance.

Social-Emotional and Behavioral

Individuals with sarcoidosis are affected by a myriad of social and emotional symptoms, although they may still be perceived as healthy by others. Having to deal with many symptoms for long periods of time leads many patients to exhibit anxiety and depression, which then affect educational performance. Fatigue is the most frequently described and debilitating symptom in adults with sarcoidosis, with 60% to 90% of patients reporting some fatigue and up to 25% of patients reporting extreme fatigue (Drent et al., 2015). Depression is particularly linked with the level of fatigue the student/patient is exhibiting. Moreover, depression in patients with sarcoidosis may be linked to cytokine imbalances (Drent et al., 2015).

Improper self-care linked to depression affects other life aspects, such as diet and exercise, contributing to the exacerbation of poor mental and physical health. Exercise limitation due to lung disease can lead to poor cognitive functioning and reduced academic engagement and performance. Patients with sarcoidosis also often suffer from anxiety associated with their reported experience of fatigue. Anxiety manifests in physical outcomes, such as increased heart rate, and in reduced cognitive and executive functioning (Drent et al., 2015). The chronic corticosteroid therapy needed to treat sarcoidosis may cause a number of psychiatric side effects, ranging from mood disorders (e.g., hypomania, mania, depression) to anxiety, delirium, and psychosis (Kenna et al., 2011).

Finally, friends, family, and health care workers may not understand and acknowledge the extent to which this disease is affecting the individual. This causes strain on relationships and families, along with possible social isolation, as the person with sarcoidosis may not choose to socialize with others. This can lead to increased stress, depression, and inattention (Drent et al., 2015).

PSYCHOEDUCATIONAL IMPLICATIONS AND SCHOOL-BASED INTERVENTIONS

Medical and Health Management

The child with sarcoidosis needs consistent support from their family, education, medical, and friend networks (Sommers, 2019). Thus, applications of the biopsychosocial model are appropriate for these children for whom many systems are affected, such as schooling, family, medical, psychological, and diet/exercise networks. Medically, considering and monitoring side effects of the medications used to treat sarcoidosis, as well as promoting appropriate healthy habits, is important.

Cognitive/Academic

Cognitive and academic concerns may emerge at any time, most likely in association with medication, stress, and fatigue. Given the potential for memory and processing issues, strategy instruction for remembering information or other approaches to improving memory, as well as frequent prompts and use of technology reminders, may be helpful. Progress monitoring and appropriate provision of support services through a 504 plan or special education may be appropriate.

Social-Emotional and Behavioral

Because these patients experience long-term anxiety and stress, a psychological intervention, such as mindfulness for stress reduction, including coping and appraisal, may be appropriate. Another effective treatment option to consider is cognitive behavior therapy, which benefits individuals with anxiety and depression and can help treat the difficult-to-manage symptoms of fatigue. Many other appropriate mind–body health treatments, such as relaxation and guided imagery, especially scripts directed at the immune system along with gratitude writing exercises, focus on physical and psychological target behaviors and are appropriate to use with individuals of all ages with these types of conditions (Maykel & Bray, 2019). Mind–body health practices allow the individual to better progress through the course of the disease and maintain an awareness of their health lifestyle so they can adjust activities as needed. Further, it is important for those diagnosed with sarcoidosis to get an adequate amount of rest, and sleeping problems sometimes related to periodic leg movements should be addressed (Drent et al., 2015). Breathing exercises and moderate physical activity, both of which can be delivered through many mind–body health techniques, benefit both physical and mental well-being (Life and Breath Foundation, 2020). Additionally, it is important to maintain healthy eating habits and consume foods that strengthen the immune system, which is implicated in sarcoidosis (Life and Breath Foundation, 2020).

CONCLUSION

Sarcoidosis is an autoimmune disease with no single cause. It can present in a multitude of ways, though most often affecting the lungs. Apart from physical manifestations, individuals affected by sarcoidosis exhibit cognitive deficits as well as depression, anxiety, and debilitating fatigue. Medications, along with mind–body health interventions, can be used to treat these individuals to improve their quality of life.

RESOURCES

Autoimmune Association. (2018). *What is sarcoidosis?* https://autoimmune.org/disease-information/sarcoidosis/

REFERENCES

Arkema, E. V., & Cozier, Y. C. (2018). Epidemiology of sarcoidosis: Current findings and future directions. *Therapeutic Advances in Chronic Disease, 9*(11), 227–240. https://doi.org/10.1177/2040622318790197

Autoimmune Association. (2018). *What is sarcoidosis?* https://autoimmune.org/disease-information/sarcoidosis/

Baculard, A., Blanc, N., Boulé, M., Fauroux, B., Chadelat, K., Boccon-Gibod, L., Tournier, G., & Clement, A. (2001). Pulmonary sarcoidosis in children: A follow-up study. *The European Respiratory Journal, 17*(4), 628–635. https://doi.org/10.1183/09031936.01.17406280

Bargagli, E., & Prasse, A. (2018). Sarcoidosis: A review for the internist. *Internal and Emergency Medicine, 13*(3), 325–331. https://doi.org/10.1007/s11739-017-1778-6

Baughman, R. P., Barriuso, R., Beyer, K., Boyd, J., Hochreiter, J., Knoet, C., Martone, F., Quadder, B., Richardson, J., Spitzer, G., Valeyre, D., & Ziosi, G. (2018). Sarcoidosis: Patient treatment priorities. *ERJ Open Research, 4*(4), Article 00141-2018. https://doi.org/10.1183/23120541.00141-2018

Baughman, R. P., Field, S., Costabel, U., Crystal, R. G., Culver, D. A., Drent, M., Judson, M. A., & Wolff, G. (2016). Sarcoidosis in America: Analysis based on health care use. *Annals of the American Thoracic Society, 13*(8), 1244–1252. https://doi.org/10.1513/AnnalsATS.201511-760OC

Chen, E. S., & Moller, D. R. (2008). Etiology of sarcoidosis. *Clinics in Chest Medicine, 29*(3), 365–377. https://doi.org/10.1016/j.ccm.2008.03.011

Drent, M., Strookappe, B., Hoitsma, E., & De Vries, J. (2015). Consequences of sarcoidosis. *Clinics in Chest Medicine, 36*(4), 727–737. https://doi.org/10.1016/j.ccm.2015.08.013

Egan, T. M. (2003). Orthotopic lung transplant for sarcoidosis. *Chest, 123*(3), 962–963. https://doi.org/10.1378/chest.123.3.962

Elfferich, M. D., Nelemans, P. J., Ponds, R. W., De Vries, J., Wijnen, P. A., & Drent, M. (2010). Everyday cognitive failure in sarcoidosis: The prevalence and the effect of anti-TNF-α treatment. *Respiration, 80*(3), 212–219. https://doi.org/10.1159/000314225

Grunewald, J., Grutters, J. C., Arkema, E. V., Saketkoo, L. A., Moller, D. R., & Müller-Quernheim, J. (2019). Sarcoidosis. *Nature Reviews Disease Primers, 5*(1), Article 45. https://doi.org/10.1038/s41572-019-0096-x

Haviland, M. G. (2016). Alexithymia. In H. S. Friedman (Ed.), *Encyclopedia of mental health* (2nd ed., pp. 47–53). https://www.sciencedirect.com/science/article/pii/B9780123970459002275

Iannuzzi, M. C., Rybicki, B. A., & Teirstein, A. S. (2007). Sarcoidosis. *The New England Journal of Medicine, 357*(21), 2153–2165. https://doi.org/10.1056/NEJMra071714

Jadotte, Y. T., Abdel Hay, R., Salphale, P., Mocellin, S., Kumar, S., Niazi, A., & Pilati, P. (2018). Interventions for cutaneous sarcoidosis. *Cochrane Database of Systematic*

Reviews, 2018(8), Article CD010817. https://doi.org/10.1002/14651858.CD010817.pub2

Kamangar, N. M., Rohani, P., & Shorr, A. F. (2022). Sarcoidosis. *Medscape*. https://emedicine.medscape.com/article/301914-overview

Kenna, H. A., Poon, A. W., de los Angeles, C. P., & Koran, L. M. (2011). Psychiatric complications of treatment with corticosteroids: Review with case report. *Psychiatry and Clinical Neurosciences, 65*(6), 549–560. https://doi.org/10.1111/j.1440-1819.2011.02260.x

Life and Breath Foundation. (2020). *Managing medications*. https://www.lifeandbreath.org/living-well-with-sarcoidosis/mental-physical-well-being/

Maykel, C. & Bray, M. A. (2019). *Promoting mind–body health in schools: Interventions for mental health professionals*. American Psychological Association.

Prasse, A. (2016). The diagnosis, differential diagnosis, and treatment of sarcoidosis. *Deutsches Ärzteblatt International, 113*(33–34), 565–574. https://doi.org/10.3238/arztebl.2016.0565

Shetty, A. K., & Gedalia, A. (2008). Childhood sarcoidosis: A rare but fascinating disorder. *Pediatric Rheumatology Online Journal, 6*(1), Article 16. https://doi.org/10.1186/1546-0096-6-16

Sommers, M. S. (2019). Sarcoidosis. In *Diseases and disorders* (6th ed.). F. A. Davis Company. https://nursing.unboundmedicine.com/nursingcentral/view/Diseases-and-Disorders/73713/all/Sarcoidosis

Trombini, G., & Trombini, E. (2012). Sarcoidosis: Psychotherapy and long-term outcome—A case report. *Case Reports in Medicine, 2012*, Article 232491. https://doi.org/10.1155/2012/232491

Ungprasert, P., Ryu, J. H., & Matteson, E. L. (2019). Clinical manifestations, diagnosis, and treatment of sarcoidosis. *Mayo Clinic Proceedings: Innovations, Quality & Outcomes, 3*(3), 358–375. https://doi.org/10.1016/j.mayocpiqo.2019.04.006

VII

MUSCULOSKELETAL DISORDERS

45

Overview of Musculoskeletal Disorders

Sai Sudha Aravala, Adeline M. Bray, Evelyn Bilias-Lolis, and Alyssa M. Bunyea

The musculoskeletal system is one of the most important systems of the human body. Its role is movement initiation and protection of the organs of the body. It provides the mechanical assistance needed to produce movements such as sitting or walking. The three major roles of this system can be described as movement, stability, and robustness or stamina in response to injury (Murphy et al., 2018). Compared with other disorders, musculoskeletal disorders are one of the leading causes of disabilities among individuals (World Health Organization, 2022). According to the Institute for Health Metrics and Evaluation (2018), musculoskeletal disease is the second most common global disability.

BODY SYSTEM INVOLVEMENT AND FUNCTIONING

The disorder is grouped into categories associated with persistent pain affecting the individual's quality of life in the work and social environment (World Health Organization, 2022). The conditions have a lifelong prevalence that increases as the individual ages. The American Academy of Orthopedic Surgeons (AAOS; 2016) viewed musculoskeletal problems in children as a worldwide issue.

When looking at the developmental aspects of the musculoskeletal system, the mesoderm layer is the primary focus. The function of the mesoderm layer is to generate connective tissue, which composes muscles (Hill, 2020). The

https://doi.org/10.1037/0000349-045
Health-Related Disorders in Children and Adolescents: A Guidebook for Educators and Service Providers, Second Edition, M. M. Perfect, C. A. Riccio, and M. A. Bray (Editors)

mesoderm layer consists of the skeletal, cardiac, and smooth muscles. The mechanism behind generation of a muscle contraction consists of the interaction of actin and myosin, a motor protein (Hill, 2020).

The formation of the mesoderm layer is one of the first steps in initiating the development of the musculoskeletal system. The early form of the mesoderm layer is called the presomitic mesoderm and provides the structure of the axial skeleton and formation of limb muscles (Kardon, 2011).

Musculoskeletal health is an aspect of physical development that is closely observed and exercised in early childhood. From the onset of early kicks and coos to an infant's growing ability to support their own head upright, the development of the musculoskeletal system is at the forefront of the developing child.

The musculoskeletal system consists of bones, joints, tendons, and muscles (AAOS, 2011). Musculoskeletal health pertains to the interconnectedness of diet, exercise, genetics, and environment on the development of a child's ability to sit, stand, walk and run (the main gait), and engage in activities of movement (Murphy et al., 2018). Skeletal growth usually starts to develop in early pregnancy (i.e., the 3rd week after conception) and continues until the bones are fully developed in puberty (Saggese et al., 2002).

Bones provide the structure for the entire body for organ and soft tissue attachment. The adult body consists of 206 bones. These bones are responsible for the following five functions: providing structural support; storing minerals (e.g., calcium) and lipids; producing red, white, and other blood cells found in the red marrow of the bone; protecting body organs; and providing the muscles leverage for movement (Shaffu & Taylor, 2018). In short, bones frame the skeletal system, protect important organs encased within this system, and serve to leverage the muscular movement (Shaffu & Taylor, 2018).

Joints are the points where two skeletal bones meet in the body (also referred to as articulation) and are classified according to their anatomical shape, position, and movement. Some joints are fibrous and immovable (e.g., those found in the cranium and teeth), others are cartilaginous and partially movable, and the large majority are synovial or freely movable (AAOS, 2011). Thus, joints are responsible for both the movement of limbs and stability (e.g., joints in the skull).

Tendons are collagen-based dense connective tissues whose function is to transmit mechanical forces to stabilize the bone frame and especially the joints. Tendons are simple tissues with one main cell type called fibroblasts and are involved in the force transmission between muscle and bone (Benjamin et al., 2008).

Finally, *muscles* afford the body with movement. There are three types of muscles in the muscular system: skeletal, smooth, and cardiac muscles. Skeletal muscles attach to the bones with the help of tendons and move voluntarily (Muscolino, 2016). Cardiac muscles, or the thick muscles of the heart, referred to as the myocardium, contract and relax in order to circulate blood in the body. Finally, smooth muscles, or involuntary muscles, function throughout the body and can be found in the stomach and digestive system, the bladder, and even behind the eyes (Muscolino, 2016).

COMMON COMPLAINTS AND INDICATORS OF DYSFUNCTION

As described thus far, musculoskeletal disorders affect an individual's ability to navigate through their daily life. As a result, the common complaints and indicators of dysfunction can vary based on the organ system that is affected. Common signs of musculoskeletal disorders can include physical abnormalities of the body, reports of pain, and muscle weakness.

Across many of the musculoskeletal diseases, visual indications of dysfunction are evident. For instance, abnormal head growth is common in both achondroplasia (Pauli, 2019) and Sotos syndrome (Tatton-Brown et al., 2022). Additionally, individuals with Charcot–Marie–Tooth disease often have foot deformities that influence their ability to walk or find proper shoes (Reilly et al., 2011). Physical signs can alert caregivers and medical professionals of possible impairment in motor abilities or indications of common symptoms associated with musculoskeletal diseases.

A common complaint of individuals with musculoskeletal problems is reported pain in different areas of the body. This is often seen in individuals with Marfan syndrome and juvenile idiopathic arthritis. Specifically, in Marfan syndrome, pain can be reported in the individual's hips due to joint problems and in their back due to a higher likelihood of a diagnosis of scoliosis (Pyeritz, 2019). Joint pain and swelling are frequent complaints in individuals with juvenile idiopathic arthritis (Barut et al., 2017).

Lastly, muscle weakness is another area of dysfunction that is often seen across musculoskeletal diseases. Weakening of the muscles can influence an individual's ability to move or their ability to engage in automatic processes for survival depending on the muscle group. Overall muscle weakness is commonly seen in neuromuscular diseases and Charcot–Marie–Tooth disease. In neuromuscular disease and muscular dystrophies, muscle weakness can be experienced throughout the body (Bertorini, 2011; Carter et al., 2018), whereas individuals with Charcot–Marie–Tooth disease specifically report weakness in the hands (Reilly et al., 2011). Weakening of the cardiovascular muscles also occurs in some musculoskeletal diseases like Marfan syndrome. The weakening of the cardiovascular muscles is more severe and can lead to death if not caught early (Velvin et al., 2015).

Overall, many of the indicators of dysfunction are characteristics that can be seen through physical examination of an individual or measures of muscle weakness. Many of the musculoskeletal disorders that will be discussed in the upcoming chapters have a genetic predisposition. Genetic testing is commonly completed through prenatal development to identify and determine abnormalities in child development (Keret et al., 2005). As a result, medical professionals can prepare expecting mothers with information to support the development of their children before their birth.

PREVIEW OF MAJOR MUSCULOSKELETAL SYSTEM CONDITIONS IN PEDIATRICS

The musculoskeletal system is subject to disorders and diseases, some of which are more difficult to detect than others. This system is made up of bones or, in other words, the human skeleton, all musculature, tendons, cartilage, ligaments, joints, and additional connective tissues. These are the parts of the system, form and function included, that can be affected. In addition to physical impairments, all of the conditions included in this part of the book present with learning and behavioral/social–emotional problems that school settings must address.

Achondroplasia

The most common type of skeletal defect is *achondroplasia* (Pauli, 2019). Achondroplasia is correlated with short stature, small limbs, and a larger than normal head (Pauli, 2019). Other associated problems with this condition include gross and fine motor and speech (expressive language and articulation) delays (Pauli, 2019). Speech language pathologists, in particular, work with these students (Pauli, 2019). See Chapter 46 by Riccio and Sohn McCormick for more information about achondroplasia.

Charcot–Marie–Tooth Disease

Charcot–Marie–Tooth disease is the most common inherited childhood neuromuscular disorder that also presents with a myriad of these similar types of psychoeducational implications (Jani-Acsadi et al., 2015). Individuals are usually diagnosed through genetic testing; however, various types of genes can contribute to the disease (Reilly et al., 2011). Common symptoms of Charcot–Marie–Tooth disease include muscle weakness and atrophy that slowly influence the function of the hands and feet (Klein, 2020). For more information about Charcot–Marie–Tooth disease, refer to Chapter 47 by Tucker and Nickels.

Juvenile Idiopathic Arthritis

Another condition that affects the musculoskeletal system is *juvenile idiopathic arthritis*. Interestingly, this is a general category and is defined by chronic inflammation of the joints with onset before 16 years (Barut et al., 2017). Systemically, juvenile idiopathic arthritis is formally defined as an autoinflammatory disease (Barut et al., 2017). Therefore, this includes such outcomes as inflammatory bowel disease and rheumatoid arthritis (Barut et al., 2017). There are various psychoeducational implications for these students, including particular needs during physical education courses (Nordal et al., 2019). Refer to Chapter 48 by Tipton-DeClue and Robinson for more information about juvenile idiopathic arthritis.

Marfan Syndrome

Another inherited condition that affects the educational process is *Marfan syndrome* (Velvin et al., 2015). Besides affecting the musculoskeletal system, Marfan syndrome also influences the cardiovascular and visual systems (Pyeritz, 2019). Early diagnosis is critical for individuals with Marfan syndrome to decrease the risk of death due to aortic dissection (Velvin et al., 2015). To learn more about Marfan syndrome, see Chapter 49 by Dale and McIntosh.

Muscular Dystrophies

Muscular dystrophies are neuromuscular disorders grouped based on similar characteristics and features (Mercuri & Muntoni, 2013). Diagnosis of muscular dystrophies occurs due to progressive muscle weakness (Carter et al., 2018). The most diagnosed type of muscular dystrophy is Duchenne muscular dystrophy (Carter et al., 2018). Symptoms related to Duchenne muscular dystrophy onset begin in early childhood (Carter et al., 2018). For more information about muscular dystrophies, please refer to Chapter 50 by Tucker and Jeune.

Osteogenesis Imperfecta

Osteogenesis imperfecta is a type of hereditary disorder that affects the skeleton but also the connective tissues. Individuals with this disorder have brittle bones along with other associated problems, such as hearing loss, neurological abnormalities, pulmonary issues, and cardiovascular abnormalities (Rodriguez Celin et al., 2018). Furthermore, cognitive and social–emotional issues present with osteogenesis imperfecta. Refer to Chapter 51 by Clark and Malecki for more details.

Sotos Syndrome

Sotos syndrome is an overgrowth disorder, with most diagnoses due to a gene mutation or deletion. Common features of the disorder include rapid bone age, specific facial features, and cognitive impairments (Tatton-Brown et al., 2022). Accompanied medical issues that can arise in individuals with Sotos syndrome include motor problems like scoliosis and hip dislocation and social and behavioral concerns (Tatton-Brown et al., 2022). See Chapter 52 by Sassu et al. to learn more about Sotos syndrome.

HEALTH CARE NEEDS AND MEDICAL SPECIALTIES

Children with musculoskeletal disorders utilize specialists to assist in motor functions, as well as language, academic, and behavioral needs. Motor functions can be divided into gross motor (e.g., walking, running, climbing) and fine motor skills (e.g., writing, coloring, cutting). Physical therapists support gross motor skills by improving the movement of the body. Children with juvenile idiopathic arthritis or Marfan syndrome may utilize physical therapists to decrease joint pain from gross motor skills like walking. Occupational therapists specialize in fine motor movements to promote daily living activities. Occupational therapists would be more useful for a child with achondroplasia who needs assistance with fine motor skills.

Students may also need specialists to support academic needs if they have lower cognitive abilities, as seen in osteogenesis imperfecta and Sotos syndrome. In a school setting, a child may qualify for an individualized education program that outlines accommodations and modifications to support their unique learning profile. More than likely, a special education teacher would work with the student to promote learning based on the child's cognitive abilities. Academic achievement assessments can inform the special education teacher on the child's strengths and weaknesses to build upon areas of weakness by utilizing their skill set.

Depending on the musculoskeletal disease, the child may also need assistance with social, emotional, and behavioral needs. In a school setting, a school psychologist can provide counseling and behavior management strategies to encourage positive social and behavioral interactions in the environment. Based on the characteristics of the disorder, students with a diagnosis of either osteogenesis imperfecta or Sotos syndrome may need the support of a school psychologist.

CONCLUSION

Overall, diseases of the musculoskeletal system impair the ability to move, think, and feel emotions, along with other outcomes such as disorders with eyesight and hearing loss. There are many school-related issues. School absenteeism, anxiety, depression, inattention, and stress are the most common occurrences with the aforementioned musculoskeletal system disorders. Thus, learning environments have to accommodate these resulting problems.

REFERENCES

American Academy of Orthopedic Surgeons. (2016). *Position statement: Children and musculoskeletal health.* https://www.aaos.org/contentassets/1cd7f41417ec4dd4b5c4c48532183b96/1170-children-and-musculoskeletal-health.pdf

Barut, K., Adrovic, A., Şahin, S., & Kasapçopur, Ö. (2017). Juvenile idiopathic arthritis. *Balkan Medical Journal, 34*(2), 90–101. https://doi.org/10.4274/balkanmedj.2017.0111

Benjamin, M., Kaiser, E., & Milz, S. (2008). Structure-function relationships in tendons: A review. *Journal of Anatomy, 212*(3), 211–228. https://doi.org/10.1111/j.1469-7580.2008.00864.x

Bertorini, T. E. (2011). *Neuromuscular disorders: Management and therapy*. Elsevier Saunders.

Carter, J. C., Sheehan, D. W., Prochoroff, A., & Birnkrant, D. J. (2018). Muscular dystrophies. *Clinics in Chest Medicine, 39*(2), 377–389. https://doi.org/10.1016/j.ccm.2018.01.004

Hill, M. A. (2020). Musculoskeletal system development. *Embryology*. https://embryology.med.unsw.edu.au/embryology/index.php/Musculoskeletal_System_Development

Institute for Health Metrics and Evaluation. (2018). *Findings from the Global Burden of Disease Study 2017*. https://www.healthdata.org/policy-report/findings-global-burden-disease-study-2017

Jani-Acsadi, A., Ounpuu, S., Pierz, K., & Acsadi, G. (2015). Pediatric Charcot–Marie–Tooth disease. *Pediatric Clinics of North America, 62*(3), 767–786. https://doi.org/10.1016/j.pcl.2015.03.012

Kardon, G. (2011). Development of the musculoskeletal system: Meeting the neighbors. *Development, 138*(14), 2855–2859. https://doi.org/10.1242/dev.067181

Keret, D., Bronshtein, M., & Wientraub, S. (2005). Prenatal diagnosis of musculoskeletal anomalies. *Clinical Orthopaedics and Related Research, 434*, 8–15. https://doi.org/10.1097/00003086-200505000-00003

Klein, C. J. (2020). Charcot–Marie–Tooth disease and other hereditary neuropathies. *Continuum, 26*(5), 1224–1256. https://doi.org/10.1212/CON.0000000000000927

Mercuri, E., & Muntoni, F. (2013). Muscular dystrophies. *The Lancet, 381*(9869), 845–860. https://doi.org/10.1016/S0140-6736(12)61897-2

Murphy, A. C., Muldoon, S. F., Baker, D., Lastowka, A., Bennett, B., Yang, M., & Bassett, D. S. (2018). Structure, function, and control of the human musculoskeletal network. *PLOS Biology, 16*(1), Article e2002811. https://doi.org/10.1371/journal.pbio.2002811

Muscolino, J. E. (2016). *The muscular system manual: The skeletal muscles of the human body* (4th ed.). Mosby.

Nordal, E., Rypdal, V., Arnstad, E. D., Aalto, K., Berntson, L., Ekelund, M., Fasth, A., Glerup, M., Herlin, T., Nielsen, S., Peltoniemi, S., Zak, M., Songstad, N. T., & Rygg, M. (2019). Participation in school and physical education in juvenile idiopathic arthritis in a Nordic long-term cohort study. *Pediatric Rheumatology, 17*(1), Article 44. https://doi.org/10.1186/s12969-019-0341-6

Pauli, R. M. (2019). Achondroplasia: A comprehensive clinical review. *Orphanet Journal of Rare Diseases, 14*(1), Article 1. https://doi.org/10.1186/s13023-018-0972-6

Pyeritz, R. E. (2019). Marfan syndrome: Improved clinical history results in expanded natural history. *Genetics in Medicine, 21*(8), 1683–1690. https://doi.org/10.1038/s41436-018-0399-4

Reilly, M. M., Murphy, S. M., & Laurá, M. (2011). Charcot–Marie–Tooth disease. *Journal of the Peripheral Nervous System, 16*(1), 1–14. https://doi.org/10.1111/j.1529-8027.2011.00324.x

Rodriguez Celin, M., Moosa, S., & Fano, V. (2018). Uncommon *IFITM5* mutation associated with severe skeletal deformity in osteogenesis imperfecta. *Annals of Human Genetics, 82*(6), 477–481. https://doi.org/10.1111/ahg.12275

Saggese, G., Baroncelli, G. I., & Bertelloni, S. (2002). Puberty and bone development. *Best Practice & Research: Clinical Endocrinology & Metabolism, 16*(1), 53–64. https://doi.org/10.1053/beem.2001.0180

Shaffu, S., & Taylor, J. (2018). Normal function of the musculoskeletal system. In P. Davey & D. Sprigings (Eds.), *Diagnosis and treatment in internal medicine* (pp. 892–893). https://doi.org/10.1093/med/9780199568741.003.0263

Tatton-Brown, K., Cole, T. R. P., & Rahman, N. (2022). Sotos syndrome. In M. P. Adam, D. B. Everman, G. M. Mirzaa, R. A. Pagon, S. E. Wallace, L. J. H. Bean, K. W. Gripp, & A. Amemiya (Eds.), *GeneReviews*. University of Washington.

Velvin, G., Bathen, T., Rand-Hendriksen, S., & Geirdal, A. Ø. (2015). Systematic review of the psychosocial aspects of living with Marfan syndrome. *Clinical Genetics, 87*(2), 109–116. https://doi.org/10.1111/cge.12422

World Health Organization. (2022). *Musculoskeletal conditions*. https://www.who.int/news-room/fact-sheets/detail/musculoskeletal-conditions

46

Achondroplasia

Cynthia A. Riccio and Anita Sohn McCormick

The most common form, and the most studied, of *dwarfing skeletal dysplasias*, or dwarfism, is achondroplasia (ACH; Pauli, 2019). ACH is associated with disproportionate short stature, limb shortening, and a larger than normal head. A function of the skeletal dysplasias, ACH is characterized by developmental motor delays that affect fine and gross motor development, as well as speech motor function (i.e., articulation; Ireland et al., 2013; Trotter et al., 2005).

ETIOLOGY

ACH is a result of an autosomal dominant transmission of a mutated fibroblast growth factor receptor three gene, or *FGFR3* on chromosome 4 (Francomano, 1995; Pauli, 2019; Wilkin et al., 1998); however, it is estimated that for 80% of cases, the mutation occurred spontaneously (i.e., neither parent was a carrier; Wilkin et al., 1998). The spontaneous mutation is more frequent in children of older fathers. Notably, once the gene has mutated, the disorder can be transmitted to future generations. Changes to *FGFR3* are known to affect both bone and neuronal development, yet the consequences are not yet fully understood (Pauli, 2019). *FGFR3* is a negative regulator of bone growth (i.e., it shortens the time frame for bone lengthening through various mechanisms). The limb shortening, for both upper and lower limbs, is called rhizomelic shortening.

https://doi.org/10.1037/0000349-046
Health-Related Disorders in Children and Adolescents: A Guidebook for Educators and Service Providers, Second Edition, M. M. Perfect, C. A. Riccio, and M. A. Bray (Editors)

Research suggests that variations in the mutation of *FGFR3* may result in milder or more severe phenotypes (Bengur et al., 2019; Spranger, 1985).

PREVALENCE AND INCIDENCE

The prevalence of ACH is approximately one in 20,000 to 30,000 births (Moffitt et al., 2011; Stevenson et al., 2012). This form of skeletal dysplasia affects more than 250,000 people worldwide (Horton et al., 2007). There are no indications of differences by gender, race/ethnicity, or culture.

SYMPTOMS

With ultrasound, the limb shortening and larger head relative to the rest of the body may be the first signs prompting further assessment before the child is born, even if there is no family history of ACH (Pauli, 2019). If not prenatally, ACH is usually identified in early infancy, not only by the limb shortening but also by the characteristic midfacial flattening, including of the nasal bridge, as well as a shorter nasal spine. The limb shortening is accompanied by reduced elbow and hip extension, resulting in restricted reach and motor functionality (Pauli, 2019). At the same time, the infant may be hypotonic (i.e., floppy) with loose ligaments in the joints (i.e., joint laxity). With increased head size and weight, the center of gravity shifts and the child has to figure out how to maintain balance when in an upright position. The delays and alternative strategies for shifting position and movement, as well as communication delays, may be key to the identification of ACH within the first 2 years of life (Ireland, Donaghey, et al., 2012). Ireland and colleagues (2013) determined that the extent of delay in motor skills is a combined function of head circumference, overall body height, and body weight, with height having greater significance in determining the age at which the infant was able to transition from lying to sitting. As the child begins to walk, they may develop swayback related to these same factors.

IMPACT ON THE STUDENT AND OUTCOMES

Medical

ACH is associated with neurological, musculoskeletal, and cardiorespiratory systems, resulting in increased rates of mortality at all ages (Fredwall et al., 2019; Hecht et al., 1987). Medical issues in children include hydrocephalus, sleep apnea, leg and spine deformities, spinal canal stenosis (narrowing), obesity, and ear infections and hearing impairment. Up to 50% of individuals with ACH undergo tube placement due to the altered facial anatomy and shortened Eustachian tubes; some may have frequent ear infections and possible hearing loss (Committee on Genetics, 1995; Trotter et al., 2005). A majority of children with ACH experience sleep-disordered breathing (Mogayzel, 1998; Tenconi et al., 2017). Although the incidence is at or less than 10%, infants with ACH are at risk for cervical cord compression and associated problems (e.g., quadriparesis, sudden infant death), and hydrocephalus (Ireland et al., 2014).

Cognitive/Academic

Many individuals with ACH are of average intelligence (Brinkmann et al., 1993; Wigg et al., 2016). At the same time, some individuals with ACH evidence developmental delays (Thompson et al., 1999), including a higher than expected co-occurrence with Down syndrome (de Azevedo Moreira et al., 2010). Regardless of cognitive ability, there are early delays in communication and motor skills, with many children with ACH evidencing delayed speech development and potentially identified with a speech sound or language disorder (Brinkmann et al., 1993). Fine motor skills may be affected as well due to the trident configuration of the fingers and persistence of a four-finger or two-finger grasp (Pauli, 2019). This can lead to problems with fatigue on pencil-and-paper tasks or other motor tasks included in the assessment process or classroom (Ireland, Donaghey, et al., 2012). Relative to same-aged peers, impairment for the group with ACH was noted by Wigg et al. (2016) in arithmetic, attention, and executive functioning, with performance ranging from impaired to within normal limits. Others have identified deficits in language and visuospatial skills, as well as arithmetic (Brinkmann et al., 1993; Thompson et al., 1999). Thus, children with ACH are at risk for a learning disability. Finally, due to physical limitations, children with ACH require more assistance in completing daily living and self-care behaviors beyond what is typically expected (Ireland et al., 2013).

Social–Emotional and Behavioral

Limited research has been conducted on the social–emotional and behavioral correlates of ACH. Given potential physical limitations and visible differences, development of peer relations may be more difficult. The early research indicated that children with ACH are prone to internalize emotions, may exhibit low self-esteem, and have a dysfunctional body image (Csapo, 1991). For children with ACH in Australia, social cognition was identified as a strength (Ireland et al., 2011). A more recent study in Japan indicated that, although children with ACH are subject to additional stressors, particularly with regard to physical inconvenience, there was no indication of psychosocial maladjustment (Nishimura & Hanaki, 2014). Furthermore, boys reported greater stress than girls with regard to peer interactions, school stressors, coping, and perceived social support. Notably, the highest school stressors scores were for junior high students, as compared with elementary or high school students (Nishimura & Hanaki, 2014).

Long term, most individuals with ACH who reach adulthood are able to function independently in social arenas and in employment settings (e.g., Gollust et al., 2003). In contrast, in adulthood, individuals with ACH were less likely to be married than the general population (Gollust et al., 2003). Further, Matsushita et al. (2019) found that for their sample, even with a range of medical interventions, ACH negatively affected quality of life.

PSYCHOEDUCATIONAL IMPLICATIONS AND SCHOOL-BASED INTERVENTIONS

Medical and Health Management

The Committee on Genetics (1995; Trotter et al., 2005) established guidelines for monitoring and supervising children with ACH. Further, systematic reviews on children with ACH have generated recommendations for monitoring of risk (Ireland, Johnson, et al., 2012; Pauli, 2019; Unger et al., 2017). Appropriate medical management for neurological as well as physical complications is needed to maintain mental and physical function (Matsushita et al., 2019). In particular, monitoring of hearing is recommended across the lifespan. In infancy, it has been recommended that upright positioning (i.e., positioning the child to sit up) be delayed as this can result in additional problems (Reynolds et al., 2001). Similarly, it is recommended to have appropriate neck supports in car seats and avoid the use of automatic swings (Pauli, 2019). Given the extent to which pain occurs in conjunction with ACH and how it increases with age (e.g., Dhiman et al., 2017), consideration of incorporating interventions and ensuring furniture that accommodates the short stature is of importance. Available treatments include therapies to suppress *FGFR3*, human growth hormones, and limb-lengthening surgeries; however, there is insufficient research regarding both positive and negative outcomes of these invasive treatments (Pauli, 2019).

Cognitive/Academic

Most children with ACH do not evidence cognitive or academic deficits. With hearing loss or co-occurring Down syndrome, however, some children may have communication issues. Seager et al. (2022) provided a systematic review of interventions to address communication issues in early years. The studies reviewed by Seager et al. were predominantly codelivered by parents and teachers, with increases in communication function. For those children with ACH who struggle in any academic areas, the evidence-based interventions for students with learning disabilities may be appropriate (for a systematic review, see McKenna et al., 2015).

At the school level, parents of children with ACH need to work together with teachers and school administrators to address their children's physical needs (Committee on Genetics, 1995; Trotter et al., 2005). One of the major considerations is ensuring appropriate accommodations for their small stature and appropriate means to complete tasks given potential physical limitations and fatigue factors (Pauli, 2019). The school needs to ensure accessibility not only for restrooms and classrooms but also for reach of materials. It is important for there to be adequate monitoring and management systems in place for both early identification and treatment of emergent problems over time (Ireland et al., 2011). A 504 plan monitoring progress would be helpful in the school setting to ensure teachers receiving the child with ACH are advised of the child's needs.

Consultation with medical personnel and active involvement of physical therapists and occupational therapists to monitor and assess the need for any physical modifications is paramount. This extends beyond furniture to how the child produces work (e.g., use of a keyboard). Speech and language services and monitoring of cognitive development and academic skill acquisition will be needed as demands in the school setting change in combination with physiological changes. In the event of hearing loss, the typical standards for habilitation are recommended (Pauli, 2019; Trotter et al., 2005). These include parent and teacher awareness, preferential seating, and use of amplification systems. Infrequently, the hearing loss will necessitate hearing aids (Tunkel et al., 2012).

Social-Emotional and Behavioral

Early on, children with ACH need to be provided with training in skills and social supports (Nishimura & Hanaki, 2014). It is important for parents and teachers to encourage socialization, beginning with preschool attendance (Trotter et al., 2005). As they age, the child with ACH needs to be able to respond to questions about their short stature, be prepared to respond if teased, and to be able to ask for help or accommodations as needed (i.e., self-determination). With the potential for low self-efficacy and school stressors, it is important that emotional functioning be monitored with supports as needed. Although contact sports and gymnastics are to be avoided, participation in swimming may provide a means to interact with peers and provide needed exercise (Pauli, 2019). Similarly, participation in extracurricular activities that do not have physical demands (e.g., school newspaper) may provide opportunities for socialization. For those children with higher levels of anxiety, cognitive-behavior-based approaches may be appropriate (Ruocco et al., 2018; van Starrenburg et al., 2017).

CONCLUSION

Consistently, across the systematic reviews on ACH (e.g., Fredwall et al., 2019; Pauli, 2019; Thompson et al., 1999), the conclusion has been that very little is known about the medical, social, or employment outcomes for individuals with ACH. Concerns have been raised with the treatment approaches currently used and the sparse research on their effectiveness with this population (Pauli,

2019). In the meantime, there is little to no research on the educational and social ramifications across the lifespan.

RESOURCES

Little People of America. https://www.lpaonline.org
KidsHealth. (2020). *Dwarfism*. https://kidshealth.org/en/parents/dwarfism.html

REFERENCES

Bengur, F. B., Ekmekci, C. G., Karaaslan, E., Gunzoz, H., & Alanay, Y. (2019). p.SER348Cys mutation in *FGFR3* gene leads to "Mild ACH/Severe HCH" phenotype. *European Journal of Medical Genetics, 63*(2), Article 103659. https://doi.org/10.1016/j.ejmg.2019.04.016

Brinkmann, G., Schlitt, H., Zorowka, P., & Spranger, J. (1993). Cognitive skills in achondroplasia. *American Journal of Medical Genetics, 47*(5), 800–804. https://doi.org/10.1002/ajmg.1320470540

Committee on Genetics. (1995). Health supervision for children with achondroplasia. *Pediatrics, 95*(3), 443–451. https://doi.org/10.1542/peds.95.3.443

Csapo, M. (1991). Psychosocial adjustment of children with short stature (achondroplasia): Social competence, behavior problems, self-esteem, family functioning, body image, and reaction to frustrations. *Behavioral Disorders, 16*(3), 219–224. https://doi.org/10.1177/019874299101600302

de Azevedo Moreira, L. M., Matos, M. A., Schiper, P. P., Carvalho, A. F. L., Gomes, I. C., Rolemberg, J. C., Ferreira de Lima, R. L. L., & Toralles, M. B. P. (2010). Co-occurrence of achondroplasia and Down syndrome: Genotype/phenotype association. *Birth Defects Research: Part A, Clinical and Molecular Teratology, 88*(4), 228–231. https://doi.org/10.1002/bdra.20653

Dhiman, N., Albaghdadi, A., Zogg, C. K., Sharma, M., Hoover-Fong, J. E., Ain, M. C., & Haider, A. H. (2017). Factors associated with health-related quality of life (HRQOL) in adults with short stature skeletal dysplasias. *Quality of Life Research, 26*(5), 1337–1348. https://doi.org/10.1007/s11136-016-1455-7

Francomano, C. A. (1995). The genetic basis of dwarfism. *The New England Journal of Medicine, 332*(1), 58–59. https://doi.org/10.1056/NEJM199501053320113

Fredwall, S. O., Maanum, G., Johansen, H., Snekkevik, H., Savarirayan, R., & Lidal, I. B. (2019). Current knowledge of medical complications in adults with achondroplasia: A scoping review. *Clinical Genetics, 97*(1), 179–197. https://doi.org/10.1111/cge.13542

Gollust, S. E., Thompson, R. E., Gooding, H. C., & Biesecker, B. B. (2003). Living with achondroplasia in an average-sized world: An assessment of quality of life. *American Journal of Medical Genetics: Part A, 120A*(4), 447–458. https://doi.org/10.1002/ajmg.a.20127

Hecht, J. T., Francomano, C. A., Horton, W. A., & Annegers, J. F. (1987). Mortality in achondroplasia. *American Journal of Human Genetics, 41*(3), 454–464. https://www.ncbi.nlm.nih.gov/pmc/articles/PMC1684180/

Horton, W. A., Hall, J. G., & Hecht, J. T. (2007). Achondroplasia. *The Lancet, 370*(9582), 162–172. https://doi.org/10.1016/S0140-6736(07)61090-3

Ireland, P. J., Donaghey, S., McGill, J., Zankl, A., Ware, R. S., Pacey, V., Ault, J., Savarirayan, R., Sillence, D., Thompson, E., Townshend, S., & Johnston, L. M. (2012). Development in children with achondroplasia: A prospective clinical cohort study. *Developmental Medicine and Child Neurology, 54*(6), 532–537. https://doi.org/10.1111/j.1469-8749.2012.04234.x

Ireland, P. J., Johnson, S., Donaghey, S., Johnston, L., Ware, R. S., Zankl, A., Pacey, V., Ault, J., Savarirayan, R., Sillence, D., Thompson, E., Townshend, S., & McGill, J. (2012). Medical management of children with achondroplasia: Evaluation of an Australasian cohort aged 0–5 years. *Journal of Paediatrics and Child Health, 48*(5), 443–449. https://doi.org/10.1111/j.1440-1754.2011.02255.x

Ireland, P. J., McGill, J., Zankl, A., Ware, R. S., Pacey, V., Ault, J., Savarirayan, R., Sillence, D., Thompson, E. M., Townshend, S., & Johnston, L. M. (2011). Functional performance in young Australian children with achondroplasia. *Developmental Medicine and Child Neurology, 53*(10), 944–950. https://doi.org/10.1111/j.1469-8749.2011.04050.x

Ireland, P. J., Pacey, V., Zankl, A., Edwards, P., Johnston, L. M., & Savarirayan, R. (2014). Optimal management of complications associated with achondroplasia. *The Application of Clinical Genetics, 7*, 117–125. https://doi.org/10.2147/TACG.S51485

Ireland, P. J., Ware, R. S., Donaghey, S., McGill, J., Zankl, A., Pacey, V., Ault, J., Savarirayan, R., Sillence, D., Thompson, E., Townshend, S., & Johnston, L. M. (2013). The effect of height, weight and head circumference on gross motor development in achondroplasia. *Journal of Paediatrics and Child Health, 49*(2), E122–E127. https://doi.org/10.1111/jpc.12078

Matsushita, M., Kitoh, H., Mishima, K., Yamashita, S., Haga, N., Fujiwara, S., Ozono, K., Kubota, T., Kitaoka, T., & Ishiguro, N. (2019). Physical, mental, and social problems of adolescent and adult patients with achondroplasia. *Calcified Tissue International, 104*(4), 364–372. https://doi.org/10.1007/s00223-019-00518-z

McKenna, J. W., Flower, A., Kim, M. K., Ciullo, S., & Haring, C. (2015). A systematic review of function-based interventions for students with learning disabilities. *Learning Disabilities Research & Practice, 30*(1), 15–28. https://doi.org/10.1111/ldrp.12049

Moffitt, K. B., Abiri, O. O., Scheuerle, A. E., & Langlois, P. H. (2011). Descriptive epidemiology of selected heritable birth defects in Texas. *Birth Defects Research: Part A, Clinical and Molecular Teratology, 91*(12), 990–994. https://doi.org/10.1002/bdra.22859

Mogayzel, P. J., Jr., Carroll, J. L., Loughlin, G. M., Hurko, O., Francomano, C. A., & Marcus, C. L. (1998). Sleep-disordered breathing in children with achondroplasia. *The Journal of Pediatrics, 132*(4), 667–671. https://doi.org/10.1016/S0022-3476(98)70358-0

Nishimura, N., & Hanaki, K. (2014). Psychosocial profiles of children with achondroplasia in terms of their short stature-related stress: A nationwide survey in Japan. *Journal of Clinical Nursing, 23*(21–22), 3045–3056. https://doi.org/10.1111/jocn.12531

Pauli, R. M. (2019). Achondroplasia: A comprehensive clinical review. *Orphanet Journal of Rare Diseases, 14*(1), 1–49. https://doi.org/10.1186/s13023-018-0972-6

Reynolds, K. K., Modaff, P., & Pauli, R. M. (2001). Absence of correlation between infantile hypotonia and foramen magnum size in achondroplasia. *American Journal of Medical Genetics, 101*(1), 40–45. https://doi.org/10.1002/ajmg.1307

Ruocco, S., Freeman, N. C., & McLean, L. A. (2018). Learning to cope: A CBT evaluation exploring self-reported changes in coping with anxiety among school children aged 5–7 years. *Educational and Developmental Psychologist, 35*(2), 67–87. https://doi.org/10.1017/edp.2018.8

Seager, E., Sampson, S., Sin, J., Pagnamenta, E., & Stojanovik, V. (2022). A systematic review of speech, language and communication interventions for children with Down syndrome from 0 to 6 years. *International Journal of Language & Communication Disorders, 57*(2), 441–463. https://doi.org/10.1111/1460-6984.12699

Spranger, J. (1985). Pattern recognition in bone dysplasias. *Progress in Clinical and Biological Research, 200,* 315–342.

Stevenson, D. A., Carey, J. C., Byrne, J. L. B., Srisukhumbowornchai, S., & Feldkamp, M. L. (2012). Analysis of skeletal dysplasias in the Utah population. *American Journal of Medical Genetics: Part A, 158A*(5), 1046–1054. https://doi.org/10.1002/ajmg.a.35327

Tenconi, R., Khirani, S., Amaddeo, A., Michot, C., Baujat, G., Couloigner, V., De Sanctis, L., James, S., Zerah, M., Cormier-Daire, V., & Fauroux, B. (2017). Sleep-disordered breathing and its management in children with achondroplasia. *American Journal of Medical Genetics: Part A, 173*(4), 868–878. https://doi.org/10.1002/ajmg.a.38130

Thompson, N. M., Hecht, J. T., Bohan, T. P., Kramer, L. A., Davidson, K., Brandt, M. E., & Fletcher, J. M. (1999). Neuroanatomic and neuropsychological outcome in school-age children with achondroplasia. *American Journal of Medical Genetics, 88*(2), 145–153. https://doi.org/10.1002/(SICI)1096-8628(19990416)88:2<145::AID-AJMG10>3.0.CO;2-B

Trotter, T. L., Hall, J. G., & the Committee on Genetics. (2005). Health supervision for children with achondroplasia. *Pediatrics, 116*(3), 771–783. https://doi.org/10.1542/peds.2005-1440

Tunkel, D., Alade, Y., Kerbavaz, R., Smith, B., Rose-Hardison, D., & Hoover-Fong, J. (2012). Hearing loss in skeletal dysplasia patients. *American Journal of Medical Genetics: Part A, 158A*(7), 1551–1555. https://doi.org/10.1002/ajmg.a.35373

Unger, S., Bonafé, L., & Gouze, E. (2017). Current care and investigational therapies in achondroplasia. *Current Osteoporosis Reports, 15*(2), 53–60. https://doi.org/10.1007/s11914-017-0347-2

van Starrenburg, M. L. A., Kuijpers, R. C. M. W., Kleinjan, M., Hutschemaekers, G. J. M., & Engels, R. C. M. E. (2017). Effectiveness of a cognitive behavioral therapy-based indicated prevention program for children with elevated anxiety levels: A randomized controlled trial. *Prevention Science, 18*(1), 31–39. https://doi.org/10.1007/s11121-016-0725-5

Wigg, K., Tofts, L., Benson, S., & Porter, M. (2016). The neuropsychological function of children with achondroplasia. *American Journal of Medical Genetics: Part A, 170*(11), 2882–2888. https://doi.org/10.1002/ajmg.a.37779

Wilkin, D. J., Szabo, J. K., Cameron, R., Henderson, S., Bellus, G. A., Mack, M. L., Kaitila, I., Loughlin, J., Munnich, A., Sykes, B., Bonaventure, J., & Francomano, C. A. (1998). Mutations in fibroblast growth-factor receptor 3 in sporadic cases of achondroplasia occur exclusively on the paternally derived chromosome. *American Journal of Human Genetics, 63*(3), 711–716. https://doi.org/10.1086/302000

47

Charcot–Marie–Tooth Disease

Jennifer Tucker and Megan Nickels

Charcot–Marie–Tooth disease (CMT) is the most common inherited childhood neuromuscular disorder (Jani-Acsadi et al., 2015). Two main types of CMT have been identified: a demyelinating form resulting from defects in the Schwann cells, causing slowed nerve conduction, and an axonal form, which presents due to abnormalities within the axon itself or its interface with Schwann cells, with normal to only slightly decreased nerve conduction speeds (Jani-Acsadi et al., 2015). The number of identified disease phenotypes continues to increase with ongoing and expanded genetic testing.

ETIOLOGY

Genetic testing has provided physicians a more accurate identification of the disease phenotype. Over 80 types of genes have been recognized as contributing to CMT (Jani-Acsadi et al., 2015; Pareyson et al., 2017). Although there are many genes implicated in the pathology of CMT, over 90% of CMT diagnoses have genetic mutations associated with peripheral myelin protein 22 gene (*PMP22*), gap junction B1 gene (*GJB1*), major peripheral myelin protein gene (*MPZ*), and either mitofusin 2 (*MFN2*) or ganglioside-induced differentiation-associated protein 1 (*GDAP1*; Pareyson et al., 2017).

CMT1 is the most prevalent type of the disease and is characterized by demyelination and slowed motor and sensory nerve conduction velocities (Jani-Acsadi et al., 2015). This type of CMT can be categorized further by its associated gene.

https://doi.org/10.1037/0000349-047
Health-Related Disorders in Children and Adolescents: A Guidebook for Educators and Service Providers, Second Edition, M. M. Perfect, C. A. Riccio, and M. A. Bray (Editors)

These subcategories of CMT1 include CMT1A, CMT1B, CMT1C, CMT1D, CMT1E, and CMT1F (Pareyson & Marchesi, 2009). CMT1A is an autosomal dominant demyelinating disease linked to *PMP22* leading to slowed nerve conduction (Jani-Acsadi et al., 2015). It is the most common form of CMT, with approximately 60% of individuals with CMT presenting with this subtype (Cornett et al., 2016). CMT1B is due to a mutation on the *MPZ* and represents a smaller percentage of individuals diagnosed with CMT1. CMT1C is associated with a mutation of the lipopolysaccharide-induced tumor necrosis factor-alpha factor gene and represents less than 1% of individuals within the larger CMT1 categorization (Jani-Acsadi et al., 2015). Significant cranial nerve involvement is unique to CMT1D. A deletion of the *PMP22* gene causes CMT1E, also known as hereditary neuropathy with pressure palsy, although this form is rarely seen in children (Jani-Acsadi et al., 2015). CMT1F is another rare clinical presentation with a similar clinical presentation to CMT1A, with some individuals experiencing cerebellar ataxia and tremor (Jani-Acsadi et al., 2015).

The second type of CMT (CMT2) includes several dominant forms of axonal neuropathies. Clinical presentation of CMT2 is like that of CMT1 except for stretch reflexes and nerve conduction velocities, which are spared. The impairments associated with CMT2 vary based on the individual genetic mutation (Jani-Acsadi et al., 2015). Of the axonal neuropathy variations of CMT, the most common is CMT2A, which is due to a genetic mutation on *MFN2* and is one of the more progressive clinical presentations (Jani-Acsadi et al., 2015). CMT2B is characterized by severe distal sensory loss placing individuals at risk for ulcers in their lower extremities. In contrast, the clinical presentation of CMT2C includes vocal cord and diaphragm paralysis (Jani-Acsadi et al., 2015). Upper extremities are severely affected in CMT2D.

Dejerine–Sottas syndrome is CMT type three. The onset begins in infancy with hypomyelinating neuropathy. The genes affected by this type of CMT may include *PMP22*, *MPZ*, or *EGR*. Nerve conduction velocities are slow in this type of CMT (Jani-Acsadi et al., 2015).

CMT4 encompasses a number of phenotypes that are recessive demyelinating or axonal neuropathies. A mutation of the *GDAP1* results in CMT4A, CMT4B is brought on by a mutation of myotubularin-related protein, and lastly, CMT4C stems from a mutation of src homology 3 domains and tetratricopeptide repeat domain protein genes (Jani-Acsadi et al., 2015).

One form of CMT, CMTX, is caused by an X-linked recessive demyelinating neuropathy and presents with some variability. The clinical presentation differs between genders, with male patients affected more severely than female patients (Jani-Acsadi et al., 2015). CMTX1 is the second most frequently diagnosed form of CMT affecting the *GJB1* (Jani-Acsadi et al., 2015).

Diagnosis of CMT is made based on clinical presentation, mode of inheritance, nerve conduction studies, and DNA testing. New tools for diagnosis and surveillance have emerged, including nerve and muscle echography and biomarkers from blood and cerebrospinal fluid; however, these are not the standard of care at this time (Pareyson et al., 2017).

PREVALENCE AND INCIDENCE

The prevalence of CMT has been reported as 10 to 28 in 100,000 individuals worldwide (Pareyson et al., 2017). Gender differences have not been documented for the larger diagnosis of CMT (Deenen et al., 2015). However, gender differences have been noted in CMT1A, which affects female individuals more often than male individuals (Colomban et al., 2014). CMT is not known to affect children based on race or ethnicity.

SYMPTOMS

Symptoms of CMT include weakness in lower extremities, decreased sensation in hands and feet, and an abnormal gait. Although some symptoms, such as unsteady gait, frequent falls, and hand weakness, are found in most individuals with CMT, symptoms may differ based on the specific genetic mutation (Cornett et al., 2016). Neuropathy in CMT affects the longest nerves first, which presents as distal limb weakness and muscle atrophy. Symptoms generally present in lower extremities prior to upper extremities. The most commonly reported early symptoms include ankle instability, frequent falls, and hand weakness (Cornett et al., 2016). Early childhood presentations may include toe walking and delayed motor development. As children grow, signs may include slow running speed, uncoordinated movements, and frequent ankle injuries (Jani-Acsadi et al., 2015). Evidence of hand weakness may not be noticed until the child begins working on independent dressing, shoe tying, and handwriting (Jani-Acsadi et al., 2015).

When looking more specifically at muscle weakness, certain patterns are recognized in children with CMT. The distal weakness in the lower extremities is most evident in the musculature of the ankle. Muscle imbalances often result in deformities in the feet, including hammer toes, high arches, and, less often, flat feet (Cornett et al., 2016; Jani-Acsadi et al., 2015). Weakness in ankle musculature is more significant in children with CMT2A and CMT4C as compared with those with CMT1A and CMTX1 (Cornett et al., 2016). Muscle weakness in the hands may be noted with muscle wasting of the hypothenar and the thenar muscles. Weakness in the hands is experienced more often by individuals with CMT1B than those with CMT1A (Cornett et al., 2016). More specifically, Cornett et al. (2016) found that individuals with CMT1A were faster on the nine-hole peg test (a fine motor assessment) than children with CMT1B, CMT2A, and CMT4C. Differences between genders were also noted with the nine-hole peg test with male children and adolescents performing faster than female children and adolescents. Children with CMT2A have been found to have significantly weaker grip strength than those with CMT1A, CMT1B, and CMTX1 (Cornett et al., 2016). Progression of the disease may lead to finger flexion contractures (Jani-Acsadi et al., 2015).

IMPACT ON THE STUDENT AND OUTCOMES

Medical

Muscle and sensory deficits affect a child's dynamic balance and gait. Gait deviations vary based on the individual and the type of CMT. Gait assessments identify the muscle imbalances and their impact on the overall gait pattern. The most common gait deviations are a wide base of support, decreased heel strike, and an inability to toe walk (Jani-Acsadi et al., 2015). Performance on functional measures such as running (Nagappa et al., 2022), long jump, and 6-minute walk test (Jani-Acsadi et al., 2015) are affected by decreased ankle strength. Children with CMT2A and CMT4C showed significantly reduced performance with strength testing of the ankle, as well as distances on the long jump and the 6-minute walk test. Balance was noted to be better in children with CMT1A and CMTX1 than those with CMT1B, CMT2A, and CMT4C as reported by Cornett et al. (2016).

Sensory deficits are typically not as severe as the motor impairments. Decreased vibration and joint position sense are revealed during sensory testing, with little to no change noted in pinprick or temperature sensation (Thomas, 1999). Sensation has been reported to be significantly reduced in children with CMT4C, and it is thought that this decreased sensation may contribute to changes in fine motor skills (Cornett et al., 2016).

Children are often referred to a neurologist with these symptoms, and nerve conduction studies, as well as electromyography testing, will provide additional insights into the underlying pathology (Jani-Acsadi et al., 2015). The clinical presentation of CMT may vary; however, all individuals experience some level of disability. A comprehensive evaluation should include a review of systems to identify oculomotor presentations, such as ptosis, optic atrophy, or glaucoma (Nagappa et al., 2022). Additional neurological signs may include diminished stretch reflexes, sensorineural hearing loss, and vocal cord or phrenic nerve paralysis (Jani-Acsadi et al., 2015). Some children experience dysautonomia with associated symptoms of urinary urgency and incontinence, orthostatic hypotension, and hyperhidrosis (Nagappa et al., 2022).

Medical management is focused on the prevention and management of range of motion and joint integrity. Interventions may include exercises, aerobics, strengthening, and orthotics. In addition, fine motor activities and splinting of upper extremities may also be beneficial (Nagappa et al., 2022).

Cognitive/Academic

Little has been documented on the cognitive implications of CMT. Selective cognitive deficits have been noted in some individuals with CMT (Kasselimis et al., 2020). These deficits were described as challenges with executive function and prominent pseudoword reading (Kasselimis et al., 2020). Additional research is warranted to understand the cognitive deficits that may present with CMT and how best to support these students in the classroom.

Auditory function is affected by both CMT1 and CMT2. Rance et al. (2012) found that although children with CMT1 and CMT2 have normal or near-normal sound detection, they do present with electrophysiological evidence of auditory neuropathy. Auditory perception was affected in most children with CMT1 (60%) and CMT2 (85%), resulting in impaired auditory processing. These deficits may present challenges in a classroom environment, as a great deal of academic material is presented through teacher interactions and lectures.

Social-Emotional and Behavioral

Children's quality of life is often influenced by their participation and engagement in school. Insights on the impact of CMT on social–emotional and behavioral domains can be found in research examining quality of life. Burns et al. (2010) found that CMT in children affected the physical domain more than emotional and social health domains. As children grow older, they may exhibit lower self-esteem and worsening emotional and behavioral difficulties (Burns et al., 2010). Taniguchi et al. (2013) reported that children with CMT1A experienced significant limitations in social and emotional domains. Appropriate assistance was often not provided to children to address these limitations, as focus is often on the musculoskeletal and neurological implications of the disease (Taniguchi et al., 2013). Social–emotional difficulties may be experienced by children in an educational setting, and appropriate supports, such as counseling, should be explored.

PSYCHOEDUCATIONAL IMPLICATIONS AND SCHOOL-BASED INTERVENTIONS

Medical and Health Management

There is no cure for CMT, although research continues, with many compounds approaching the clinical trial stage (Pareyson et al., 2017). Medical management focuses on disease surveillance, management of symptoms, and anticipation of disease progression (Jani-Acsadiet al., 2015). CMTPedS is a validated scoring system used to assess the impact of CMT and is a helpful tool for documenting disease progression (Cornett et al., 2017).

A multidisciplinary team best addresses symptoms and functional limitations. Members of the multidisciplinary team often include the neurologist, physical therapist, orthopedist, occupational therapist, and others as deemed appropriate by the team (Jani-Acsadi et al., 2015). The orthopedist will monitor joint deformities and associated pain and will collaborate with team members to establish a plan of care with the goal of maintaining both mobility and quality of life (Jani-Acsadi et al., 2015). Physical and occupational therapists will address functional limitations through therapeutic exercise, stretching, balance activities, gait training, and activity modifications (McCorquodale et al., 2016). Surgery such as osteotomies, joint fusions, or tendon lengthening may be necessary to treat skeletal deformities and muscle imbalances. Pharmaceutical treatments are not available currently but are under investigation (Pareyson & Marchesi, 2009). Genetic research and clinical trials will provide valuable insights into the identification and medical management of CMT in childhood.

Cognitive/Academic

Lidström et al. (2012) found that improved coordination and utilization of computer technologies, such as a tablet, laptop, or audio recording, may increase educational opportunities for children with physical disabilities and compensate for handwriting difficulties. More recently, Yiu et al. (2022) recommended adapted keyboard setting to reduce errors, word prediction, and text to talk as helpful technologies for children with CMT. In addition, they recommended splinting and adaptive equipment as needed to promote independence with activities of daily living. Children should be monitored closely and referred for further assessment if auditory processing issues are suspected. Children with auditory processing issues may benefit from preferential seating in the classroom or FM listening devices (Rance et al., 2012).

Social–Emotional and Behavioral

Mobility impairments affect a child's ability to not only navigate the school environment but also participate in learning and social experiences. Children may require ankle foot orthoses and assistive devices, such as a walker or Lofstrand crutches, for ambulation (Jani-Acsadi et al., 2015). Gait becomes an energy-demanding activity resulting in fatigue. A wheelchair may offer mobility with energy conservation but may be perceived as a barrier to full inclusion. Schools are often equipped with the environmental features to promote physical participation; however, children with mobility impairments who lack appropriate assistive devices often report continuing to experience barriers to learning and social experiences (Gcaza & Lorenzo, 2008). Pain and fatigue are frequent complaints of children with CMT. If these are new complaints or are increasing, it is important to communicate with the family to ensure follow-up with the medical team. Energy-conservation techniques can be employed, and the education team can collaborate to determine if any additional adjustments are needed to reduce mobility demands throughout the day and conserve energy for academic tasks.

CONCLUSION

Children with CMT present with lower physical, psychological, and social well-being than the overall pediatric population. The impact on psychological, social–emotional, and behavioral domains increases with progression of the disease (Burns et al., 2010). Supporting children with CMT in educational settings may require changing accommodations over the course of their childhood and adolescence to ensure that they reach their greatest potential.

RESOURCES

Charcot–Marie–Tooth Association. PO Box 105, Glenolden, PA 19036, 1-800-606-2682. The Charot–Marie–Tooth Association offers a wide array of resources for individuals living with CMT.

National Institute of Neurological Disorders and Stroke, National Institutes of Health. PO Box 5801, Bethesda, MD 20892, 1-800-352-9424. The National Institutes of Health provide evidence-based resources for neurological conditions, including CMT.

National Institute of Neurological Disorders and Stroke. (2018). *Charcot–Marie–Tooth disease fact sheet*. National Institutes of Health. https://www.ninds.nih.gov/Disorders/Patient-Caregiver-Education/Fact-Sheets/Charcot-Marie-Tooth-Disease-Fact-Sheet

REFERENCE

Burns, J., Ryan, M. M., & Ouvrier, R. A. (2010). Quality of life in children with Charcot–Marie–Tooth disease. *Journal of Child Neurology, 25*(3), 343–347. https://doi.org/10.1177/0883073809339877

Colomban, C., Micallef, J., Lefebvre, M. N., Dubourg, O., Gonnaud, P. M., Stojkovic, T., Jouve, E., Blin, O., Pouget, J., & Attarian, S. (2014). Clinical spectrum and gender differences in a large cohort of Charcot–Marie–Tooth type 1A patients. *Journal of the Neurological Sciences, 336*(1–2), 155–160. https://doi.org/10.1016/j.jns.2013.10.029

Cornett, K. M. D., Menezes, M. P., Bray, P., Halaki, M., Shy, R. R., Yum, S. W., Estilow, T., Moroni, I., Foscan, M., Pagliano, E., Pareyson, D., Laurá, M., Bhandari, T., Muntoni, F., Reilly, M. M., Finkel, R. S., Sowden, J., Eichinger, K. J., Herrmann, D. N., . . . Burns, J. (2016). Phenotypic variability of childhood Charcot–Marie–Tooth disease. *JAMA Neurology, 73*(6), 645–651. https://doi.org/10.1001/jamaneurol.2016.0171

Cornett, K. M. D., Menezes, M. P., Shy, R. R., Moroni, I., Pagliano, E., Pareyson, D., Estilow, T., Yum, S. W., Bhandari, T., Muntoni, F., Laura, M., Reilly, M. M., Finkel, R. S., Eichinger, K. J., Herrmann, D. N., Bray, P., Halaki, M., Shy, M. E., & Burns, J. (2017). Natural history of Charcot–Marie–Tooth disease during childhood. *Annals of Neurology, 82*(3), 353–359. https://doi.org/10.1002/ana.25009

Deenen, J. C., Horlings, C. G., Verschuuren, J. J., Verbeek, A. L., & van Engelen, B. G. (2015). The epidemiology of neuromuscular disorders: A comprehensive overview of the literature. *Journal of Neuromuscular Diseases, 2*(1), 73–85. https://doi.org/10.3233/JND-140045

Gcaza, S., & Lorenzo, T. (2008). Discovering the barriers that stop children with disabilities from being children: The impact of lack of access to mobility devices—A human rights perspective. *South African Journal of Occupational Therapy, 38*(1), 16–21.

Jani-Acsadi, A., Ounpuu, S., Pierz, K., & Acsadi, G. (2015). Pediatric Charcot–Marie–Tooth disease. *Pediatric Clinics of North America, 62*(3), 767–786. https://doi.org/10.1016/j.pcl.2015.03.012

Kasselimis, D., Karadima, G., Angelopoulou, G., Breza, M., Tsolakopoulos, D., Potagas, C., Panas, M., & Koutsis, G. (2020). Evidence for cognitive deficits in X-linked Charcot–Marie–Tooth disease. *Journal of the International Neuropsychological Society, 26*(3), 294–302. https://doi.org/10.1017/S1355617719001188

Lidström, H., Almqvist, L., & Hemmingsson, H. (2012). Computer-based assistive technology device for use by children with physical disabilities: A cross-sectional study. *Disability and Rehabilitation: Assistive Technology, 7*(4), 287–293. https://doi.org/10.3109/17483107.2011.635332

McCorquodale, D., Pucillo, E. M., & Johnson, N. E. (2016). Management of Charcot–Marie–Tooth disease: Improving long-term care with a multidisciplinary approach. *Journal of Multidisciplinary Healthcare, 9*, 7–19. https://doi.org/10.2147/JMDH.S69979

Nagappa, M., Sharma, S., & Taly, A. B. (2022). Charcot–Marie–Tooth. *StatPearls*. StatPearls Publishing. https://www.ncbi.nlm.nih.gov/books/NBK562163/

Pareyson, D., & Marchesi, C. (2009). Diagnosis, natural history, and management of Charcot–Marie–Tooth disease. *Lancet Neurology, 8*(7), 654–667. https://doi.org/10.1016/S1474-4422(09)70110-3

Pareyson, D., Saveri, P., & Pisciotta, C. (2017). New developments in Charcot–Marie–Tooth neuropathy and related diseases. *Current Opinion in Neurology, 30*(5), 471–480. https://doi.org/10.1097/WCO.0000000000000474

Rance, G., Ryan, M. M., Bayliss, K., Gill, K., O'Sullivan, C., & Whitechurch, M. (2012). Auditory function in children with Charcot–Marie–Tooth disease. *Brain, 135*(5), 1412–1422. https://doi.org/10.1093/brain/aws085

Taniguchi, J. B., Elui, V. M., Osório, F. L., Hallak, J. E., Crippa, J. A., Machado-de-Sousa, J. P., Kebbe, L. M., Lourenço, C. M., Scarel-Caminaga, R. M., & Marques, W., Jr. (2013). Quality of life in patients with Charcot–Marie–Tooth disease type 1A. *Arquivos de Neuro-Psiquiatria, 71*(6), 392–396. https://doi.org/10.1590/0004-282X20130045

Thomas, P. K. (1999). Overview of Charcot–Marie–Tooth disease type 1A. *Annals of the New York Academy of Sciences, 883*(1), 1–5. https://doi.org/10.1111/j.1749-6632.1999.tb08560.x

Yiu, E. M., Bray, P., Baets, J., Baker, S. K., Barisic, N., de Valle, K., Estilow, T., Farrar, M. A., Finkel, R. S., Haberlová, J., Kennedy, R. A., Moroni, I., Nicholson, G. A., Ramchandren, S., Reilly, M. M., Rose, K., Shy, M. E., Siskind, C. E., Yum, S. W., . . . Burns, J. (2022). Clinical practice guideline for the management of paediatric Charcot–Marie–Tooth disease. *Journal of Neurology, Neurosurgery, and Psychiatry, 93*(5), 530–538. https://doi.org/10.1136/jnnp-2021-328483

48

Juvenile Idiopathic Arthritis

Rebecca J. Tipton-DeClue and Eric L. Robinson

Juvenile idiopathic arthritis (JIA), formally known as juvenile rheumatoid arthritis, is a general category for chronic inflammation of the joints that begins before 16 years of age and persists for at least 6 weeks (Cron et al., 2013; Malattia & Martini, 2014).

The diagnostic criteria for JIA have been updated three times since 1995 to develop criteria that would create similar groups of children with arthritis and to help classify research studies related to epidemiology, outcomes, and therapy. In 1997, the International League of Associations for Rheumatology created five criteria for classification of JIA in the United States, with the intention to separate childhood-onset arthritis by causal mechanisms and treatment strategies (Petty et al., 1998). These include (a) systemic arthritis, (b) polyarthritis or polyarticular JIA, (c) oligoarthritis, (d) enthesitis-related arthritis, and (e) psoriatic arthritis. Systemic JIA is considered an autoinflammatory disease, whereas the other types are considered autoimmune diseases.

The JIA umbrella includes juvenile-onset ankylosing spondylitis, psoriatic arthritis, inflammatory bowel disease, juvenile-onset adult-type (seropositive) rheumatoid arthritis, and Still's disease (seronegative chronic arthritis) but excludes other causes of chronic arthritis, including sarcoidosis, Sjögren's syndrome, systemic lupus erythematosus, Lyme disease, dermatomyositis, and other diseases that can present as chronic arthritis in childhood (Cron et al., 2013; Malattia & Martini, 2014). It is important to note that JIA is a diagnosis of exclusion, that is, a diagnosis reached by a process of elimination instead of examination or testing. Thus, each of the five categories likely represents

https://doi.org/10.1037/0000349-048
Health-Related Disorders in Children and Adolescents: A Guidebook for Educators and Service Providers, Second Edition, M. M. Perfect, C. A. Riccio, and M. A. Bray (Editors)

multiple distinct diseases (Cron et al., 2013; Prakken et al., 2011), with some children changing categories over time and some children presenting with symptoms that are not fully described by any one category (Nordal et al., 2011).

ETIOLOGY

For the five classifications of JIA, despite significant research, all remain idiopathic, or of unknown etiology (Malattia & Martini, 2014; Petty et al., 2004). Although JIA is believed to have a genetic influence, progress identifying the genes has been slow (Prahalad & Glass, 2008). For example, genetics studies encoding the human leukocyte antigens have been confirmed and replicated, but genetic variants other than human leukocyte antigens can also influence vulnerability (Prahalad & Glass, 2008).

PREVALENCE AND INCIDENCE

Prevalence estimates for JIA are widely debated (Manners & Bower, 2002), with rates varying based on genetic and environmental risk factors. Accounting for all five subtypes, JIA is currently thought to affect approximately one in 1,000 children (Cron et al., 2013), making it the most common rheumatic condition of childhood (Donn, 2015) and a frequent cause of short- and long-term disability worldwide.

SYMPTOMS

The hallmark symptom of JIA is inflammation of the joints. Depending on the type of JIA, the joint inflammation may be in the extremities, such as in the hips, plantar fascia, and fingers. Secondary symptoms include a pinkish rash, fatigue, a low-grade fever, and spinal pain. Diagnostic characteristics; sex differences; treatment, including pharmacological; and affected populations of each subtype are described in Table 48.1.

IMPACT ON THE STUDENT AND OUTCOMES

The impact of JIA on students is dependent on the type and severity of the disease. It is important to note that JIA does not typically have a direct impact on a student's education in that the disease does not interfere with academic subjects. Instead, JIA can lead to a student missing a significant amount of school, which affects their ability to maintain course assignments and support from their teacher. Specific medical, social–emotional, and behavioral outcomes are discussed next.

TABLE 48.1. Juvenile Idiopathic Arthritis Diagnostic Categories and Descriptions

Category	Systemic arthritis	Polyarthritis or polyarticular JIA	Oligoarthritis	Enthesitis-related arthritis	Psoriatic arthritis
Etiology	Unknown	Unknown	Possible genetic predisposition	Unknown	Possible genetic if family history of psoriasis
Prevalence	10% to 20% of all JIA	17% of all JIA; more likely in female individuals	50% of all JIA	10% to 20% of all JIA; more common in male individuals	18% of all JIA; affects male and female individuals equally
Symptoms	May be monophasic, polycyclic, or persistent; may include evanescent salmon-pink rash; may include various other systemic syndromes.	With RF negative, may include growth failure, fatigue, low grade fever; typically asymmetric joints; frequent co-occurrence of temporomandibular joint syndrome. With RF positive, onset is earlier than 16 years of age, with five or more joints (both large and small) affected.	Affects no more than four joints, most likely in the lower limbs; asymmetric onset prior to 6 years of age; high antinuclear antibodies.	Arthritis and enthesitis (inflammation of tendons or ligaments at insertion points with two or more of the following: sacroiliac joint tenderness, inflammatory spinal pain, spondyloarthropathy, inflammatory bowel disease) impacts lower extremities more frequently, like the hip, insertion of the Achilles, plantar fascia, and tarsals.	Presence or family history of psoriasis results in inflammation of fingers and toes or fingernail abnormalities and joint inflammation.
Additional medical concerns	33% will have permanent musculoskeletal damages that may affect mobility; possible pulmonary complications.	With RF positive, may develop pulmonary lesions, cardiac valvular lesions, and amyloidosis; least likely to remit.	For 30%, vision may be affected due to iridocyclitis of anterior uveitis.	Causes lower levels of mobility and overall physical health compared with other JIA types; remission occurs in 44% of cases; sacroiliitis occurs in 35% of cases; female individuals have poorer outcomes than male individuals, with increased pain and decreased mobility.	Vision may be affected due to chronic uveitis; arthritic symptoms may remit with early onset associated with lower rates of remission.

(*continues*)

TABLE 48.1. Juvenile Idiopathic Arthritis Diagnostic Categories and Descriptions (*Continued*)

Category	Systemic arthritis	Polyarthritis or polyarticular JIA	Oligoarthritis	Enthesitis-related arthritis	Psoriatic arthritis
Cognitive/ academic concerns	No specific concerns; academic success might be impacted by absences during school year.	No specific concerns; academic success might be impacted by absences during school year.	No specific concerns; academic success might be impacted by absences during school year.	No specific concerns; academic success might be impacted by absences during school year.	No specific concerns; academic success might be impacted by absences during school year.
Social-emotional and behavioral concerns	No specific concerns; restricted mobility may impact participation in physical education and athletics.	No specific concerns; restricted mobility may impact participation in physical education and athletics.	No specific concerns; restricted mobility may impact participation in physical education and athletics.	No specific concerns; restricted mobility may impact participation in physical education and athletics.	No specific concerns; restricted mobility may impact participation in physical education and athletics.
Treatment approaches	Various medications, most commonly steroid or other anti-inflammatory medications; physical therapy.	Various medications, most commonly steroid or other anti-inflammatory medications; physical therapy; with RF positive, may require corticosteroid injections; antirheumatic drugs.	Various medications, most commonly steroid or other anti-inflammatory medications; may require corticosteroid injections; treatment to address psoriasis as well; physical therapy.	Treatment is based on the presentation of symptoms but typically includes physical therapy and treatment with steroids.	Various medications, most commonly steroid or other anti-inflammatory medications; physical therapy.

Note. See the following for more information on categories of JIA and accompanying characteristics: Cron et al., 2013; Feldmann et al., 2005; Petty et al., 2004; Prakken et al., 2011; Ravelli and Martini, 2007; Sikora and Grom, 2011; Stoll et al., 2006; Wallace et al., 2005. JIA = juvenile idiopathic arthritis; RF = rheumatoid factor.

Medical

Long-term outcomes for students with JIA can include functional impairments, psychosocial differences, and ongoing complications of disease (Wallace, 2006). Though over one third of patients achieve remission, certain subtypes of JIA are associated with more difficult longitudinal outcomes, and current treatments of JIA are not fully developed (Packham & Hall, 2002; Wallace, 2006).

Social–Emotional and Behavioral

Although all categories of JIA are burdensome, none are associated with increased social or emotional problems (Feldmann et al., 2005). Some evidence indicates that children with JIA have more internalizing symptoms when compared with their peer group but not greater symptoms for externalizing issues or poor self-concept (LeBovidge et al., 2003). Further evidence suggests that children with JIA might be at higher risk for sleep disturbances (Ward et al., 2017), which could result in daytime sleepiness. Care of a child with JIA also may impact the daily life of families. For example, the number of missed work hours among parents with a child with JIA is estimated to be 2.78 times greater than parents of children with no medical needs (Rasu et al., 2015).

PSYCHOEDUCATIONAL IMPLICATIONS AND SCHOOL-BASED INTERVENTIONS

The psychoeducational implications of JIA are driven by the type and severity of the disease. Students who miss a considerable amount of school may need additional support through special education assistance or homebound services to maintain academic progress. School-based interventions are also guided by seriousness of the disease and may involve purposeful social plans between the student with JIA and their peer group to maintain social interactions and support. Information on medical and health management, cognitive/academic impact, and social–emotional interventions is covered next.

Medical and Health Management

Currently, a combination of pharmacological interventions, physical therapy, occupational therapy, and family training (Hashkes & Laxer, 2005; Janow et al., 2016) is considered best practice for treatment of JIA. There is a range of pharmacological treatments (see Table 48.1) for children with JIA, with a steroid intervention being most common.

Cognitive/Academic

JIA is not associated with cognitive impairment (Feldmann et al., 2005), and there are no specific academic challenges related to the disease. Depending on the severity of the disease, which can lead to school absences, a child with JIA should be monitored by school officials, including the school psychologist, to determine the potential academic impact of missing school. In cases when a child with JIA is struggling academically, a multidisciplinary team consisting of a parent or guardian, school psychologist, school nurse, administrator, teachers, occupational therapist, and/or physical therapist should be able to address a child's psychoeducational needs. Professional services through Section 504 of the Americans With Disabilities Act (504 Services) should consider challenges including chronic tardiness and difficulty with a traditional physical education class. Children with JIA may need a variety of supports, ranging from extra time to physically move between classes, extra time to turn in assignments, rest periods or breaks to stretch throughout the school day, and possibly adaptive equipment to assist in note-taking (Anzilotti, 2020). For children with more comprehensive educational needs, special education eligibility can be pursued through the Individuals With Disabilities Education Act, likely qualifying under the Other Health Impairment category.

Social–Emotional and Behavioral

JIA is not associated with increased social or emotional problems (Feldmann et al., 2005). Although there are limited data that children with JIA have more internalizing symptoms, no evidence shows poor self-concept (LeBovidge et al., 2003). Each child with JIA, though, should be viewed individually, and their teachers should be made aware of potential internalizing behaviors. If symptoms develop, the teacher should inform school officials, including the school psychologist, and an intervention plan can be created. An important, yet indirect, social–emotional intervention to benefit a child with JIA is for school officials, including the school psychologist, to become a great resource for their parents. As Rasu and colleagues (2015) reported, parents with a child with JIA miss an estimated 2.78 times more work hours than parents of a child without JIA, due primarily to appointments, hospital visits, and so on. Therefore, the school psychologist can benefit a child with JIA by providing parents community resources that include respite care, support groups, and child care options.

CONCLUSION

To summarize, JIA is a general category for chronic inflammation of the joints that begins before 16 years of age and persists for at least 6 weeks. It impacts approximately one in 1,000 students. There are five classifications of JIA, and treatment, typically a combination of pharmacological and physical therapies, ranges depending on the classification. There is no known direct cognitive or academic impact for children with JIA, but limited mobility, school absences, and possible sleep disturbances might occur. The school psychologist, along with the school nurse, should monitor children with JIA and, depending on the severity, might create an individualized education program and provide services with a 504 plan under the Other Health Impairment category.

RESOURCES

Arthritis Foundation. (n.d.). *Juvenile idiopathic arthritis (JIA)*. https://www.arthritis.org/about-arthritis/types/juvenile-idiopathic-arthritis-jia/

Brescia, A. C. (2021). *Juvenile idiopathic arthritis*. KidsHealth. https://kidshealth.org/en/parents/jra.html

REFERENCES

Anzilotti, A. M. (2020). *Juvenile idiopathic arthritis (JIA) special needs factsheet (for schools)*. KidsHealth. https://kidshealth.org/en/parents/jia-factsheet.html

Cron, R. Q., Weiser, P., & Beukelman, T. (2013). Juvenile idiopathic arthritis. In R. R. Rich, T. A. Fleisher, W. T. Shearer, H. W. Schroeder Jr., A. J. Frew, & C. M Weyand (Eds.), *Clinical immunology: Principles and practice* (4th ed., pp. 637–647). Elsevier.

Donn, R. (2015). Etiology and pathogenesis of juvenile idiopathic arthritis. In M. C. Hochberg, A. J. Silman, J. S. Smolen, M. E. Weinblatt, & M. H. Weisman (Eds.), *Rheumatology* (6th ed., pp. 845–850). Elsevier. https://doi.org/10.1016/B978-0-323-09138-1.00102-9

Feldmann, R., Weglage, J., Roth, J., Foell, D., & Frosch, M. (2005). Systemic juvenile rheumatoid arthritis: Cognitive function and social adjustment. *Annals of Neurology, 58*(4), 605–609. https://doi.org/10.1002/ana.20626

Hashkes, P. J., & Laxer, R. M. (2005). Medical treatment of juvenile idiopathic arthritis. *JAMA, 294*(13), 1671–1684. https://doi.org/10.1001/jama.294.13.1671

Janow, G., Schanberg, L. E., Setoguchi, S., Hasselblad, V., Mellins, E. D., Schneider, R., Kimura, Y., & the CARRA Legacy Registry Investigators. (2016). The systemic juvenile idiopathic arthritis cohort of the Childhood Arthritis and Rheumatology Research Alliance Registry: 2010–2013. *The Journal of Rheumatology, 43*(9), 1755–1762. https://doi.org/10.3899/jrheum.150997

LeBovidge, J. S., Lavigne, J. V., Donenberg, G. R., & Miller, M. L. (2003). Psychological adjustment of children and adolescents with chronic arthritis: A meta-analytic review. *Journal of Pediatric Psychology, 28*(1), 29–39. https://doi.org/10.1093/jpepsy/28.1.29

Malattia, C., & Martini, A. (2014). Juvenile idiopathic arthritis. In N. R. Rose & I. R. Mackay (Eds.), *The autoimmune diseases* (5th ed., pp. 525–536). Elsevier. https://doi.org/10.1016/B978-0-12-384929-8.00037-X

Manners, P. J., & Bower, C. (2002). Worldwide prevalence of juvenile arthritis—Why does it vary so much? *The Journal of Rheumatology, 29*(7), 1520–1530.

Nordal, E., Zak, M., Aalto, K., Berntson, L., Fasth, A., Herlin, T., Lahdenne, P., Nielsen, S., Straume, B., Rygg, M., & the Nordic Study Group of Pediatric Rheumatology. (2011). Ongoing disease activity and changing categories in a long-term Nordic cohort study of juvenile idiopathic arthritis. *Arthritis and Rheumatism, 63*(9), 2809–2818. https://doi.org/10.1002/art.30426

Packham, J. C., & Hall, M. A. (2002). Long-term follow-up of 246 adults with juvenile idiopathic arthritis: Functional outcome. *Rheumatology, 41*(12), 1428–1435. https://doi.org/10.1093/rheumatology/41.12.1428

Petty, R. E., Southwood, T. R., Baum, J., Bhettay, E., Glass, D. N., Manners, P., Maldonado-Cocco, J., Suarez-Almazor, M., Orozco-Alcala, J., & Prieur, A. M. (1998). Revision of the proposed classification criteria for juvenile idiopathic arthritis: Durban, 1997. *The Journal of Rheumatology, 25*(10), 1991–1994. https://pubmed.ncbi.nlm.nih.gov/9779856/

Petty, R. E., Southwood, T. R., Manners, P., Baum, J., Glass, D. N., Goldenberg, J., He, X., Maldonado-Cocco, J., Orozco-Alcala, J., Prieur, A. M., Suarez-Almazor, M. E., Woo, P., & the International League of Associations for Rheumatology. (2004). International League of Associations for Rheumatology classification of juvenile idiopathic arthritis: Second revision, Edmonton, 2001. *The Journal of Rheumatology, 31*(2), 390–392. https://pubmed.ncbi.nlm.nih.gov/14760812/

Prahalad, S., & Glass, D. N. (2008). A comprehensive review of the genetics of juvenile idiopathic arthritis. *Pediatric Rheumatology Online Journal, 6*(1), Article 11. https://doi.org/10.1186/1546-0096-6-11

Prakken, B., Albani, S., & Martini, A. (2011). Juvenile idiopathic arthritis. *The Lancet, 377*(9783), 2138–2149. https://doi.org/10.1016/S0140-6736(11)60244-4

Rasu, R. S., Cline, S. K., Shaw, J. W., Hayes, O., Agbor Bawa, W., & Cifaldi, M. A. (2015). Impact of JIA on parents' work absences. *Rheumatology, 54*(7), 1177–1185. https://doi.org/10.1093/rheumatology/keu414

Ravelli, A., & Martini, A. (2007). Juvenile idiopathic arthritis. *The Lancet, 369*(9563), 767–778. https://doi.org/10.1016/S0140-6736(07)60363-8

Sikora, K. A., & Grom, A. A. (2011). Update on the pathogenesis and treatment of systemic idiopathic arthritis. *Current Opinion in Pediatrics, 23*(6), 640–646. https://doi.org/10.1097/MOP.0b013e32834cba24

Stoll, M. L., Zurakowski, D., Nigrovic, L. E., Nichols, D. P., Sundel, R. P., & Nigrovic, P. A. (2006). Patients with juvenile psoriatic arthritis comprise two distinct populations. *Arthritis and Rheumatism, 54*(11), 3564–3572. https://doi.org/10.1002/art.22173

Wallace, C. A. (2006). Current management of juvenile idiopathic arthritis. *Best Practice & Research Clinical Rheumatology, 20*(2), 279–300. https://doi.org/10.1016/j.berh.2005.11.008

Wallace, C. A., Huang, B., Bandeira, M., Ravelli, A., & Giannini, E. H. (2005). Patterns of clinical remission in select categories of juvenile idiopathic arthritis. *Arthritis and Rheumatism, 52*(11), 3554–3562. https://doi.org/10.1002/art.21389

Ward, T. M., Beebe, D. W., Chen, M. L., Landis, C. A., Ringold, S., Pike, K., & Wallace, C. A. (2017). Sleep disturbances and neurobehavioral performance in juvenile idiopathic arthritis. *The Journal of Rheumatology, 44*(3), 361–367. https://doi.org/10.3899/jrheum.160556

49

Marfan Syndrome

Brittany A. Dale and David E. McIntosh

First described in 1896 by Antoine Bernard-Jean Marfan, Marfan syndrome is an autosomal dominant genetic disorder of the connective tissue caused by defects of the fibrillin-1 gene located on chromosome 15. This mutation results in a defective protein, fibrillin. Fibrillin is a constituent of microfibrils, which can (in certain tissues) combine with elastin to form elastic fibers.

ETIOLOGY

Marfan syndrome is most commonly inherited but can be the result of a mutation in the affected gene of an individual with no family history of the disorder. Because the disorder is autosomal dominant, individuals with Marfan syndrome have a 50% risk of transmitting the disorder to their children; however, spontaneous mutation is the cause of approximately 25% of diagnosed cases (Giarelli et al., 2010).

PREVALENCE AND INCIDENCE

According to the Marfan Foundation, one in 5,000 people in the United States are affected by Marfan syndrome. Marfan syndrome affects both sexes and all ethnic groups equally. Diagnosis of Marfan syndrome can occur at any age; however, early diagnosis is critical in preventing cardiovascular death due to

https://doi.org/10.1037/0000349-049
Health-Related Disorders in Children and Adolescents: A Guidebook for Educators and Service Providers, Second Edition, M. M. Perfect, C. A. Riccio, and M. A. Bray (Editors)

common aortic complications. Research has indicated that the average age of diagnosis is approximately 19 (Groth et al., 2015), although it often goes undiagnosed due to the variability in clinical presentation. Currently, physicians follow the Ghent nosology when diagnosing Marfan syndrome, which may include genetic testing (Loeys et al., 2010). Using the updated Ghent criteria, diagnosis is based on the degree of the person's aortic root dilation (i.e., widening of the aorta where it connects with the heart) and ectopia lentis (i.e., displacement of the eye lens) with or without identified gene mutations. These criteria result in identifying approximately 95% of Marfan cases (Loeys et al., 2010).

SYMPTOMS

Although all body systems can be affected by the connective tissue defects seen in Marfan syndrome, the most common abnormalities occur in the musculoskeletal, ocular, and cardiovascular systems. The clinical presentation of symptoms may vary immensely due to a large number of fibrillin-gene mutations documented in this population. The most severe symptoms, however, are often associated with the cardiovascular system, specifically the aorta. Aortic root dilation is the most common cardiovascular problem found in a pediatric Marfan population, and preventative medication management is a common practice (Mueller et al., 2013). This aortic dilation puts these individuals at higher risk for aortic dissection (i.e., tearing), the most common cause of death in this population (Giarelli et al., 2010).

The most common ocular manifestations include ectopia lentis (dislocation of the lens), myopia (nearsightedness), and amblyopia (lazy eye). Individuals with Marfan syndrome may also present with an abnormally flat cornea, hypoplastic iris or hypoplastic ciliary muscle, and an increased axial length of the globe (Ryan-Krause, 2002). After the age of 40, cataracts and acute glaucoma are common, and surgical repair of dislocated lenses may be warranted. Acute or chronic glaucoma also may occur before adulthood.

IMPACT ON THE STUDENT AND OUTCOMES

Medical

Individuals with Marfan syndrome are commonly described as tall and slender. Fingers and toes (arachnodactyly) and arms and legs (dolichostenomelia) are often longer than usual. Joint laxity (loose joints), hypotonia, and flexion contractures (drawing together of muscles around the joints that results in deformities) are also highly prevalent. Scoliosis (abnormal curvature of the spine) and pectus deformities (protrusion or indentation of the sternum) are common. Overcrowded teeth caused by narrow jaws and mouths may require dental surgery. These physical aspects of Marfan syndrome vary among patients and are often a significant cause of chronic pain within the population (Velvin et al., 2015). As patients with Marfan syndrome age, they have a higher risk for rapid aortic root dilation and referral to surgery (Hoskoppal et al., 2018). Advances in medical technology, understanding of the syndrome, and aortic surgery have resulted in increased life expectancy for individuals with Marfan syndrome, with many living into their 70s (Goldfinger et al., 2017).

Cognitive/Academic

Little research has been conducted on the educational and psychological features or presence of other disorders (e.g., learning disabilities, attention-deficit/hyperactivity disorder [ADHD], depression) that may be associated with Marfan syndrome. According to educational resources published by the Marfan Foundation (2013), physicians reported a perceived higher incidence of ADHD. Although not a direct assessment of these comorbid disorders, one study indicated 24% of children diagnosed with Marfan syndrome who participated in a health-related quality of life study self-reported a neurodevelopmental disorder (i.e., ADHD or learning disability; Handisides et al., 2019).

According to the Marfan Foundation (2013), Marfan syndrome does not cause cognitive disabilities. Historical research (Hofman et al., 1988) supports this claim and reported average cognitive ability in a sample of children. More current research on adults with Marfan syndrome found no differences on various tests of cognitive ability and neuropsychological functioning compared with the standardization samples of the tests (Rand-Hendriksen et al., 2007); however, reduced visuomotor coordination was seen on a pegboard test, suggesting some aspects of functioning can be affected by the visual impairments seen in individuals with Marfan syndrome.

Social-Emotional and Behavioral

Researchers have reported a broad range of psychiatric comorbidity among children and adolescents with chronic health conditions, ranging from 7% to 40% (Pao & Bosk, 2011). These children not only have to deal with typical adjustment to life stressors (e.g., school demands, friendships) but also must account for the impact of their chronic condition on their daily lives. Level of pain in children with Marfan syndrome should be closely monitored, as research indicates early onset of pain symptoms is related to worsening mental health function in adulthood (Speed et al., 2017). Being proactive regarding a child's physical symptoms related to Marfan syndrome could prevent future mental health problems.

Given the visible physical characteristics of Marfan syndrome, children with the disorder may experience more psychological distress compared with their peers due to feeling less attractive and having regulated physical activities (e.g., avoiding unnecessary strain on the cardiovascular system due to sports). Research has indicated that teenagers believed they would experience improved self-image and better physical functioning if they did not have the medical condition (Schneider et al., 1990). Researchers also found that teenagers are often unaware of the reproductive ramifications of having a heritable genetic disorder (Schneider et al., 1990), which could affect their perception of a future family. Moreover, research has indicated that stress level is higher in parents of children with chronic health conditions compared with parents of healthy children (Cousino & Hazen, 2013).

PSYCHOEDUCATIONAL IMPLICATIONS AND SCHOOL-BASED INTERVENTIONS

Medical and Health Management

Principals, teachers, school psychologists, school counselors, and other school professionals should be aware of all students diagnosed with Marfan syndrome and their potential need for intensive medical care. It is common for some children to simultaneously receive treatment from a cardiologist, dentist, ophthalmologist, speech therapist, and physical therapist, and frequent absences due to medical appointments are common. Teachers may need to develop lessons in advance if a child needs to be hospitalized for an extended period of time, and in some cases, homebound education might be necessary. Educational and health plans may include accommodations for modified or alternative physical education and should discuss how the educational team will address extended absences due to medical complications (Schilling & Getch, 2018).

Given the strain on the cardiovascular system and risk of aortic dissection in students with Marfan syndrome, physical activities, such as sports and exercise, are discouraged. Adolescents, however, may not adhere to the recommendations of their cardiologists and may participate in more physical activity than suggested (Schneider et al., 1990). School nurses, psychologists, teachers, and counselors should monitor teenagers with Marfan syndrome more closely for compliance with medical recommendations. Other medical accommodations could address fatigue, which commonly occurs with heart conditions. Students may be provided with extended time to transition between classes, unlimited visits to the nurse's office, rest periods during the day, and extra books for home and school to reduce the strain of carrying around a heavy backpack. Accommodations for visual impairments are also standard in children with Marfan syndrome.

Adolescents with Marfan syndrome also need to be aware of chronic disease management as they approach adulthood and move away from their parents. Self-management skills may need to be taught to this population while they are still in the school environment. Giarelli et al. (2008) indicated that independently managing a chronic health condition involves adhering to treatment guidelines, seeking information about the disorder, and practicing health promotion, which is arguably a prerequisite to self-care and self-advocacy. School-based transition teams need to be aware of these self-advocacy needs and include related goals in transition plans for students with Marfan syndrome.

Cognitive/Academic

Teachers should be aware of the impact multiple absences can have on a child's academic achievement in the classroom. If a child with Marfan syndrome is falling behind compared with peers, quality of instruction and attendance should be considered prior to making a referral for a special education evaluation. When conducting psychoeducational evaluations of suspected disabilities in school-aged children with Marfan syndrome, school psychologists must consider how the motor and physical functioning of the child might affect test results. Specifically, school psychologists must take into consideration any uncorrected visual limitations of the child with Marfan syndrome when interpreting results of standardized tests. Due to the potential visual complications of Marfan syndrome, children may require materials in large print, or they may need preferential seating within the classroom.

Social–Emotional and Behavioral

School psychologists and school counselors are in unique positions to facilitate adaptation and psychological well-being in the school environment. For example, counseling may be needed for depression caused by physical and social complications, death of a parent who was afflicted with the syndrome, or adjustment issues that may arise after an initial diagnosis.

School-wide intervention and in-service presentations may be necessary to educate school personnel and classmates about Marfan syndrome. Specifically, as children with Marfan syndrome exhibit distinct physical differences, they may be subjected to bullying at school (Marfan Foundation, 2013). To educate others and reduce stigma, classmates of children with Marfan syndrome may benefit from classroom or school-wide presentations about chronic health conditions. Research also suggests that school personnel are often unprepared to address the needs of children with chronic health conditions. Schilling and Getch (2018) reported that only 44% of surveyed special education directors received formal training in meeting the needs of students with chronic health conditions, and they argued that more in-service training in this area is necessary. These trainings may be necessary for schools with students diagnosed with Marfan syndrome.

School personnel should also acknowledge the strain raising a child with Marfan syndrome may place on the parents. Parent training programs show promise in improving the overall family quality of life of those who have children with chronic health conditions. Kieckhefer and colleagues (2014) implemented a 7-week parent training program for families with children diagnosed with chronic physical health conditions. They found improved parental self-efficacy, increased parent coping, decreased depressive symptoms, and overall greater family quality of life for those who attended the training and argued that intervention can occur in a non-disease-specific manner (Kieckhefer et al., 2014). With the low incidence of Marfan syndrome within school communities, these findings indicate parents could receive supportive services within a chronic disease management context and potentially relate to other parents with similar coping needs.

CONCLUSION

Collaboration is an essential component of enhancing the functioning of a child with Marfan syndrome in the school environment. School psychologists, school counselors, principals, and teachers need to be in constant communication with the affected child's parents, and when necessary, the child's medical team, to ensure their educational programming adequately addresses the child's individualized needs.

RESOURCES

Marfan Foundation. https://www.marfan.org/. Offers resources and online communities for children and teens.

Marfan Foundation (2013). *Need-to-know information for the teacher: Raising awareness of Marfan syndrome and related disorders.* https://marfan.org/resource-library/need-to-know-information-for-the-teacher/

Marfan Foundation. (n.d.). *Parent toolkit.* https://www.marfan.org/event/parent-toolkit

REFERENCES

Cousino, M. K., & Hazen, R. A. (2013). Parenting stress among caregivers of children with chronic illness: A systematic review. *Journal of Pediatric Psychology, 38*(8), 809–828. https://doi.org/10.1093/jpepsy/jst049

Giarelli, E., Bernhardt, B. A., Mack, R., & Pyeritz, R. E. (2008). Adolescents' transition to self-management of a chronic genetic disorder. *Qualitative Health Research, 18*(4), 441–457. https://doi.org/10.1177/1049732308314853

Giarelli, E., Bernhardt, B. A., & Pyeritz, R. E. (2010). Self-surveillance by adolescents and young adults transitioning to self-management of a chronic genetic disorder. *Health Education & Behavior, 37*(1), 133–150. https://doi.org/10.1177/1090198109331670

Goldfinger, J. Z., Preiss, L. R., Devereux, R. B., Roman, M. J., Hendershot, T. P., Kroner, B. L., Eagle, K. A., & the GenTAC Registry Consortium. (2017). Marfan syndrome and quality of life in the GenTAC Registry. *Journal of the American College of Cardiology, 69*(23), 2821–2830. https://doi.org/10.1016/j.jacc.2017.04.026

Groth, K. A., Hove, H., Kyhl, K., Folkestad, L., Gaustadnes, M., Vejlstrup, N., Stochholm, K., Østergaard, J. R., Andersen, N. H., & Gravholt, C. H. (2015). Prevalence, incidence, and age at diagnosis in Marfan syndrome. *Orphanet Journal of Rare Diseases, 10*(1), Article 153. https://doi.org/10.1186/s13023-015-0369-8

Handisides, J. C., Hollenbeck-Pringle, D., Uzark, K., Trachtenberg, F. L., Pemberton, V. L., Atz, T. W., Bradley, T. J., Cappella, E., De Nobele, S., Groh, G. K., Hamstra, M. S., Korsin, R., Levine, J. C., Lindauer, B., Liou, A., Neal, M. K. M., Markham, L. W., Morrison, T., Mussatto, K. A., . . . Lacro, R. V. (2019). Health-related quality of life in children and young adults with Marfan syndrome. *The Journal of Pediatrics, 204*, 250–255. https://doi.org/10.1016/j.jpeds.2018.08.061

Hofman, K. J., Bernhardt, B. A., Pyeritz, R. E., Opitz, J. M., & Reynolds, J. F. (1988). Marfan syndrome: Neuropsychological aspects. *American Journal of Medical Genetics, 31*(2), 331–338. https://doi.org/10.1002/ajmg.1320310210

Hoskoppal, A., Menon, S., Trachtenberg, F., Burns, K. M., De Backer, J., Gelb, B. D., Gleason, M., James, J., Lai, W. W., Liou, A., Mahony, L., Olson, A. K., Pyeritz, R. E., Sharkey, A. M., Stylianou, M., Wechsler, S. B., Young, L., Levine, J. C., Tierney, E. S. S., . . . Bradley, T. J. (2018). Predictors of rapid aortic root dilation and referral for aortic surgery in Marfan syndrome. *Pediatric Cardiology, 39*(7), 1453–1461. https://doi.org/10.1007/s00246-018-1916-6

Kieckhefer, G. M., Trahms, C. M., Churchill, S. S., Kratz, L., Uding, N., & Villareale, N. (2014). A randomized clinical trial of the Building on Family Strengths program: An education program for parents of children with chronic health conditions. *Maternal and Child Health Journal, 18*(3), 563–574. https://doi.org/10.1007/s10995-013-1273-2

Loeys, B. L., Dietz, H. C., Braverman, A. C., Callewaert, B. L., De Backer, J., Devereux, R. B., Hilhorst-Hofstee, Y., Jondeau, G., Faivre, L., Milewicz, D. M., Pyeritz, R. E., Sponseller, P. D., Wordsworth, P., & De Paepe, A. M. (2010). The revised Ghent nosology for the Marfan syndrome. *Journal of Medical Genetics, 47*(7), 476–485. https://doi.org/10.1136/jmg.2009.072785

Marfan Foundation. (2013). *Need-to-know information for the teacher: Raising awareness of Marfan syndrome and related disorders*. https://marfan.org/resource-library/need-to-know-information-for-the-teacher/

Mueller, G. C., Stark, V., Steiner, K., von Kodolitsch, Y., Rybczynski, M., Weil, J., & Mir, T. S. (2013). Impact of age and gender on cardiac pathology in children and adolescents with Marfan syndrome. *Pediatric Cardiology, 34*, 991–998. https://doi.org/10.1007/s00246-012-0593-0

Pao, M., & Bosk, A. (2011). Anxiety in medically ill children/adolescents. *Depression and Anxiety, 28*(1), 40–49. https://doi.org/10.1002/da.20727

Rand-Hendriksen, S., Sørensen, I., Holmström, H., Andersson, S., & Finset, A. (2007). Fatigue, cognitive functioning and psychological distress in Marfan syndrome, a pilot study. *Psychology Health and Medicine, 12*(3), 305–313. https://doi.org/10.1080/13548500600580824

Ryan-Krause, P. (2002). Identify and manage Marfan syndrome in children. *The Nurse Practitioner, 27*(10), 26–36. https://doi.org/10.1097/00006205-200210000-00008

Schilling, E. J., & Getch, Y. Q. (2018). School reentry services for students with chronic health conditions: An examination of regional practices. *Psychology in the Schools, 55*(9), 1027–1040. https://doi.org/10.1002/pits.22154

Schneider, M. B., Davis, J. G., Boxer, R. A., Fisher, M., & Friedman, S. B. (1990). Marfan syndrome in adolescents and young adults: Psychosocial functioning and knowledge. *Journal of Developmental and Behavioral Pediatrics, 11*(3), 122–127. https://doi.org/10.1097/00004703-199006000-00005

Speed, T. J., Mathur, V. A., Hand, M., Christensen, B., Sponseller, P. D., Williams, K. A., & Campbell, C. M. (2017). Characterization of pain, disability, and psychological burden in Marfan syndrome. *American Journal of Medical Genetics: Part A, 173*(2), 315–323. https://doi.org/10.1002/ajmg.a.38051

Velvin, G., Bathen, T., Rand-Hendriksen, S., & Geirdal, A. Ø. (2015). Systematic review of the psychosocial aspects of living with Marfan syndrome. *Clinical Genetics, 87*(2), 109–116. https://doi.org/10.1111/cge.12422

50

Muscular Dystrophies

Jennifer Tucker and Megan Jeune

Muscular dystrophies are a group of neuromuscular disorders with similar features. Duchenne muscular dystrophy (DMD) is the most common and is a terminal condition characterized by progressive muscular damage, muscle weakness, loss of functional mobility, and respiratory and cardiac impairments (Birnkrant et al., 2018; Leigh et al., 2018). While the life expectancy has lengthened with improved medical management, it remains shortened at only 20 to 30 years. Clinical presentations for the distinct types of muscular dystrophies vary; however, diagnosis and medical management have improved, resulting in longer lifespans than previous generations. Thus, it is critical to provide comprehensive multidisciplinary care to maximize quality of life.

ETIOLOGY

A mutation in the dystrophin gene results in insufficient amounts of dystrophin, which is a protein critical for normal muscle activity that enables optimal function of the myofibers in muscles (Birnkrant et al., 2018; Leigh et al., 2018). The lack of dystrophin leads to muscle damage. As the muscle tissue is broken down, it is replaced with fibrotic tissue and fat (Leigh et al., 2018). Becker muscular dystrophy (BMD) is a variant of DMD. Differences between BMD and DMD result from the amount of dystrophin available. In DMD there is an absence of dystrophin; however, with BMD, an abnormal version of dystrophin

https://doi.org/10.1037/0000349-050
Health-Related Disorders in Children and Adolescents: A Guidebook for Educators and Service Providers, Second Edition, M. M. Perfect, C. A. Riccio, and M. A. Bray (Editors)

results in a reduction in overall functionality. Both DMD and BMD are X-linked disorders typically affecting male individuals, although female individuals may be mildly affected and carriers of the genes. Emery–Dreifuss muscular dystrophy (EDMD) also results from an X-linked recessive trait or is inherited as an autosomal dominant trait. As with DMD and BDM, boys are more frequently diagnosed with EDMD. Facioscapulohumeral dystrophy (FSHD) is an autosomal disorder seen in both male and female individuals that generally appears in late childhood or adolescence but can appear at any point. Early onset FSHD is an autosomal dominant disorder resulting in a complex disease process consisting of large deletions of *D4Z4* repeats (Mah & Chen, 2018). Myotonic dystrophy (DM) type 1 is caused by a mutation of the dystrophia myotonica gene and has five clinical phenotypes: (a) premutation, (b) mild adult DM, (c) classical adult DM, (d) childhood-onset DM, and (e) congenital DM. Onset can occur at any age; however, the literature on clinical presentation and natural history of the disease in children is limited (Ho et al., 2015). Thirty-one types of limb-girdle muscular dystrophies (LGMDs) have been identified, eight of which are autosomal dominant and 23 of which are autosomal recessive type, with the most severe types presenting during childhood. Autosomal recessive and severe childhood autosomal recessive muscular dystrophy (SCARMD) are both used to describe a type of muscular dystrophy like DMD with progressive weakening of muscles in the arms, legs, and hips. Like DMD, symptoms of SCARMD are typically seen in young children aged 2 to 6 years, and life expectancy is hypothesized to be between 20 and 30 years. Unlike DMD, both sexes are equally afflicted by SCARMD. Advances in genetic testing and research offer ongoing insights into the etiology of the diverse types of muscular dystrophy.

PREVALENCE AND INCIDENCE

The prevalence of muscular dystrophies, as a diagnosis category, has been reported as between 19.8 and 25.1 per 100,000 (Theadom et al., 2014). The incidence and prevalence of the specific types of muscular dystrophy vary, with some being more common than others (Table 50.1).

DMD, the most common form of muscular dystrophy, affects 15.9 per 100,000 births each year in the United States (Leigh et al., 2018; Ryder et al., 2017). EDMD, a slowly progressive disease (although rapid onset has been documented), impacts limb, facial, spine, and heart muscles, affecting 0.1 to 1.9 per 100,000 individuals (Theadom et al., 2014). Another common form is FSHD, affecting one out of 15,000 to one out of 20,000 individuals (Tawil et al., 2015). Early onset FSHD is seen in a small percentage (4%–21%) of the overall population of individuals with FSHD and approximately half of the individuals with pediatric FSHD (Mah & Chen, 2018). DM type 1 affects skeletal muscle and smooth muscle as well as the eyes, heart, endocrine system, and central nervous system, with a reported prevalence of one in 8,000 individuals (Ho et al., 2015).

TABLE 50.1. Additional Types of Muscular Dystrophies

Type	Incidence	Etiology	Symptoms
Facioscapulohumeral dystrophy (FSHD)	1 in 15,000 to 1 in 20,000 (Tawil et al., 2015)	Autosomal disorder	Facial weakness, shoulder girdle weakness, developmental delay, and/or dysphagia (Goselink et al., 2018; Mah & Chen, 2018)
Myotonic dystrophy (DM) type 1	1 in 8,000 (Ho et al., 2015)	Caused by a mutation of the dystrophia myotonica gene, 5 clinical phenotypes	Weakness, respiratory complications, cognitive deficits, and incontinence, but may be subtle, leading to delayed diagnosis
Emery–Dreifuss muscular dystrophy (EDMD)	1 in 100,000	Resulting from X-linked recessive trait or inherited as an autosomal dominant trait	Atrophy of affected muscles in upper and lower limbs, contractures of joints (e.g., elbows, Achilles tendons), and cardiomyopathy
Limb-girdle muscular dystrophy (LGMD)	1 in 14,500 to 1 in 123,000	31 types identified: 8 autosomal dominant and 23 autosomal recessive types	Progressive muscle weakening of voluntary muscles in the hip and shoulder, resulting in severe physical weakness and shortened lifespan (Nigro & Savarese, 2014)
Autosomal recessive and severe child autosomal recessive muscular dystrophy (SCARMD)	Varied	Autosomal recessive	Progressive weakening of muscles in the arms, legs, and hips

SYMPTOMS

Symptoms of DMD present in boys ages 2 to 5 years and consist of delayed motor milestones, toe walking, difficulty with running and climbing stairs, and hypertrophy of the calf muscles (Birnkrant et al., 2018; Leigh et al., 2018; Yiu & Kornberg, 2015). Gowers's sign, an abnormal pattern of rising from the floor reflective of lower extremity muscle weakness, is a characteristic movement pattern (Birnkrant et al., 2018). Like DMD, BMD begins with proximal weakness in both the upper and lower extremities, but the progression of BMD is slower and less predictable than DMD. Primary symptoms of BMD include the proximal weakness that alters gait patterns and may not appear until childhood or adolescence. Individuals with BMD may use a wide base of support or toe walk. The cardiac and respiratory muscles also may be affected and weaken over time. These signs prompt a referral to a neurologist for evaluation and diagnosis. Diagnosis is made through genetic testing and muscle biopsy and often takes up to a year (Leigh et al., 2018). Once a diagnosis has been made, the family should be referred for genetic counseling and testing. Female carriers also need to be referred for evaluations (Birnkrant et al., 2018). Currently, newborn testing does not include testing for DMD.

Early-onset FSHD symptoms differ from DMD and BMD and include facial weakness, shoulder girdle weakness, developmental delay, and/or dysphagia (Goselink et al., 2018; Mah & Chen, 2018). The facial weakness may present with facial asymmetry or difficulty with drinking through a straw or blowing activities. Scapular muscle weakness causes bilateral scapular winging, which may be asymmetrical. In addition, the scapular weakness and instability poses challenges for overhead activities and lifting. Muscle wasting may also alter the appearance of the upper extremities (Goselink et al., 2018; Mul et al., 2016). Trunk musculature is also affected by FSHD, resulting in postural changes, challenges with balance, and difficulty getting up from lying down. Last, the lower extremity musculature may decline in strength as well. Functional skills such as getting up from a chair and ascending stairs are challenging due to the lower extremity weakness. Individuals with childhood-onset FSHD may experience significant hearing loss (Hamel & Tawil, 2018). It is important to note that in addition to weakness, most individuals with FSHD also experience pain and fatigue (Goselink et al., 2018; Mul et al., 2016). As with other forms of muscular dystrophies, the respiratory muscles may be impacted, and pulmonary function should be monitored carefully (Tawil et al., 2015).

Children with LGMD experience progressive muscle weakening of voluntary muscles in the hip and shoulder, resulting in severe physical weakness and shortened lifespan (Nigro & Savarese, 2014). Although the disorders primarily result in deterioration of proximal limb muscles, systemic deterioration often manifests throughout the child's musculature, with cardiac issues also present.

Congenital DM presents with severe hypotonia and weakness at birth. In addition, babies often experience respiratory complications. Mortality for the first year of life may be 30% to 40% (Ho et al., 2015). Childhood-onset DM appears during the 1st decade of life. Symptoms include weakness, respiratory complications, cognitive deficits, and incontinence. The onset may be unclear with vague symptoms, resulting in a delayed diagnosis.

Individuals with DM exhibit with distal muscle weakness, visual impairments, sleep disorders, cognitive deficits, respiratory complications, and psychosocial challenges. A significant percentage of children with DM type 1 have at least one psychiatric disorder, such as anxiety or attention-deficit disorders (Ho et al., 2015). Respiratory complications (e.g., sleep breathing disorders, frequent infections, weak cough, pneumonia) are common in childhood-onset DM. Visual impairments may include strabismus and/or reduced acuity. Children may also experience cognitive deficits and speech delays (Ho et al., 2015).

IMPACT ON THE STUDENT AND OUTCOMES

Medical

The initial symptoms of DMD of significant motor delay, abnormal gait, Gowers's sign, and decreased balance emerge in boys between the ages of 2 and 5 years (Birnkrant et al., 2018; Leigh et al., 2018; Yiu & Kornberg, 2015). Global delay, raised serum creatinine kinase, and raised liver enzymes may be seen in a small percentage of boys with DMD (Yiu & Kornberg, 2015). Deterioration of strength becomes more marked at 6 years of age, and if untreated, many children are wheelchair dependent for mobility by 11 to 12 years of age (Yiu & Kornberg, 2015). The changes in strength and resulting muscle imbalances often lead to scoliosis.

Cardiopulmonary impairments also emerge as a component of DMD (Birnkrant et al., 2018; Yiu & Kornberg, 2015). A small percentage (25%) of children under the age of 6 will present with persistent tachycardia. After the age of 10 there is evidence of cardiomyopathy, which later affects approximately one third of boys by 14 years of age and all boys by 18 years of age (Yiu & Kornberg, 2015). Cardiac complications are the primary cause of mortality in this population; therefore, individuals with DMD should be closely monitored by a cardiologist.

All individuals with DMD experience restrictive lung disease (Birnkrant et al., 2018; Yiu & Kornberg, 2015). Vital capacity increases throughout early childhood, peaking around the age of 12, after which it declines (Birnkrant et al., 2018; Yiu & Kornberg, 2015). Sleep disorders are associated with pulmonary impairments and are experienced throughout the lifespan. Respiratory function may also be affected by scoliosis and the structural restrictions on the lungs (Yiu & Kornberg, 2015). Although the life expectancy has lengthened with improved medical management, it remains shortened at only 20 to 30 years.

Progressive muscle weakness leads to medical complications most often seen in cardiopulmonary impairments and chronic pain. For example, most individuals with FSHD also experience pain and fatigue (Goselink et al., 2018; Mul et al., 2016). Like other forms of muscular dystrophies, the respiratory muscles may also be affected, and pulmonary function should be monitored carefully (Tawil et al., 2015). Likewise, individuals with DM (refer to Table 50.1) exhibit with distal muscle weakness, visual impairments (e.g., strabismus, reduced acuity), sleep disorders, and respiratory complications (e.g., sleep breathing disorders, frequent infections, weak cough, pneumonia). Similarly, symptoms of EDMD are described as a triad: atrophy of affected muscles in upper and lower limbs, contractures of joints (e.g., elbows, Achilles tendons), and cardiomyopathy developing after the

2nd decade of life. While there are many distinct types of LGMD, the clinical presentation remains consistent with the other types of muscular dystrophy described previously, with systemic and progressive muscle weakening resulting in severe physical weakness, cardiac issues, and shortened lifespan (Nigro & Savarese, 2014).

Finally, the autosomal recessive and SCARMD describe a type of muscular dystrophy like DMD with progressive weakening of muscles in the arms, legs, and hips. Symptoms of SCARMD are typically seen in young children aged 2 to 6, and life expectancy is estimated to be between 20 and 30 years (refer to Table 50.1). Children afflicted with SCARMD are usually wheelchair bound by their midteens.

Cognitive/Academic

Children with DMD present with intellectual disabilities, which may affect their success in the classroom. Intellectual impairments are also associated with DMD, as the average IQ of the DMD population is 85, which is one standard deviation below population norms (Yiu & Kornberg, 2015). As with DMD, boys with BMD may have mild learning disabilities (Emery, 2002). Ferrero and Rossi (2022) examined the literature on cognitive levels and neuropsychiatric disorders in individuals with BMD. They found that symptoms in both domains may be present in a significant percentage of individuals with BMD and stressed the importance of cognitive and mental health screenings. The Mini-Mental State Examination (Folstein et al., 1975) was shown to be a good cognitive screening assessment for DMD patients over the age of 9 years (Nardes et al., 2020). Unlike the progressive symptoms, their intellectual skills do not decline over time. In the school setting, accommodations to address motor impairments may be needed.

Social-Emotional and Behavioral

In addition to decreased cognitive ability (Yiu & Kornberg, 2015), individuals with DMD have increased incidences of attention-deficit/hyperactivity disorder (32%), autism spectrum disorder (15%), and anxiety (27%; Banihani et al., 2015). Further, boys with DMD and BMD may evidence behavioral disabilities (Emery, 2002). Psychosocial interventions are beneficial for children and their families as they navigate a lifelong disease.

PSYCHOEDUCATIONAL IMPLICATIONS AND SCHOOL-BASED INTERVENTIONS

Medical and Health Management

Currently, corticosteroids are the primary pharmacologic treatment for DMD. Use of corticosteroids has been beneficial in terms of gaining and maintaining strength. Research suggests that long-term use of corticosteroids may prolong independent ambulation, slow the progression of cardiorespiratory impairments, and decrease the risk of scoliosis (Yiu & Kornberg, 2015).

Disease surveillance and symptom management remain the primary focus across the lifespan. As respiratory impairments increase, individuals with DMD or other muscular dystrophies may require the use of noninvasive intermittent positive pressure support and at late stages may opt for full-time ventilation (Birnkrant et al., 2018; Yiu & Kornberg, 2015). Beta-blockers and angiotensin-converting enzyme inhibitors may be prescribed to address cardiac abnormalities (Yiu & Kornberg, 2015).

Referrals to orthopedics and physical therapy address range of motion, strength, and mobility. Spinal fusion surgery may be needed if the scoliosis is resulting in additional respiratory compromise (Yiu & Kornberg, 2015). To maintain bone health, calcium and vitamin D supplements may be prescribed. Life expectancy for individuals with muscular dystrophies has increased, especially for those with DMD. Thus, it is imperative that comprehensive multidisciplinary care be in place to help the individual and their family navigate the disease process across their lifespan.

Medical management of muscular dystrophies should include ongoing disease surveillance with a focus on monitoring for complications. Referrals to specialists could include pulmonology, ophthalmology, and otolaryngology. An orthopedist will determine if the individual would benefit from a surgical scapular fixation. Similarly, there is no pharmacologic treatment for DM type 1. Medical management requires a multidisciplinary team monitoring the disease, managing complications, and addressing impairments to improve quality of life (Ho et al., 2015).

Cognitive/Academic

The needs for children with muscular dystrophies change over time in response to disease progression. It is important to address not only the physical needs but also the cognitive supports necessary to ensure learning and participation in school settings. As stated previously, the Mini-Mental State Examination may be used as a cognitive screening tool for children with DMD over the age of 9 years (Nardes et al., 2020). Scores on the Mini-Mental State Examination stabilize and plateau between the ages of 9 and 10 years, which contributes to its reliability and sensitivity as a screening tool for cognitive impairments. Specifically, a score less than 21 is a good screening test for intellectual disabilities and provides justification for further neuropsychological or educational testing (Nardes et al., 2020). Children benefit from comprehensive neuropsychological or educational psychological assessment to identify challenges and necessary interventions to ensure success.

Ongoing assessments of posture and mobility will benefit students to ensure comfort and facilitate the highest levels of participation. Children may enter the school system as independent ambulators and later transition to manual or power wheelchairs. Physical fatigue leads to cognitive fatigue; therefore, teachers and therapists need to collaborate to ensure that the child maintains as much independence as possible without adding an additional burden. Children with FSHD, for example, will be affected by muscular weakness, pain, and fatigue. It is important to avoid overhead activities such as writing on a whiteboard. Lifting also is challenging, so a child may be best served by having a set of books at home and one at school to avoid the need for carrying them throughout the day. Ensuring that seating provides necessary postural support will assist with trunk weakness.

Providing accommodations to ensure participation in learning and social experiences in an academic setting will add to their quality of life across the lifespan. Hearing screenings should be conducted regularly to ensure that any hearing loss is identified. Accommodations for hearing loss may be necessary to ensure the child's success in school. Muscle weakness may require adaptations for handwriting and other fine motor tasks to make them less demanding. Language delays have been documented as early as preschool in boys with DMD (Chieffo et al., 2022). Therefore, children may also need speech therapy services to address speech delays (Chieffo et al., 2022; Ho et al., 2015).

Social-Emotional and Behavioral

As with any chronic medical condition, the clinical presentation is not limited to physical symptoms but also may include social–emotional and behavioral challenges. Ferrero and Rossi (2022) recommended both neurodevelopmental and neuropsychological assessments at the time of diagnosis. Based on their insights of the increased incidence of cognitive and neuropsychiatric impairments in individuals with BMD, it is suggested that cognitive rehabilitation and behavioral management be an additional and key component of the interprofessional team.

Depression and anxiety are experienced by many individuals with muscular dystrophies. Higher incidences of internalizing symptoms, autism spectrum disorder, attention-deficit/hyperactivity disorder, and social impairments have been reported in individuals with muscular dystrophy as compared with the general population (Tesei et al., 2020). More specifically, individuals with DM experience psychosocial challenges, and a significant percentage of children with DM type 1 have at least one psychiatric disorder (e.g., anxiety, attention-deficit/hyperactivity disorder; Ho et al., 2015). Tesei et al. (2020) reported a link between these disorders and coping strategies employed by children and their families. Therefore, children and families may benefit from psychosocial services focused on adjustment and coping strategies.

Donaldson et al. (2021) found that psychosocial challenges were increasingly experienced during the transition periods in the education of a child with DMD/BMD. More specifically, this population of students often had limited postsecondary education, were unemployed, and lived at home. The authors suggested that expanding school supports such as paraprofessionals and related services, including physical and occupational therapies, may improve educational outcomes. In addition to these needed rehabilitative services, adolescents with DMD/BMD frequently underutilize vocational rehabilitation services (Donaldson et al., 2021). A tool that might assist with the complex issues that arise during transition is the DMD Transition Toolkit (Trout et al., 2018). This toolkit provides a transition readiness assessment and comprehensive checklist to assist with the complex needs of this population (Trout et al., 2018). Psychosocial support and services are an integral component of the health care team (Colvin et al., 2018; Donaldson et al., 2021). Collaboration between school and medical social workers will ensure that during this time of transition all areas are addressed, promoting the most positive outcomes for the students.

CONCLUSION

Muscular dystrophy describes a number of neuromuscular disorders. All types of muscular dystrophy affect strength, mobility, and respiratory and other systems at varying rates of disease progression. These symptoms present challenges in educational settings and may prevent a child with muscular dystrophy from reaching their full academic potential. Understanding the physiological implications is essential to provide appropriate accommodations. Recent medical advances have extended lifespans; therefore, support throughout education is critical for learning and quality of life during childhood and beyond.

RESOURCES

Muscular Dystrophy Association. https://www.mda.org/

Muscular Dystrophy Association. (n.d.). *School accommodation recommendations.* https://www.mda.org/sites/default/files/Guide_SchoolAccommodations-DMD2.pdf

Anzilotti, A. W. (2020). *Muscular dystrophy.* KidsHealth. https://kidshealth.org/en/parents/muscular-dystrophy.html

Gavin, M. L. (2020). *Muscular dystrophy factsheet (for schools).* KidsHealth. https://kidshealth.org/en/parents/md-factsheet.html

REFERENCES

Banihani, R., Smile, S., Yoon, G., Dupuis, A., Mosleh, M., Snider, A., & McAdam, L. (2015). Cognitive and neurobehavioral profile in boys with Duchenne muscular dystrophy. *Journal of Child Neurology, 30*(11), 1472–1482. https://doi.org/10.1177/0883073815570154

Birnkrant, D. J., Bushby, K., Bann, C. M., Apkon, S. D., Blackwell, A., Brumbaugh, D., Case, L. E., Clemens, P. R., Hadjiyannakis, S., Pandya, S., Street, N., Tomezsko, J., Wagner, K. R., Ward, L. M., Weber, D. R., & the DMD Care Considerations Working Group. (2018). Diagnosis and management of Duchenne muscular dystrophy, Part 1: Diagnosis, and neuromuscular, rehabilitation, endocrine, and gastrointestinal and nutritional management. *The Lancet Neurology, 17*(3), 251–267. https://doi.org/10.1016/S1474-4422(18)30024-3

Chieffo, D. P. R., Moriconi, F., Mastrilli, L., Lino, F., Brogna, C., Coratti, G., Altobelli, M., Massaroni, V., Norcia, G., Ferraroli, E., Lucibello, S., Pane, M., & Mercuri, E. (2022). Language development in preschool Duchenne muscular dystrophy boys. *Brain Sciences, 12*(9), Article 1252. https://doi.org/10.3390/brainsci12091252

Colvin, M. K., Poysky, J., Kinnett, K., Damiani, M., Gibbons, M., Hoskin, J., Moreland, S., Trout, C. J., & Weidner, N. (2018). Psychosocial management of the patient with Duchenne muscular dystrophy. *Pediatrics, 142*(Suppl. 2), S99–S109. https://doi.org/10.1542/peds.2018-0333L

Donaldson, A., Guntrum, D., Ciafaloni, E., & Statland, J. (2021). Achieving life milestones in Duchenne/Becker muscular dystrophy: A retrospective analysis. *Neurology: Clinical Practice, 11*(4), 311–317. https://doi.org/10.1212/CPJ.0000000000000970

Emery, A. E. (2002). The muscular dystrophies. *The Lancet, 359*(9307), 687–695. https://doi.org/10.1016/S0140-6736(02)07815-7

Ferrero, A., & Rossi, M. (2022). Cognitive profile and neuropsychiatric disorders in Becker muscular dystrophy: A systematic review of literature. *Neuroscience and Biobehavioral Reviews, 137*, Article 104648. https://doi.org/10.1016/j.neubiorev.2022.104648

Folstein, M. F., Folstein, S. E., & McHugh, P. R. (1975). "Mini-mental state". A practical method for grading the cognitive state of patients for the clinician. *Journal of Psychiatric Research, 12*(3), 189–198. https://doi.org/10.1016/0022-3956(75)90026-6

Goselink, R. J. M., Schreuder, T. H. A., van Alfen, N., de Groot, I. J. M., Jansen, M., Lemmers, R. J. L. F., van der Vliet, P. J., van der Stoep, N., Theelen, T., Voermans, N. C., van der Maarel, S. M., van Engelen, B. G. M., & Erasmus, C. E. (2018). Facioscapulohumeral dystrophy in childhood: A nationwide natural history study. *Annals of Neurology, 84*(5), 627–637. https://doi.org/10.1002/ana.25326

Hamel, J., & Tawil, R. (2018). Facioscapulohumeral muscular dystrophy: Update on pathogenesis and future treatments. *Neurotherapeutics, 15*(4), 863–871. https://doi.org/10.1007/s13311-018-00675-3

Ho, G., Cardamone, M., & Farrar, M. (2015). Congenital and childhood myotonic dystrophy: Current aspects of disease and future directions. *World Journal of Clinical Pediatrics, 4*(4), 66–80. https://doi.org/10.5409/wjcp.v4.i4.66

Leigh, F., Ferlini, A., Biggar, D., Bushby, K., Finkel, R., Morgenroth, L. P., & Wagner, K. R. (2018). Neurology care, diagnostics, and emerging therapies of the patient with Duchenne muscular dystrophy. *Pediatrics, 142*(Suppl. 2), S5–S16. https://doi.org/10.1542/peds.2018-0333C

Mah, J. K., & Chen, Y. W. (2018). A pediatric review of facioscapulohumeral muscular dystrophy. *Journal of Pediatric Neurology, 16*(4), 222–231. https://doi.org/10.1055/s-0037-1604197

Mul, K., Lassche, S., Voermans, N. C., Padberg, G. W., Horlings, C. G., & van Engelen, B. G. (2016). What's in a name? The clinical features of facioscapulohumeral muscular dystrophy. *Practical Neurology, 16*(3), 201–207. https://doi.org/10.1136/practneurol-2015-001353

Nardes, F., Araújo, A. P. D. Q. C., Ribeiro, M. G., Bittar, M., & Gomes, H. F. (2020). The Mini-Mental State Examination (MMSE) as a cognitive screening tool in Duchenne muscular dystrophy. *Annals of Child Neurology, 28*(2), 57–65. https://doi.org/10.26815/acn.2020.00052

Nigro, V., & Savarese, M. (2014). Genetic basis of limb-girdle muscular dystrophies: The 2014 update. *Acta Myologica, 33*(1), 1–12.

Ryder, S., Leadley, R. M., Armstrong, N., Westwood, M., de Kock, S., Butt, T., Jain, M., & Kleijnen, J. (2017). The burden, epidemiology, costs and treatment for Duchenne muscular dystrophy: An evidence review. *Orphanet Journal of Rare Diseases, 12*(1), Article 79. https://doi.org/10.1186/s13023-017-0631-3

Tawil, R., Kissel, J. T., Heatwole, C., Pandya, S., Gronseth, G., & Benatar, M. (2015). Evidence-based guideline summary: Evaluation, diagnosis, and management of facioscapulohumeral muscular dystrophy: Report of the Guideline Development, Dissemination, and Implementation Subcommittee of the American Academy of Neurology and the Practice Issues Review Panel of the American Association of Neuromuscular & Electrodiagnostic Medicine. *Neurology, 85*(4), 357–364. https://doi.org/10.1212/WNL.0000000000001783

Tesei, A., Nobile, M., Colombo, P., Civati, F., Gandossini, S., Mani, E., Molteni, M., Bresolin, N., & D'Angelo, G. (2020). Mental health and coping strategies in families of children and young adults with muscular dystrophies. *Journal of Neurology, 267*(7), 2054–2069. https://doi.org/10.1007/s00415-020-09792-6

Theadom, A., Rodrigues, M., Roxburgh, R., Balalla, S., Higgins, C., Bhattacharjee, R., Jones, K., Krishnamurthi, R., & Feigin, V. (2014). Prevalence of muscular dystrophies: A systematic literature review. *Neuroepidemiology, 43*(3–4), 259–268. https://doi.org/10.1159/000369343

Trout, C. J., Case, L. E., Clemens, P. R., McArthur, A., Noritz, G., Ritzo, M., Wagner, K. R., Vroom, E., & Kennedy, A. (2018). A transition toolkit for Duchenne muscular dystrophy. *Pediatrics, 142*(Suppl. 2), S110–S117. https://doi.org/10.1542/peds.2018-0333M

Yiu, E. M., & Kornberg, A. J. (2015). Duchenne muscular dystrophy. *Journal of Paediatrics and Child Health, 51*(8), 759–764. https://doi.org/10.1111/jpc.12868

51

Osteogenesis Imperfecta

Kelly N. Clark and Christine K. Malecki

Osteogenesis imperfecta (OI) is a hereditary disorder that primarily impacts the ability to grow strong bones and other connective tissues. Also known as *brittle bone disease,* OI is caused by genetic defects related to Type I collagen, including abnormalities in collagen structure, production, quantity, and functioning (Forlino et al., 2011). OI has eight clinical types, based on variations in inheritance of the disorder and phenotypical presentation (i.e., specific clinical symptoms, severity of symptomatology). These are detailed in Table 51.1 with information on the etiology, form of transmission, and key characteristics.

ETIOLOGY

In most cases, OI is caused by inherited mutations in two genes (*COL1A1* and *COL1A2*) that are involved in the synthesis of Type 1 collagen (Majorana et al., 2010). Mutations in these genes may cause qualitative (i.e., structural) and/or quantitative (i.e., amount of collagen produced) defects in collagen synthesis. Because collagen fibers form the essential building blocks of connective tissues such as bones, ligaments, and tendons (Frey et al., 1998), defects in collagen structure and functioning result in low bone mass among individuals with OI. Consequently, OI is characterized by increased fragility of bones, deformities of bones, and growth deficiencies, among other symptoms (Forlino et al., 2011). OI occurs primarily through autosomal dominant inheritance (i.e., gene mutation

https://doi.org/10.1037/0000349-051
Health-Related Disorders in Children and Adolescents: A Guidebook for Educators and Service Providers, Second Edition, M. M. Perfect, C. A. Riccio, and M. A. Bray (Editors)

TABLE 51.1. Classification of OI Types

Type	Severity	Genetic mutation	Inheritance	Key characteristics
I	Mildest form; nondeforming	*COL1A1* (premature stop codon)	Autosomal dominant	• Most common form (50% of affected) • Minimal bone deformity; fractures decrease after puberty and into adulthood • Near normal stature • Hearing loss and blue sclera common • DI is rare
II	Most severe form; lethal	*COL1A1* or *COL1A2* (glycine substitution)	Autosomal dominant; autosomal recessive (rare)	• Perinatal lethal (in utero, infancy) • Bones damaged from intrauterine fractures • Large, soft skull • Underdeveloped respiratory system • Darkly shaded sclera
III	Most severe form; nonlethal	*COL1A1* or *COL1A2* (glycine substitution)	Autosomal dominant; autosomal recessive (uncommon)	• Fractures common • Very short stature (typically shorter than 3.5 feet) • Curved spine; large skull; triangular face • DI is common • Blue-/gray-/purple-tinted sclera • Hearing loss
IV	Mildly severe	*COL1A1* or *COL1A2* (glycine substitution)	Autosomal dominant	• Broad variability spanning from phenotypes similar to Type I to Type III (variability in DI, scleral discoloration, hearing loss, and stature) • Fractures common but physical movement (e.g., walking, sitting, standing) possible
V	Moderately severe	Unknown	Autosomal dominant	• Similar to Type IV in variability of fractures • Callus formation where bones have fractured or spontaneous formation
VI	Moderately severely deforming	Unknown	Autosomal recessive	• Extremely rare • Mineralization defect in bones • Similar to Type IV
VII	Moderately deforming	*CRTAP*	Autosomal recessive	• Variability in phenotypic expression; some more severe resemble Type II, whereas others resemble Type IV • Short stature; short leg and arm bones • Deformity of hip bone may cause limp
VIII	Severely deforming	*LEPRE1*	Autosomal recessive	• Similar to Types II and III • Significant growth deficiency • Under-mineralized bones

Note. Data from Forlino et al. (2011), Majorana et al. (2010), Osteogenesis Imperfecta Foundation (2015), Van Dijk and Sillence (2014). DI = dentinogenesis imperfecta (i.e., weakened teeth, possible tooth discoloration).

inherited from only one parent causes OI); however, OI also may be inherited through autosomal recessive (i.e., gene mutation must be inherited from both parents to cause OI) or spontaneous de novo patterns. More severe cases of OI may be diagnosed prenatally, although OI is usually diagnosed in infancy or childhood, with bone fractures being the most common reason for referral. OI should be differentially diagnosed from other bone diseases (e.g., idiopathic juvenile osteoporosis, hypophosphatasia) by a physician (Marr et al., 2017).

PREVALENCE AND INCIDENCE

OI is a rare condition, affecting approximately six to seven per 100,000 people worldwide. OI occurs equally among male and female individuals, as well as across all racial/ethnic groups (Osteogenesis Imperfecta Foundation, 2015).

SYMPTOMS

Mutations in *COL1A1* and/or *COL1A2* produce a wide variety of symptom severity through their phenotypic expression (Forlino et al., 2011). OI is characterized by low bone mass, fragile bones, and skeletal deformities; therefore, children with OI are highly susceptible to recurrent bone fractures, even after experiencing little trauma or impact to the bone (Forlino et al., 2011). Bone deformities may include bowing of the legs, curved spine, barrel-shaped chest, and triangular facial structure (Johns Hopkins Medicine, n.d.). Joint hypermobility and loose joints also may occur in individuals with OI (Majorana et al., 2010). An additional primary feature of OI is growth deficiency that may result in short stature (Hill et al., 2014). Type I is the mildest form of OI, with affected children typically not experiencing bone fractures until they begin walking; further, Type I is the most common form of OI (i.e., 50% of those affected; Osteogenesis Imperfecta Foundation, 2015). In addition to skeletal defects, children with OI also experience abnormalities in other connective tissues. The white part of the eye, or sclera, may have a blue or grayish tint (Majorana et al., 2010), although scleral discoloration varies within and across OI types. Although not present in Type I OI, other OI types may include *dentinogenesis imperfecta*, a disorder of tooth development caused by weakened dentin formation within the teeth; when present, the first set of teeth is likely to be more severely affected than permanent teeth (Majorana et al., 2010). See Table 51.1 for more detailed characteristics.

IMPACT ON THE STUDENT AND OUTCOMES

Children with OI may experience a variety of medical, cognitive/academic, and social–emotional and behavioral outcomes associated with their diagnosis. These outcomes are described in the following sections.

Medical

In addition to fractures and bone deformity that may require medical intervention, many individuals with OI, particularly Types I through IV, experience progressive hearing loss (Majorana et al., 2010). Research has suggested that hearing loss typically begins in early adulthood and about 50% to 60% of individuals with OI experience hearing loss by age 50; however, about 5% to 9% of individuals with OI experience hearing loss beginning in childhood (Starr et al., 2010). Many individuals with OI experience vestibular dysfunction (e.g., vertigo) caused by defects in the bones of the middle ear, which may be surgically corrected (Forlino et al., 2011). Other characteristics of OI include neurological abnormalities (e.g., hydrocephalus, macrocephaly) and pulmonary/cardiovascular abnormalities (e.g., recurrent pneumonia, heart failure, rib cage deformities; Forlino et al., 2011). Difficulties with muscle tone may be evident in children with OI, as well as easily bruised skin (Johns Hopkins Medicine, n.d.). The most severe cases of OI involve nonviable births, with miscarriages occurring during pregnancy due to in utero fracture or respiratory difficulties, or death during infancy (Hill et al., 2014). Individuals with mild and moderate forms of OI can expect a normal lifespan, whereas those with severe forms may have a life expectancy of 20 to 30 years (Starr et al., 2010).

Cognitive/Academic

Youth with OI have normal cognitive ability, despite physical limitations (Osteogenesis Imperfecta Foundation, 2005; Starr et al., 2010). Therefore, children with OI are fully capable of accessing the general education curriculum with modifications to their environments and/or accommodations. Widmann and colleagues (2002) found that all participating adults with OI had graduated high school, 80% attended some college, and 57% obtained a college or postgraduate degree. Although employment rates of adults with OI were similar to the general population, the unemployment rate among adults with OI was slightly higher. Employment status was significantly associated with the ability to ambulate independently, as nearly half of wheelchair users had never obtained employment (Widmann et al., 2002).

Social–Emotional and Behavioral

Despite the variety of adverse medical outcomes that youth with OI may face, they can achieve expected social–emotional functioning with appropriate supports and modifications. Those with milder forms of OI may experience a psychological burden related to having an *invisible illness* (i.e., a disability that is not readily apparent to others at first sight), and others may not recognize the need to accommodate bone fragility (Johns Hopkins Medicine, n.d.). This is particularly true during childhood, as peers may not fully understand another child's bone fragility. Social integration difficulties may be further compounded by limited participation of children with OI in common physical activities (e.g., playing on the playground, contact sports; Johns Hopkins Medicine, n.d.). Children experiencing short stature and/or skeletal deformities caused by OI may be ostracized by peers. When OI symptoms preclude the child's ability to perform routine activities independently, they may be ostracized further for relying heavily on the support of others to function. As a result, children with mild, moderate, and severe forms of OI may experience feelings of social isolation and/or social anxiety (Marr et al., 2017).

In addition to potential social isolation, youth with OI are vulnerable to emotional difficulties revolving around fears and anxieties of experiencing a fracture or receiving medical intervention (e.g., X-ray, cast, surgery). Using an interview-based qualitative approach with children diagnosed with OI and their caregivers, Marr and colleagues (2017) revealed several themes around fear from the child (e.g., activities that previously caused a bone fracture, needles, operations, early death) and parents (e.g., dropping off the child at daycare or school, safety hazards that could cause a fracture). Anxiety experienced by parents could exacerbate the child's fears of fractures; additionally, caregivers may become overprotective of the child in efforts to prevent fractures, inadvertently creating a state of learned helplessness and overdependence within the child (Marr et al., 2017).

PSYCHOEDUCATIONAL IMPLICATIONS AND SCHOOL-BASED INTERVENTIONS

Within the educational setting, youth diagnosed with OI may benefit from a variety of accommodations and interventions. Although these supports should be individualized at the student level, a summary of potential supports is presented next.

Medical and Health Management

Medical treatment of OI in childhood is centered on preventing fractures, reducing skeletal deformities, providing appropriate pain relief, and facilitating motor functioning (Hill et al., 2014). Until recently, medical research suggested no viable pharmacological treatment for OI (Frey et al., 1998); however, bisphosphonate therapy has since proven to be an effective treatment for youth with moderate to severe OI. Bisphosphonates reduce bone resorption (i.e., transfer of calcium from connective tissue to the blood stream) by decreasing the functioning of osteoclasts, which are the cells that are primarily responsible for bone resorption (Hill et al., 2014). As a result, bisphosphonate-treated youth have increased bone density and mass, improved vertebral structure, and reduced bone fractures (Forlino et al., 2011). Although not yet supported through randomized clinical trials, qualitative research has suggested that bisphosphonate therapy may improve motor functioning and muscular strength and reduce pain among youth with OI (Hill et al., 2014). Ongoing clinical trials of children with OI Types I, III, and IV have supported the efficacy of growth hormone treatment for significantly accelerating linear growth, with associated effects on skeletal and muscular mass and strength in children with milder forms of OI (Forlino et al., 2011; Marr et al., 2017).

Bone fractures and skeletal deformities may be ameliorated through surgical placement of intramedullary rods to stabilize the bone (Johns Hopkins Medicine, n.d.). Rodding is often a critical factor for not only preventing fracture and deformity but also supporting ambulation and increased range of motion as limbs are more appropriately aligned (Marr et al., 2017). Surgery is most beneficial when combined with physical/occupational therapy designed to improve gross motor abilities and independent functioning (Forlino et al., 2011). Hydrotherapy (i.e., gentle water-based exercises) may be an ideal physical activity for youth with OI due to lower risk of injury. Youth with OI may benefit from a variety of assistive devices to prevent fractures and improve mobility (e.g., braces, wheelchairs; Johns Hopkins Medicine, n.d.). In the school setting, the physical environment may be modified to allow for safe navigation (e.g., ramp/ elevator access) to lower risk of falls, as well as special transportation services. Adaptive physical education may be beneficial to prevent injury and promote gentle movement. A crisis plan should be developed by a multidisciplinary team that proactively prevents potential injury and also prepares educators for safe and responsive management of injury (e.g., fractures).

Children with OI may require continued monitoring of audiological functioning, and some may benefit from the use of FM systems or other personal listening devices. Youth with OI may have greater susceptibility to viral and bacterial infections (e.g., common cold, flu); thus, children with OI should maintain good hygiene (e.g., handwashing) and learning environments should be disinfected (e.g., use of antibacterial wipes) to limit infections. Ongoing dental care is another important factor, as youth with OI may require dental procedures, including braces, surgery, and capping teeth to maintain oral health (Johns Hopkins Medicine, n.d.).

Cognitive/Academic

Students diagnosed with OI may require a variety of school-based supports and services for them to fully access the educational environment. There is strong consensus that children with OI should be educated in the general education setting to the greatest extent possible (Osteogenesis Imperfecta Foundation, 2005). Children with OI may be eligible for early intervention and/or early childhood services from birth to age 5. To ensure that children with OI are educated in the least restrictive environment, it is often necessary to provide them with appropriate supplementary supports and services. This is important to provide the best opportunity for children with OI to develop socially, emotionally, and behaviorally alongside typical peers. Modifications for classroom learning such as assistive technologies, adaptive materials (e.g., scissors, writing utensils), and homebound instruction during medical absences should be allowed for the student so they can best demonstrate their capabilities. Supports for youth with OI should be individualized to their specific needs, strengths, and challenges, with modifications to the support plan as the child's needs change over time.

Social-Emotional and Behavioral

Children with OI and their families may benefit from mental health services provided by a psychologist, social worker, or other mental health professional. These services may target feelings of anxiety, depression, and stress and also may address parents' fatigue related to caring for a child with OI (Marr et al., 2017). Additionally, caregivers may experience anxieties related to accusations of child abuse at emergency rooms, particularly in milder presentations of OI (Starr et al., 2010); thus, families should carry documentation of an OI diagnosis (Johns Hopkins Medicine, n.d.). Coordination of care within a multidisciplinary team, as well as access to social support, benefits, charities, and other funding sources for assistive devices and equipment and other needs, is important. Consistent school–family–health care communication is essential, and education of school staff and peers may also be supportive. Psychological assessment and intervention are essential across the lifespan of a person affected by OI, as coping and adjusting to this lifelong condition may cause a variety of mental health concerns in the individual with OI, as well as in caregivers and other immediate family members (Marr et al., 2017).

CONCLUSION

Coordination of care between the home and school settings is essential to support youth with OI. School psychologists, social workers, physical and occupational therapists, and others may be integral team members in monitoring the global functioning of a child with OI and providing accommodations and intervention. When provided with appropriate supports, children with OI can access the educational environment and develop academically, socially, and emotionally to lead a full and productive life.

RESOURCES

Brittle Bone Society. (2015). *Information on osteogenesis imperfecta for primary schools.* http://redbridgeserc.org/uploads/factsheets/103884_Advice_For_Primary_Schools_revised.pdf

Johns Hopkins Medicine. (n.d.). *Osteogenesis imperfecta.* https://www.hopkinsmedicine.org/healthlibrary/conditions/bone_disorders/osteogenesis_imperfecta_in_children_85,P00123

MedlinePlus. (2016). *Osteogenesis imperfecta*. National Library of Medicine. https://medlineplus.gov/osteogenesisimperfecta.html
Osteogenesis Imperfecta Foundation. https://oif.org/

REFERENCES

Forlino, A., Cabral, W. A., Barnes, A. M., & Marini, J. C. (2011). New perspectives on osteogenesis imperfecta. *Nature Reviews Endocrinology, 7*(9), 540–557. https://doi.org/10.1038/nrendo.2011.81

Frey, G., Palmer, D., & Bounds, R. (1998). Osteogenesis imperfecta. In L. E. Phelps (Ed.), *Health-related disorders in children and adolescents: A guidebook for understanding and educating* (pp. 488–493). American Psychological Association.

Hill, C. L., Baird, W. O., & Walters, S. J. (2014). Quality of life in children and adolescents with osteogenesis imperfecta: A qualitative interview-based study. *Health and Quality of Life Outcomes, 12*(1), Article 54. https://doi.org/10.1186/1477-7525-12-54

Johns Hopkins Medicine. (n.d.). *Osteogenesis imperfecta*. https://www.hopkinsmedicine.org/healthlibrary/conditions/bone_disorders/osteogenesis_imperfecta_in_children_85,P00123

Majorana, A., Bardellini, E., Brunelli, P. C., Lacaita, M., Cazzolla, A. P., & Favia, G. (2010). Dentinogenesis imperfecta in children with osteogenesis imperfecta: A clinical and ultrastructural study. *International Journal of Paediatric Dentistry, 20*(2), 112–118. https://doi.org/10.1111/j.1365-263X.2010.01033.x

Marr, C., Seasman, A., & Bishop, N. (2017). Managing the patient with osteogenesis imperfecta: A multidisciplinary approach. *Journal of Multidisciplinary Healthcare, 10*, 145–155. https://doi.org/10.2147/JMDH.S113483

Osteogenesis Imperfecta Foundation. (2005). *Preparing to send a child with OI to school*. https://oif.org/wp-content/uploads/2019/08/Education__Preparing_to_Send_Child_to_School.pdf

Osteogenesis Imperfecta Foundation. (2015). *OI types*. https://oif.org/informationcenter/about-oi/

Starr, S. R., Roberts, T. T., & Fischer, P. R. (2010). Osteogenesis imperfecta: Primary care. *Pediatrics, 31*(8), e54–e64. https://doi.org/10.1542/pir.31-8-e54

Van Dijk, F. S., & Sillence, D. O. (2014). Osteogenesis imperfecta: Clinical diagnosis, nomenclature and severity assessment. *American Journal of Medical Genetics: Part A, 164*(6), 1470–1481. https://doi.org/10.1002/ajmg.a.36545

Widmann, R. F., Laplaza, F. J., Bitan, F. D., Brooks, C. E., & Root, L. (2002). Quality of life in osteogenesis imperfecta. *International Orthopaedics, 26*(1), 3–6. https://doi.org/10.1007/s002640100292

52

Sotos Syndrome

Kari A. Sassu, Aarti P. Bellara, Michelle Levine-Schmitt,
Emily L. Winter, Katherine R. Nelson, Alyssa M. Bunyea,
Cindy C. Labbe, Elana S. Volfinzon, and Adeline M. Bray

Sotos syndrome is a congenital overgrowth disorder associated with medical, educational, and social–emotional effects. The overgrowth in particular is associated with advanced bone age, macrocephaly (i.e., head circumference that measures two standard deviations larger than the average for the given sex and age), distinctive craniofacial features (e.g., high-bossed forehead; prominent narrow jaw; long, narrow face), and intellectual disability (Albores-Gallo et al., 2017; Baujat & Cormier-Daire, 2007; Lane, Van Herwegen, & Freeth, 2019). Sotos syndrome affects multiple systems.

ETIOLOGY

Of Sotos syndrome cases, 90% are the result of mutations of the *NSD1* gene (nuclear receptor binding SET domain protein 1), which is expressed in the brain, kidney, skeletal muscle, and spleen. It has been suggested that it is involved in positive and negative transcription (Lane et al., 2016). The remaining 10% of individuals with Sotos syndrome meet the clinical criteria and are given the diagnosis of Sotos-like or Sotos syndrome 2 (Lane et al., 2016). For these individuals, the causes have not been fully determined (Waggoner et al., 2005).

Typical defects in *NSD1* with Sotos syndrome include mutations and deletions (Baujat & Cormier-Daire, 2007). The *NSD1* gene is located on chromosome 5q35 and codes for histone methyltransferases that are a part of

https://doi.org/10.1037/0000349-052
Health-Related Disorders in Children and Adolescents: A Guidebook for Educators and Service Providers, Second Edition, M. M. Perfect, C. A. Riccio, and M. A. Bray (Editors)

transcriptional regulation (Baujat & Cormier-Daire, 2007). These mutations lead to the phenotype of this syndrome marked mainly by accelerations in bone growth. The *NSD1* gene also is implicated in childhood acute myeloid leukemia, neuroblastoma, and glioma (Berdasco et al., 2009; Jaju et al., 2001).

PREVALENCE AND INCIDENCE

The incidence of Sotos syndrome is estimated at one in every 14,000 births (Lane et al., 2016; Tatton-Brown et al., 2019). The likelihood of an individual having Sotos syndrome is low compared with other chromosomal abnormality disorders. Comparatively, the estimated rate for an individual to have Down syndrome is one in every 700 births, making it the most common genetic abnormality disorder in the United States (Berry-Kravis et al., 2019). The fragile X syndrome incidence rate is roughly one in every 4,000 to 5,000 births (Berry-Kravis et al., 2019). Given the rarity of Sotos syndrome and the likelihood of misdiagnosis, it is understandable that no empirical studies across racial and/or ethnic groups were found. Factors related to misdiagnoses and overlapping characteristics have led some to conclude that the true incidence may actually be higher than is typically quoted in the scientific literature.

SYMPTOMS

As noted, Sotos syndrome is an overgrowth disorder. Advanced growth is noted throughout childhood with height often above the 97th percentile between 2 and 6 years old (Baujat & Cormier-Daire, 2007). In the neonatal period, about 65% of infants are jaundiced at birth (Lane et al., 2016; Tatton-Brown et al., 2019). About 75% of neonates may also experience congenital hypotonia (i.e., underdeveloped muscle tone) and lax joints (Lane et al., 2016; Tatton-Brown et al., 2019), which may delay motor skills in early development. These, together with rapid bone growth and delays in meeting developmental milestones, may lead to the diagnosis of Sotos or Sotos-like syndrome in early childhood.

IMPACT ON THE STUDENT AND OUTCOMES

Medical

Sotos syndrome is accompanied by various medical factors, and the extent to which these occur varies across individuals with the syndrome. Some of these are related to bone growth. For example, research suggests a relatively high incidence of scoliosis in individuals with Sotos, occurring in about 30% of *NSD1*-positive cases (Tatton-Brown et al., 2019). Although scoliosis cases are not usually severe enough to require a brace or surgical intervention, some treatments may be needed.

About 15% of individuals with an *NSD1* pathogenic variant also have anomalies of the kidneys and urinary system (Tatton-Brown et al., 2019). Upper respiratory problems are frequent, often leading to some degree of hearing loss. Seizures are found in nearly 50% of patients, with roughly half of these being febrile (Baujat & Cormier-Daire, 2007). Absence, tonic–clonic, myoclonic, and partial complex seizures all have been reported (Tatton-Brown et al., 2019). Sotos and other related syndromes often are associated with neoplasms; however, one study estimated malignancy risk to be lower than 2.2% (Baujat & Cormier-Daire, 2007).

Cognitive/Academic

The majority of individuals with Sotos syndrome present with an intellectual disability, ranging from mild to severe, and commonly display delays in expressive language and motor development during infancy (Baujat & Cormier-Daire, 2007; Lane, Van Herwegen, & Freeth, 2019; Mouridsen & Hansen, 2002). Although Sotos has been studied extensively within the medical field, considerably less attention has been directed toward the neuropsychological features of the syndrome (Mouridsen & Hansen, 2002; Sarimski, 2003). It should be noted that research around cognitive impairments related to Sotos syndrome reflect bias and imperfect research methodology (i.e., a reliance on case studies, lack of control groups), which affect the generalizability of the findings (Mouridsen & Hansen, 2002).

Learning disabilities and more general academic difficulties are common among those with Sotos syndrome as well (Lane, Milne, & Freeth, 2019). A systematic review of the literature suggests the common profile of an individual with Sotos syndrome includes relative strengths in verbal abilities and visuospatial memory and relative weaknesses in nonverbal reasoning abilities and quantitative reasoning (Lane, Milne, & Freeth, 2019).

Academically, studies have noted that most students require assistance with numeracy, with trends suggesting a greater ability in literacy after controlling for intelligence (Lane et al., 2016). On average, relative academic strengths may include reading, writing, and receptive and expressive language skills (Park et al., 2014; Sarimski, 2003).

Social-Emotional and Behavioral

Individuals with Sotos syndrome frequently experience several common social and behavioral characteristics. In school, students' difficulties with peer group relationships and lack of awareness of social cues are commonly observed. Other typical concerns include phobias, difficulty with social interactions, and aggressive tendencies (Lane et al., 2016).

Given these concerns, it is not surprising there is a high prevalence of symptomatology common to autism spectrum disorder (ASD) in individuals with Sotos syndrome, as well as attention-deficit/hyperactivity disorder and anxiety (Lane et al., 2016, 2017). In addition, children with Sotos syndrome may display difficulty with overall language structure and pragmatic language skills, restricted interests, and repetitive behaviors, a profile consistent with a diagnosis of ASD (Lane et al., 2017; Sheth et al., 2015). Social impairment emerges as a more marked characteristic of children with both Sotos and ASD as compared with other aspects of ASD-like repetitive behavior and difficulty with communication, although a preference for routine and repetitive language was found in one study (Sheth et al., 2015).

Children with Sotos have been found to display increased instances of phobias, separation anxiety, and generalized anxiety in new situations as compared with other same-aged children with intellectual disabilities, which may negatively affect social functioning (Rutter & Cole, 1991). Further, research has found that children with Sotos syndrome displayed an increased risk for self-injury and physical aggression as compared with other groups with intellectual disorder (Sheth et al., 2015). This finding is consistent with other research suggesting higher reported rates of tantrums and aggression in individuals with Sotos than in their typically developing same-aged peers (Lane et al., 2016). It should be noted that children with Sotos tend to be larger than their same-aged peers; therefore, their behavior may be perceived as more problematic and less age appropriate than it would be in children whose size is consistent with their chronological age (Lane et al., 2016). These associated challenges interfere with overall academic and social–emotional functioning as well as mental health (Sheth et al., 2015).

PSYCHOEDUCATIONAL IMPLICATIONS AND SCHOOL-BASED INTERVENTIONS

Medical and Health Management

Given the multitude of challenges these children may face, the coordinated efforts of medical professionals, parents, teachers, and specialists often are required in order to maximize the child's outcomes. As medical factors vary with each individual, medical treatment and intervention plans are created based on the assessed needs of a particular individual. Pediatric follow-ups and referrals to appropriate specialists are crucial during infancy to allow detection and management of possible clinical events or co-occurring conditions attributable to the syndrome (e.g., scoliosis, seizures, renal and cardiac anomalies) later in life. Early childhood interventions such as infant stimulation, occupational therapy, and adaptive physical education may help to mediate some of the physical challenges associated with the syndrome.

Those with Sotos often display hypotonia, which may delay motor skills in infants and young children (MedlinePlus, 2021). Physical and occupational therapies may be required within and/or outside of the school setting. Children with Sotos syndrome may need physical therapy to maximize mobility, treat scoliosis, and reduce the risk of later onset orthopedic problems (Tatton-Brown et al., 2019). Other physical challenges include those involving speech, language, and speech–motor coordination (MedlinePlus, 2021). For example, children with Sotos syndrome may have a stutter, a monotone voice, and/or problems with creating sounds. Speech therapy and intervention may be recommended to address these challenges. Schools can take part in treatment by fostering a structured environment where affected children are able to practice these skills with minimal distraction from others in the environment (Holla & Prasad, 2011).

Programs and therapies such as infant stimulation, occupational therapy, and adaptive physical education may prove necessary in early childhood to aid in overcoming motor function and speech delays. They may also play a significant role in the nurturing of a child (Baujat & Cormier-Daire, 2007). These programs can be integrated into the school setting, where teachers can provide further support when these problems present and interfere with the child's behavior, functioning, and learning. The medical team can work with parents and teachers to create appropriate methods for working with children with Sotos (Baujat & Cormier-Daire, 2007).

Cognitive/Academic

Individuals with Sotos syndrome show difficulties with learning, speech, and behavior, largely affecting the child's educational experience (Tatton-Brown et al., 2019). A psychologist often works closely with parents, teachers, and other members of the school team to develop appropriate and effective methods to accommodate the child's learning, behavioral, social, and emotional needs. Given the variability in overall cognitive abilities of those with Sotos syndrome, it is critical to assess the individual's strengths and weaknesses in order to design effective support plans that appropriately address individual needs (Varley & Crnic, 1984). Developmental screenings should be performed on a frequent basis to evaluate the presence and extent of intellectual, physical, and psychomotor delays or disabilities to help recommend the appropriate interventions (Institute of Medicine Committee on Nervous System Disorders in Developing Countries, 2001). To support children with Sotos syndrome academically, it is important to understand the cognitive profile common to the syndrome and to recognize individual differences. In addition to establishing the level of cognitive delay, it is important to consider language development. For many children with Sotos ages 3 to 5, developmental preschool through the local school district is recommended. Over time, information derived from ongoing assessments and interventions may be helpful in informing school-based modifications and emphasizing areas of strength through instructional methods (e.g., use of visuals, verbal prompts). As is critical to the success of all children with special needs, specialized academic programming should be based on the individual student's unique needs and abilities and should capitalize on the child's strengths in addressing challenges.

Social–Emotional and Behavioral

Assessment of social–emotional functioning for children with Sotos should also be included in a comprehensive evaluation. Compared with typically developing children, those with Sotos syndrome show higher rates of behavioral problems (Lane et al., 2016). Although a spectrum of behavioral disorders is associated with Sotos syndrome, some of the most common behavioral problems that have been reported in the literature include aggression, tantrums, anxiety, and attention-deficit/hyperactivity disorder and ASD symptomatology (Gajre et al., 2015; Lane et al., 2017). A variety of options may prove helpful in aiding these children's social and behavioral skills development. These include specialized academic instruction/programming and applied behavior analysis (ABA; Tatton-Brown et al., 2019). ABA strategies often are employed to reduce a range of maladaptive behaviors in children, including those with Sotos syndrome (Tatton-Brown et al., 2019). Research suggests that students demonstrate success when teachers utilize strategies based in ABA, such as prompting, fading, performance feedback, and generalization, not only in behavioral areas but also to improve reading, literacy, and mathematics (Solis et al., 2016; Zoder-Martell et al., 2016).

Intervention is not limited to behavioral or ABA approaches. In discussing future implications of his research, Sarimski (2003) suggested that counseling for children with Sotos syndrome should focus on social skills instruction and facilitating peer interactions. Further, researchers have suggested that families consider developing a close consultative relationship with a developmental pediatrician and potentially a pediatric psychiatrist for any significant social–emotional and behavioral concerns that may compromise the safety of the child (Tatton-Brown et al., 2019).

CONCLUSION

Sotos syndrome is a complex disorder that may present with myriad challenges across multiple domains. For many children with Sotos syndrome, the characteristic early developmental delays, intellectual impairment, and overgrowth can create adjustment difficulties and challenges that persist in the school setting. Although there is no standard course of treatment for Sotos syndrome, efforts are usually directed toward the specific symptoms and associated challenges. The complexity of Sotos syndrome emphasizes the importance of well-designed and thoughtful educational and therapeutic interventions as well as the coordinated efforts required to deliver these appropriately.

RESOURCES

Sotos Syndrome Support Association. (n.d.). *Awareness and understanding through education and support*. https://sotossyndrome.org/wp-content/uploads/SSSAbro_Apr.pdf

MedlinePlus. (2021). *Sotos syndrome*. National Library of Medicine. https://medlineplus.gov/genetics/condition/sotos-syndrome/

Lane, C., & Freeth, M. (2018). *Sotos syndrome: An educational guide*. Child Growth Foundation. https://childgrowthfoundation.org/wp-content/uploads/2018/07/Sotos-Syndrome-Educational-Guide.pdf

Genetic Education Materials for School Success. (2015). *Sotos syndrome*. New England Regional Genetics Network. https://www.negenetics.org/gemss/conditions/sotos-syndrome

REFERENCES

Albores-Gallo, L., Fritsche-García, L., Miranda-Aguirre, A. P., & Avila-Acosta, M. (2017). Brief report: Macrocephaly phenotype and psychiatric comorbidity in a clinical sample of Mexican children and adolescents with autism spectrum disorders. *Journal of Autism and Developmental Disorders, 47*(9), 2911–2917. https://doi.org/10.1007/s10803-017-3175-4

Baujat, G., & Cormier-Daire, V. (2007). Sotos syndrome. *Orphanet Journal of Rare Diseases, 2*(1), Article 36. https://doi.org/10.1186/1750-1172-2-36

Berdasco, M., Ropero, S., Setien, F., Fraga, M. F., Lapunzina, P., Losson, R., Alaminos, M., Cheung, N.-K., Rahman, N., & Esteller, M. (2009). Epigenetic inactivation of the Sotos overgrowth syndrome gene histone methyltransferase *NSD1* in human neuroblastoma and glioma. *Proceedings of the National Academy of Sciences, 106*(51), 21830–21835. https://doi.org/10.1073/pnas.0906831106

Berry-Kravis, E., Myers, K., & Roizen, N. J. (2019). Down syndrome and fragile X syndrome. In M. L. Batshaw, N. J. Roizen & L. Pellegrino (Eds.), *Children with disabilities* (7th ed., pp. 265–284). Brookes.

Gajre, M. P., Mhatre, P., & Vijaykumar, R. (2015). Sotos syndrome with developmental co-ordination disorder; report of a case. *Journal of Taibah University Medical Sciences, 10*(2), 234–237. https://doi.org/10.1016/j.jtumed.2014.05.007

Holla, R. G., & Prasad, A. N. (2011). Sotos syndrome. *Medical Journal Armed Forces India, 67*(3), 288–290. https://doi.org/10.1016/S0377-1237(11)60067-1

Institute of Medicine Committee on Nervous System Disorders in Developing Countries. (2001). *Neurological, psychiatric, and developmental disorders: Meeting the challenge in the developing world*. National Academy Press. https://doi.org/10.17226/10111

Jaju, R. J., Fidler, C., Haas, O. A., Strickson, A. J., Watkins, F., Clark, K., Cross, N. C. P., Cheng, J.-F., Aplan, P. D., Kearney, L., Boutlwood, J., & Wainscoat, J. S. (2001). A novel gene, *NSD1*, is fused to *NUP98* in the t(5;11)(q35;p15.5) in de novo childhood acute myeloid leukemia. *Blood, 98*(4), 1264–1267. https://doi.org/10.1182/blood.V98.4.1264

Lane, C., Milne, E., & Freeth, M. (2016). Cognition and behaviour in Sotos syndrome: A systematic review. *PLOS ONE, 11*(2), Article e0149189. https://doi.org/10.1371/journal.pone.0149189

Lane, C., Milne, E., & Freeth, M. (2017). Characteristics of autism spectrum disorder in Sotos syndrome. *Journal of Autism and Developmental Disorders, 47*(1), 135–143. https://doi.org/10.1007/s10803-016-2941-z

Lane, C., Milne, E., & Freeth, M. (2019). The cognitive profile of Sotos syndrome. *Journal of Neuropsychology, 13*(2), 240–252. https://doi.org/10.1111/jnp.12146

Lane, C., Van Herwegen, J., & Freeth, M. (2019). Parent-reported communication abilities of children with Sotos syndrome: Evidence from the Children's Communication Checklist-2. *Journal of Autism and Developmental Disorders, 49*(4), 1475–1483. https://doi.org/10.1007/s10803-018-3842-0

MedlinePlus. (2021). *Sotos syndrome*. National Library of Medicine. https://medlineplus.gov/genetics/condition/sotos-syndrome/

Mouridsen, S. E., & Hansen, M. B. (2002). Neuropsychiatric aspects of Sotos syndrome: A review and two case illustrations. *European Child & Adolescent Psychiatry, 11*(1), 43–48. https://doi.org/10.1007/s007870200007

Park, S. H., Lee, J. E., Sohn, Y. B., & Ko, J. M. (2014). First identified Korean family with Sotos syndrome caused by a novel intragenic mutation in *NSD1*. *Annals of Clinical and Laboratory Science, 44*(2), 228–231. https://pubmed.ncbi.nlm.nih.gov/24795065/

Rutter, S. C., & Cole, T. R. P. (1991). Psychological characteristics of Sotos syndrome. *Developmental Medicine and Child Neurology, 33*(10), 898–902. https://doi.org/10.1111/j.1469-8749.1991.tb14799.x

Sarimski, K. (2003). Behavioural and emotional characteristics in children with Sotos syndrome and learning disabilities. *Developmental Medicine and Child Neurology, 45*(3), 172–178. https://doi.org/10.1111/j.1469-8749.2003.tb00926.x

Sheth, K., Moss, J., Hyland, S., Stinton, C., Cole, T., & Oliver, C. (2015). The behavioral characteristics of Sotos syndrome. *American Journal of Medical Genetics: Part A, 167*(12), 2945–2956. https://doi.org/10.1002/ajmg.a.37373

Solis, M., El Zein, F., Vaughn, S., McCulley, L. V., & Falcomata, T. S. (2016). Reading comprehension interventions for students with autism spectrum disorders: An alternating treatments comparison. *Focus on Autism and Other Developmental Disabilities, 31*(4), 284–299. https://doi.org/10.1177/1088357615583464

Tatton-Brown, K., Cole, T. R., & Rahman, N. (2019). Sotos syndrome. In M. P. Adam, D. B. Everman, G. M. Mirzaa, et al. (Eds.), *GeneReviews*. University of Washington. https://www.ncbi.nlm.nih.gov/books/NBK1479/

Varley, C. K., & Crnic, K. (1984). Emotional, behavioral, and cognitive status of children with cerebral gigantism. *Journal of Developmental and Behavioral Pediatrics, 5*(3), 132–134. https://doi.org/10.1097/00004703-198406000-00006

Waggoner, D. J., Raca, G., Welch, K., Dempsey, M., Anderes, E., Ostrovnaya, I., Alkhateeb, A., Kamimura, J., Matsumoto, N., Schaeffer, G. B., Martin, C. L., & Das, S. (2005). *NSD1* analysis for Sotos syndrome: Insights and perspectives from the clinical laboratory. *Genetics in Medicine, 7*(8), 524–533. https://doi.org/10.1097/01.GIM.0000178503.15559.d3

Zoder-Martell, K. A., Dieringer, S. T., & Dufrene, B. A. (2016). Introduction to the special issue: The use of applied behavioral analysis to address student academic referral concerns. *Psychology in the Schools, 53*(1), 5–7. https://doi.org/10.1002/pits.21882

VIII

MIXED/MULTISYSTEM DISORDERS

53

Overview of Mixed/ Multisystem Disorders

Cynthia A. Riccio

Mixed/multisystem disorders, as might be apparent from that label, are disorders that present and impact functioning across biological systems. These disorders are most often inherited and have differential and heterogeneous effects on the individuals affected. Each of the chapters in this part is concerned with a specific disorder or group of disorders. The overview here highlights what is known about each, with more information and details available in the specific chapters. A key finding across all of these is the variability in presentation necessitating that treatment be based on the signs and symptoms present in each individual.

BODY SYSTEM INVOLVEMENT AND FUNCTIONING

The multiple systems involved vary depending on the disorder. For each of the disorders or cluster of disorders in this section, two or more of the systems discussed in previous sections (i.e., the cardiac and circulatory system, the central nervous system [CNS], the digestive system, the endocrine and reproductive system, the respiratory system, and the musculoskeletal system) are affected. For example, with CHARGE syndrome, CNS effects specific to the visual system as well as the auditory system are frequent, as well as cardiac defects and alterations to growth and development. Another example would be fragile X syndrome, with CNS effects evident in high frequencies of seizure disorders, digestive issues, ocular defects, and visual problems. The structures and systems involved are

https://doi.org/10.1037/0000349-053
Health-Related Disorders in Children and Adolescents: A Guidebook for Educators and Service Providers, Second Edition, M. M. Perfect, C. A. Riccio, and M. A. Bray (Editors)

described in the respective chapters. The extent to which each system is affected is driven by the genetic transmission of the disorder or genetic anomaly.

COMMON COMPLAINTS AND INDICATORS OF DYSFUNCTION

Many of these conditions, with the exception of pediatric cancer, have associated distinctive facial characteristics, and the children affected are often identified at birth. Health conditions, including cardiac defects, may also be evident at birth and warrant medical intervention. Less immediately obvious are the effects on physical, cognitive, and social–emotional development, with mild to more severe delays in growth and effects on cognition and behavior. For those children not identified at birth, delays in meeting language, social, and motor milestones may become evident in early childhood, most often before they enter kindergarten. In milder cases, the impacts on cognitive/academic and social/behavioral functioning will warrant school-based intervention.

PREVIEW OF MULTIPLE BODY SYSTEMS DISORDERS AND SPECIALTIES IN PEDIATRICS

CHARGE Syndrome

Hartshorne and Slavin (Chapter 54) share the research and evidence base on *CHARGE syndrome*. The letters of the name identify the congenital features evident at birth and provide insight into the multiple systems that may be affected. For example, the failure of fissures in the eye to close (coloboma of the eye) is observable at birth, as are some heart defects. With multiple systems affected, integrated behavioral health could include pediatric specialists in ear/nose/throat disorders, cardiology, audiology, ophthalmology, and urology, as well as professionals to deal with the developmental issues and parent concerns.

Cornelia de Lange Syndrome

Cornelia de Lange syndrome is another developmental disorder affecting multiple systems to varying degrees. The severity of the condition and the associated signs and symptoms can vary widely but may include distinctive facial characteristics, growth delays, intellectual disability, and limb defects. Jimenez and Riccio (Chapter 55) discuss the immediate signs and symptoms of Cornelia de Lange syndrome that most often lead to diagnosis (Deardorff et al., 2016), as well as the prognosis and supports needed.

Fragile X Syndrome

Although *fragile X syndrome* is classified as an intellectual disability disorder by the American Academy of Pediatrics, it is also associated with seizure disorders, connective tissue abnormalities, and gastrointestinal problems (Kidd et al., 2014). The extent to which problems present depends on the extent to which the gene involved is compromised and the sex of the child. The variations of fragile X are covered in Chapter 56 by Theodore et al. In addition to medical issues associated with fragile X, many with the syndrome have intellectual disability, some with milder effects, and female individuals may evidence specific learning disabilities. Further complicating development of individuals with this syndrome, the child may exhibit significant behavioral and emotional problems.

Lysosomal Storage Disorders

Lysosomal storage disorders are a group of disorders that can affect multiple body organs, including the brain, bones, and muscle. Lysosomes carry the enzymes in cells that break down lipids and sugars to help cells function. The resulting damage can affect multiple body organs, including the brain, bones, and muscle. There are a vast number of lysosomal storage disorders with genetic transmission. The most common of these include Fabry disease, Gaucher disease, Niemann–Pick disease, Pompe disease, Tay–Sachs disease, and the mucopolysaccharidosis diseases. Symptoms vary depending on the specific enzymes missing and the systems and organs affected. Fairchild and Islas provide an overview of all but mucopolysaccharidosis in Chapter 57, as well as the medical, educational, and behavior correlates and supports needed.

Mucopolysaccharidosis Diseases

With *mucopolysaccharidosis diseases,* one or more of the 11 enzymes needed to break down mucopolysaccharides, a specific group of lysosomes called glycosaminoglycans are either absent or not functioning properly. This condition is inherited with variations based on the specific enzymes affected. Because these lysosomes are involved in bone, tendons, cartilage, the corneas of the eye, connective tissue, and lubrication of joints, multiple systems are affected (National Institute of Neurological Disorders and Stroke, 2022). Further, as levels increase over time (i.e., reach toxic levels), there are potential effects on organ and system functioning, including brain development and function. Tureaud et al. (Chapter 58) provide more detail regarding the mechanism of inheritance and the symptoms that lead to diagnosis, as well as the cognitive, educational, and social–emotional correlates of this group of disorders. They also provide information on evidence-based treatments and resources for mental health practitioners involved in providing support.

Neurocutaneous Disorders

Neurocutaneous disorders include a constellation of multisystem disorders associated with both cutaneous and CNS lesions (Ullrich, 2016). The most common features of those under the neurocutaneous syndrome label include hereditary or genetic origin; involvement of the nervous system, skin, and visual system; and progressive evolution of lesions in childhood and adolescence, as well as disorganized tissue or malformations (i.e., hamartomas) and a tendency for malignant transformations. Many, but not all, neurocutaneous disorders are associated with brain tumors, including neurofibromatosis, tuberous sclerosis complex, and Von Hippel Landau disease.

There are many neurocutaneous disorders. The most common are neurofibromatosis (Perdue et al.; Chapter 59), Sturge–Weber syndrome (Jimenez & Hynd; Chapter 62), and tuberous sclerosis (Riccio & Sun; Chapter 63). In the disorders covered in these individual chapters, and likely common across other neurocutaneous disorders, the impact of the disorder is multifaceted and idiosyncratic depending on the extent of the visible markings or stigmata as well as the underlying locations of the tumors—or in the case of tuberous sclerosis, the tubers—which can affect any part of the CNS and its function.

Pediatric Cancer

Pediatric cancer is the result of the rapid growth and multiplication of abnormal cells in the body. Other than leukemia (see Chapter 5 by Theodore et al.), the most common childhood cancers are lymphoma; brain, bone, and kidney cancers; and cancer of the nerve cells. The invasion of malignant cells destroys the body's healthy tissue and may affect other organs and tissues, thus affecting multiple systems. Because initial symptoms are often attributed to benign causes, the diagnosis is often delayed. Not only the disease itself but the medical interventions (e.g., radiation, chemotherapy, loss of a limb) as well can have an impact on the child and their family. In Chapter 60, Theodore et al. review the issues associated with pediatric cancer and the subsequent effect not only on physical well-being but also on cognitive and academic functioning and social–emotional/behavioral outcomes.

Smith–Magenis Syndrome

Smith–Magenis syndrome is a chromosome deletion syndrome (i.e., some part of 17-p is missing) that affects the production of a key gene and protein needed for activation of other genes, particularly those associated with circadian rhythms. Although it is not clearly understood how this one gene and the protein affect other systems, individuals with Smith–Magenis syndrome present not only with sleep disturbance but also with specific facial characteristics, short stature, vision and hearing problems, and curvature of the spine. Developmental delays and mild to moderate intellectual disability are also common. Van Haneghan et al. (Chapter 61) review the signs, symptoms, and progression from perspectives of medical issues, educational problems, behavioral/social–emotional outcomes, and needed supports.

HEALTH CARE NEEDS AND MEDICAL SPECIALTIES

The need for individualized planning to meet the needs of those with these and any other disorders that impact multiple body systems is critical. With multiple systems affected and interactions among physical health, cognitive/educational outcome, and social–emotional/behavioral issues, a team of integrated behavioral health service providers is needed. At the very least, the primary care physician and any specialists currently working with the child need to be involved in care and support planning. At the same time, service providers in the community (e.g., physical therapy, occupational therapy, respiratory therapy, family therapy and parent services) may be needed, as many school districts lack sufficient resources to address the needs of these students and their families. Educators, counselors, and mental health professionals need to be involved to ensure and provide needed educational and social–emotional support within the school setting.

REFERENCES

Deardorff, M. A., Clark, D. M., & Krantz, I. D. (2016). Cornelia de Lange syndrome. In M. P. Adam, D. B. Everman, G. M. Mirzaa, et al. (Eds.), *GeneReviews*. University of Washington, Seattle. http://www.ncbi.nlm.nih.gov/books/NBK1104

Kidd, S. A., Lachiewicz, A., Barbouth, D., Blitz, R. K., Delahunty, C., McBrien, D., Visootsak, J., & Berry-Kravis, E. (2014). Fragile X syndrome: A review of associated medical problems. *Pediatrics, 134*(5), 995–1005. https://doi.org/10.1542/peds.2013-4301

National Institute of Neurological Disorders and Stroke. (2022, July 25). *Mucopolysaccharidoses fact sheet*. National Institutes of Health. https://www.ninds.nih.gov/health-information/disorders/mucopolysaccharidoses

Ullrich, N. J. (2016). Neurocutaneous syndromes and brain tumors. *Journal of Child Neurology, 31*(12), 1399–1411. https://doi.org/10.1177/0883073815604220

54

CHARGE Syndrome

Timothy S. Hartshorne and Lillian J. Slavin

CHARGE is an acronym suggested by a team of geneticists in 1980 (Pagon et al., 1981). Each letter stands for an anomaly initially identified as characteristic of the syndrome: C—coloboma (missing piece) of the eye, H—heart defects, A—atresia of the choana (passages in the back of the nose), R—restriction in growth and/or development, G—genital hypoplasia, and E—ear anomalies including shape and function.

ETIOLOGY

In the majority of cases, CHARGE syndrome is caused by an autosomal dominant mutation to the chromodomain helicase DNA binding protein 7 (*CHD7*) gene on the long arm of chromosome 8. In most cases, this is by de novo, or spontaneous, mutation, meaning the parents do not carry the mutation. If one parent does, there is a 50% chance their offspring will have CHARGE. Prior to the identification of the gene in 2004, CHARGE was known as an association because the typical anomalies occurred more often than by chance but a cause had not been identified (Hefner, 2021). Approximately 70% of clinically diagnosed patients with CHARGE test positive for the *CHD7* mutation.

Funding: This research did not receive any funding from agencies in the public, commercial, or not-for-profit sectors.

https://doi.org/10.1037/0000349-054
Health-Related Disorders in Children and Adolescents: A Guidebook for Educators and Service Providers, Second Edition, M. M. Perfect, C. A. Riccio, and M. A. Bray (Editors)

PREVALENCE AND INCIDENCE

The prevalence of CHARGE is estimated by various studies to be one in 8,500 to 35,000. A study in the Netherlands where, because of its small size, virtually every child in the country can be identified, found an incidence of one in 15,000 to 17,000 (Janssen et al., 2012). There does not appear to be a difference in male/female ratio or differences between countries of origin. Survival can be challenging during the first 4 years of life, but after that life expectancy is likely near normal (Hefner & Fassi, 2017).

SYMPTOMS

The clinical diagnosis of CHARGE has been refined several times, generally in terms of major and minor characteristics (Hale et al., 2016). Of importance are the sensory organs and systems, as it is common that individuals have deficient sight, hearing, smell, taste, touch, balance, and proprioception. Neurological findings include hypoplastic or missing semicircular canals in the inner ear and cerebellum differences. The prefrontal cortex also may be affected, per executive dysfunction challenges (T. S. Hartshorne et al., 2007). Gastrointestinal problems, particularly with swallow and motility issues, can be serious (Blake & Hudson, 2017).

CHARGE is a highly variable phenotype. It is hard to describe typical CHARGE symptoms or outcomes. One individual might graduate from college, and another might require 24/7 care. Each of the anomalies can vary as well, such that one person might have virtually no hearing in one ear but much more in the other, another person may have near normal hearing, and yet another is totally deaf in both ears.

IMPACT ON THE STUDENT AND OUTCOMES

Early intervention is essential for optimal growth and development. Medical issues need to be addressed as early as possible. Attention to cognitive and social/emotional development will lead to better outcomes.

Medical

The major medical issues that lead to mortality are heart malformations and gastrointestinal issues. Nearly every kind of heart malformation can be found in CHARGE, but as in every issue, not every person with CHARGE has a heart problem (Thangappan et al., 2021). The entire gastrointestinal process can be affected, from an unsafe swallow to constipation. Slow motility is common (Blake & Hudson, 2017). Individuals with CHARGE are extremely medically complicated; they frequently experience illness and difficulties related to otology, rhinology, breathing, feeding, sleeping, neurodevelopment, endocrinology, the heart, the musculoskeletal system, and the immune system (T. S. Hartshorne et al., 2021).

Cognitive/Academic

Individuals with CHARGE commonly experience developmental delays across numerous areas (e.g., social skills, adaptive behavior, cognition), which are thought to be secondary to the sensory and medical impairments present at birth (Salem-Hartshorne & Jacob, 2005). Many children with CHARGE stay academically on level until around third or fourth grade, when the tasks become more abstract and conceptual. Some continue to do well through college and even graduate school. Others will need special education support.

Social-Emotional and Behavioral

Socially, most children with CHARGE are very motivated for contact with others but develop social skills very slowly (T. S. Hartshorne, 2021). The sensory impairments can be a major factor in this, and sometimes other children will avoid a peer with obvious physical impairments. Many young adults report problems finding and maintaining friendships, along with challenges in finding employment.

A behavioral phenotype has been suggested that includes low normal intelligence, goal-directed behavior, social interest but with immature social skills, repetitive behaviors, sensation seeking, and problems with self-regulation and shifting attention (T. S. Hartshorne et al., 2017). Behavioral problems are not inevitable but are very common. In addition to sleep problems, aggression, tactile defensiveness, and anxiety, including obsessions, sensory issues have been identified as an interference with quality of life for adolescents and adults with CHARGE (N. Hartshorne et al., 2016).

PSYCHOEDUCATIONAL IMPLICATIONS AND SCHOOL-BASED INTERVENTIONS

As with everything else, there is a wide disparity among children with CHARGE and their academic performance, with sensory impairments being a major contributor.

Medical and Health Management

As CHARGE can affect every sensory system and is associated with significant medical, communicative, social, motor, and behavioral difficulties, a multidisciplinary team approach is needed to adequately address medical and psychoeducational needs across settings. It is recommended that educational team members collaborate with medical professionals to fully understand the needs of each individual, as it is their responsibility to manage medical complications at school. Further, educational team members must understand the severity of medical issues and that they will always take precedence over educational considerations. Additionally, challenging behavior exhibited at school—and at home—should be considered to have a medical component. Medical complications, especially those that create pain (e.g., ear infection, impacted tooth), should be ruled out in the presence of sudden, atypical behavior prior to attempting to alter the behavior using another methodology.

Cognitive/Academic

Due to the complexity of CHARGE, it can sometimes be challenging for school teams to view the student as a whole rather than the sum of their symptoms. One method of helping school teams understand the student is to develop a personal passport (Brown, 2004), which is a document that outlines who the individual is, their likes and dislikes, their method of communication, and their goals. As parents are the experts on their child, they should be treated as equal team members and should be pivotal in the development of the personal passport—and any individualized education program or transition plan.

In addition to viewing the student holistically, school teams must understand that individuals with CHARGE are often truly multiply sensory impaired. Such sensory impairment profoundly affects the way these students can access information from their environments. A top priority of educational teams should be to ensure individuals with CHARGE are presented material through multiple sensory pathways, particularly those that the individual prefers. In order to understand how the individual best accesses sensory information, functional hearing and vision assessments should be conducted. Information gained by the occupational therapist and physical therapist should also be considered. This sensory profile of the individual will assist the team in structuring the individual's environment.

Vision loss can be addressed through numerous environmental accommodations (e.g., large print, braille, angled work surface, consideration of lighting, minimizing visual clutter). Hearing loss can be addressed via assistive technology (e.g., amplification system, hearing aids), medical interventions (e.g., cochlear implant, bone-anchored hearing aids), environmental accommodations (e.g., minimizing unnecessary auditory information), and teaching sign language. Residual vision and hearing will be maximized by the minimization of visual and auditory distractions in educational materials and the classroom. Vestibular and proprioceptive issues can be addressed by providing ample opportunities for movement, stimulating the vestibular and proprioceptive systems (e.g., rocking, swinging, deep pressure), and providing seating accommodations that reduce the effort required by the individual to maintain an appropriate posture (e.g., lying on side, chairs with arms). For elaboration on suggestions to address sensory needs of individuals with

CHARGE in schools, see Griffin et al. (2004), Lewis and Lowther (2001), and Smith et al. (2010).

Because individuals with CHARGE receive reduced information from their environment through their sensory systems and spend the first several years of their lives in and out of the hospital, they miss opportunities to learn and develop that their typically developing peers receive automatically. It is important that these delays be seen as such: *delays*. Individuals with CHARGE have a great capacity to learn and develop when provided with appropriate access to their environment and the opportunity to learn directly (Smith et al., 2010). They should be taught concepts explicitly utilizing multiple sensory channels whenever possible. The potential of individuals with CHARGE should never be underestimated. When they are challenged, their growth and learning can be significant.

Communication can be very challenging given their multiple sensory impairments and structural abnormalities (e.g., choanal atresia, cleft lip). Often, behavior is their method of communication, especially as they are initially developing their communicative abilities. Thus, behavior should always be interpreted as communication (Griffin et al., 2004; Smith et al., 2010). Professionals working with individuals with CHARGE should attempt to understand the behavior and what it could be communicating, especially pain behaviors. However, simply learning behavioral cues is not sufficient in terms of establishing effective communication. *Total communication* is the most frequently recommended tool for developing functional communication in individuals with CHARGE (Griffin et al., 2004; Lewis & Lowther, 2001; Smith et al., 2010). The goal of total communication is to create as many strategies for communication as possible for the child. Thus, numerous avenues for communication should be made available (e.g., oral language, sign language, gestures, pictures, touch and object cues, calendar systems).

Social-Emotional and Behavioral

With limited options to communicate with those around them, individuals with CHARGE are often left with no choice but to communicate their wants and needs via their behavior. The major sources of problem behavior in individuals with CHARGE are believed to be pain, sensory issues, and anxiety (T. S. Hartshorne et al., 2017). Whenever an individual with CHARGE is exhibiting problematic behavior, professionals should first consider if the behavior is truly problematic (i.e., not simply annoying), try to ascertain what the individual is attempting to communicate with their behavior, and then try to address the behavior.

Recognizing behavior as adaptive, communicative, and/or responsive to internal states does not change the sometimes-challenging ways in which the behavior is exhibited: Self-stimulatory behavior, maladaptive routines, tics, and obsessive-compulsive behavior are just a few common examples (Smith et al., 2010). However, behavior should not be changed without giving the individual another way of communicating the same want or need or addressing the source of the complaint. In addressing the three main sources of problem behavior, professionals should rule out pain/medical complications, provide consistent sensory input using suggestions found in the previous section, and attempt to reduce anxiety. One prominent method of reducing anxiety in individuals with CHARGE is developing a comprehensive, individualized, daily calendar system (T. S. Hartshorne et al., 2017). Such a calendar system helps individuals anticipate and plan their day, as well as build their receptive and expressive communication.

CONCLUSION

Individuals with CHARGE present with a complex clinical profile, which can be challenging to accommodate in a medical or educational setting. Medical and educational professionals should collaborate whenever possible to ensure consistent treatment across settings and promote a deeper understanding of the individual. A collaborative multidisciplinary team approach to service provision is essential for improving outcomes.

RESOURCES

CHARGE Syndrome Foundation. (n.d.). *Education professional packet.* https://www.chargesyndrome.org/for-professionals/education-professional-packet/

Sense. (n.d.). *CHARGE syndrome.* https://www.sense.org.uk/get-support/information-and-advice/conditions/charge-syndrome/

Hefner, M., & Davenport, S. (2002). *Management manual for parents.* CHARGE Syndrome Foundation. https://www.chargesyndrome.org/for-families/resources/publications/management-manual-for-parents/

CHARGE Syndrome Foundation. https://www.chargesyndrome.org/

National Center on Deaf-Blindness. https://nationaldb.org/

Ward, C., & Patterson, M. (2011). *Why I am me: All about CHARGE syndrome.* CHARGE Syndrome Australia. https://www.chargesyndrome.org.au/store/why-i-am-me/

REFERENCES

Blake, K. D., & Hudson, A. S. (2017). Gastrointestinal and feeding difficulties in CHARGE syndrome: A review from head-to-toe. *American Journal of Medical Genetics: Part C, Seminars in Medical Genetics, 175*(4), 496–506. https://doi.org/10.1002/ajmg.c.31586

Brown, D. M. (2004). "Knowing the child"—Personal passports. *California Deafblind Services reSources, 11*(4). http://www.cadbs.org/newsletter/

Griffin, H. C., Davis, M. L., & Williams, S. C. (2004). CHARGE syndrome: Educational and technological interventions. *RE:view, 35*(4), 149–158.

Hale, C. L., Niederriter, A. N., Green, G. E., & Martin, D. M. (2016). Atypical phenotypes associated with pathogenic CHD7 variants and a proposal for broadening

CHARGE syndrome clinical diagnostic criteria. *American Journal of Medical Genetics: Part A, 170*(2), 344–354. https://doi.org/10.1002/ajmg.a.37435

Hartshorne, N., Hudson, A., MacCuspie, J., Kennert, B., Nacarato, T., Hartshorne, T., & Blake, K. (2016). Quality of life in adolescents and adults with CHARGE syndrome. *American Journal of Medical Genetics: Part A, 170*(8), 2012–2021. https://doi.org/10.1002/ajmg.a.37769

Hartshorne, T. S. (2021). Behavior in CHARGE syndrome. In T. S. Hartshorne, M. A. Hefner, & K. D. Blake (Eds.), *CHARGE syndrome* (2nd ed., pp. 413–424). Plural Publishing.

Hartshorne, T. S., Hefner, M. A., & Blake, K. D. (Eds.). (2021). *CHARGE syndrome* (2nd ed.). Plural Publishing.

Hartshorne, T. S., Nicholas, J., Grialou, T. L., & Russ, J. M. (2007). Executive function in CHARGE syndrome. *Child Neuropsychology, 13*(4), 333–344. https://doi.org/10.1080/09297040600850944

Hartshorne, T. S., Stratton, K. K., Brown, D., Madhavan-Brown, S., & Schmittel, M. C. (2017). Behavior in CHARGE syndrome. *American Journal of Medical Genetics: Part C, Seminars in Medical Genetics, 175*(4), 431–438. https://doi.org/10.1002/ajmg.c.31588

Hefner, M. A. (2021). Introduction. In T. S. Hartshorne, M. A. Hefner, & K. D. Blake (Eds.), *CHARGE syndrome* (2nd ed., pp. xi–xv). Plural Publishing.

Hefner, M. A., & Fassi, E. (2017). Genetic counseling in CHARGE syndrome: Diagnostic evaluation through follow up. *American Journal of Medical Genetics: Part C, Seminars in Medical Genetics, 175*(4), 407–416. https://doi.org/10.1002/ajmg.c.31589

Janssen, N., Bergman, J. E. H., Swertz, M. A., Tranebjaerg, L., Lodahl, M., Schoots, J., Hofstra, R. M., van Ravenswaaij-Arts, C. M., & Hoefsloot, L. H. (2012). Mutation update on the *CHD7* gene involved in CHARGE syndrome. *Human Mutation, 33*(8), 1149–1160. https://doi.org/10.1002/humu.22086

Lewis, C., & Lowther, J. (2001). CHARGE association: Symptoms, behaviour and intervention. *Educational Psychology in Practice, 17*(1), 69–77. https://doi.org/10.1080/02667360120039997

Pagon, R. A., Graham, J. M., Jr., Zonana, J., & Yong, S. L. (1981). Coloboma, congenital heart disease, and choanal atresia with multiple anomalies: CHARGE association. *The Journal of Pediatrics, 99*(2), 223–227. https://doi.org/10.1016/S0022-3476(81)80454-4

Salem-Hartshorne, N., & Jacob, S. (2005). Adaptive behavior in children with CHARGE syndrome. *American Journal of Medical Genetics: Part A, 133A*(3), 262–267. https://doi.org/10.1002/ajmg.a.30546

Smith, K. G., Smith, I. M., & Blake, K. (2010). CHARGE syndrome: An educators' primer. *Education & Treatment of Children, 33*(2), 289–314. https://doi.org/10.1353/etc.0.0093

Thangappan, K., Hatton, A., & Morales, D. L. S. (2021). Cardiovascular system in CHARGE. In T. S. Hartshorne, M. A. Hefner, & K. D. Blake (Eds.), *CHARGE syndrome* (2nd ed., pp. 175–185). Plural Publishing.

55

Cornelia de Lange Syndrome

Emily M. Jimenez and Cynthia A. Riccio

Cornelia de Lange syndrome (CdLS) is a complex malformation syndrome, initially termed Brachmann–de Lange syndrome, first identified by Brachmann in 1916 and later again by Cornelia de Lange in 1933 (Boyle et al., 2015). It is now recognized as one of the cohesinopathies (Barbero, 2013; Dorsett & Ström, 2012). CdLS is a heterogeneous condition with multiple congenital anomalies and a large range of associated symptoms that are physical, behavioral, and cognitive in nature (Ajmone et al., 2014). The severity of each of these symptom categories varies according to the individual and genes affected, ranging from mild to severe.

ETIOLOGY

CdLS is the result of genetic mutations, with 65% of individuals with CdLS diagnosis having a mutation in one of the cohesin complex-associated genes (*NIPBL*, *SMC1A*, *SMC3*, *RAD21*, or *HDAC8*; Ajmone et al., 2014). CdLS has an autosomal dominant or X-linked method of inheritance; however, in many cases, the mutation is spontaneous (i.e., there is no family history; Genetic and Rare Diseases Information Center, 2021). All the mutations affect proteins or enzymes of the cohesion pathway, which is involved in chromosome segregation, DNA repair, and gene regulation (Barbero, 2013).

https://doi.org/10.1037/0000349-055
Health-Related Disorders in Children and Adolescents: A Guidebook for Educators and Service Providers, Second Edition, M. M. Perfect, C. A. Riccio, and M. A. Bray (Editors)

PREVALENCE AND INCIDENCE

CdLS is rare in occurrence, with the current estimate for prevalence at one in 10,000 to 30,000 births (Ajmone et al., 2014; MedlinePlus, 2022); however, others report it at 0.5 to 10 in 100,000 (Boyle et al., 2015). The condition may be underdiagnosed or misdiagnosed if symptom presentation is mild or the combination of symptoms is unable to be attributed to CdLS (Boyle et al., 2015).

SYMPTOMS

The most recognizable symptoms of CdLS are usually the dysmorphic facial features (i.e., arched eyebrows, long and curly eyelashes, eyelid drooping, thick and posteriorly rotated ears, flattened midface, thin upper lip). Excessive hair growth, cleft palate (an opening in the roof of the mouth), dental anomalies, seizures, heart problems, hearing, and vision problems may also be present (Basile et al., 2007; Boyle et al., 2015; Mulder et al., 2017). Additional physical abnormalities also may include microcephaly (smaller than average head size), shortened arms, reduced hand size, or other defects of the upper body (Ajmone et al., 2014). Thus, there are multiple phenotypes of CdLS.

IMPACT ON THE STUDENT AND OUTCOMES

Medical

Gastrointestinal and renal problems are frequently associated with CdLS and can result in frequent hospital stays throughout the child's life (Bull et al., 1993). Further, 20% of those with CdLS develop epilepsy. Common physical characteristics requiring clinical involvement include delay in growth pre- and postnatally, as well as musculoskeletal malformations, most frequently occurring as reduced limb size (Basile et al., 2007). Additional orthopedic complications include incomplete elbow extension, hip dysplasia, scoliosis, and early onset of osteoporosis (Jackson et al., 1993). Dysmorphic facial features may require medical or surgical intervention early in the child's life, depending on the severity. In addition, hearing loss occurs in a majority of individuals with CdLS. Lastly, individuals born with a cleft palate (an opening in the roof of the mouth), seizure presentation, heart problems, and vision problems all usually require medical intervention (Boyle et al., 2015).

Cognitive/Academic

Many individuals with CdLS present with intellectual disabilities, generally ranging from moderate to profound intellectual impairment (Ajmone et al., 2014); however, cases of CdLS with normal intellectual ability have been cited in the literature (e.g., Ajmone et al., 2014; Basile et al., 2007; Boyle et al., 2015).

The area of functioning most often impaired is communication (Sarimski, 2002), which is considered a critical area for these children developmentally (Ajmone et al., 2014). Both verbal and nonverbal speech and communication problems have been identified in individuals with a CdLS diagnosis, with 44% to 53% of patients significantly delayed for speech when younger, 61% to 67% of whom are described as limited talkers and 33% as fully nonverbal (Goodban, 1993).

Social-Emotional and Behavioral

Despite the communication deficits, most children with CdLS do not evidence social impairments; however, some may be diagnosed with autism spectrum disorder when repetitive, restricted behavior is present (Bell et al., 2018; Oliver et al., 2008). Other typical behavioral issues associated with CdLS include hyperactivity, aggression, attention problems, compulsions, and social anxiety (Basile et al., 2007; Moss et al., 2008; Sloneem et al., 2009). The physical features associated with CdLS can cause social anxiety concerns later on in adolescence (Nelson et al., 2017; Oliver et al., 2008). Self-injurious behavior may also be present and may take the form of self-biting, head banging, pulling out hair, and so on, often in conjunction with increased gastrointestinal problems or pain from other associated disorders if the individual is nonverbal and unable to express this discomfort in other ways (Sloneem et al., 2009).

PSYCHOEDUCATIONAL IMPLICATIONS AND SCHOOL-BASED INTERVENTIONS

Medical and Health Management

With significant medical conditions, as well as musculoskeletal problems, integrated care with monitoring of physical status is important. Medical management often occurs in response to symptoms, and it is recommended that identification of potential issues be investigated at the time of diagnosis and monitored thereafter (Kline et al., 2007). This monitoring of symptoms can also occur in the schools by school professionals in order to best inform the medical team of what behaviors and symptoms look like in a natural setting. The severity of the symptoms may affect the child's stamina, ability to form social relations with peers, and ability to attenuate to classroom material in a highly stimulating environment.

Cognitive/Academic

Communication is likely an area that will require intervention in the classroom setting for these children. Pragmatic interventions for developmental language disorder focus on grammar and vocabulary (Jensen de López et al., 2022). The most appropriate intervention for a given child depends on their baseline functioning. Another suggestion is for the implementation of augmentative and alternative communication interventions (Sevcik et al., 2008). Even for those whose cognitive ability is not compromised, there is the likelihood of learning disabilities (Boyle et al., 2015), with appropriate supports needed through special education. One approach to improving academic performance is self-directed strategy instruction, which is supported by research for a range of academic deficits (Cuenca-Carlino et al., 2016; Limpo & Alves, 2014). Physical and occupational therapy may be appropriate, as well as accommodations for any physical limitations. This may consist of work on joint contractures, hip complications, scoliosis treatment, and therapy to improve overall orthotic use (Jackson et al., 1993). For individuals with intellectual disability, supervised living and working situations in adulthood are likely.

Based on longitudinal study of individuals with CdLS, this syndrome is associated with a complex pattern of change and stability not only at the group level but at the individual level as well (Cochran et al., 2019). As such, appropriate interventions will need to be determined on a case-by-case basis, with ongoing monitoring at an individual level to ensure that needs are met appropriately.

Social-Emotional and Behavioral

In the school setting, appropriate behavioral management consistent with other children who display similar target behaviors is needed. For those with autistic features, interventions for children with autism may be appropriate (see Tiede & Walton, 2019). Addressing social interaction and externalizing behaviors will be most problematic with children who do not have communication skills, highlighting the importance of early intervention in children with CdLS (Seager et al., 2022; Tiede & Walton, 2019). As noted by Cochran et al. (2019), behavioral changes over time are not consistent across individuals. As such, monitoring of these changes is needed, with frequent adjustment to goals and interventions.

CONCLUSION

CdLS is a complex disorder that may co-occur with multiple other disorders. Medical issues, as well as impaired communication, difficulties meeting academic expectations, and dysregulation of their own behavior socially and when frustrated, provide multiple challenges when meeting the needs of these children. Taken together, an integrated model of care, with communication between parents, medical professionals, and school personnel, is important.

RESOURCES

MedlinePlus. (2022). *Cornelia de Lange syndrome*. National Library of Medicine. https://medlineplus.gov/genetics/condition/cornelia-de-lange-syndrome/

Genetic and Rare Diseases Information Center. (2021). *Cornelia de Lange syndrome*. National Center for Advancing Translational Sciences. https://rarediseases.info.nih.gov/diseases/10109/cornelia-de-lange-syndrome (available in Spanish)

National Organization for Rare Disorders. (2020). *Rare disease database: Cornelia de Lange syndrome*. https://rarediseases.org/rare-diseases/cornelia-de-lange-syndrome/

CdLS Foundation. https://www.cdlsusa.org/

REFERENCES

Ajmone, P. F., Rigamonti, C., Dall'Ara, F., Monti, F., Vizziello, P., Milani, D., Cereda, A., Selicorni, A., & Costantino, A. (2014). Communication, cognitive development and behavior in children with Cornelia de Lange syndrome (CdLS): Preliminary results. *American Journal of Medical Genetics: Part B, Neuropsychiatric Genetics, 165*(3), 223–229. https://doi.org/10.1002/ajmg.b.32224

Barbero, J. L. (2013). Genetic basis of cohesinopathies. *The Application of Clinical Genetics, 6*, 15–23. https://doi.org/10.2147/TACG.S34457

Basile, E., Villa, L., Selicorni, A., & Molteni, M. (2007). The behavioural phenotype of Cornelia de Lange syndrome: A study of 56 individuals. *Journal of Intellectual Disability Research, 51*(9), 671–681. https://doi.org/10.1111/j.1365-2788.2007.00977.x

Bell, L., Oliver, C., Wittkowski, A., Moss, J., & Hare, D. (2018). Attenuated behaviour in Cornelia de Lange and fragile X syndromes. *Journal of Intellectual Disability Research, 62*(6), 486–495. https://doi.org/10.1111/jir.12481

Boyle, M. I., Jespersgaard, C., Brøndum-Nielsen, K., Bisgaard, A.-M., & Tümer, Z. (2015). Cornelia de Lange syndrome. *Clinical Genetics, 88*(1), 1–12. https://doi.org/10.1111/cge.12499

Bull, M. J., Fitzgerald, J. F., Heifetz, S. A., & Brei, T. J. (1993). Gastrointestinal abnormalities: A significant cause of feeding difficulties and failure to thrive in Brachmann–de Lange syndrome. *American Journal of Medical Genetics, 47*(7), 1029–1034. https://doi.org/10.1002/ajmg.1320470720

Cochran, L., Welham, A., Oliver, C., Arshad, A., & Moss, J. F. (2019). Age-related behavioural change in Cornelia de Lange and Cri du Chat syndromes: A seven year follow-up study. *Journal of Autism and Developmental Disorders, 49*(6), 2476–2487. https://doi.org/10.1007/s10803-019-03966-6

Cuenca-Carlino, Y., Freeman-Green, S., Stephenson, G. W., & Hauth, C. (2016). Self-regulated strategy instruction for teaching multi-step equations to middle school students struggling in math. *The Journal of Special Education, 50*(2), 75–85. https://doi.org/10.1177/0022466915622021

Dorsett, D., & Ström, L. (2012). The ancient and evolving roles of cohesin in gene expression and DNA repair. *Current Biology, 22*(7), R240–R250. https://doi.org/10.1016/j.cub.2012.02.046

Genetic and Rare Diseases Information Center. (2021). *Cornelia de Lange syndrome*. National Center for Advancing Translational Sciences. https://rarediseases.info.nih.gov/diseases/10109/cornelia-de-lange-syndrome

Goodban, M. T. (1993). Survey of speech and language skills with prognostic indicators in 116 patients with Cornelia de Lange syndrome. *American Journal of Medical Genetics, 47*(7), 1059–1063. https://doi.org/10.1002/ajmg.1320470725

Jackson, L., Kline, A. D., Barr, M. A., & Koch, S. (1993). de Lange syndrome: A clinical review of 310 individuals. *American Journal of Medical Genetics, 47*(7), 940–946. https://doi.org/10.1002/ajmg.1320470703

Jensen de López, K. M., Kraljević, J. K., & Bang Struntze, E. L. (2022). Efficacy, model of delivery, intensity and targets of pragmatic interventions for children with developmental language disorder: A systematic review. *International Journal of Language & Communication Disorders, 57*, 764–781. https://doi.org/10.1111/1460-6984.12716

Kline, A. D., Krantz, I. D., Sommer, A., Kliewer, M., Jackson, L. G., FitzPatrick, D. R., Levin, A. V., & Selicorni, A. (2007). Cornelia de Lange syndrome: Clinical review, diagnostic and scoring systems, and anticipatory guidance. *American Journal of Medical Genetics: Part A, 143A*(12), 1287–1296. https://doi.org/10.1002/ajmg.a.31757

Limpo, T., & Alves, R. A. (2014). Implicit theories of writing and their impact on students' responses to a SRSD intervention. *British Journal of Educational Psychology, 84*(4), 571–590. https://doi.org/10.1111/bjep.12042

MedlinePlus. (2022). *Cornelia de Lange syndrome*. National Library of Medicine. https://medlineplus.gov/genetics/condition/cornelia-de-lange-syndrome/

Moss, J. F., Oliver, C., Berg, K., Kaur, G., Jephcott, L., & Cornish, K. (2008). Prevalence of autistic spectrum disorder phenomenology in Cornelia de Lange and Cri du Chat syndromes. *American Journal on Mental Retardation, 113*(4), 278–291. https://doi.org/10.1352/0895-8017(2008)113[278:POASPI]2.0.CO;2

Mulder, P. A., Huisman, S. A., Hennekam, R. C., Oliver, C., van Balkom, I. D., & Piening, S. (2017). Behaviour in Cornelia de Lange syndrome: A systematic review. *Developmental Medicine and Child Neurology, 59*(4), 361–366. https://doi.org/10.1111/dmcn.13361

Nelson, L., Crawford, H., Reid, D., Moss, J., & Oliver, C. (2017). An experimental study of executive function and social impairment in Cornelia de Lange syndrome. *Journal of Neurodevelopmental Disorders, 9*(1), Article 33. https://doi.org/10.1186/s11689-017-9213-x

Oliver, C., Arron, K., Sloneem, J., & Hall, S. (2008). Behavioural phenotype of Cornelia de Lange syndrome: Case-control study. *The British Journal of Psychiatry, 193*(6), 466–470. https://doi.org/10.1192/bjp.bp.107.044370

Sarimski, K. (2002). Analysis of intentional communication in severely handicapped children with Cornelia-de-Lange syndrome. *Journal of Communication Disorders, 35*(6), 483–500. https://doi.org/10.1016/S0021-9924(02)00117-X

Seager, E., Sampson, S., Sin, J., Pagnamenta, E., & Stojanovik, V. (2022). A systematic review of speech, language and communication interventions for children with Down syndrome from 0 to 6 years. *International Journal of Language & Communication Disorders, 57*(2), 441–463. https://doi.org/10.1111/1460-6984.12699

Sevcik, R. A., Barton-Hulsey, A., & Romski, M. (2008). Early intervention, AAC, and transition to school for young children with significant spoken communication disorders and their families. *Seminars in Speech and Language, 29*(2), 92–100. https://doi.org/10.1055/s-2008-1079123

Sloneem, J., Arron, K., Hall, S. S., & Oliver, C. (2009). Self-injurious behaviour in Cornelia de Lange syndrome: 2. Association with environmental events. *Journal of Intellectual Disability Research, 53*(7), 590–603. https://doi.org/10.1111/j.1365-2788.2009.01183.x

Tiede, G., & Walton, K. M. (2019). Meta-analysis of naturalistic developmental behavioral interventions for young children with autism spectrum disorder. *Autism, 23*(8), 2080–2095. https://doi.org/10.1177/1362361319836371

56

Fragile X Syndrome

Lea A. Theodore, Adeline M. Bray, Lydia Rumpf, Sai Sudha Aravala, and Justina Petrullo

One of the most common causes of intellectual disabilities, fragile X syndrome (FXS), is an inherited genetic disorder where the bottom of the X chromosome is pinched off. Although the disorder is diagnosed in both male and female individuals, FXS occurs more frequently in boys, who also experience more severe symptoms. This is because female individuals have two X chromosomes, providing girls with an additional layer of protection should damage occur to one of their X chromosomes. Boys, however, only have one X chromosome, which if impaired, increases the likelihood of FXS and further explains their symptom severity.

ETIOLOGY

FXS is the result of mutations in the *FMR1* gene, which is located on the X chromosome. The *FMR1* gene makes a protein, fragile X mental retardation protein, that is needed for normal brain development. Children diagnosed with FXS do not have enough of this protein. As an inherited condition, the fragile X gene may be passed down from generation to generation. A permutation in the *FMR1* gene of a mother results in having offspring with a 50% chance of also inheriting the altered gene, whereas fathers with FXS may only pass the gene to their daughters. Children who inherit the mutated gene will either be diagnosed with FXS or become a carrier, meaning that they may pass this affected gene to their children (Hunter et al., 2014).

https://doi.org/10.1037/0000349-056
Health-Related Disorders in Children and Adolescents: A Guidebook for Educators and Service Providers, Second Edition, M. M. Perfect, C. A. Riccio, and M. A. Bray (Editors)

PREVALENCE AND INCIDENCE

Although the exact prevalence and incidence rates are not known, boys are 2 times more likely to be diagnosed with FXS. More specifically, it is estimated that one in 2,500 to 4,000 boys and one in 7,000 to 8,000 girls are diagnosed with FXS. Notably, women are 4 times more likely to be carriers of FXS. Finally, this syndrome has been found in all races and ethnic groups (Raspa et al., 2017).

SYMPTOMS

Children with FXS experience a range of developmental and learning problems, as well as physical anomalies. Symptoms associated with FXS include intellectual disabilities, delays in reaching developmental milestones, learning problems, sensory integration difficulties, anxiety, attention problems, seizures, and autismlike behaviors such as lack of eye contact and hand flapping. Physical features of children with FXS include a large head, long and narrow face, large ears, prominent forehead and chin, loose joints, and flat feet.

IMPACT ON THE STUDENT AND OUTCOMES

Medical Outcomes

FXS is classified as an intellectual disability disorder by the American Academy of Pediatrics (Kidd et al., 2014). Common medical outcomes include seizures and those related to connective tissue abnormalities, such as otitis media (OM) and gastrointestinal problems (Kidd et al., 2014). OM is a common but chronic condition in which the middle ear is infected, often resulting in a loss of hearing during critical periods of development. Children diagnosed with FXS are at greater risk for otitis media, middle ear infections, and hearing loss, all of which are common in many genetic disorders. Further, children with FXS are more likely than their peers without FXS to develop OM during early childhood development (Harmes et al., 2013). Ocular disorders are also common in most children with FXS. Children with visual problems are more likely to have comorbid ocular issues, including refractive errors (Alanay et al., 2007) and strabismus (i.e., abnormal alignment of the eyes), which is most prevalent in boys. Children with FXS may also experience sleep issues, with approximately 50% having some form of a sleeping disorder (Kronk et al., 2009). Congenital malformations also may be present but are considered rare (Kidd et al., 2014).

Cognitive/Academic Outcomes

FXS is a genetically based disorder that results in fairly severe intellectual and developmental disabilities. As mentioned previously, FXS occurs primarily in boys (Murphy, 2009); however, many girls diagnosed with FXS exhibit learning disabilities despite not having an intellectual disorder (Mazzocco, 2001). Further, girls with FXS are more likely to have solid verbal skills and fairly good visual perception, whereas executive functioning skills tend to be weak, resulting in impairments in working memory and attention. Girls with FXS also experience difficulty with math and number sense (Murphy, 2009). Notably, individuals with FXS often exhibit similar behavioral characteristics of individuals with autism spectrum disorder (ASD; Harris et al., 2008).

Academically, children with FXS struggle with reading and language skills, in particular, phonemic awareness. Cognitively, working memory, sequential processing, and attention are most likely to be affected. Boys diagnosed with both FXS and ASD have more deleterious outcomes with respect to language development overall, which affects reading as well as other academic domains, including spelling, written language, and math. Further, boys with FXS display global academic deficits, but most notably in the area of mathematics (Klusek et al., 2015). Compared with girls with FXS, boys more commonly experience cognitive deficiencies and demonstrate substantially weaker executive functioning, along with poor short-term memory and reduced visuospatial and visuomotor skills. These deficits culminate in a poorer prognosis with respect to academic and social functioning vis-à-vis their female counterparts (Murphy, 2009).

Social-Emotional and Behavioral

FXS provides challenges to children diagnosed with the disorder, as well as the individuals around them. This has the potential to profoundly impact multiple areas of their lives, including making friends, engaging in recreational activities, and interacting with others, all essential for developing a good quality of life. Individuals with FXS have particular difficulty making friends because they exhibit atypical social behavior that is consistent with ASD (DaWalt et al., 2019).

Developing friendships has been found to be instrumental in supporting emotional and behavioral difficulties while enhancing interactions and prosocial behaviors with peers (Frolli et al., 2015). By addressing social and emotional development in children with FXS, language skills increased, autism behaviors decreased, and adaptive behaviors beneficial to socialization were enhanced. It has been surmised that the enhanced cognitive and behavioral functioning is the result of the maturation of certain brain systems responsible for control of attention (Frolli et al., 2015). The aforementioned results provide optimism and hope to children growing up with this disorder.

Four major behavioral issues exhibited in both genders with FXS include anxiety, hyperarousal, inattention, and impulsiveness. Approximately 73% of preteens exhibit difficulty with distractibility and maintaining attention, which is believed to correspond to the high attention-deficit disorder rate in this population of students (Cornish et al., 2004). Socially, children with FXS experience a great deal of difficulty making and maintaining friendships due to their state of hyperarousal. These children tend to be anxious and have difficulty with changes in routine. Throughout the day, hyperactivity, inattention, anxiety, and noncompliance are typically evidenced. Therefore, forming social relationships with peers and adults is challenging and an issue well-suited for intervention.

PSYCHOEDUCATIONAL IMPLICATIONS AND SCHOOL-BASED INTERVENTIONS

Students with FXS experience myriad health-related issues, but cognitive, academic, and social–emotional functioning also matter. All of these need to be addressed by health professionals as well as school psychologists in the schools. Next are the concerns and school-based interventions that may be provided.

Medical and Health Management

Children and adolescents diagnosed with FXS experience myriad medical issues. Specifically, they are at greater risk for cardiac disorders; ear, nose, and throat disorders; gastrointestinal disorders; neurological disorders; ocular disorders; sleep problems; congenital malformations; and growth issues. Clearly, medical problems are more common in children with FXS and span a wide range of physical problems. With respect to heart-related problems, children may experience low muscle tone, which may result in mitral valve prolapse and an overall weakening of aortic vessels. Children with FXS are more susceptible to OM, beginning in their 1st year of life. If left untreated, OM could lead to hearing loss as well as speech- and language-related disorders. Recurrent sinusitis is a common problem, likely related to the facial structure or connective tissue issues that result in OM. Gastrointestinal issues such as diarrhea, constipation, gastroesophageal reflux, and chronic urinary tract infections are common medical problems that children with FXS experience. Children with FXS typically have a high threshold for pain, thus reducing the likelihood that they will tell a parent of pain. Neurologically, seizures occur at a greater frequency, with approximately 20% of boys diagnosed with epilepsy (Kidd et al., 2014). Children with FXS are also at greater risk for vision problems, including strabismus, ptosis, nystagmus, and myopia/hyperopia. Difficulty sleeping, loud snoring, and obstructive sleep apnea are common sleep problems, whereas congenital malformations, such as congenital heart defects and cleft lip or palate are less likely to be manifested in children with FXS. Finally, with respect to growth, an examination of measurement curves indicates that boys tend to be taller in stature than their typically developing peers, while their weight may be higher in childhood but decrease to more normal ranges during adolescence. In contrast, no difference in height or weight was evidenced in girls with FXS (Kidd et al., 2014). Psychopharmacological interventions are often the first line of treatment used to manage problematic behavioral symptoms of children with FXS (Finucane et al., 2013).

The wide range of medical issues that children with FXS may experience should be carefully monitored by the child's pediatrician and/or other specialists who may need to work with the child. Clearly, early identification of any problem will help place the child on a better trajectory toward appropriate treatment and good health. Thus, the pediatrician treating a child with FXS needs to be vigilant in looking for and asking about the aforementioned issues and symptoms, with referrals to appropriate specialists for further evaluation if necessary (Kidd et al., 2014).

Cognitive/Academic

Professionals providing early intervention supports should focus on improving and strengthening the phonological awareness of children with FXS. Phonological awareness has been linked to general reading ability, and research suggests promising outcomes for children with FXS enrolled in intervention programs such as the HeadSprout Early Reading Program (Adlof et al., 2018). Children with FXS are often cheerful and cooperative, making the implementation of such interventions relatively easy and practical. It may also be useful to pair interventions, educational instruction, and directions with visual stimuli. A comprehensive, informed approach is necessary when providing useful interventions to FXS children and their families.

Social-Emotional and Behavioral

FXS comes with difficult personal, familial, and educational challenges. Children with FXS may struggle to navigate social situations and meet educational demands, and they often present behavioral problems in school and home settings (Moskowitz et al., 2011). Families of children with FXS may struggle to manage symptoms and may be unaware of the myriad services available to their child. By providing feasible techniques and interventions for parents, school personnel and health care providers may help alleviate a wide range of frustration for both children with FXS and those individuals providing them support. Parents and caregivers of children with FXS should seek appropriate and comprehensive assessment for their children, which will assist parents in gaining access to useful services and allow support providers to develop evidence-based intervention plans that target specific areas of need. These evaluations should be conducted as soon as possible, as results provide access to early intervention services and individualized education programs (Nash et al., 2019). These services provide children and families with a network of support from many professionals, including psychiatrists, behavioral analysts, speech pathologists, occupational therapists, school psychologists, and special education teachers.

Although these medical interventions may be useful, parents and health care professionals also should consider the use of home- and school-based behavioral interventions for children with FXS. Awareness of the significant overlap in symptoms and behaviors in children with FXS and children with ASD should trigger the use of behavioral interventions in dealing with various issues. Behavioral interventions should be implemented early to maximize growth and prepare children with FXS for challenges that may arise in school settings, such as transitions, demanding tasks, and dealing with self-injurious behaviors (Schwarte, 2008). Employing behavioral techniques that are idiosyncratic to the individual circumstances and behaviors of the child and based on a thorough evaluation and functional behavioral assessment will lead to interventions designed to target specific areas of difficulty. Providing a sense of structure and routine in school and home settings may help alleviate distress in children with FXS and their families (Moskowitz & Jones, 2015).

CONCLUSION

Children with FXS experience a range of developmental and learning problems, as well as physical anomalies. Symptoms associated with FXS include intellectual disabilities, delays in reaching developmental milestones, learning problems, sensory integration difficulties, anxiety, attention problems, seizures, and autismlike behaviors. Thus, knowledge of evidence-based treatments and strategies, as well as clear communication among all individuals working with the child, is crucial to supporting children diagnosed with FXS and their families.

RESOURCES

Caravajal, I. F., & Aldridge, D. (2011). *Understanding fragile X syndrome: A guide for families and professionals*. Jessica Kingsley Publishers.

Griffin, E. (2005). *Fragile X, fragile hope: Finding joy in parenting a special needs child*. Emerald Books.

REFERENCES

Adlof, S. M., Klusek, J., Hoffmann, A., Chitwood, K. L., Brazendale, A., Riley, K., Abbeduto, L. J., & Roberts, J. E. (2018). Reading in children with fragile X syndrome: Phonological awareness and feasibility of intervention. *American Journal on Intellectual and Developmental Disabilities, 123*(3), 193–211. https://doi.org/10.1352/1944-7558-123.3.193

Alanay, Y., Ünal, F., Turanlı, G., Alikaşifoğlu, M., Alehan, D., Akyol, U., Belgin, E., Şener, C., Aktaş, D., Boduroğlu, K., Utine, E., Volkan-Salancı, B., Özusta, Ş., Genç, A., Başar, F., Sevinç, Ş., & Tunçbilek, E. (2007). A multidisciplinary approach to the management of individuals with fragile X syndrome. *Journal of Intellectual Disability Research, 51*(2), 151–161. https://doi.org/10.1111/j.1365-2788.2006.00942.x

Cornish, K. M., Turk, J., Wilding, J., Sudhalter, V., Munir, F., Kooy, F., & Hagerman, R. (2004). Annotation: Deconstructing the attention deficit in fragile X syndrome: A developmental neuropsychological approach. *Journal of Child Psychology and*

Psychiatry, 45(6), 1042–1053. https://doi.org/10.1111/j.1469-7610.2004.t01-1-00297.x

DaWalt, L. S., Usher, L. V., Greenberg, J. S., & Mailick, M. R. (2019). Friendships and social participation as markers of quality of life of adolescents and adults with fragile X syndrome and autism. *Autism, 23*(2), 383–393. https://doi.org/10.1177/1362361317709202

Finucane, B., Haas-Givler, B., & Simon, E. W. (2013). Knowledge and perceptions about fragile X syndrome: Implications for diagnosis, intervention, and research. *Intellectual and Developmental Disabilities, 51*(4), 226–236. https://doi.org/10.1352/1934-9556-51.4.226

Frolli, A., Piscopo, S., & Conson, M. (2015). Developmental changes in cognitive and behavioural functioning of adolescents with fragile-X syndrome. *Journal of Intellectual Disability Research, 59*(7), 613–621. https://doi.org/10.1111/jir.12165

Harmes, K. M., Blackwood, R. A., Burrows, H. L., Cooke, J. M., Van Harrison, R., & Passamani, P. P. (2013). Otitis media: Diagnosis and treatment. *American Family Physician, 88*(7), 435–440. https://www.aafp.org/afp/2013/1001/p435.html

Harris, S. W., Hessl, D., Goodlin-Jones, B., Ferranti, J., Bacalman, S., Barbato, I., Tassone, F., Hagerman, P. J., Herman, H., & Hagerman, R. J. (2008). Autism profiles of males with fragile X syndrome. *American Journal on Mental Retardation, 113*(6), 427–438. https://doi.org/10.1352/2008.113:427-438

Hunter, J., Rivero-Arias, O., Angelov, A., Kim, E., Fotheringham, I., & Leal, J. (2014). Epidemiology of fragile X syndrome: A systematic review and meta-analysis. *American Journal of Medical Genetics: Part A, 164*(7), 1648–1658. https://doi.org/10.1002/ajmg.a.36511

Kidd, S. A., Lachiewicz, A., Barbouth, D., Blitz, R. K., Delahunty, C., McBrien, D., Visootsak, J., & Berry-Kravis, E. (2014). Fragile X syndrome: A review of associated medical problems. *Pediatrics, 134*(5), 995–1005. https://doi.org/10.1542/peds.2013-4301

Klusek, J., Hunt, A. W., Mirrett, P. L., Hatton, D. D., Hooper, S. R., Roberts, J. E., & Bailey, D. B. (2015). Reading and phonological skills in boys with fragile X syndrome. *Journal of Autism and Developmental Disorders, 45*(6), 1699–1711. https://doi.org/10.1007/s10803-014-2328-y

Kronk, R., Dahl, R., & Noll, R. (2009). Caregiver reports of sleep problems on a convenience sample of children with fragile X syndrome. *American Journal of Intellectual Developmental Disabilities, 114*, 383–392. https://doi.org/10.1352/1944-7588-114.6.383

Mazzocco, M. M. (2001). Math learning disability and math LD subtypes: Evidence from studies of Turner syndrome, fragile X syndrome, and neurofibromatosis type 1. *Journal of Learning Disabilities, 34*(6), 520–533. https://doi.org/10.1177/002221940103400605

Moskowitz, L. J., Carr, E. G., & Durand, V. M. (2011). Behavioral intervention for problem behavior in children with fragile X syndrome. *American Journal on Intellectual and Developmental Disabilities, 116*(6), 457–478. https://doi.org/10.1352/1944-7558-116.6.457

Moskowitz, L. J., & Jones, E. A. (2015). Uncovering the evidence for behavioral interventions with individuals with fragile X syndrome: A systematic review. *Research in Developmental Disabilities, 38*, 223–241. https://doi.org/10.1016/j.ridd.2014.12.011

Murphy, M. M. (2009). A review of mathematical learning disabilities in children with fragile X syndrome. *Developmental Disabilities Research Reviews, 15*(1), 21–27.

Nash, R., Riley, C., Gilbertson, K., Paramsothy, P., Raspa, M., Wheeler, A., Dziuban, E. J., & Peacock, G. (2019). A description of the educational setting among individuals with fragile X syndrome. *American Journal on Intellectual and Developmental Disabilities, 124*(1), 57–76. https://doi.org/10.1352/1944-7558-124.1.57

Raspa, M., Wheeler, A. C., & Riley, C. (2017). Public health literature review of fragile X syndrome. *Pediatrics, 139*(Suppl. 3), S153–S171. https://doi.org/10.1542/peds.2016-1159C

Schwarte, A. R. (2008). Fragile X syndrome. *School Psychology Quarterly, 23*(2), 290–300. https://doi.org/10.1037/1045-3830.23.2.290

57

Lysosomal Storage Disorders

Allison Fairchild and Melina Islas

The lysosome, which was described by De Duve et al. in 1955, is an organelle with many important functions, including innate immunity and cell division; however, lysosomes may sometimes be the target of dysfunction, which leads to disruption of these important functions. To date, more than 50 lysosomal storage disorders (LSDs) have been identified as a result of the wide range of dysfunctions. Although there is currently no cure for these disorders, research has led to a rapid increase in medical treatments and therapies (Parkinson-Lawrence et al., 2010).

ETIOLOGY

LSDs are a group of more than 50 diverse metabolic disorders caused by genetic deficits (i.e., missing enzymes) in lysosomal acid hydrolase, receptor, activator, membrane, or transporter proteins. Specific LSDs may be determined depending on the type of deficits in the lysosomal enzymes, cofactors, and transporters (Kadali et al., 2014), and they are typically categorized by the type of substrate stored. These issues cause progressive accumulation of substrates, which in turn results in the deterioration of cell and tissue functioning (Wang et al., 2011). They are single-gene disorders (Beck, 2018) and typically inherited in an autosomal recessive manner, with the exception of Fabry, Hunter, and Danon diseases, which are linked to the X chromosome (Wang et al., 2011).

https://doi.org/10.1037/0000349-057
Health-Related Disorders in Children and Adolescents: A Guidebook for Educators and Service Providers, Second Edition, M. M. Perfect, C. A. Riccio, and M. A. Bray (Editors)

PREVALENCE AND INCIDENCE

Individual LSDs are considered to be relatively rare. They often are undiagnosed or misdiagnosed (Platt et al., 2012). Therefore, it is difficult to determine an exact prevalence rate. It is estimated that the occurrence ranges from one in 1,500 to 7,000 live births (Reuser et al., 2011). Data suggest that these disorders are more common in male than in female individuals (Kadali et al., 2014). Some disorders are more prevalent within specific populations. For example, there is a higher prevalence of Gaucher and Tay–Sachs in Ashkenazi Jewish populations (Boustany, 2013).

SYMPTOMS

The diversity in LSDs results in a wide range of clinical presentations with highly heterogeneous symptoms that mainly depend on which enzyme the individual is missing (see Table 57.1). Symptoms may present as early as infancy but typically emerge in childhood or adolescence. Common symptoms include acroparesthesia (i.e., feelings of burning, tingling, prickling, or numbness in the extremities), diminished sweating, and complaints of stomach/digestion issues (Aldenhoven et al., 2009). Less common in children are symptoms of kidney dysfunction, left ventricular hypertrophy, and stroke. In some of the more common LSDs like Fabry disease and Gaucher disease, individuals present with musculoskeletal manifestations. These often include joint stiffness and contractures, stunted growth, and bone density abnormalities (Aldenhoven et al., 2009). Signs and symptoms of LSDs are reported more in boys than in girls. For example, acroparesthesia and gastrointestinal problems presented in almost 20% more boys than girls in a sample of individuals diagnosed with an LSD; however, kidney dysfunction appeared to be more common in girls than in boys (Pintos-Morell & Beck, 2009).

IMPACT ON THE STUDENT AND OUTCOMES

Medical

Physical symptoms of LSDs can be seen in multiple tissues and organs; manifestations can be complex and vary depending on which specific disorder is present. Typically, medical issues in those with LSDs include pulmonary and cardiac problems, deafness, blindness, movement problems, and bone abnormalities (Marques & Saftig, 2019). Medical problems related to the central nervous system can be the most debilitating and impactful on overall health (Parenti, 2009).

Cognitive/Academic

Two common cognitive impacts of LSDs include neuronal storage deficits and neural cell death, which lead to rapid cognitive decline in individuals with

TABLE 57.1. Specific Lysosomal Storage Disorders and Symptoms

Disease	Frequency	Defining features
Gaucher disease	1:50,000 to 100,000	Enlarged liver and spleen, low red blood cell count, easy bruising, lung disease, bone abnormalities (e.g., bone pain, fractures, arthritis), abnormal eye movements, seizures, and brain damage (MedlinePlus, 2022)
Pompe disease	1:40,000	Muscle weaknesses, poor muscle tone, enlarged liver, heart defects, delayed motor skills, and abnormally large heart (MedlinePlus, 2016)
Metachromatic leukodystrophy	1:40,000 to 160,000	Progressive deterioration of cognitive functions and motor skills (e.g., the ability to walk), loss of sensation in the extremities, incontinence, seizures, paralysis, inability to speak, blindness, and hearing loss (MedlinePlus, 2021a)
Krabbe disease	1:100,000	Muscle weakness, difficulty with feeding, fever, stiff posture, delayed mental and physical development, progressive muscle weakening, vision loss, and seizures (MedlinePlus, 2018)
Mucopolysacchari-dosis II, aka Hunter syndrome	1:100,000 to 170,000 in male individuals	Large head, buildup of fluid in the brain, enlarged liver and spleen, soft pouching around the belly button, thick skin, hearing loss, and heart valve patterns; occurs almost exclusively in male individuals (MedlinePlus, 2008)
GM1 gangliosidosis	1:100,000 to 200,000	Developmental regression, exaggerated startle reactions, enlarged liver and spleen, skeletal abnormalities, seizures, profound intellectual disability, loss of vision, clouding of the cornea, "cherry red spot" in eye, and enlarged and weakened heart muscles (MedlinePlus, 2013)
Mucopolysacchari-dosis IV, aka Morquio syndrome	1:200,000 to 300,000	Skeletal abnormalities (e.g., short stature; knock knees; abnormalities of the ribs, chest, spine, hips, and wrists), clouding of the cornea, hearing loss, upper respiratory infections, coarse facial features, and mildly enlarged liver (MedlinePlus, 2019)
Tay-Sachs disease	20,000 cases per year	Seizures, vision and hearing loss, intellectual disability, paralysis, "cherry red spot" in eye, weakened muscles, loss of motor skills, and exaggerated startle response (MedlinePlus, 2021b)

these disorders. The brain is especially vulnerable to LSDs, due to its limited capacity for regeneration (Boustany, 2013). Children with Niemann–Pick disease Type C experience a regression in speech and aphasia, where they forget the words to use for objects. They lose their ability to concentrate and will experience deficits in short-term memory. Speech and language deficits are also common in Pompe disease, which also decreases an individual's cognitive functioning (Spiridigliozzi et al., 2017). Other LSDs that involve the central nervous system cause intellectual disability. Martin et al. (2008) found that intelligence tests do not adequately assess the cognitive functioning of children with LSDs due to the wide range of neurological, sensory, and somatic involvement that influences the results.

Social-Emotional and Behavioral

Although there is clearly a myriad of cognitive and health deficits involved in LSDs, behavioral and psychiatric manifestations further complicate the diagnosis of these conditions due to the potential for severe presentation. Several LSDs have unique social–emotional and behavioral impacts, but some manifestations are consistent across many of the disorders (Staretz-Chacham et al., 2010). Behavioral symptoms may look similar to behavior observed in students with autism spectrum disorder (e.g., increased sensitivity to touch, self-mutilation, mouthing or biting of objects). Restlessness, hyperactivity, and anxious tendencies also may be present. School-aged individuals with LSDs may exhibit aggression or destructive outbursts. During adolescence, acute psychosis, paranoid delusions, hallucinations, and disorganized behavior and thoughts may emerge. Mood disorders, such as depression and bipolar disorder, may also be present (Staretz-Chacham et al., 2010). Cole et al. (2007) reported on an analysis of 184 patients in the United Kingdom with Fabry disease and found that 46% of the patients participating in the study suffered from clinically significant depression and 28% suffered from severe clinical depression.

PSYCHOEDUCATIONAL IMPLICATIONS AND SCHOOL-BASED INTERVENTIONS

Medical and Health Management

With no cure available for LSDs, treatments generally seek to stabilize organ functions or attempt to slow the progression of the disorder. Because these disorders affect multiple bodily systems, individuals sometimes need surgery to prevent complications or need multiple medical devices, such as orthoses, hearing aids, or special glasses. Enzyme replacement therapy is an example of a treatment that slows the progression of LSDs and even improves some organ function (Beck, 2018). Enzyme replacement therapy works by inserting enzymes (produced from genetically modified cells retrieved from animals, humans, plants, or eggs) intravenously on a weekly or biweekly basis. Substrate reduction is another option for treatment of LSDs that works by slowing the production of storage material instead of breaking it down. This approach is carried out by taking an oral medication; however, substrate reduction is clinically approved for only two LSDs (Gaucher disease and Niemann–Pick disease Type C; Beck, 2018). Chaperone therapy is a pharmacological treatment option that can be combined with enzyme replacement therapy for optimal results; however, currently it is only available in Europe due to insufficient clinical evidence (Beck, 2018). Gene therapy is a promising treatment because LSDs are well known as single-gene disorders. In vivo gene therapy involves the direct injection of a gene into an organ, whereas ex vivo gene therapy involves a hematopoietic stem cell transplant that delivers enzymes to the deficient area. Gene therapy is also under review and, thus, not readily available to patients despite promising results in areas such as behavior, attention, and sleep (Beck, 2018).

Despite the promising emergence of new treatment options, youth with LSDs will likely have many absences and will need accommodations in school due to the symptoms of LSDs (e.g., fatigue, pain, gastrointestinal issues). Seizures are common with some LSDs, which may require that a school nurse be closely involved with the child and their teacher so that all parties know what to do in the event that the student has a seizure on campus. Depending on the frequency of seizures, a paraprofessional may need to be assigned to the student to provide individual supervision.

Cognitive/Academic

Many, if not all, symptoms of LSDs will affect individuals in one way or another in the academic setting. Children with LSDs will likely meet eligibility for special education or 504 services. A 504 plan ensures that students with disabilities receive accommodations that provide them equal access to their education, and a student receiving special education has been identified as having a disability that adversely affects their education. Students found eligible for special education receive an individualized education program that ensures specialized instruction and related services. To address the effects of short-term memory loss and motor impairments in students with an LSD, a peer may be designated as a scribe for this student, written assignments should be substituted with nonwritten assignment options, and frequently used items should be labeled for when memory fails (Gartin et al., 2013). The student will likely need to work with an occupational therapist due to regression in motor skills. In the classroom, teachers can accommodate the loss in motor skills by ensuring that larger walking paths are available and providing extra transition times for the student (Gartin et al., 2013). A speech–language pathologist also may be needed as some students experience dysarthria (i.e., when the muscles around the mouth impair the student from forming words) and aphasia. Because intelligence tests may not adequately assess cognitive skills in students with LSDs, nonverbal cognitive assessments that involve minimal motor skills should be used rather than tests that rely on language.

Social–Emotional and Behavioral

Many of these conditions are progressive over time and tend to cause regression of certain skills that a child once had (e.g., speech, memory, cognitive abilities). For example, a student with impacted speech will have a difficult time verbalizing their thoughts and/or have motor difficulties with speech and may opt to disengage from conversation or verbal demands. In addition, symptoms of muscle weakness and physical abnormalities will make it difficult for the child with an LSD to participate regularly in sports, recess, or physical education classes, further creating social barriers for the child. This can be highly frustrating for the student; however, the social–emotional consequences can be lessened by providing accommodations in the classroom, where it is important to keep the student involved socially and educationally to prevent social isolation. The child's educational plan may include an agreement wherein the child may be excused from class to spend time in a resource classroom when they are becoming emotionally aroused.

In addition, the school counselor or school psychologist may provide emotional support to the student and the family. Hamlet et al. (2011) found that 88% of school counselors reported primarily addressing the social–emotional needs of students with chronic illness. The supports and accommodations included participating in group counseling, educating the students' classmates on their condition in a therapeutic manner, and keeping students in a routine as much as possible. Identification and connection with a support group is essential for parents of a student with a progressive and fatal disease, such as an LSD. Although the most valuable interventions for the student with an LSD will come from their medical team and may include medical management, supportive therapy has been found to be variably effective for alleviation of some clinical problems associated with some LSDs (Staretz-Chacham et al., 2010).

CONCLUSION

Due to the wide range of disorders and symptoms that fall under the LSD umbrella, children with LSDs are often undiagnosed or misdiagnosed. However, medical advancements and research have allowed for the discovery of effective treatments of these disorders. In the schools, the involvement of a variety of professionals is necessary, such as physicians, school psychologists, occupational and physical therapists, and speech therapists. Services from these professionals, as well as appropriate accommodations in the classroom and school, are needed to allow students with LSDs to function and succeed in school.

RESOURCES

Genetic Education Materials for School Success. 10 West Edge Drive, Suite 101, Durham, NH 03284. https://www.gemssforschools.org/

National Gaucher Foundation. 5410 Edson Lane #220, Rockville, MD 20852. https://www.gaucherdisease.org/

National Institutes of Health: MedlinePlus. 9000 Rockville Pike, Bethesda, MD 20892. https://medlineplus.gov/genetics/

National Organization for Rare Disorders. 55 Kenosia Avenue, Danbury, CT 06810. https://rarediseases.org

REFERENCES

Aldenhoven, M., Sakkers, R. J. B., Boelens, J., de Koning, T. J., & Wulffraat, N. M. (2009). Musculoskeletal manifestations of lysosomal storage disorders. *Annals of the Rheumatic Diseases, 68*(11), 1659–1665. https://doi.org/10.1136/ard.2008.095315

Beck, M. (2018). Treatment strategies for lysosomal storage disorders. *Developmental Medicine and Child Neurology, 60*(1), 13–18. https://doi.org/10.1111/dmcn.13600

Boustany, R.-M. N. (2013). Lysosomal storage diseases—The horizon expands. *Nature Reviews Neurology, 9*(10), 583–598. https://doi.org/10.1038/nrneurol.2013.163

Cole, A. L., Lee, P. J., Hughes, D. A., Deegan, P. B., Waldek, S., & Lachmann, R. H. (2007). Depression in adults with Fabry disease: A common and under-diagnosed problem. *Journal of Inherited Metabolic Disease, 30*(6), 943–951. https://doi.org/10.1007/s10545-007-0708-6

Gartin, B. C., Murdick, N. L., Cooley, J., & Barnett, S. (2013). Teaching children with Niemann–Pick disease. *Physical Disabilities: Education and Related Services, 32*(2), 38–50. https://doi.org/10.14434/pders.v32i2.12995

Hamlet, H. S., Gergar, P. G., & Schaefer, B. A. (2011). Students living with chronic illness: The school counselor's role. *Professional School Counseling, 14*(3), 202–210. https://doi.org/10.1177/2156759X1101400304

Kadali, S., Kolusu, A., Gummadi, M. R., & Undamatla, J. (2014). The relative frequency of lysosomal storage disorders: A medical genetics referral laboratory's experience from India. *Journal of Child Neurology, 29*(10), 1377–1382. https://doi.org/10.1177/0883073813515075

Marques, A. R. A., & Saftig, P. (2019). Lysosomal storage disorders—Challenges, concepts and avenues for therapy: Beyond rare diseases. *Journal of Cell Science, 132*(2), Article jcs221739. https://doi.org/10.1242/jcs.221739

Martin, H. R., Poe, M. D., Reinhartsen, D., Pretzel, R. E., Roush, J., Rosenberg, A., Dusing, S. C., & Escolar, M. L. (2008). Methods for assessing neurodevelopment in lysosomal storage diseases and related disorders: A multidisciplinary perspective. *Acta Paediatrica, 97*(s457), 69–75. https://doi.org/10.1111/j.1651-2227.2008.00651.x

MedlinePlus. (2008). *Mucopolysaccharidosis type II*. National Library of Medicine. https://medlineplus.gov/genetics/condition/mucopolysaccharidosis-type-ii/

MedlinePlus. (2013). *GM1 gangliosidosis*. National Library of Medicine. https://medlineplus.gov/genetics/condition/gm1-gangliosidosis/

MedlinePlus. (2016). *Pompe disease*. National Library of Medicine. https://medlineplus.gov/genetics/condition/pompe-disease/

MedlinePlus. (2018). *Krabbe disease*. National Library of Medicine. https://medlineplus.gov/genetics/condition/krabbe-disease/

MedlinePlus. (2019). *Mucopolysaccharidosis type IV*. National Library of Medicine. https://medlineplus.gov/genetics/condition/mucopolysaccharidosis-type-iv/

MedlinePlus. (2021a). *Metachromatic leukodystrophy*. National Library of Medicine. https://medlineplus.gov/genetics/condition/metachromatic-leukodystrophy/

MedlinePlus. (2021b). *Tay–Sachs disease*. National Library of Medicine. https://medlineplus.gov/genetics/condition/tay-sachs-disease/

MedlinePlus. (2022). *Gaucher disease*. National Library of Medicine. https://medlineplus.gov/genetics/condition/gaucher-disease/

Parenti, G. (2009). Treating lysosomal storage diseases with pharmacological chaperones: From concept to clinics. *EMBO Molecular Medicine, 1*(5), 268–279. https://doi.org/10.1002/emmm.200900036

Parkinson-Lawrence, E. J., Shandala, T., Prodoehl, M., Plew, R., Borlace, G. N., & Brooks, D. A. (2010). Lysosomal storage disease: Revealing lysosomal function and physiology. *Physiology, 25*(2), 102–115. https://doi.org/10.1152/physiol.00041.2009

Pintos-Morell, G., & Beck, M. (2009). Fabry disease in children and the effects of enzyme replacement treatment. *European Journal of Pediatrics, 168*(11), 1355–1363. https://doi.org/10.1007/s00431-009-0937-9

Platt, F. M., Boland, B., & van der Spoel, A. C. (2012). The cell biology of disease: Lysosomal storage disorders: The cellular impact of lysosomal dysfunction. *The Journal of Cell Biology, 199*(5), 723–734. https://doi.org/10.1083/jcb.201208152

Reuser, A. J., Verheijen, F. W., Bali, D., van Diggelen, O. P., Germain, D. P., Hwu, W.-L., Lukacs, Z., Mühl, A., Olivova, P., Piraud, M., Wuyts, B., Zhang, K., & Keutzer, J. (2011). The use of dried blood spot samples in the diagnosis of lysosomal storage disorders—Current status and perspectives. *Molecular Genetics and Metabolism, 104*(1–2), 144–148. https://doi.org/10.1016/j.ymgme.2011.07.014

Spiridigliozzi, G. A., Keeling, L. A., Stefanescu, M., Li, C., Austin, S., & Kishnani, P. S. (2017). Cognitive and academic outcomes in long-term survivors of infantile-onset Pompe disease: A longitudinal follow-up. *Molecular Genetics and Metabolism, 121*(2), 127–137. https://doi.org/10.1016/j.ymgme.2017.04.014

Staretz-Chacham, O., Choi, J. H., Wakabayashi, K., Lopez, G., & Sidranksy, E. (2010). Psychiatric and behavioral manifestations of lysosomal storage disorders. *American Journal of Medical Genetics, 153B*(7), 1253–1265. https://doi.org/10.1002/ajmg.b.31097

Wang, R. Y., Bodamer, O. A., Watson, M. S., Wilcox, W. R., & ACMG Work Group on Diagnostic Confirmation of Lysosomal Storage Diseases. (2011). Lysosomal storage diseases: Diagnostic confirmation and management of presymptomatic individuals. *Genetics in Medicine, 13*(5), 457–484. https://doi.org/10.1097/GIM.0b013e318211a7e1

58

Mucopolysaccharide Disorders

Carolyn Tureaud, Taylor-Kristen Myers, and Michelle M. Perfect

Mucopolysaccharide (MPS) disorders are a subset of hereditary-based lysosomal storage disorders (see Chapter 57 by Fairchild and Islas on lysosomal storage disorders). Lysosomes are enzyme-containing cell structures that are crucial in the degradation of various proteins. Disturbances within the breakdown process of certain proteins may not only be detrimental to the overall function of the cell but can also be the cause of cognitive impairment, skeletal deformity, and global developmental delay within a person (Filocamo et al., 2018).

ETIOLOGY

The conditions grouped as MPS disorders all have similar causation. Children with these disorders possess extremely dangerous levels of toxic cellular waste within their body tissues. This toxicity is due to missing or deficient enzymes sanctioned with riding cells of specific proteins during lysosomal degradation or cell breakdown. The progressive buildup of certain sulfates left over from the cells' inability to fully dispose of proteins can produce a variety of complications in the child, including cell destruction (Tomatsu et al., 2013). MPS disorders are genetic in nature and inherited via an autosomal recessive gene. Hunter

The work on this chapter was supported in part by the Institute of Education Sciences, U.S. Department of Education, through Grant R305B160003. The opinions expressed are those of the authors and do not represent views of the Institute or the U.S. Department of Education.

https://doi.org/10.1037/0000349-058
Health-Related Disorders in Children and Adolescents: A Guidebook for Educators and Service Providers, Second Edition, M. M. Perfect, C. A. Riccio, and M. A. Bray (Editors)

syndrome (MPS II) is the only one that is recessively sex-linked; hence, it is predominantly expressed in male individuals. There are several subdivisions of MPS disorders, all uniquely influenced by different genes and enzyme deficiencies (Filocamo et al., 2018). Please see Table 58.1 for a listing of subtypes along with the underlying genetic etiology, featuring gene mutations.

TABLE 58.1. Subdivisions of Mucopolysaccharide Disorders

Type of MPS	Prevalence	Time of onset	Gene mutation	Symptoms
Hurler (MPS IH)	About one out of every 100,000 newborns. Both male and female children are affected in the same way (Lehtonen et al., 2018); about 0.7 per 100,000 in the United States (Puckett et al., 2021)	Onset as early as infancy, diagnosable at 6 months	*IDUA* gene mutation	Bone and joint disease, developmental delays, hydrocephalus, and cardiovascular irregularities
Hurler–Scheie (MPS IH/S)	One in 115,000	Onset as early as age 3	*IDUA* gene mutation	"Coarse facial features, joint stiffness, short stature, clouding of the corneas, abnormally enlarged liver and spleen (hepatosplenomegaly), and skeletal and cardiac abnormalities" (NORD, 2017)
Scheie (MPS IS)	One in 500,000 (Neufeld & Muenzer, 2019)	Onset as early as age 5	*IDUA* gene mutation	"Carpal tunnel syndrome, and backward flow of blood into the heart (aortic regurgitation)" (NORD, 2017)
Hunter syndrome (MPS II)	Primarily in male individuals; accounts for about one in 100,000 to 170,000; 0.7 per 100,000 in the United States (Puckett et al., 2021)	Onset as early as age 2	*IDS* gene mutation	Cognitive delay, coarseness of voice, sleep apnea, large head (macrocephaly), hernias, carpal tunnel, and knock knees (genu valgum)
Sanfilippo syndrome (MPS IIIA, IIIB, IIIC, and IIID)	One in 24,000 to 70,000; 0.71 per 100,000 in the United States (Puckett et al., 2021)	Onset as early as age 2	*GNS, HGSNA, NAGLU,* and *SGSH* gene mutations	Dementia, loss of mobility, skeletal abnormalities, seizures, behavioral disturbances (i.e., pica, hyperactivity, and temper tantrums)

Type of MPS	Prevalence	Time of onset	Gene mutation	Symptoms
Morquio (MPS IVA and IVB)	One in 200,000; 0.38 per 100,000 in the United States	Onset in early childhood	*GALNS* and *GLB1* gene mutation	Skeletal abnormalities, hypermobility, odontoid hypoplasia
Maroteaux-Lamy syndrome (MPS VI)	Estimated to occur in one case in 250,000 to 600,000 individuals	Onset as early as birth	*ARSB* gene mutation	Short stature, degenerative joint disease, and blindness
Sly syndrome (MPS VII)	Fewer than one in 250,000 (Yu, 2017)	Onset as early as infancy	*GUSB* gene mutation	Skeletal abnormalities, hernias, clouding of the corneas, hydrocephalus, short stature, heart disease, coarse facial features, and abnormal accumulation of fluid in various tissues of the body (hydrops fetalis; NORD, 2017)
Hyaluronidase deficiency (MPS IX)	Extremely rare, current prevalence of this type is currently unknown	Onset as early as age 1	*HYAL1* gene mutation	Short stature, cleft palate, soft-tissue masses, frequent ear infections (Zielonka et al., 2017)

Note. MPS = mucopolysaccharide; NORD = National Organization for Rare Disorders.

PREVALENCE AND INCIDENCE

Accurate reflections of these disorders within the general population are difficult to ascertain, due to under- and misdiagnosis (for subtype estimates, see Table 58.1). All MPS disorders combined are estimated to affect one in 25,000 births (Tomatsu et al., 2013), with incidence rates computed to be 0.98 per 100,000 in the United States and ranging from 1.53 to 4.8 per 100,000 worldwide (Puckett et al., 2021). The condition can be inherited by people of all races and ethnicities. In an epidemiological study in the United States, the prevalence of all MPS disorders was estimated to be 2.67 per 1,000,000 (Puckett et al., 2021).

SYMPTOMS

Within the MPS clinical spectrum, the nature and severity of symptoms vary. Core symptoms of each subtype can range from skeletal abnormalities to blindness. What remains consistent across the subdivisions of MPS disorders is the neurodegenerative and progressive worsening of symptoms over time. MPS disorder gravely affects organ system function, and depending on the severity of impact, life expectancy of individuals can be significantly affected.

IMPACT ON THE STUDENT AND OUTCOMES

MPS I, MPS II, and MPS III are known to have different medical, behavioral, and cognitive outcomes, which vary from mild to severe. Progressive degradation is common for several subtypes, and some observe achievement of milestones and then rapidly deteriorate.

Medical

Shortened lifespans are common, and mortality may occur within the first 10 years of life after receiving a diagnosis of MPS I and within the first 2 decades for MPS II or MPS III (Cross & Hare, 2013). Children who are diagnosed with Hurler syndrome (MPS IH) have substandard motor-related capabilities, though delays may be minimized with increased practice opportunities and access to treatments (Dusing et al., 2006). Without medical intervention, children with either MPS I or MPS III may experience enlarged regions of the brain such as the basal ganglia and corpus callosum. Brain atrophy may occur in youth with all subtypes of MPS III (Shapiro et al., 2017). MPS III diagnosis suggests children will have the capability to walk before reaching 18 months of age; however, like MPS I, their range of movement becomes more restricted and uncoordinated starting in early preschool years (Malm & Månsson, 2010).

Cognitive/Academic

As hearing impairments are common in students with MPS I, significant language difficulties may be found among those with MPS IH. Cognitive functioning has also been assessed to be significantly delayed, with peaks in ability during preschool ages and an accelerated worsening of abilities through years after (Shapiro et al., 2017). About a quarter of those with MPS II have an attenuated form, which presents without the cognitive impairment and is not progressive (Shapiro, Rudser, et al., 2016). Youth with MPS III present significant delayed language acquisition, and evidence from research has suggested that before 18 months, there is no appearance of word utterances, although some children are capable of short sentences (two to three words; Malm & Månsson, 2010). These language delays, and other behaviors associated with autism spectrum disorder, often contribute to misdiagnosis or late diagnosis of MPS IIID. MPS IIIB subtype is characterized by dementia attributable to the accumulation of heparan sulfate in the central nervous system. In one study in the Netherlands, only 39 of the 69 patients between the ages of 4 months and 6 years diagnosed with MPS III could be evaluated for developmental level as the rest of the participants were assessed to be developmentally below 3 months (Valstar et al., 2011).

Social-Emotional and Behavioral

As MPS disorders include a wide variety of different subdivisions, behavioral and social–emotional outcomes of these children also may vary. Socially, children with an MPS disorder who are immunocompromised are more likely to suffer more acutely because of possible medical treatment complications that then lead to fewer social opportunities. Pitt et al. (2009) found that among those with MPS 1H who received a bone marrow transplant, preschoolers with MPS 1H were at greater risk for poor adaptive and social skills compared with elementary-aged youth, whereas those older than 12 years were rated more poorly in adaptive functioning. Children with an MPS disorder who were under 12 years of age were found to participate less in community-based activities, such as sports, music groups, and peer interactions, than those without an MPS disorder. Individuals older than 12 with an MPS disorder reported fewer home-based peer interactions than their younger counterparts, despite no variations in socializing activities within families based on medical status (Pitt et al., 2009). Further, Lehtonen et al. (2018) found that parental ratings of children with MPS 1H revealed higher rates of socialization difficulties than the normative samples, whereas parent ratings did not reflect them to be more likely to be at risk in internalizing and externalizing symptoms.

Children with an MPS disorder have frequent disturbances in fearfulness and sleep; however, children with severe MPS II differ because of their experiences with frequent challenging behaviors (Cross & Hare, 2013). Although those with attenuated MPS II do not show deficits in disruptive behaviors—and in fact, some show improvement—there is evidence of diminished sense of self-worth as they reach adolescence (Shapiro, Rudser, et al., 2016). MPS III is connected to severe behavioral problems, such as restlessness, aggression, hyperactivity, inappropriate language, emotional outbursts, and sensory sensitivity (Cross & Hare, 2013; Escolar et al., 2017; Valstar et al., 2011). In addition, children with MPS IIIA and IIIB often may not exhibit the typical startle response and show less fear than their same-aged peers (Shapiro, King, et al., 2016). For instance, in a study comparing MPS IIIA and MPS IIIB with MPS IH, individuals with MPS III were more likely to pace around an unfamiliar room and touch a scary mask. Those with MPS IIIB were also slightly more likely to approach a stranger (Shapiro, King, et al., 2016). Sleep deficiencies in MPS 1H (Lehtonen et al., 2018), MPS II, and particularly MPS III have been characterized by delayed sleep latency, nighttime awakenings, insomnia symptoms, and irregular sleep schedules (e.g., daytime sleep; Cross & Hare, 2013; Escolar et al., 2017; Shapiro et al., 2017).

PSYCHOEDUCATIONAL IMPLICATIONS AND SCHOOL-BASED INTERVENTIONS

With early detection of the condition and treatment before age 2, children experience greater learning gains. However, many of the treatments only slow progression of the disease and are not curative. Students may be eligible for several categories within the Individuals With Disabilities Education Act, including multiple disabilities due to motor impairments, intellectual disabilities, language delays, and/or the potential for being deaf and hard of hearing (Eisengart et al., 2021). There may be justification for a one-to-one aide or shared paraprofessional for students with MPS disorders, particularly those with more severe forms of the disease, to allow them access to instruction so that they can benefit from meaningful participation in inclusive classrooms.

Medical and Health Management

As there is no cure for MPS, the currently available treatments only slow or curtail progression of the disease. Youth may require hearing aids. At home, students with trouble breathing may utilize a continuous or bilevel positive airway pressure device for nighttime hypoxia (Berger et al., 2013). Enzyme replacement therapy has been used as a treatment for less chronic forms of MPS I (MPS IH-S or MPS IS). However, as the enzymes do not pass the blood–brain barrier, it is not considered a first-line treatment (Eisengart et al., 2018). Rather, hematopoietic cell transplant, which is obtained either from bone marrow or stem cells from a donor, has been used with MPS IH because it mitigates the soft tissue destruction (Eisengart et al., 2018). Melatonin has been used to regulate sleep–wake cycles that contribute to difficulties in daytime functioning (Escolar et al., 2017; Shapiro et al., 2017).

School nurses and other health care assistants should be involved in any services delivered at school. Further, although potentially relevant for all health-related conditions, given the complexity of MPS disorders, families should be reminded and encouraged to invite health care providers or a representative knowledgeable about the medical condition and the student's course of the disorder to individualized education program meetings. School personnel should also seek a release of information to obtain updated medical records and consult with the various specialists (e.g., cardiologists for cardiac involvement, pulmonologists for respiratory issues or sleep disordered breathing, orthopedic and behavioral pediatricians).

Given the decline in motor ability and pain management, both occupational and physical therapy are likely necessary components of intervention (Dusing et al., 2006; Eisengart et al., 2018). Individuals with MPS II (Hunter syndrome) often require surgery to correct carpal tunnel or hernia. In addition to therapy targeting balance and strength, many of these students will likely need adapted physical education. Specific accommodations or assistive technologies may include adaptations to utensils, supportive shoes, easily removable clothing, and locomotive modifications for safe mobility. Malm and Månsson (2010) noted that even for youth with MPS III (Sanfilippo syndrome) who can walk, it is typically recommended that they utilize a wheelchair due to the likelihood of becoming fatigued when outdoors.

Cognitive/Academic

Despite the known developmental delays in cognition and communication, few studies have examined nonmedical-based interventions. Although research-based interventions for students with learning disabilities or intellectual impairment may be applicable, the rates of decline observed in this population warrant more frequent monitoring of learning gains and skill maintenance (Eisengart et al., 2018). Therefore, it is recommended that school psychologists consider administering curriculum-based measurements that track academic performance over time or conducting annual screenings for intellectual functioning and academic achievement. Intensive speech and language services are needed to support the student's communication. Because MPS disorders are progressive, it is important to monitor cognitive skills more frequently. In a review of cognitive measures that have been utilized in this population, researchers found that various version of the Bayley Scales of Infant Development, Wechsler Scales, Differential Abilities Scales, and the Kaufman Assessment Battery for Children have been utilized, with recommendations for the Differential Abilities Scales and Kaufman Assessment Battery given the low floor of these instruments (Janzen et al., 2017).

Social-Emotional and Behavioral

Individualized education programs may include goals related to developmentally appropriate self-care and life skills, accompanied by specially designed instruction and services to address adaptive functioning difficulties. Patient advocacy groups revealed that children with MPS IVA/VI encounter challenges of adequate maintenance of their independence and social bias (Akyol et al., 2019). Due to research indicating lower social engagement and skills, interventions should both target social skills development and increase opportunities for participation in extracurricular activities. Collaborations with a sleep specialist or sleep interventions may be needed to support behavioral management. A functional behavior assessment inclusive of sleep diaries and symptom logs (individualized to the student) might be useful to identify contributing factors that are not immediately observable (e.g., sleep disordered breathing, circadian rhythm disruption; Perfect et al., 2020). Supporting families to manage aggression, encouraging caregivers to connect with other families who have children with an MPS disorder, offering coping skill development for families, and providing opportunities for respite are important (Somanadhan & Larkin, 2016).

CONCLUSION

Almost all types of MPS disorders need medical intervention in some way. However, because there is no cure, the existing therapies can only delay or stop the illness from progressing. Furthermore, even though treatments may slow the loss of abilities, many children with an MPS disorder nevertheless have substantial motor and verbal impairments.

RESOURCES

Hunter's Hope Foundation. PO Box 643, Orchard Park, NY 14127; 716-667-1200; 877-984-HOPE (4673). http://www.huntershope.org

National MPS Society. PO Box 14686, Durham, NC 27709-4686; 877-MPS(677)-1001; 919-806-0101. http://www.mpssociety.org

REFERENCES

Akyol, M. U., Alden, T. D., Amartino, H., Ashworth, J., Belani, K., Berger, K. I., Borgo, A., Braunlin, E., Eto, Y., Gold, J. I., Jester, A., Jones, S. A., Karsli, C., Mackenzie, W., Marinho, D. R., McFadyen, A., McGill, J., Mitchell, J. J., Muenzer, J., . . . Scarpa, M. (2019). Recommendations for the management of MPS IVA: Systematic evidence- and consensus-based guidance. *Orphanet Journal of Rare Diseases, 14*(1), Article 137. https://doi.org/10.1186/s13023-019-1074-9

Berger, K. I., Fagondes, S. C., Giugliani, R., Hardy, K. A., Lee, K. S., McArdle, C., Scarpa, M., Tobin, M. J., Ward, S. A., & Rapoport, D. M. (2013). Respiratory and sleep disorders in mucopolysaccharidosis. *Journal of Inherited Metabolic Disease, 36*(2), 201–210. https://doi.org/10.1007/s10545-012-9555-1

Cross, E. M., & Hare, D. J. (2013). Behavioural phenotypes of the mucopolysaccharide disorders: A systematic literature review of cognitive, motor, social, linguistic and behavioural presentation in the MPS disorders. *Journal of Inherited Metabolic Disease, 36*(2), 189–200. https://doi.org/10.1007/s10545-012-9572-0

Dusing, S. C., Thorpe, D., Rosenberg, A., Mercer, V., & Escolar, M. L. (2006). Gross motor abilities in children with Hurler syndrome. *Developmental Medicine and Child Neurology, 48*(11), 927–930. https://pubmed.ncbi.nlm.nih.gov/17044963/

Eisengart, J. B., Esler, A. N., Ellinwood, N. M., Hudock, R. L., King, K. E., Klein, T. L., Lee, C., Morton, J., Stephens, K., Ziegler, R., & O'Neill, C. (2021). Issues of COVID-19-related distance learning for children with neuronopathic mucopolysaccharidoses. *Molecular Genetics and Metabolism, 134*(1–2), 68–76. https://doi.org/10.1016/j.ymgme.2021.06.012

Eisengart, J. B., Rudser, K. D., Xue, Y., Orchard, P., Miller, W., Lund, T., Van der Ploeg, A., Mercer, J., Jones, S., Mengel, K. E., Gökce, S., Guffon, N., Giugliani, R., de Souza, C., Shapiro, E. G., & Whitley, C. B. (2018). Long-term outcomes of systemic therapies for Hurler syndrome: An international multicenter comparison. *Genetics in Medicine, 20*(11), 1423–1429. https://doi.org/10.1038/gim.2018.29

Escolar, M. L., Jones, S. A., Shapiro, E. G., Horovitz, D. D. G., Lampe, C., & Amartino, H. (2017). Practical management of behavioral problems in mucopolysaccharidoses disorders. *Molecular Genetics and Metabolism, 122*(Suppl.), 35–40. https://doi.org/10.1016/j.ymgme.2017.09.010

Filocamo, M., Tomanin, R., Bertola, F., & Morrone, A. (2018). Biochemical and molecular analysis in mucopolysaccharidoses: What a paediatrician must know. *Italian Journal of Pediatrics, 44*(Suppl. 2), Article 129. https://doi.org/10.1186/s13052-018-0553-2

Janzen, D., Delaney, K. A., & Shapiro, E. G. (2017). Cognitive and adaptive measurement endpoints for clinical trials in mucopolysaccharidoses types I, II, and III: A review of the literature. *Molecular Genetics and Metabolism, 121*(2), 57–69. https://doi.org/10.1016/j.ymgme.2017.05.005

Lehtonen, A., Rust, S., Jones, S., Brown, R., & Hare, D. (2017). Social functioning and behaviour in mucopolysaccharidosis IH [Hurlers syndrome]. *JIMD Reports, 39*, 75–81. https://doi.org/10.1007/8904_2017_47

Malm, G., & Månsson, J. E. (2010). Mucopolysaccharidosis type III (Sanfilippo disease) in Sweden: Clinical presentation of 22 children diagnosed during a 30-year period. *Acta Paediatrica, 99*(8), 1253–1257. https://doi.org/10.1111/j.1651-2227.2010.01800.x

National Organization for Rare Disorders. (2017). *Mucopolysaccharidoses*. https://rarediseases.org/rare-diseases/mucopolysaccharidoses/

Neufeld, E. F., & Muenzer, J. (2019). The mucopolysaccharidoses. In D. L. Valle, S. Antonarakis, A. Ballabio, A. L. Beaudet, & G. A. Mitchell. (Eds.), *The online metabolic and molecular bases of inherited disease*. McGraw Hill. https://ommbid.mhmedical.com/content.aspx?bookid=2709&sectionid=225544161

Perfect, M. M., Frye, S. S., & Williams, S. B. H. (2020). The mind–body connection in sleep health: Conducting assessments and interventions in school settings. In C. Maykel & M. Bray (Eds.), *Promoting mind–body health in schools: Interventions for mental health professionals* (pp. 335–353). American Psychological Association. https://doi.org/10.1037/0000157-023

Pitt, C., Lavery, C., & Wager, N. (2009). Psychosocial outcomes of bone marrow transplant for individuals affected by mucopolysaccharidosis I Hurler disease: Patient social competency. *Child: Care, Health and Development, 35*(2), 271–280. https://doi.org/10.1111/j.1365-2214.2008.00918.x

Puckett, Y., Mallorga-Hernández, A., & Montaño, A. M. (2021). Epidemiology of mucopolysaccharidoses (MPS) in United States: Challenges and opportunities. *Orphanet Journal of Rare Diseases, 16*(1), Article 241. https://doi.org/10.1186/s13023-021-01880-8

Shapiro, E. G., Jones, S. A., & Escolar, M. L. (2017). Developmental and behavioral aspects of mucopolysaccharidoses with brain manifestations—Neurological signs and symptoms. *Molecular Genetics and Metabolism Reports, 122*(Suppl.), 1–7. https://doi.org/10.1016/j.ymgme.2017.08.009

Shapiro, E., King, K., Ahmed, A., Rudser, K., Rumsey, R., Yund, B., Delaney, K., Nestrasil, I., Whitley, C., & Potegal, M. (2016). The neurobehavioral phenotype in mucopolysaccharidosis type IIIB: An exploratory study. *Molecular Genetics and Metabolism Reports, 6*, 41–47. https://doi.org/10.1016/j.ymgmr.2016.01.003

Shapiro, E. G., Rudser, K., Ahmed, A., Steiner, R. D., Delaney, K. A., Yund, B., King, K., Kunin-Batson, A., Eisengart, J., & Whitley, C. B. (2016). A longitudinal study of emotional adjustment, quality of life and adaptive function in attenuated MPS II. *Molecular Genetics and Metabolism Reports, 7*, 32–39. https://doi.org/10.1016/j.ymgmr.2016.03.005

Somanadhan, S., & Larkin, P. J. (2016). Parents' experiences of living with, and caring for children, adolescents and young adults with mucopolysaccharidosis (MPS). *Orphanet Journal of Rare Diseases, 11*(1), Article 138. https://doi.org/10.1186/s13023-016-0521-0

Tomatsu, S., Fujii, T., Fukushi, M., Oguma, T., Shimada, T., Maeda, M., Kida, K., Shibata, Y., Futatsumori, H., Montaño, A. M., Mason, R. W., Yamaguchi, S., Suzuki, Y., & Orii, T. (2013). Newborn screening and diagnosis of mucopolysaccharidoses. *Molecular Genetics and Metabolism, 110*(1–2), 42–53. https://doi.org/10.1016/j.ymgme.2013.06.007

Valstar, M. J., Marchal, J. P., Grootenhuis, M., Colland, V., & Wijburg, F. A. (2011). Cognitive development in patients with mucopolysaccharidosis type III (Sanfilippo syndrome). *Orphanet Journal of Rare Diseases, 6*(1), Article 43. https://doi.org/10.1186/1750-1172-6-43

Yu, C. (2017). Lysosomal storage disorders: Mucopolysaccharidoses. In U. Garg & L. D. Smith (Eds.), *Biomarkers in inborn errors of metabolism* (pp. 191–209). Elsevier. https://doi.org/10.1016/B978-0-12-802896-4.00006-7

Zielonka, J., Joseph, J., Sikora, A., Hardy, M., Ouari, O., Vasquez-Vivar, J., Cheng, G., Lopez, M., & Kalyanaraman, B. (2017). Mitochondria-targeted triphenylphosphonium-based compounds: Syntheses, mechanisms of action, and therapeutic and diagnostic applications. *Chemical Reviews, 117*(15), 10043–10120. https://doi.org/10.1021/acs.chemrev.7b00042

59

Neurofibromatosis

Elizabeth Perdue, Lindsey J. Carnes, and Cynthia A. Riccio

The neurofibromatoses (NFs) are classified as neurocutaneous disorders due to the genetically transmitted presentation of hyperpigmentation of the skin (Crawford & Schorry, 2006; Hersh & Committee on Genetics, 2008; National Institute of Neurological Disorders and Stroke [NINDS], 2022). As with other neurocutaneous disorders, NFs involve both the nervous system and function as well as the skin, with associated symptoms emerging over the individual's lifetime as the disorder manifests. Scientists have categorized the disorder as neurofibromatosis Type 1 (NF1 or von Recklinghausen), neurofibromatosis Type 2 (NF2), and schwannomatosis (NINDS, 2022; Ullrich, 2016). Only NF1 and NF2 present during the developmental period.

ETIOLOGY

The NF gene is autosomal dominant, such that if either parent has the defective gene, each child born to that parent has a 50% chance of inheriting it. The NF1 gene is located at chromosome 17q11.2 (NINDS, 2022; Ullrich, 2016). The NF2 gene is transmitted similarly; however, the chromosome affected is 22q (Ullrich, 2016). Although most affected persons inherit the disorder, between 30% and 50% of new cases arise spontaneously through genetic mutation; the mutated gene then can be passed on to later generations. With this mutation, proteins that coordinate cell division and growth are affected (Julian et al., 2014). Due to the cellular-level abnormalities,

https://doi.org/10.1037/0000349-059
Health-Related Disorders in Children and Adolescents: A Guidebook for Educators and Service Providers, Second Edition, M. M. Perfect, C. A. Riccio, and M. A. Bray (Editors)

multiple organ systems can be affected. Organ systems such as the skin, nervous system, bones, and eyes are commonly afflicted by NF complications (Hirbe & Gutmann, 2014).

PREVALENCE AND INCIDENCE

NF1 is the more common type and occurs in approximately one in 3,000 to 4,000 individuals in the United States (NINDS, 2022). It occurs across racial and ethnic groups, affecting male and female individuals equally. In contrast, NF2 is rare, occurring in one out of 25,000 individuals (NINDS, 2022). In both cases, transmission is autosomal dominant. Due to the rarity of NF2 occurrences, the focus of this text is on NF1.

SYMPTOMS

NF primarily affects the development and growth of neural (nerve) cell tissues (NINDS, 2022). NF1 is characterized by café au lait spots or macules, with six or more macules, often present at birth or during infancy and almost always by 10 years of age (Hersh & Committee on Genetics, 2008). These are usually most pronounced on the trunk, with the size of the macules increasing as the child ages (Ullrich, 2016). There may be freckling in skinfolds that present by about 5 years of age. Neurofibromas that appear as small bumps under the skin may be present as well. The number and size of these increase with age and can involve multiple nerves (plexiform neurofibromas; Sampson et al., 2019); in some cases, neurofibromas may become malignant. Small bumps on the iris (Lisch nodules) are another sign of NF1; however, these are not necessarily large enough to be seen and do not affect vision. NF1 further presents as tumors of the central and peripheral nervous system, bone abnormalities (e.g., scoliosis), and lesions of the vascular and viscera systems (Sampson et al., 2019). A clinical diagnosis of NF1 results when any two of these symptoms are present based on the National Institutes of Health (1988) Consensus Development Conference on Neurofibromatosis.

The course of NF1 is not predictable, although it usually stabilizes by adulthood (Sampson et al., 2019). In many cases, symptoms are mild and individuals with NF1 live normal and productive lives. The effect of NF1 depends on the number of tumors and neurofibromas, as well as their location and the subsequent impact on surrounding tissues. In some cases, however, NF1 can be severely debilitating and involve the optic and cochlear nerves (Hersh & Committee on Genetics, 2008; NINDS, 2022). A tumor on the optic nerve (optic glioma) is likely to affect vision, whereas one on the cochlear nerve can affect hearing and auditory processing (Gutmann et al., 2017).

IMPACT ON THE STUDENT AND OUTCOMES

Medical

When neurofibromas result in pain, disfiguration, or in the case of malignancy, medical intervention may be needed (Sampson et al., 2019). In cases where the cochlear nerve may be affected, with subsequent impairment to hearing, consideration of a cochlear implant or brain stem implant may be appropriate (Vincent et al., 2008). In more severe forms, cardiac problems (e.g., hypertension) may necessitate medical intervention (Ullrich, 2016; Williams et al., 2009). Research suggests a high frequency of orthopedic complications in NF1, with up to 25% evidencing orthopedic problems (Crawford & Schorry, 2006). These problems may result in fine and gross motor impairments, interfering with independent daily living skills (Hyman et al., 2005).

Individuals with NF1 are also more likely to develop tumors in both the central and peripheral nervous systems (Gutmann et al., 2017; Hirbe & Gutmann, 2014). Leukemia, breast cancer, and brain tumors are especially prevalent. Approximately 15% to 20% of children with NF1 will experience optic pathway gliomas. Brainstem gliomas are often observed in older children. These neurological tumors may require shunting, surgical resection, or chemotherapy (Gutmann et al., 2017; Hirbe & Gutmann, 2014).

Cognitive/Academic

Some type of cognitive impairment is the most common neurological complication of NF1 in childhood and often the major concern of the parent of a child with the disorder (North et al., 2002). The extent of neurocognitive deficits is associated with the severity of NF1 (Krab et al., 2009). As a result, NF1 has no specific cognitive pattern (Levine et al., 2006). Although intellectual disability is not a common feature of NF1, there is a high frequency of associated learning disabilities (Beaussart et al., 2018), communication disorders, and subsequent special education placement. Approximately 30% to 65% of children experience deficits in both receptive and expressive language (Williams et al., 2009). Watt et al. (2008) found that 67% to 75% of children in their study evidenced difficulty with one or more reading subskills; learning disability in math was less frequent. With academic underachievement, there is risk of failure to complete high school and subsequent limitations on career choice (North et al., 2002).

Social-Emotional and Behavioral

Children with NF1 are at increased risk of developing emotional and behavioral problems (Noll et al., 2007). The presence of comorbidity, particularly with attention-deficit/hyperactivity disorder (Hyman et al., 2005) and/or autism spectrum disorder (Chisholm et al., 2018), is frequent among children with

NF1. Research suggests that children with more severe and visible NF symptoms may be at risk for a myriad of psychological difficulties, including low self-esteem (Counterman et al., 1995). Children with physical deformities, including those associated with NF, have difficulties in forming friendships and are often rejected by peers.

PSYCHOEDUCATIONAL IMPLICATIONS AND SCHOOL-BASED INTERVENTIONS

For children with NF1, support from parents and teachers is important for healthy adjustment; however, it may be difficult to persuade some parents that their youngsters need special attention. In an effort to maximize a child's sense of normalcy and adequacy, parents and teachers may inadvertently ignore a child's emotional distress. Therefore, psychologists, physicians, and other professionals who work with children should consider assessing the need for supportive and preventive services, particularly at ages where appearance and competence are crucial developmental issues. Numerous resources, practical recommendations, and interventions are included at the end of this chapter, and a brief overview is provided in the following sections regarding medical and health management, cognitive/academic concerns, and social–emotional and behavioral difficulties.

Medical and Health Management

Given that medical difficulties associated with NF1 can be variable, recommendations for health management can also vary. Generally, health education is warranted, with appropriate consideration of the individual's age (Ferner et al., 2007). Monitoring of disease progression and complications as well as genetic counseling services are also recommended (Ferner et al., 2007). Hirbe and Gutmann (2014) reiterated the utilization of pharmacological interventions for concerns including pain. Overall, collaboration among key individuals in multiple settings (e.g., medical, educational, home) for children with NF1 is imperative in maintaining consistent medical management and safety.

Cognitive/Academic

Neurocognitive deficits are not uncommon among individuals with NF1. For children within the school setting, accommodations for learning difficulties should be considered, and students would ideally be supported by a multidisciplinary team to promote academic success (Hirbe & Gutmann, 2014). An evidence-based approach to address specific academic difficulties is self-regulated strategy development (Limpo & Alves, 2014). The student's development and progress should be continually monitored; significant assistance and intervention associated with executive functioning and working memory abilities are common among individuals, particularly children, with NF1 (Ferner et al., 2007; Hyman et al., 2005). Research supports the use of programs for executive functioning, especially metacognitive skills, to improve academic outcomes (Otero et al., 2014; Riccio & Gomes, 2013).

Social-Emotional and Behavioral

Individuals with NF1 vary in the reporting of daily difficulties, especially as NFs are considered heterogeneous diseases. While some individuals report relatively typical lives, others experience severe social and emotional concerns, including cosmetic disfigurement, neurologic dysfunction, psychological distress, and disability (Vranceanu et al., 2013). Social support and counseling are often recommended as self-esteem is often negatively affected within this youth population (Ferner et al., 2007; Krab et al., 2009). Teachers and parents can assist in modeling social behaviors. Overall, individuals with NF report lower quality of life as compared with the typical population, with variation dependent upon factors such as socioeconomic status and visibility and severity of disease. Additionally, although a diminished quality of life is reported for children and adolescents who have NF1 diagnoses, research supports the benefits of strong family relationships on the individual's reported quality of life and psychological adjustment (Graf et al., 2006). Interventions to support family structure may be warranted in specific cases. Further, those who seek treatment from NF specialists reported significantly greater enjoyment of life (Vranceanu et al., 2013). This emphasizes the importance of medical intervention and support.

NF1 is frequently associated with co-occurring academic and social–emotional problems, as well as attention-deficit/hyperactivity disorder. Pharmacological intervention may be considered for behavior management (Ferner et al., 2007). Peer reactions to the NF1 stigmata can often be negative. Direct individual and group intervention (e.g., counseling, modeling) needs to be multifaceted to address academic issues, social issues, emotional concerns, and attention problems, as well as any medical complications. Cognitive behavior therapy may be appropriate (Eiraldi et al., 2016; Ruocco et al., 2018; van Starrenburg et al., 2017) to address both internalizing and externalizing problems and develop coping skills. Mindfulness approaches have garnered support as a school-based treatment to address stress and may be effective for children with NF1 (McKeering & Hwang, 2019; Schonert-Reichl et al., 2015).

Given the complexities of NF1, collaboration across disciplines with differing interventions provided in concert is paramount in effective intervention (Riccio et al., 2010). Due to the neurodevelopmental changes associated with NF1, early identification and progress monitoring are needed to ensure appropriate educational interventions are in place (Hyman et al., 2005).

CONCLUSION

NF1 is a complex disease that can be significantly debilitating, particularly to youths. As with many diseases, the presentation of NF1 can vary by individual, affecting a variety of day-to-day functioning domains, including general health, medical management, cognition and learning, emotions, and behavior. Still, numerous NF1 resources are available to provide support and intervention strategies for individuals, parents, educators, and medical teams.

RESOURCES

KidsHealth. (2022). *Neurofibromatosis Type 1*. https://kidshealth.org/en/parents/nf.html

Children's Tumor Foundation. (2017). *The NF parent guidebook: How to help children with learning challenges associated with neurofibromatosis Type 1*. https://www.ctf.org/images/uploads/NF_Parent_Guidebook_CTF_web.pdf

Children's Tumor Foundation. (n.d.). *Understanding NF*. https://www.ctf.org/understanding-nf/nf1 (available in English, Spanish, French, and Arabic)

St. Louis Children's Hospital. (n.d.). *App recommendations*. Washington University. https://nfcenter.wustl.edu/nicoles-nook-summer-app-recommendations/

National Institute of Neurological Disorders and Stroke. (2022). *Neurofibromatosis fact sheet*. National Institutes of Health. https://www.ninds.nih.gov/Disorders/Patient-Caregiver-Education/Fact-Sheets/Neurofibromatosis-Fact-Sheet (available in English and Spanish)

Genetics Education Materials for School Success. (2015). *Neurofibromatosis 1*. New England Regional Genetics Network. https://www.negenetics.org/gemss/conditions/neurofibromatosis-1 (available in English and Spanish)

REFERENCES

Beaussart, M. L., Barbarot, S., Mauger, C., & Roy, A. (2018). Systematic review and meta-analysis of executive functions in preschool and school-age children with neurofibromatosis Type 1. *Journal of the International Neuropsychological Society, 24*(9), 977–994. https://doi.org/10.1017/S1355617718000383

Chisholm, A. K., Anderson, V. A., Pride, N. A., Malarbi, S., North, K. N., & Payne, J. M. (2018). Social function and autism spectrum disorder in children and adults with neurofibromatosis Type 1: A systematic review and meta-analysis. *Neuropsychology Review, 28*(3), 317–340. https://doi.org/10.1007/s11065-018-9380-x

Counterman, A. P., Saylor, C. F., & Pai, S. (1995). Psychological adjustment of children and adolescents with neurofibromatosis. *Children's Health Care, 24*(4), 223–234. https://doi.org/10.1207/s15326888chc2404_2

Crawford, A. H., & Schorry, E. K. (2006). Neurofibromatosis update. *Journal of Pediatric Orthopedics, 26*(3), 413–423. https://doi.org/10.1097/01.bpo.0000217719.10728.39

Eiraldi, R., Power, T. J., Schwartz, B. S., Keiffer, J. N., McCurdy, B. L., Mathen, M., & Jawad, A. F. (2016). Examining effectiveness of group cognitive-behavioral therapy for externalizing and internalizing disorders in urban schools. *Behavior Modification, 40*(4), 611–639. https://doi.org/10.1177/0145445516631093

Ferner, R. E., Huson, S. M., Thomas, N., Moss, C., Willshaw, H., Evans, D. G., Upadhyaya, M., Towers, R., Gleeson, M., Steiger, C., & Kirby, A. (2007). Guidelines for the diagnosis and management of individuals with neurofibromatosis 1. *Journal of Medical Genetics, 44*(2), 81–88. https://doi.org/10.1136/jmg.2006.045906

Graf, A., Landolt, M. A., Mori, A. C., & Boltshauser, E. (2006). Quality of life and psychological adjustment in children and adolescents with neurofibromatosis Type 1. *The Journal of Pediatrics, 149*(3), 348–353. https://doi.org/10.1016/j.jpeds.2006.04.025

Gutmann, D. H., Ferner, R. E., Listernick, R. H., Korf, B. R., Wolters, P. L., & Johnson, K. J. (2017). Neurofibromatosis Type 1. *Nature Reviews Disease Primers, 3*(1), Article 17004. https://doi.org/10.1038/nrdp.2017.4

Hersh, J. H., & the Committee on Genetics. (2008). Health supervision for children with neurofibromatosis. *Pediatrics, 121*(3), 633–642. https://doi.org/10.1542/peds.2007-3364

Hirbe, A. C., & Gutmann, D. H. (2014). Neurofibromatosis Type 1: A multidisciplinary approach to care. *Lancet Neurology, 13*(8), 834–843. https://doi.org/10.1016/S1474-4422(14)70063-8

Hyman, S. L., Shores, A., & North, K. N. (2005). The nature and frequency of cognitive deficits in children with neurofibromatosis Type 1. *Neurology, 65*(7), 1037–1044. https://doi.org/10.1212/01.wnl.0000179303.72345.ce

Julian, N., Edwards, N. E., DeCrane, S., & Hingtgen, C. M. (2014). Neurofibromatosis 1: Diagnosis and management. *The Journal for Nurse Practitioners, 10*(1), 30–35. https://doi.org/10.1016/j.nurpra.2013.07.001

Krab, L. C., Oostenbrink, R., de Goede-Bolder, A., Aarsen, F. K., Elgersma, Y., & Moll, H. A. (2009). Health-related quality of life in children with neurofibromatosis Type 1: Contribution of demographic factors, disease-related factors, and behavior. *The Journal of Pediatrics, 154*(3), 420–425.e1. https://doi.org/10.1016/j.jpeds.2008.08.045

Levine, T. M., Materek, A., Abel, J., O'Donnell, M., & Cutting, L. E. (2006). Cognitive profile of neurofibromatosis Type 1. *Seminars in Pediatric Neurology, 13*(1), 8–20. https://doi.org/10.1016/j.spen.2006.01.006

Limpo, T., & Alves, R. A. (2014). Implicit theories of writing and their impact on students' responses to a SRSD intervention. *British Journal of Educational Psychology, 84*, 571–590. https://doi.org/10.1111/bjep.12042

McKeering, P., & Hwang, Y.-S. (2019). A systematic review of mindfulness-based school interventions with early adolescents. *Mindfulness, 10*(4), 593–610. https://doi.org/10.1007/s12671-018-0998-9

National Institute of Neurological Disorders and Stroke. (2022). *Neurofibromatosis fact sheet*. https://www.ninds.nih.gov/Disorders/Patient-Caregiver-Education/Fact-Sheets/Neurofibromatosis-Fact-Sheet

National Institutes of Health. (1988). Neurofibromatosis: Conference statement: National Institutes of Health Consensus Development Conference. *Archives of Neurology, 45*(5), 575–578. https://pubmed.ncbi.nlm.nih.gov/3128965/

Noll, R. B., Reiter-Purtill, J., Moore, B. D., Schorry, E. K., Lovell, A. M., Vannatta, K., & Gerhardt, C. A. (2007). Social, emotional, and behavioral functioning of children with NF1. *American Journal of Medical Genetics: Part A, 143A*(19), 2261–2273. https://doi.org/10.1002/ajmg.a.31923

North, K., Hyman, S., & Barton, B. (2002). Cognitive deficits in neurofibromatosis 1. *Journal of Child Neurology, 17*(8), 605–612. https://doi.org/10.1177/088307380201700811

Otero, T. M., Barker, L. A., & Naglieri, J. A. (2014). Executive function treatment and intervention in schools. *Applied Neuropsychology: Child, 3*(3), 205–214. https://doi.org/10.1080/21622965.2014.897903

Riccio, C. A., & Gomes, H. (2013). Interventions for executive function deficits in children and adolescents. *Applied Neuropsychology: Child, 2*(2), 133–140. https://doi.org/10.1080/21622965.2013.748383

Riccio, C. A., Sullivan, J. R., & Cohen, M. J. (2010). *Neuropsychological assessment and intervention for childhood and adolescent disorders*. Wiley. https://doi.org/10.1002/9781118269954

Ruocco, S., Freeman, N. C., & McLean, L. A. (2018). Learning to cope: A CBT evaluation exploring self-reported changes in coping with anxiety among school children aged 5–7 years. *Educational and Developmental Psychologist, 35*(2), 67–87. https://doi.org/10.1017/edp.2018.8

Sampson, J., Thompson, H. L., & Parilo, D. M. W. (2019). Caring for children with neurofibromatosis Type 1. *Nursing, 49*(4), 30–36. https://doi.org/10.1097/01.NURSE.0000554214.17051.d9

Schonert-Reichl, K. A., Oberle, E., Lawlor, M. S., Abbott, D., Thomson, K., Oberlander, T. F., & Diamond, A. (2015). Enhancing cognitive and social–emotional development through a simple-to-administer mindfulness-based school program for elementary school children: A randomized controlled trial. *Developmental Psychology, 51*(1), 52–66. https://doi.org/10.1037/a0038454

Ullrich, N. J. (2016). Neurocutaneous syndromes and brain tumors. *Journal of Child Neurology, 31*(12), 1399–1411. https://doi.org/10.1177/0883073815604220

van Starrenburg, M. L. A., Kuijpers, R. C. M. W., Kleinjan, M., Hutschemaekers, G. J. M., & Engels, R. C. M. E. (2017). Effectiveness of a cognitive behavioral therapy-based indicated prevention program for children with elevated anxiety levels: A randomized controlled trial. *Prevention Science, 18*(1), 31–39. https://doi.org/10.1007/s11121-016-0725-5

Vincent, J. L., Kahn, I., Snyder, A. Z., Raichle, M. E., & Buckner, R. L. (2008). Evidence for a frontoparietal control system revealed by intrinsic functional connectivity. *Journal of Neurophysiology, 100*(6), 3328–3342. https://doi.org/10.1152/jn.90355.2008

Vranceanu, A. M., Merker, V. L., Park, E., & Plotkin, S. R. (2013). Quality of life among adult patients with neurofibromatosis 1, neurofibromatosis 2 and schwannomatosis: A systematic review of the literature. *Journal of Neuro-Oncology, 114*(3), 257–262. https://doi.org/10.1007/s11060-013-1195-2

Watt, S. E., Shores, A., & North, K. N. (2008). An examination of lexical and sublexical reading skills in children with neurofibromatosis Type 1. *Child Neuropsychology, 14*(5), 401–418. https://doi.org/10.1080/09297040701595505

Williams, V. C., Lucas, J., Babcock, M. A., Gutmann, D. H., Korf, B., & Maria, B. L. (2009). Neurofibromatosis Type 1 revisited. *Pediatrics, 123*(1), 124–133. https://doi.org/10.1542/peds.2007-3204

60

Pediatric Cancer

Lea A. Theodore, Melissa A. Bray, Lauren Gammie, Cassandra Odell, Larissa Hoefler, Kerrilyn Surdi, Lydia Rumpf, and Alyssa Perri Elias

Pediatric cancer results from the rapid growth and multiplication of abnormal cells in the body. These cancer cells typically form tumors, or masses of abnormal cells, which may travel to other parts of the body, where they continue to grow at exponential rates, forming new tumors. This deluge of malignant cells destroys the body's healthy tissues and may affect other organs and tissues throughout the body. As cancer cells grow, they require more of the body's nutrients, which weakens children's overall immune system, limits their strength, and destroys organs and bones. Pediatric cancer is rare, accounting for approximately 1% of newly diagnosed cancers (American Cancer Society, 2018). The most common childhood cancers include leukemia; lymphoma; brain, bone, and kidney cancer; and cancer of the nerve cells. Since presenting symptoms resemble other benign conditions, a cancer diagnosis is often delayed. Once a cancer diagnosis has been made, it is imperative that parents seek out treatment from a pediatric oncologist.

ETIOLOGY

Although the cause of childhood cancers is largely unknown, most cancers are thought to develop as a result of genetic mutations that result in uncontrollable cell growth. Unfortunately, there is no prevention for these genetic transmutations because they are random and unpredictable. Several risk factors for the

https://doi.org/10.1037/0000349-060
Health-Related Disorders in Children and Adolescents: A Guidebook for Educators and Service Providers, Second Edition, M. M. Perfect, C. A. Riccio, and M. A. Bray (Editors)

development of pediatric cancer have also been posited, including medical conditions, problems with development in the womb, exposure to infections, exposure to radiation, and previous cancer treatments. However, environmental factors, such as exposure to toxic substances, are not probable causes of childhood cancer.

PREVALENCE AND INCIDENCE

Cancer in children is rare, accounting for approximately 1% of newly diagnosed cancers (Siegel et al., 2018). Prior to age 15, one out of 408 children will receive a cancer diagnosis, and one out of 285 will be diagnosed with cancer before the age of 20 (Howlader et al., 2017). Among children between the ages of 1 and 14 years old, the most common cancers include acute lymphocytic leukemia, brain and central nervous system tumors, neuroblastomas, and non-Hodgkin lymphoma. The most common cancers diagnosed in adolescents aged 15 to 19 years include Hodgkin lymphoma, thyroid cancer, brain and central nervous system tumors, and testicular germ cell tumors (Siegel et al., 2018). There is a greater incidence rate for childhood cancer in male children, but this difference dissipates during adolescence, with male and female adolescents exhibiting an equal incidence of cancer. With respect to race and ethnicity, White and Latinx children have the highest incidence rates for cancer, and African American and Asian American/Pacific Islander children and adolescents have the lowest rates (Pan et al., 2010).

SYMPTOMS

Symptoms associated with childhood cancer are similar to those of other illnesses and conditions. Common presenting indicators and red flags associated with a cancer diagnosis include excessive bruising and bleeding; fatigue; joint pain; unexplained weight loss; night sweats; headaches, particularly those that occur in the morning; nausea; vomiting; ashen pallor; unexplained irritability; increasing head circumference; vision problems; gait issues; constant infections; and lumps or masses on the body (Fragkandrea et al., 2013).

IMPACT ON THE STUDENT AND OUTCOMES

Pediatric cancer has both short- and long-term impacts on children; that is, cancer affects a child's physical, social–emotional, cognitive, and academic development. Given the medical treatment of cancer, children often miss a great deal of school, which affects their education and socialization with peers, placing their social skills at a different level than their same-aged fellow students. All of these issues have the potential to significantly impact the quality of life for children with cancer. Thus, it is imperative for child's teachers and other school personnel to work collaboratively with the family to develop appropriate scholastic and medical plans for the child and address the issues mentioned previously. Importantly, school personnel should be made aware of the fact that although cancer treatment may be completed, children with pediatric cancer are likely to continue to struggle with academic, cognitive, social–emotional, and medical issues (Irwin & Elam, 2011).

Medical

Despite remitting cancer, cancer treatments have the potential to cause later health problems in children surviving cancer. Due to new advances in medicine and technology, the survival rates of childhood cancer have increased to a 5-year survival rate of approximately 80% (American Cancer Society, 2018). As more children survive, physicians are seeing higher rates of late effects of cancer treatments in adulthood. Medical outcome data show that 60% to 90% of child cancer survivors will develop chronic health-related conditions and 20% to 80% of survivors will experience life-threatening conditions during adulthood (Howlader et al., 2017). Adverse late effects of treatment include, but are not limited to, issues with organs, muscles, and tissues; reproductive problems; digestive issues; hearing, vision, and dental problems; attenuated growth and development; cognitive, academic, and social and emotional functioning; psychological adjustment; and greater risk of developing a second cancer (Physician Data Query, 2019). The intensity of latent treatment effects is dependent on multiple factors, including type of cancer, treatment employed (e.g., surgery, chemotherapy, radiation, stem cell transplants, targeted therapy), and patient-related factors (e.g., child's sex, health prior to diagnosis, family history, age of diagnosis and treatment; Physician Data Query, 2019). In order to minimize long-term negative effects, doctors recommend regular and yearly follow-up visits with a pediatric oncologist to improve children's overall health and quality of life.

Cognitive/Academic

Academically, children undergoing cancer treatment fall increasingly behind in reading, spelling, and mathematics. This academic regression is typically indicative not of a skill deficiency but rather of a diminished degree of skill attainment due to missed school, health distractors, and emotional stressors. Inadequate academic performance is heavily influenced by the secondary side effects of cancer treatments (e.g., fatigue and missed school days). Learning problems may also occur due to a lapse in the acquisition of academic skills (Armstrong et al., 1999). Children who undergo cancer treatment at younger ages typically have the most difficulty with focused and sustained attention, as well as problems in selective attention, cognitive flexibility, processing speed, and executive functioning (Brinkman et al., 2016).

Social-Emotional and Behavioral

Children with cancer often struggle with socialization. These social adjustment difficulties typically present as social withdrawal and deficits in social skills. Many children have deficits in nonverbal reasoning that make it difficult to understand and navigate social situations (Semrud-Clikeman & Ellison, 2009). Emotionally, childhood cancer survivors struggle with multiple issues, including perception of their physical appearance and changes to their bodies; concerns regarding cancer reoccurrence; worries about new health problems; feelings of resentment for having to go through treatment; anxiety regarding differential treatment by their peers; and apprehension about future events, such as getting married and having children (American Cancer Society, 2017). In light of the aforementioned psychosocial issues, it is not surprising that some children are diagnosed with internalizing and/or externalizing disorders or posttraumatic stress disorders while battling cancer. Risk factors for impaired social and emotional functioning that may persist in survivors include low cognitive and adaptive functioning, living in single-parent families, having a chaotic family environment, and being of low socioeconomic status (Semrud-Clikeman & Ellison, 2009).

PSYCHOEDUCATIONAL IMPLICATIONS

Building a cohesive understanding of the experiences a child with cancer will face is an important component of supporting children and their well-being. Emotionally, children will need sensitive responses to their changing moods and feelings. Children diagnosed with cancer often share with others that their illness makes them feel lonely and isolated, confused, and different from children without cancer (Crossland, 2002). Parents, siblings, and others affected by the child's diagnosis often experience similar feelings of anger, distress, and confusion. To address these issues, it is important to encourage open communication, promote the use of support services offered, and help the family recognize that modifications will need to be made to manage the effects of the disease. Helping the child and those affected by the cancer diagnosis is encouraged to ameliorate feelings of isolation and provide support in managing treatment. Promoting positivity regarding the child's perceptions and future outlook should be a primary focus in working with children with cancer. Moreover, children with cancer are more likely to experience academic burdens; changes in relationships with peers; feelings of inferiority (e.g., disappointment, disgust, failure); and limited opportunities to participate in school, athletics, and extracurricular activities (Boles et al., 2017). Fostering the maintenance of friendships and encouraging children to attend social events, education, athletics, and other activities children enjoyed prior to their illness will help reinforce their overall sense of well-being (Li & Wendt, 1998).

If the child is hospitalized or cannot attend school, parents and educators are encouraged to explore the availability of hospital school programs or homebound tutoring (Li & Wendt, 1998). Removing children from school will limit their typical school-day activities and may adversely affect their academic and psychosocial development (Butler et al., 2008). Academically, continuing to provide necessary instruction to ensure the child is maintaining appropriate levels of academic skills is important, not only for educational purposes but also for enhancing self-esteem and improving social relationships (Vance & Eiser, 2002). Technological methods, such as Zoom and FaceTime, are recommended to promote communication with the child's classmates and school environment. Providing opportunities that allow the child to feel involved with the experiences of their peers may positively support the child's development of social interactions and feelings of belonging.

When children reach a point where they can return to school, several reentry strategies should be considered by parents and teachers to help support a successful transition. Such strategies include providing classmates with short intervention sessions focused on learning about cancer, ways it develops, and how it is treated. This facilitates school reentry, enhances the self-esteem of the child with cancer, promotes peer acceptance, increases positive social interactions, and decreases levels of depression.

SCHOOL-BASED INTERVENTIONS

Dynamic communication between health care providers, educational personnel, and family members promotes seamless coordination among and between individuals working with the child diagnosed with cancer. Health care providers communicate the medical needs of the child; parents tend to the needs of the child; and school personnel adjust to meet the child's needs, maintain alliance with parents, and tactfully manage peer expectations and reactions regarding the child's diagnosis. School psychologists are ideally suited to serve as a liaison in a multidisciplinary system, coordinating and facilitating smooth interactions between distinct ecological systems.

Problem-solving therapy for parents has been found to enhance their ability to resolve problems and decrease symptoms of depression and anxiety, which may allow caregivers to better care for their children (Law et al., 2014). This type of therapy may also help improve parents' ability to cope with challenges, thereby enhancing their self-efficacy. When accompanying the child to medical treatments, parents should prepare the child and discuss what to expect, provide soothing distractions from painful procedures by singing or playing music, and support and validate the child's experiences.

As mentioned previously, children with cancer are at increased risk of experiencing academic and learning problems as well as social and emotional issues and physical problems. As such, these children are entitled to services under the Individuals With Disabilities Education Act, typically under Other Health Impairment. An individualized plan developed to meet the child's unique needs may provide specialized placement, psychological services such as supportive counseling, adaptive physical education, speech/language and physical and occupational therapy, and transportation services.

Cancer treatment may also cause deficits in fine motor speed, processing speed, and visual motor integration. Technological support can be especially beneficial in enhancing learning using auditory and language-based processes, including technological advances such as audiobooks and computer voice recognition software (Armstrong et al., 1999). Physical problems after cancer treatment may affect children's ability to navigate through a school building and perform in the classroom. Schools may need to accommodate children's physical needs by providing two sets of books—one set kept at school and one set kept at the child's home—to assist with weakness during treatment. A child who is fatigued and weak from cancer treatment may need to be excused from physical education classes and have opportunities to rest during the day. It might also be beneficial to arrange for shorter school days and allow extra time to transition between classes and other activities. Additional accommodations that might be useful include moving a child's locker closer to the classroom, providing access to an elevator, allowing extra time to complete assignments and take tests, providing oral exams when necessary, minimizing the amount of written work required, and permitting the use of a calculator. Children with cancer may also have dietary problems, such as inconsistent or irregular appetite and thirst needs. Accommodations such as allowing the child to carry a water bottle throughout the school day, providing long-term bathroom passes, and allowing a longer lunch period with extra snacks throughout the school day will help address these issues (Root et al., 2016).

CONCLUSION

Pediatric cancer is a rare childhood illness that often goes undetected due to similarity of presenting symptoms with other benign conditions. The exact cause of childhood cancer is unknown and thus not preventable. Children diagnosed with cancer experience myriad social–emotional, behavioral, academic, and medical side effects, which may have lifelong ramifications. Knowledge of evidence-based treatments and strategies and clear communication among all individuals working with the child are crucial to supporting children, from diagnosis to remittance.

RESOURCES

Hoffman, R. I. (2013). *Educating the child with cancer: A guide for parents and teachers* (2nd ed.). American Childhood Cancer Organization. This is a resource for families and schools designed to promote communication and understanding between parents, educators, and medical professionals, thereby enhancing collaboration and treatment across contexts.

Leukemia & Lymphoma Society. (n.d.). *The Trish Greene Back to School Program for Children With Cancer*. https://www.lls.org/trish-greene-back-school-program-children-cancer. This program offers information and resources for parents and educators to support academic development, including transitioning back to school.

St. Jude's "Together." (2019). *School support*. St. Jude Children's Research Hospital. https://together.stjude.org/en-us/for-families/school.html. This website offers information regarding classroom accommodations, homebound services, advocating for a child with cancer, and supporting connections between children and their classmates.

American Cancer Society. (2017). *Helping your child manage school during cancer treatment*. https://www.cancer.org/treatment/children-and-cancer/when-your-child-has-cancer/during-treatment/keeping-up-with-schoolwork.html. This website provides information and recommendations for homebound instruction, hospitalized or clinic-based schools, attending school during cancer treatment, and support services for 504 plans/individualized education programs.

REFERENCES

American Cancer Society. (2017). *Late effects of childhood cancer treatment*. https://www.cancer.org/treatment/children-and-cancer/when-your-child-has-cancer/late-effects-of-cancer-treatment.html

American Cancer Society. (2018). *Facts & figures 2018*. https://www.cancer.org/research/cancer-facts-statistics/all-cancer-facts-figures/cancer-facts-figures-2018.html

Armstrong, F. D., Blumberg, M. J., & Toledano, S. R. (1999). Neurobehavioral issues in childhood cancer. *School Psychology Review, 28*(2), 194–203. https://doi.org/10.1080/02796015.1999.12085957

Boles, J. C., Winsor, D. L., Mandrell, B., Gattuso, J., West, N., Leigh, L., & Grissom, S. M. (2017). Student/patient: The school perceptions of children with cancer. *Educational Studies, 43*(5), 549–566. https://doi.org/10.1080/03055698.2017.1312288

Brinkman, T. M., Li, C., Vannatta, K., Marchak, J. G., Lai, J. S., Prasad, P. K., Kimberg, C., Vuotto, S., Di, C., Srivastava, D., Robison, L. L., Armstrong, G. T., & Krull, K. R. (2016). Behavioral, social, and emotional symptom comorbidities and profiles in adolescent survivors of childhood cancer: A report from the Childhood Cancer Survivor Study. *Journal of Clinical Oncology, 34*(28), 3417–3425. https://doi.org/10.1200/JCO.2016.66.4789

Butler, R. W., Copeland, D. R., Fairclough, D. L., Mulhern, R. K., Katz, E. R., Kazak, A. E., Noll, R. B., Patel, S. K., & Sahler, O. J. Z. (2008). A multicenter, randomized clinical trial of a cognitive remediation program for childhood survivors of a pediatric malignancy. *Journal of Consulting and Clinical Psychology, 76*(3), 367–378. https://doi.org/10.1037/0022-006X.76.3.367

Crossland, A. (2002). Efficacy beliefs and the learning experiences of children with cancer in the hospital setting. *Alberta Journal of Educational Research, 48*(1), 5–19. https://eric.ed.gov/?id=EJ649441

Fragkandrea, I., Nixon, J. A., & Panagopoulou, P. (2013). Signs and symptoms of childhood cancer: A guide for early recognition. *American Academy of Family Physicians, 88*(3), 185–192. https://pubmed.ncbi.nlm.nih.gov/23939697/

Howlader, N., Noone, A. M., Krapcho, M., Miller, D., Bishop, K., Kosary, C. L., Yu, M., Ruhl, J., Tatalovich, Z., Mariotto, A., Lewis, D. R., Chen, H. S., Feuer, E. J., & Cronin, K. A. (Eds.). (2017). *SEER cancer statistics review, 1975–2014*. National Cancer Institute. https://seer.cancer.gov/csr/1975_2014/

Irwin, M. K., & Elam, M. (2011). Are we leaving children with chronic illness behind? *Physical Disabilities: Education & Related Services, 30*(2), 67–80. https://eric.ed.gov/?id=EJ955447

Law, E. F., Fisher, E., Fales, J., Noel, M., & Eccleston, C. (2014). Systematic review and meta-analysis of parent and family-based interventions for children and adolescents with chronic medical conditions. *Journal of Pediatric Psychology, 39*(8), 866–886. https://doi.org/10.1093/jpepsy/jsu032

Li, C.-Y., & Wendt, R. N. (1998). Cancer (childhood). In L. Phelps (Ed.), *Health-related disorders in children and adolescents* (pp. 114–120). American Psychological Association. https://doi.org/10.1037/10300-016

Pan, I. J., Daniels, J. L., & Zhu, K. (2010). Poverty and childhood cancer incidence in the United States. *Cancer Causes & Control, 21*(7), 1139–1145. https://doi.org/10.1007/s10552-010-9528-3

Physician Data Query. (2019). *Late effects of treatment for childhood cancer (PDQ)—Patient version*. National Cancer Institute. https://www.cancer.gov/types/childhood-cancers/late-effects-pdq

Root, M. M., Bray, M. A., Maykel, C., Cross, K., Shankar, N. L., & Theodore, L. A., (2016). Students with cancer: Presenting issues and effective solutions. *International Journal of School & Educational Psychology, 4*(1), 25–33. https://doi.org/10.1080/21683603.2016.1130549

Semrud-Clikeman, M., & Ellison, P. A. T. (2009). Neuropsychological correlates of childhood and adolescent internalized disorders: Mood and anxiety disorders. In M. Semrud-Clikeman & P. A. T. Ellison (Eds.), *Child neuropsychology* (2nd ed., pp. 181–224). Springer. https://doi.org/10.1007/978-0-387-88963-4_9

Siegel, R. L., Miller, K. D., & Jemal, A. (2018). Cancer statistics, 2018. *CA: A Cancer Journal for Clinicians, 68*(1), 7–30. https://doi.org/10.3322/caac.21442

Vance, Y. H., & Eiser, C. (2002). The school experience of the child with cancer. *Child: Care, Health and Development, 28*(1), 5–19. https://doi.org/10.1046/j.1365-2214.2002.00227.x

61

Smith–Magenis Syndrome

James P. Van Haneghan, Abigail Baxter, and Harvey N. Switzky

Smith–Magenis syndrome (SMS) is rare autosomal deletion disorder involving deletion or mutation of genetic material on the short arm of chromosome 17 in an area labeled as 17p11.2 (Smith et al., 1982). SMS has a variety of physical, behavioral, and cognitive sequelae that have a profound impact on school, social, and family contexts. In this chapter, we describe SMS and examine the many challenges faced by children and their caregivers.

ETIOLOGY

The genetic locus of the disorder is the retinoic acid induced gene 1 (*RAI1*) that affects circadian rhythms and brain and craniofacial development (Edelman et al., 2007). The *RAI1* gene effects appear to be the common denominator, but other genetic deletions in the 17p11.2 area are connected to variations in the phenotypical manifestations of the disorder (Edelman et al., 2007). The disorder can be diagnosed through a variety of higher resolution genetic techniques, such as fluorescence in situ hybridization and chromosome microarray analysis. These approaches, along with *RAI1* sequencing when there is no 17p11.2 deletion, can help identify variants of the disorder (Vilboux et al., 2011). The syndrome can be diagnosed prenatally through amniocentesis (Fan & Farrell, 1994), but the deletion has no clear cause. It is unrelated to parental age or other parental characteristics, although there have been cases of mothers showing mosaicism (i.e., evidence of the deletion in some cells but not others; Zori et al., 1993). Several

https://doi.org/10.1037/0000349-061
Health-Related Disorders in Children and Adolescents: A Guidebook for Educators and Service Providers, Second Edition, M. M. Perfect, C. A. Riccio, and M. A. Bray (Editors)

authors (e.g., Gropman et al., 2006) have suggested that parental genetic testing could help clarify if there is any parental genetic connection.

PREVALENCE AND INCIDENCE

First identified in the early 1980s, SMS has an estimated incidence of at least one in 25,000 (Greenberg et al., 1991), although Stratton et al. (1986) suggested that the rate could be higher. Approximately 10% of cases are related to *RAI1* gene mutations rather than deletions in 17p11.2 (Edelman et al., 2007). New techniques for identification and the clear role of *RAI1* should lead to more precise identification of the disorder. For example, Yeetong et al. (2016) reported how an unexplained case of an adult with phenotypical features of SMS without a deletion in 17p11.2 was identified to have the more recently discovered *RAI1* mutation variant.

SYMPTOMS

Although some elements of SMS appear early in development, the earliest signs are difficult to differentiate from other disorders where there is failure to thrive (Gropman et al., 2006). For example, Gropman et al. (2006) found that infants with SMS were hypotonic, lethargic, and had feeding problems. They also reported that several of the infants had undergone genetic testing because they were suspected of having Down syndrome. Gropman et al. reported that the more difficult symptoms of SMS emerge during the toddler and preschool years.

The syndrome has physical and psychological manifestations. Underlying variation in the amount and type of genotypic array appears to be associated with differences in the severity and presence of some characteristics (Edelman et al., 2007). For example, Edelman et al. (2007) reported different configurations of manifestations for those with the *RAI1* mutation rather than the deletion. The most frequent manifestations in the literature are developmental delay, stereotypies, self-injury, sleep disturbance, eye abnormalities, hoarse voice, oral/motor dysfunction, hyperactivity, short stature, hearing loss, dental abnormalities, and scoliosis.

Among the physical manifestations, facial features are particularly prominent. The front-to-back length of the head is shortened in proportion to the head breadth (brachycephaly), there is incomplete development in the midface area (above the mouth and below the forehead; i.e., midface hypoplasia), the bridge of the nose is broad and flat, and there are malformations of the ears and epicanthal folds (i.e., extra folds of skin on the part of the eye where the upper and lower lids meet on the portion nearest the nose). The distinctiveness of these facial features appears to increase with age and vary according to the genetic defect (deletion vs. mutation; Edelman et al., 2007). Along with the facial features, there have been reports of shortened limbs, fingers, toes (brachydactyly) and shortened stature.

Hearing and visual problems are common (Edelman et al., 2007). Finucane et al. (1993) reported strabismus (i.e., turning inward or outward of the eye) in all 10 cases in their report. All but their youngest patients were myopic (i.e., nearsighted), some severely so. Further, there is a greater risk for retinal detachment because of extreme myopia and susceptibility to head trauma (e.g., head banging, trauma associated with aggression and hyperactivity). They reported retinal detachments in three out of the 10 cases (Finucane et al., 1993). Hearing loss has been reported in over half the cases and may be associated in some individuals with SMS with chronic otitis media (i.e., middle ear infections; Brendal et al., 2017). Malformations or malpositioning of the ears is common as well (Finucane et al., 1993). Brendal et al. (2017) reported fluctuating and progressive hearing loss in individuals with SMS. In addition, they reported hyperacusis (i.e., abnormal sensitivity to normal sound levels).

IMPACT ON THE STUDENT AND OUTCOMES

Medical

Disordered sleep is common and appears related to problems in the cycle of melatonin production. Instead of increased melatonin being produced in the evenings to facilitate sleeping, production increases during the day and is lower at night (De Leersnyder et al., 2003). Further, individuals with SMS tend to have obesity problems that appear to be related to food satiety issues similar to those in Prader–Willi syndrome (Alaimo et al., 2015).

Cognitive/Academic

SMS is a complex disorder because the medical and physical issues create and exacerbate cognitive and behavioral issues. Edelman et al. (2007) reported that intellectual impairment is positively correlated with deletion size and that individuals with the *RAI1* mutation tend to have less intellectual impairment. Oromotor dysfunction and craniofacial abnormalities can create feeding and expressive communication issues. Adding to communication problems are ear infections that disrupt language development. These all contribute to academic difficulties (Martin et al., 2006). Executive and sequential processing difficulties create problems in attending and learning for individuals with SMS, whereas visual reasoning tasks, without motor components, seem to be a relative strength (Dykens et al., 1997). People with SMS often have attentional difficulties, display impulsivity, and have difficulty staying on task.

Social-Emotional and Behavioral

Aside from the cognitive impacts of language disruption, the inability to communicate can lead to frustration and problem behaviors. For example, hyperacusis makes the child more edgy and can contribute to behavioral outbursts. Sleep problems contribute to learning and behavioral problems in a variety of ways. A tired child has difficulty learning, is less regulated, and is subject to behavioral problems. Alaimo et al. (2015) reported more frequent and more severe problems for individuals with SMS in three categories of behaviors: self-injury, stereotypy, and aggressive/destructive behaviors. Stereotypies, self-injurious behavior, and communication problems sometimes lead to a diagnosis of autism spectrum disorder (ASD). Laje, Morse, et al. (2010) reported that because of communication problems, the majority of individuals with SMS are likely to have an ASD diagnosis. Additionally, lower pain sensitivity makes self-injurious behavior harder to extinguish. See Edelman et al. (2007) for further detail on the variations among subgroups with different deletions.

PSYCHOEDUCATIONAL IMPLICATIONS AND SCHOOL-BASED INTERVENTIONS

Medical and Health Management

Based on the connection of medical and health issues to academic, social, and behavioral outcomes, early multidisciplinary interventions are important to ameliorate some of the sequelae that arise from core medical issues. Medical treatment for ear infections, audiological testing, and other aspects of the system that subsumes typical language and communication are crucial to address. Further, it is important to address dental- and vision-related issues (Poisson et al., 2015).

Because of the impact of sleep on so many aspects of children's lives and those around them, sleep problems need to be addressed. Over the last decade, interventions to improve sleep through changing melatonin levels have been studied. Melatonin-based interventions have shown mixed results, with some anecdotal positive cases (e.g., Been, 2003). A rigorous single-case study by Wheeler et al. (2005) found no impact. De Leersnyder et al. (2003) found that a combination of a β_1-adrenergic antagonist in the morning with doses of melatonin in the evening improved sleep. The medication tasimelteon has been examined (e.g., Hull et al., 2017) and found to have a positive impact on sleep and potentially aberrant behavior. Along with drug interventions, many anecdotally reported practices for arranging sleep environments purport to help children's sleep and reduce the time parents are awake, but these have not been systematically studied (e.g., enclosed beds).

Cognitive/Academic

The attentional difficulties associated with SMS make it important to collect a variety of data to make judgments about intellectual capacity and achievement. It may be difficult to determine whether poor performance was a function of attentional problems in the situation or due to underlying intellectual capacity. As noted, auditory and speech-related issues can create challenges for educating children with SMS. Some anecdotal reports have indicated success teaching sign language to improve communication (Gropman et al., 2006). Executive functioning (Wilde & Oliver, 2017) and sequential processing (Dykens et al., 1997) have been identified as significant deficit areas in SMS. Udwin et al. (2001) suggested taking advantage of relative strengths noted by Dykens et al. (1997) in long-term memory, as well as considering weaknesses, when designing instruction. Based on the strengths and weaknesses noted, instruction that limits cognitive load, allows for overlearning, is highly structured, and provides visual prompts may help keep the child with SMS on task.

Social–Emotional and Behavioral

Poisson et al. (2015) recommended comprehensive treatment plans that go beyond the use of psychotropic medication, which has been found to be of limited effectiveness (Laje, Bernert, et al., 2010) with one class (benzodiazepines) having a potentially deleterious impact. There are no studies of using standard medications for attention-deficit/hyperactivity disorder. Laje, Bernert, et al. (2010) reported that six of seven classes of medication were not rated as effective in treating attention-deficit/hyperactivity disorder in children with SMS. Poisson et al. mentioned reported use of methylphenidate for increasing attention and helping with alertness given disordered sleep, but Laje, Bernert, et al. found that parents of children with SMS who were prescribed methylphenidate or other stimulants reported no impact on symptomatology.

There is minimal evidence concerning the use of applied behavior analysis in individuals with SMS. Given some of the success in working with individuals with ASD, coupled with the presence of ASD diagnoses in many children with SMS, this is surprising. Hodnett et al. (2018) reported the first systematic applied behavior analysis study of two individuals with SMS. They reported success in using extinction and differential reinforcement of other behaviors with two individuals with SMS. Their successes merit further investigation, and they pointed out that future work needs to consider the constellation of other factors that can affect successful implementation (e.g., sleep, language, and speech issues).

Taylor and Oliver (2008) observed that problem behaviors were associated with lack of adult caregiver attention. Given the high prevalence of behavioral issues and the lack of sleep, parenting a child with SMS is demanding (Foster et al., 2010). These demands can exhaust parents, especially when such problems are intractable and not well regulated through pharmaceutical interventions (Laje, Bernert, et al., 2010). Foster et al. (2010) reported that parents who find positives in their experience show better coping and that parents who are anxious about their situation benefit from counseling. There is a clear need for additional work that focuses not only on the child but also on family, school, and social systems in which the child is embedded. Only with a comprehensive perspective can combinations of medical and behavioral interventions to reduce problem behaviors be implemented. Further, sleep-deprived parents may be less effective in addressing behavioral problems, further exacerbating their potential impact.

CONCLUSION

Since the identification of SMS, the body of evidence surrounding this disorder has grown. Some progress has been made in understanding the locus of the genetic defects, addressing some aspects of the disorder (e.g., sleep), and making efforts to put some systematic evidence together concerning what may or may not work in treating aspects of SMS.

RESOURCES

Parents and Researchers Interested in Smith–Magenis Syndrome. https://www.prisms.org/

Parents and Researchers Interested in Smith–Magenis Syndrome. (n.d.). *International partners*. https://www.prisms.org/awareness/international-partners/

REFERENCES

Alaimo, J. T., Barton, L. V., Mullegama, S. V., Wills, R. D., Foster, R. H., & Elsea, S. H. (2015). Individuals with Smith–Magenis syndrome display profound neurodevelopmental behavioral deficiencies and exhibit food-related behaviors equivalent to Prader–Willi syndrome. *Research in Developmental Disabilities, 47*, 27–38. https://doi.org/10.1016/j.ridd.2015.08.011

Been, J. V. (2003). Improvement of sleep disturbances and behaviour in Smith–Magenis syndrome with morning melatonin [Electronic response to de Leersnyder et al., "Beta-adrenergic antagonists and melatonin reset the clock and restore sleep in a circadian disorder, Smith-Magenis syndrome"]. *Journal of Medical Genetics, 40*. https://jmg.bmj.com/content/improvement-sleep-disturbances-and-behaviour-smith-magenis-syndrome-morning-melatonin

Brendal, M. A., King, K. A., Zalewski, C. K., Finucane, B. M., Introne, W., Brewer, C. C., & Smith, A. C. M. (2017). Auditory phenotype of Smith–Magenis syndrome. *Journal of Speech, Language, and Hearing Research, 60*(4), 1076–1087. https://doi.org/10.1044/2016_JSLHR-H-16-0024

De Leersnyder, H., Bresson, J. L., de Blois, M. C., Souberbielle, J. C., Mogenet, A., Delhotal-Landes, B., Salefranque, F., & Munnich, A. (2003). β_1-adrenergic antagonists and melatonin reset the clock and restore sleep in a circadian disorder, Smith–Magenis syndrome. *Journal of Medical Genetics, 40*(1), 74–78. https://doi.org/10.1136/jmg.40.1.74

Dykens, E. M., Finucane, B. M., & Gayley, C. (1997). Brief report: Cognitive and behavioral profiles in persons with Smith–Magenis syndrome. *Journal of Autism and Developmental Disorders, 27*(2), 203–211. https://doi.org/10.1023/A:1025800126086

Edelman, E. A., Girirajan, S., Finucane, B., Patel, P. I., Lupski, J. R., Smith, A. C. M., & Elsea, S. H. (2007). Gender, genotype, and phenotype differences in Smith–Magenis syndrome: A meta-analysis of 105 cases. *Clinical Genetics, 71*(6), 540–550. https://doi.org/10.1111/j.1399-0004.2007.00815.x

Fan, Y.-S., & Farrell, S. A. (1994). Prenatal diagnosis of interstitial deletion of 17(p11.2p11.2) (Smith–Magenis syndrome) [Letter to the editor]. *American Journal of Medical Genetics, 49*(2), 253–254. https://doi.org/10.1002/ajmg.1320490220

Finucane, B. M., Jaeger, E. R., Kurtz, M. B., Weinstein, M., & Scott, C. I., Jr. (1993). Eye abnormalities in the Smith–Magenis contiguous gene deletion syndrome. *American Journal of Medical Genetics, 45*(4), 443–446. https://doi.org/10.1002/ajmg.1320450409

Foster, R. H., Kozachek, S., Stern, M., & Elsea, S. H. (2010). Caring for the caregivers: An investigation of factors related to well-being among parents caring for a child with Smith–Magenis syndrome. *Journal of Genetic Counseling, 19*(2), 187–198. https://doi.org/10.1007/s10897-009-9273-5

Greenberg, F., Guzzetta, V., Montes de Oca-Luna, R., Magenis, R. E., Smith, A. C. M., Richter, S. F., Kondo, I., Dobyns, W. B., Patel, P. I., & Lupski, J. R. (1991). Molecular analysis of the Smith–Magenis syndrome: A possible contiguous-gene syndrome associated with del(17)(p11.2). *American Journal of Human Genetics, 49*(6), 1207–1218.

Gropman, A. L., Duncan, W. C., & Smith, A. C. M. (2006). Neurologic and developmental features of the Smith–Magenis syndrome (del 17p11.2). *Pediatric Neurology, 34*(5), 337–350. https://doi.org/10.1016/j.pediatrneurol.2005.08.018

Hodnett, J., Scheithauer, M., Call, N. A., Mevers, J. L., & Miller, S. J. (2018). Using a functional analysis followed by differential reinforcement and extinction to reduce challenging behaviors in children with Smith–Magenis syndrome. *American Journal on Intellectual and Developmental Disabilities, 123*(6), 558–573. https://doi.org/10.1352/1944-7558-123.6.558

Hull, J. T., Polymeropoulos, C., Cho, Y., Xiao, C., & Polymeropoulos, M. H. (2017). Tasimelteon improves sleep quality and behavior in individuals with Smith–Magenis syndrome (SMS) in an open-label study. *Sleep Medicine, 40*(Suppl. 1), Article e139. https://doi.org/10.1016/j.sleep.2017.11.406

Laje, G., Bernert, R., Morse, R., Pao, M., & Smith, A. C. (2010). Pharmacological treatment of disruptive behavior in Smith–Magenis syndrome. *American Journal of Medical Genetics: Part C. Seminars in Medical Genetics, 154C*(4), 463–468. https://doi.org/10.1002/ajmg.c.30282

Laje, G., Morse, R., Richter, W., Ball, J., Pao, M., & Smith, A. C. M. (2010). Autism spectrum features in Smith–Magenis syndrome. *American Journal of Medical Genetics: Part C. Seminars in Medical Genetics, 154C*(4), 456–462. https://doi.org/10.1002/ajmg.c.30275

Martin, S. C., Wolters, P. L., & Smith, A. (2006). Adaptive and maladaptive behavior in children with Smith–Magenis syndrome. *Journal of Autism and Developmental Disorders, 36*(4), 541–552. https://doi.org/10.1007/s10803-006-0093-2

Poisson, A., Nicolas, A., Cochat, P., Sanlaville, D., Rigard, C., de Leersnyder, H., Franco, P., Des Portes, V., Edery, P., & Demily, C. (2015). Behavioral disturbance and treatment strategies in Smith–Magenis syndrome. *Orphanet Journal of Rare Diseases, 10*(1), Article 111. https://doi.org/10.1186/s13023-015-0330-x

Smith, A. C. M., McGavran, L., & Waldstein, G. (1982). Deletion of the 17 short arm in two patients with facial clefts. *American Journal of Human Genetics, 34,* Article 410A.

Stratton, R. F., Dobyns, W. B., Greenberg, F., DeSana, J. B., Moore, C., Fidone, G., Runge, G. H., Feldman, P., Sekhon, G. S., Pauli, R. M., Ledbetter, D. H., Opitz, J. M., & Reynolds, J. F. (1986). Interstitial deletion of (17)(p11. 2p11. 2): Report of six additional patients with a new chromosome deletion syndrome. *American Journal of Medical Genetics, 24*(3), 421–432. https://doi.org/10.1002/ajmg.1320240305

Taylor, L., & Oliver, C. (2008). The behavioural phenotype of Smith–Magenis syndrome: Evidence for a gene–environment interaction. *Journal of Intellectual Disability Research, 52*(10), 830–841. https://doi.org/10.1111/j.1365-2788.2008.01066.x

Udwin, O., Webber, C., & Horn, I. (2001). Abilities and attainment in Smith–Magenis syndrome. *Developmental Medicine and Child Neurology, 43*(12), 823–828. https://pubmed.ncbi.nlm.nih.gov/11769269/

Vilboux, T., Ciccone, C., Blancato, J. K., Cox, G. F., Deshpande, C., Introne, W. J., Gahl, W. A., Smith, A. C., & Huizing, M. (2011). Molecular analysis of the retinoic acid induced 1 gene (*RAI1*) in patients with suspected Smith–Magenis syndrome without the 17p11.2 deletion. *PLOS ONE, 6*(8), Article e22861. https://doi.org/10.1371/journal.pone.0022861

Wheeler, B., Taylor, B., Simonsen, K., & Reith, D. M. (2005). Melatonin treatment in Smith–Magenis syndrome. *Sleep, 28*(12), 1609–1610. https://doi.org/10.1093/sleep/28.12.1609

Wilde, L., & Oliver, C. (2017, August). Brief report: Contrasting profiles of everyday executive functioning in Smith–Magenis syndrome and Down syndrome. *Journal of Autism and Developmental Disorders, 47*(8), 2602–2609. https://doi.org/10.1007/s10803-017-3140-2

Yeetong, P., Vilboux, T., Ciccone, C., Boulier, K., Schnur, R. E., Gahl, W. A., Huizing, M., Laje, G., & Smith, A. C. M. (2016). Delayed diagnosis in a house of correction: Smith–Magenis syndrome due to a de novo nonsense *RAI1* variant. *American Journal of Medical Genetics: Part A, 170*(9), 2383–2388. https://doi.org/10.1002/ajmg.a.37602

Zori, R. T., Lupski, J. R., Heju, Z., Greenberg, F., Killian, J. M., Gray, B. A., Driscoll, D. J., Patel, P. I., & Zackowski, J. L. (1993). Clinical, cytogenetic, and molecular evidence for an infant with Smith–Magenis syndrome born from a mother having a mosaic 17p11.2p12 deletion. *American Journal of Medical Genetics, 47*(4), 504–511. https://doi.org/10.1002/ajmg.1320470414

62

Sturge–Weber Syndrome

Emily M. Jimenez and George W. Hynd

Although Sturge–Weber syndrome (SWS) is a relatively rare congenital disorder, individuals with this syndrome are often recognized when encountered due to what is referred to as a port-wine birthmark on the face. This is one of the most observable and distinguishing features of SWS, which contributes to social–emotional challenges in addition to the high variability of medical complexity seen with this disorder.

ETIOLOGY

The original description of the syndrome was first introduced by William Allen Sturge, an English physician and archaeologist, in 1879. He presented a case of contralateral partial epilepsy caused, he believed, by an intracranial angioma (a benign tumor of the vascular wall). Notably, he described his young patient as having a visible facial angioma. Somewhat later, Siegfried Kalischer (1897), a German neurologist, provided the first pathologic study, but it was left up to Parkes Weber, an English dermatologist, in 1929 to identify the intracranial calcifications that were associated with the seizures frequently seen in the syndrome. In recognition of the contributions by Sturge and Weber, this disorder became known as Sturge–Weber syndrome.

SWS is not a heritable disorder. Rather, it is believed to result from a somatic mosaic mutation in the *GNAQ* (G protein subunit alpha Q) gene. This mutation is believed to manifest during early fetal development and may contribute to

https://doi.org/10.1037/0000349-062
Health-Related Disorders in Children and Adolescents: A Guidebook for Educators and Service Providers, Second Edition, M. M. Perfect, C. A. Riccio, and M. A. Bray (Editors)

abnormal blood vessel growth in the brain, resulting in consequences for the function of adjacent cells. This mutation is thought to occur sporadically and for no known reason (Huang et al., 2017).

INCIDENCE AND PREVALENCE

SWS is incredibly rare and is estimated to occur in one of every 20,000 to 50,000 live births. Additionally, approximately three in 1,000 babies are born with a port-wine stain birthmark, but only 6% of those babies have the neurological symptoms (developmental delays) associated with SWS (National Organization for Rare Disorders, 2021).

SYMPTOMS

This disorder is characterized by the port-wine stain on the upper third of the face, eyelid, or scalp. Most frequently, the port-wine stain (actually a cutaneous capillary malformation) is unilateral and most visible on the upper third of the face, although it is occasionally bilateral and there is considerable variation in the distribution of this most notable characteristic. For diagnosis, a triad of features is often considered: the facial port-wine stain or birthmark, the leptomeningeal angiomas (various cerebral malformations and tumors of the inner two meninges, the arachnoid, and the pia mater), and glaucoma (increased pressure in the eye).

Some literature indicates that SWS should be organized into three different subtypes, described as follows. Type 1 is described as having the neurological symptoms, the skin presentation of the port-wine stain, and frequent seizures. Type 2 is described as having the port-wine stain birthmark and no neurological symptoms. Notably, individuals in Type 1 or Type 2 may also have glaucoma. Type 3, which may be diagnosed later in life due to the emergence of neurological symptoms only, manifests with no skin abnormalities due to port-wine stains and no presence of glaucoma (Lowe et al., 2017; National Organization for Rare Disorders, 2021).

IMPACT ON THE STUDENT AND OUTCOMES

Medical

Not infrequently, the syndrome may be diagnosed during the 1st year of life due to the emergence of partial and/or generalized secondary seizures. The seizures are most often associated with calcifications that occur in abnormal development of the arachnoid and pia mater or the leptomeninges; however, the resulting cerebral calcifications may not be visible by magnetic resonance imaging or computed tomography scans until after 6 months to a year (Volpe et al., 2017). When seizures are present, they often increase in both frequency and severity as the child matures. The seizures are also increasingly associated with other challenging medical, developmental, and behavioral outcomes. These outcomes are discussed further in the following sections. Additionally, there is some evidence that the port-wine stain common with this diagnosis can predict the development of epilepsy, with bilateral port-wine stains corresponding with a higher risk of epilepsy. No increased risk of epilepsy has been associated with unilateral port-wine stains (Juhász, 2016). It has also been noted that the involvement of the upper eyelid and forehead in the presentation of the port-wine stain results in an increased risk for neurological problems (Waelchli et al., 2014).

Cognitive/Academic

The presence or absence of seizures is the primary indicator for the severity of impact an SWS diagnosis will have on the child's life. With seizures, Type 1 or 3 depending on the presence of a port-wine stain, SWS will affect not only the child's social outcomes but also their neurocognitive status. Seizure onset before 1 year of age has a particularly strong impact on global cognitive functioning in children with SWS (Luat et al., 2018). A reduction in global cognitive functioning can result in greater school difficulties and require more modifications in a traditional school environment. The type of cognitive deficit that the seizures cause is influenced heavily by the age of onset and the laterality, or the side of the brain onset occurs, of the seizures (Luat et al., 2018). Seizure presentation develops in approximately 75% to 80% of the one in 20,000 to 50,000 patients with SWS, and of those up to 93% have bilateral cerebral involvement (Lo et al., 2012).

Further, seizure onset before 7 months in age and frontal lobe involvement in seizures have both been connected with more severe motor deficits (Luat et al., 2018). The overall profile of a child with SWS and seizure presentation has been rated more similar to children with epilepsy than to children with SWS and no seizures, who were more similar to the control group. Children with SWS and seizures were described by their teachers as having increased behavior problems, poorer global academic outcomes, and poorer cognitive development in comparison with the control population (Raches et al., 2012).

Social-Emotional and Behavioral

SWS also affects the child socially and emotionally, most notably due to the port-wine stain being an aesthetic skin abnormality that is often in very visible areas of the body and face. Particularly, larger port-wine stains have been associated with an increase in mood and social problems in children (Chapieski et al., 2000). Children with SWS also generally exhibit problems with social skills, overall mood, and compliance (Chapieski et al., 2000). The presence of a port-wine stain has been connected with overall poorer quality of life for the child, which can extend all the way into adulthood (Hagen et al., 2017). Those who were most at risk for psychological problems with an SWS diagnosis also had lower full-scale IQ scores, greater chance of seizure disorders or related seizure presentation, and a greater frequency of seizures (Chapieski et al., 2000).

PSYCHOEDUCATIONAL IMPLICATIONS AND SCHOOL-BASED INTERVENTIONS

Medical and Health Management

Most medical and health-related needs for these children in schools will be related to their seizures, if present. The 504 plan or individualized education program (IEP) developed for the child with SWS may include needs specific to the epileptic symptoms, including implementation of a seizure action plan. Many will likely be on antiepileptic drugs but even still may have seizure presentation in the classroom or school environment. Attention should be paid to the school's seizure protocol and the development of a seizure action plan, and the school nurse should be notified of this possible need for intervention if a seizure does occur.

Cognitive/Academic

Additionally, school professionals should be mindful of possible cognitive deficits and the need for academic intervention or support this may require. The severity of cognitive deficit is closely related to the presence of seizures, with more cognitive abnormalities seen in children with SWS who have seizures as a symptom. Regarding seizures, the most common outcome the child may experience is inattentiveness in their classroom environment. Special education services may be beneficial for a child with SWS for these reasons. Children with SWS and seizures are referred for special education services about 10 times as often as children with only SWS (Raches et al., 2012). These cognitive deficits may require interventions such as visual aids, additional time for work completion, reteaching/preteaching of new material, and intervention specific to the area(s) of cognitive functioning impacted, which are unique to the individual (Seaman, 2016). Another intervention for improving academic performance is self-directed strategy instruction, the use of which is supported by research for a wide range of academic difficulties in children (Cuenca-Carlino et al., 2016; Limpo & Alves, 2014).

Social-Emotional and Behavioral

Those who are caring for individuals with SWS may notice possible negative impacts on the child's emotional health (Hagen et al., 2017). In the classroom setting, professionals should be aware that the child's social interactions may be negatively affected by this diagnosis and that this may be an area in need of intervention. It may be helpful for the school to incorporate social skills training, allow the child to be paired with a peer at lunch, or educate the other children in the class of the reasons for the presence of the birthmark or medical needs the child may have. Positive self-image development may also be a therapeutic goal for children who have undergone dramatic life changes or social rejection as a result of their SWS diagnosis. Resources for appropriate social–emotional well-being (e.g., counseling, classroom-based intervention programs) should be provided as necessary, and all classroom-based interventions should be dependent on the child's level of openness and comfort discussing their diagnosis.

CONCLUSION

Despite the rarity of SWS, its unique physical presentation often makes it easy to identify. The triad of primary symptoms associated with this diagnosis make treatment and patient outcomes highly variable for each individual with SWS. The port-wine stain birthmark can present unique social–emotional challenges, seizure presentation can result in increased monitoring and doctor's visits, and the presence of glaucoma can cause additional vision concerns and modifications. Additionally, there is great variation in the levels of cognitive ability among patients with SWS. The presence or absence of seizures is the primary indicator for the severity of impact an SWS diagnosis will have on the child's life and should be considered when working with individuals with this diagnosis.

RESOURCES

Sturge–Weber Foundation. (n.d.). *Understanding Sturge–Weber.* https://sturge-weber.org/new-to-swf/understanding-sturge-weber.html

National Organization for Rare Disorders. (2021). *Sturge–Weber syndrome.* https://rarediseases.org/rare-diseases/sturge-weber-syndrome/

MedlinePlus. (2018). *Sturge–Weber syndrome.* National Library of Medicine. https://medlineplus.gov/genetics/condition/sturge-weber-syndrome/

Sturge–Weber Foundation. (n.d.). *Educational documents and websites.* https://sturge-weber.org/for-patients/educational-resources/educational-documents.html (some resources available in Spanish)

REFERENCES

Chapieski, L., Friedman, A., & Lachar, D. (2000). Psychological functioning in children and adolescents with Sturge–Weber syndrome. *Journal of Child Neurology, 15*(10), 660–665. https://doi.org/10.1177/088307380001501004

Cuenca-Carlino, Y., Freeman-Green, S., Stephenson, G. W., & Hauth, C. (2016). Self-regulated strategy instruction for teaching multi-step equations to middle school students struggling in math. *The Journal of Special Education, 50*(2), 75–85. https://doi.org/10.1177/0022466915622021

Hagen, S. L., Grey, K. R., Korta, D. Z., & Kelly, K. M. (2017). Quality of life in adults with facial port-wine stains. *Journal of the American Academy of Dermatology, 76*(4), 695–702. https://doi.org/10.1016/j.jaad.2016.10.039

Huang, L., Couto, J. A., Pinto, A., Alexandrescu, S., Madsen, J. R., Greene, A. K., Sahin, M., & Bischoff, J. (2017). Somatic *GNAQ* mutation is enriched in brain endothelial cells in Sturge–Weber syndrome. *Pediatric Neurology, 67,* 59–63. https://doi.org/10.1016/j.pediatrneurol.2016.10.010

Juhász, C. (2016). Predicting and preventing epilepsy in Sturge–Weber syndrome? *Pediatric Neurology Briefs, 30*(11), Article 43. https://doi.org/10.15844/pedneurbriefs-30-11-3

Kalischer, S. (1897). Demonstration des gerhirns eines kindes mit telangiectasie der linksseitigen gesichts: Kopfhaut und hirnoberflache [Demonstration of the brain of a child with telangiectasia of the left side of the face: Scalp and cerebral surface]. *Berlin Wochenschur, 34,* Article 1059.

Limpo, T., & Alves, R. A. (2014). Implicit theories of writing and their impact on students' responses to a SRSD intervention. *British Journal of Educational Psychology, 84*(4), 571–590. https://doi.org/10.1111/bjep.12042

Lo, W., Marchuk, D. A., Ball, K. L., Juhász, C., Jordan, L. C., Ewen, J. B., Comi, A., & the Brain Vascular Malformation Consortium National Sturge–Weber Syndrome Workgroup. (2012). Updates and future horizons on the understanding, diagnosis, and treatment of Sturge–Weber syndrome brain involvement. *Developmental Medicine and Child Neurology, 54*(3), 214–223. https://doi.org/10.1111/j.1469-8749.2011.04169.x

Lowe, J., Than, C., & Rai, V. (2017). Sturge–Weber syndrome Type 3 in a 44 year old woman: A case report & review of the literature. *Neurology, 88*(16 Suppl.), Article 183.

Luat, A. F., Behen, M. E., Chugani, H. T., & Juhász, C. (2018). Cognitive and motor outcomes in children with unilateral Sturge–Weber syndrome: Effect of age at seizure onset and side of brain involvement. *Epilepsy & Behavior, 80,* 202–207. https://doi.org/10.1016/j.yebeh.2018.01.012

National Organization for Rare Disorders. (2021). *Sturge–Weber syndrome.* https://rarediseases.org/rare-diseases/sturge-weber-syndrome/

Raches, D., Hiscock, M., & Chapieski, L. (2012). Behavioral and academic problems in children with Sturge–Weber syndrome: Differences between children with and without seizures. *Epilepsy & Behavior, 25*(3), 457–463. https://doi.org/10.1016/j.yebeh.2012.06.004

Seaman, J. (2016). *Interventions for cognitive and academic deficits: A compendium of accommodations and instructional strategies corresponding to Woodcock–Johnson III Cognitive and Achievement clusters.* Intervention Central. https://psych.hsd.ca/Interventions%20for%20Cognitive%20and%20Academic%20Deficits.pdf

Sturge, W. A. (1879). A case of partial epilepsy, apparently due to a lesion of the vasomotor centers of the brain. *Transactions of the Clinical Society of London, 12,* 162–167.

Volpe, J., Inder, T., Darras, B., de Vries, L. S., du Plessis, A., Neil, J., & Perlman, J. (2017). *Neurology of the newborn* (6th ed.). Elsevier.

Waelchli, R., Aylett, S. E., Robinson, K., Chong, W. K., Martinez, A. E., & Kinsler, V. A. (2014). New vascular classification of port-wine stains: Improving prediction of Sturge–Weber risk. *British Journal of Dermatology, 171*(4), 861–867. https://doi.org/10.1111/bjd.13203

Weber, P. F. (1929). A note on the association of extensive haemangiomatosus naevus of the skin with cerebral (meningeal) haemangioma, especially cases of facial vascular naevus with contralateral hemiplegia. *Proceedings of the Royal Society of Medicine, 22,* 431–442. https://doi.org/10.1177/003591572902200422

63

Tuberous Sclerosis Complex

Cynthia A. Riccio and Huilin Linda Sun

Tuberous sclerosis complex (TSC), once called Bourneville's disease, is one of the most frequently occurring neurocutaneous disorders. Because the skin and the central nervous system originate from the same type of tissue, called ectoderm, in fetal development, some neurocutaneous disorders such as TSC affect both the skin and the brain (Ullrich, 2016). Like neurofibromatosis Type 1 and Sturge–Weber syndrome, TSC is characterized by flesh-colored or red-brown spots or stigmata of the skin called facial angiofibromas, previously known as adenoma sebaceum (Jacks & Witman, 2015), as well as other types of skin lesions (Northrup et al., 2013).

The complex's name comes from potato-like lesions or tubers in the cerebral cortex (Curatolo et al., 2015). Cortical tubers are benign malformations that result from disordered neuron migration and differentiation in fetal development (Ullrich, 2016). Other types of tumors caused by TSC are subependymal nodules, which are located in the walls of the ventricles, and subependymal giant cell astrocytomas, which can block the flow of fluids in the brain and cause hydrocephalus (National Institute of Neurological Disorders and Stroke [NINDS], 2022; Ullrich, 2016). Because of the high variability in the location, number, and type of lesions in the brain and the body, individuals with TSC have a wide variation in symptoms and difficulties (Northrup et al., 2013).

https://doi.org/10.1037/0000349-063
Health-Related Disorders in Children and Adolescents: A Guidebook for Educators and Service Providers, Second Edition, M. M. Perfect, C. A. Riccio, and M. A. Bray (Editors)

ETIOLOGY

TSC is caused by mutations in the genes *TSC1* and *TSC2*. The *TSC1* gene is on chromosome 9q34.3 and encodes the production of hamartin, and the *TSC2* gene is on chromosome 16p13.3 and encodes tuberin (NINDS, 2022). Hamartin and tuberin are tumor-suppressing proteins involved in the suppression of a kinase, mTOR; the malfunction of these proteins leads to growths of benign tumors in a number of organ systems (van Eeghen et al., 2012). Although TSC can be inherited and in that case is autosomal dominant, most cases are the result of spontaneous mutations of the *TSC1* or *TSC2* gene. In rare situations, parents without TSC may transmit the disorder to their offspring via gonadal mosaicism; a portion of their reproductive cells may carry the mutation, and the affected areas may be transmitted to the fetus (NINDS, 2022).

PREVALENCE AND INCIDENCE

It is estimated that 25,000 to 40,000 individuals in the United States are affected by TSC, with an estimated incidence of one in 6,000 live births and prevalence of one in 20,000 (Volpi et al., 2019). TSC occurs in all racial, ethnic, and gender groups (NINDS, 2022). Genetic testing for the mutations that inactivate the hamartin and tuberin proteins may help diagnosis.

SYMPTOMS

TSC can cause a number of skin conditions; some appear early on, whereas others develop in middle childhood and later. These include skin areas with no pigmentation most frequently on the trunk and limbs (amelanotic naevus), rough patches of skin in the lower back area (shagreen patch), fleshy outgrowth of tissue (subungual fibroma), elevated lesions on the forehead or scalp (fibrous cephalic plaques), and café au lait spots (Northrup et al., 2013). Facial angiofibromas may appear between ages 2 and 5. Similarly, hypomelanotic macules present in children under 5 and are considered an early visible indicator of TSC. These lesions can look like "ash-leaf spots"; they also may be oval or polygonal-shaped hypopigmented patches up to several centimeters in size (Jacks & Witman, 2015). Angiofibromas, on the other hand, are rarer in younger children but increase over time to 75% occurrence in children above age 9. They may look like skin-colored or red-brown dome-shaped papules. The shagreen patches commonly appear before children turn 10. TSC is progressive in that the characteristic lesions are not commonly identified in children under the age of 2 years, unless severe or if TSC is diagnosed by genetic testing. They look like a plaque patch with a bumpy surface (Northrup et al., 2013).

Growth of tumors may occur in various organ systems, causing heart, kidney, lung, and cognitive problems. When the brain is involved, symptoms may include seizures, headache, nausea, vomiting, lethargy, or visual disturbance. Retinal hamartomas (lesions) and retinal achromic patches (hypopigmentation) may not cause significant vision damage but are considered unique characteristics of TSC (Northrup et al., 2013). Usually, children are diagnosed between the ages of 11 and 15 years or when they show medical symptoms. In many cases the lesions are found after the onset of seizures (Chu-Shore et al., 2010). TSC could cause mortality if hydrocephalus or kidney disorders are triggered by growth of tumors (Curatolo et al., 2015).

IMPACT ON THE STUDENT AND OUTCOMES

Medical

Although TSC shares similarities with other chronic illnesses and disabilities, its high variability in symptoms and outcomes even within a family poses uncertainty for prediction of outcomes (Zaroff et al., 2004). The occurrence of seizure disorders in up to 95% of those with TSC is a lifelong medical concern (Chu-Shore et al., 2010). The seizures may begin as infantile spasms and evolve over time into a seizure disorder (Mettin et al., 2014). Episodes of seizure may cause setbacks when they result in loss of skills and learning progress. Difficulty with communication, eating, sleep, and energy level may persist following seizures; bone fractures may also occur during seizure-related falls (McDonald et al., 2019). Tumors in the brain may result in increased intracranial pressure and frequent headaches. Surgery may be necessary when a subependymal giant cell astrocytoma in the brain causes fluid blockage or hydrocephalus (NINDS, 2022; Ullrich, 2016).

Light sensitivity and vision problems such as double vision may occur (Curatolo et al., 2015). Some children with TSC may have sleep difficulties, for which melatonin and sleep hygiene recommendations were found to be helpful (Zaroff et al., 2004). TSC also affects other organs and may cause medical complications involving the heart, lungs, skin, and kidneys. Visible skin conditions may develop over time.

Cognitive/Academic

Children with TSC exhibit significant variations in cognitive abilities. There is a high frequency of intellectual, behavioral, and psychosocial impairments associated with TSC, now described as TSC-associated neuropsychiatric disorders (Toldo et al., 2019). These problems related to TSC are underaddressed compared with medical concerns (de Vries et al., 2015).

The tumors in the brain are most likely to cause disability (van Eeghen et al., 2012). For children with infantile spasms, marked improvement in cognitive abilities has been found when spasms are controlled. At the most severe presentation of TSC, children may show a decline in cognition from 12 to 36 months of age; intellectual disability may be the impetus for evaluation and subsequent diagnosis of TSC (Jeste et al., 2014).

In academic areas, reading, writing, spelling, and math difficulties have been found in children with TSC regardless of intellectual disability status (Toldo et al., 2019). For children with TSC who have average general intelligence, cognitive weaknesses may exist in specific areas influencing school functioning. Approximately 30% of children without intellectual deficits show developmental delay, dyspraxia, dyscalculia, speech delay, visuospatial problems, and memory problems (Zaroff et al., 2004). Children with TSC and average intelligence may be perceived as unmotivated by adults who are not aware of these difficulties (de Vries et al., 2015).

Social-Emotional and Behavioral

Many children with TSC have difficulties with communication, behaviors, and social skills. Aggressive behaviors were observed in up to 66% of children with TSC and associated neuropsychiatric disorders (de Vries et al., 2015; Wilde et al., 2018). Children with higher seizure frequency, mixed seizure disorder, and low adaptive skills are especially likely to show behavioral problems. Unlike many children with other types of intellectual disabilities and co-occurring behavioral problems, children with TSC may have normal strength and ambulatory skills. This could pose physical difficulty for adults when managing the child's aggressive or injurious behaviors (Zaroff et al., 2004).

Although externalizing behaviors are frequent, internalizing issues are also elevated compared with the general population regardless of the intellectual level of the child (de Vries et al., 2007). Extreme shyness, anxiety, depressed mood, and elevated risk (27%) of self-injurious behaviors have been found (Toldo et al., 2019). Self-injury has a high persistence rate; risk of self-injury is significantly associated with pediatric pain and lack of self-help skills (Wilde et al., 2018).

The co-occurrence of autism spectrum disorder (ASD) among individuals with TSC is well above what is expected in the general population (Jeste et al., 2014). Risk factors for ASD include cognitive decline or regression early in development, epilepsy, infantile spasms, and *TSC2* gene mutation (Vignoli et al., 2015). TSC-related vision problems may result in delays in social development because early social interactions are heavily mediated by eye gaze (Jeste et al., 2014). As visually mediated social delays occur as early as 6 months of age, before language delays or restricted behaviors, they are considered another marker for early diagnosis or intervention. Children with TSC and ASD symptoms have difficulties in social responsiveness, reciprocal social interaction, communicative language, and restricted or repetitive behaviors, possibly related to cognitive deficits in the areas of self-regulation and cognitive flexibility (Wilde et al., 2018).

TSC also has a high level of co-occurrence with attention-deficit/hyperactivity disorder. Tumors or seizures may alter development of the frontal lobe, the brain area related to executive function. Although children with TSC are not characterized by a specific neuropsychological profile, they are known to have various difficulties. Children with TSC may have problems with inattention, impulsivity, disinhibition, and irritability. Comorbidity between intellectual disabilities, ASD, and attention-deficit/hyperactivity disorder is also possible. Moreover, some antiepileptic medication may have side effects that aggravate attention problems or agitation (Toldo et al., 2019).

Parenting stress is especially elevated when children with TSC show challenging behaviors and pervasive needs, with no respite from caregiving responsibilities (Kopp et al., 2008). Many parents reported the need for constant supervision of their children with TSC regardless of the children's age (McDonald et al., 2019). Parents can be hypervigilant about crisis, which leads to overestimation of threat. They may set aside future planning and family activities to meet the immediate needs of their child with TSC and thus feel guilty for the lack of time spent on their typically developing children.

PSYCHOEDUCATIONAL IMPLICATIONS AND SCHOOL-BASED INTERVENTIONS

Medical and Health Management

Seizure control is crucial to the well-being of children with TSC (Jambaqué et al., 2000). For medical examination, brain imaging every 1 to 3 years is recommended to monitor growth of subependymal giant cell astrocytomas (Zaroff et al., 2004). Pain management and medications need to be coordinated across medical staff working with the child and family members. An extended school year, homebound services, or reduced school hours may help children who have limited stamina and who may regress without consistent support. When hospitalization is needed, interdisciplinary planning should take place before the hospitalization and continue after the child transitions back to school.

Cognitive/Academic

Within the school setting, the child with TSC may benefit from special education, 504 services, or other support services (van Eeghen et al., 2012; Zaroff et al., 2004). Regular monitoring of academic progress will help to identify the child's strengths, as well as weaknesses, and inform educational programming. Individualized education programs may be developed to include academic content and goals that match the child's current cognitive level. Teaching one skill or concept at a time, providing ample practice opportunities, reteaching materials, using direct and concrete language, and preparing visual aids or manipulatives may help children meet academic goals. Chunking academic tasks and providing regular breaks may reduce fatigue in children with TSC. For children with adaptive skill deficits, instruction in life skills, communication, and social skills may facilitate autonomy. Physical and occupational therapy may facilitate motor skill development. Strategies such as self-monitoring, self-talk, help-seeking, relaxation, and mindfulness may help children develop executive functioning skills. Depending on the individual, small-group intervention, testing accommodations, speech–language therapy, occupational therapy, and physical therapy may be appropriate (de Vries et al., 2015; Zaroff et al., 2004). Children may benefit from comprehensive evaluations at milestones (e.g., diagnosis, school entry, transitions) to monitor how their functioning changes over time (Zaroff et al., 2004).

Social-Emotional and Behavioral

As noted, children with TSC may present with significant behavioral problems. Functional behavioral analysis may uncover the cause of children's problem behaviors and provide specific ways to prevent problem behaviors and increase appropriate behaviors. School psychologists may assist with behavioral intervention plan development. Consistent with positive behavioral supports, praise and reinforcement should be provided when children show appropriate behaviors. In addition, pain management, functional communication skills training, activity schedules, and monitoring may reduce self-injurious behaviors (Eden et al., 2014).

To facilitate social adjustment, early intervention targeting social skills, possibly through applied behavior analysis techniques, may be appropriate. For the child who is frequently absent, virtual visits with peers can be encouraged for socialization, entertainment, and help with schoolwork. Further, internalizing symptoms such as feelings of isolation, depression, and anxiety about returning to school should be monitored. To address potential stigma, peers of children with TSC should be informed about the noncontagious nature of the disorder; a schoolwide awareness-raising plan may address concerns with all types of chronic illness and disabilities. Given potential additional burdens on parents and siblings, participation in family support groups is recommended for family members of children with TSC (Zaroff et al., 2004). Multidisciplinary support teams involving medical and school personnel may help plan family services for children with TSC.

CONCLUSION

As with many chronic health disorders, it is imperative to consider each child with TSC as an individual and engage in appropriate assessment activities to identify needed supports. Further, communication between medical personnel, family, and school staff is critical to ensure integrated care. Regardless of intellectual ability, children with TSC are at risk for medical complications, educational difficulties, and adjustment problems. The extent to which supports are provided early on will contribute to the child's long-term outcome (Zaroff et al., 2004).

RESOURCES

National Institute of Neurological Disorders and Stroke. (2022). *Tuberous sclerosis fact sheet.* https://www.ninds.nih.gov/Disorders/Patient-Caregiver-Education/Fact-Sheets/Tuberous-Sclerosis-Fact-Sheet

Tuberous Sclerosis Alliance. https://www.tsalliance.org/ (available in Spanish)

REFERENCES

Chu-Shore, C. J., Major, P., Camposano, S., Muzykewicz, D., & Thiele, E. A. (2010). The natural history of epilepsy in tuberous sclerosis complex. *Epilepsia, 51*(7), 1236–1241. https://doi.org/10.1111/j.1528-1167.2009.02474.x

Curatolo, P., Moavero, R., & de Vries, P. J. (2015). Neurological and neuropsychiatric aspects of tuberous sclerosis complex. *Lancet Neurology, 14*(7), 733–745. https://doi.org/10.1016/S1474-4422(15)00069-1

de Vries, P. J., Hunt, A., & Bolton, P. F. (2007). The psychopathologies of children and adolescents with tuberous sclerosis complex (TSC): A postal survey of U.K. families. *European Child & Adolescent Psychiatry, 16*(1), 16–24. https://doi.org/10.1007/s00787-006-0570-3

de Vries, P. J., Whittemore, V. H., Leclezio, L., Byars, A. W., Dunn, D., Ess, K. C., Hook, D., King, B. H., Sahin, M., & Jansen, A. (2015). Tuberous sclerosis associated neuropsychiatric disorders (TAND) and the TAND Checklist. *Pediatric Neurology, 52*(1), 25–35. https://doi.org/10.1016/j.pediatrneurol.2014.10.004

Eden, K. E., de Vries, P. J., Moss, J., Richards, C., & Oliver, C. (2014). Self-injury and aggression in tuberous sclerosis complex: Cross syndrome comparison and associated risk markers. *Journal of Neurodevelopmental Disorders, 6*(1), Article 10. https://doi.org/10.1186/1866-1955-6-10

Jacks, S. K., & Witman, P. M. (2015). Tuberous sclerosis complex: An update for dermatologists. *Pediatric Dermatology, 32*(5), 563–570. https://doi.org/10.1111/pde.12567

Jambaqué, I., Chiron, C., Dumas, C., Mumford, J., & Dulac, O. (2000). Mental and behavioural outcome of infantile epilepsy treated by vigabatrin in tuberous sclerosis patients. *Epilepsy Research, 38*(2–3), 151–160. https://doi.org/10.1016/S0920-1211(99)00082-0

Jeste, S. S., Wu, J. Y., Senturk, D., Varcin, K., Ko, J., McCarthy, B., Shimizu, C., Dies, K., Vogel-Farley, V., Sahin, M., & Nelson, C. A., III. (2014). Early developmental trajectories associated with ASD in infants with tuberous sclerosis complex. *Neurology, 83*(2), 160–168. https://doi.org/10.1212/WNL.0000000000000568

Kopp, C. M. C., Muzykewicz, D. A., Staley, B. A., Thiele, E. A., & Pulsifer, M. B. (2008). Behavior problems in children with tuberous sclerosis complex and parental stress. *Epilepsy & Behavior, 13*(3), 505–510. https://doi.org/10.1016/j.yebeh.2008.05.010

McDonald, A., Goodwin, J., Roberts, S., Fish, L., Vaughan, B., Cooper, A., & Cadwgan, J. (2019). "We've made the best of it. But we do not have a normal life": Families' experiences of tuberous sclerosis complex and seizure management. *Journal of Intellectual Disability Research, 63*(8), 947–956. https://doi.org/10.1111/jir.12609

Mettin, R. R., Merkenschlager, A., Bernhard, M. K., Elix, H., Hirsch, W., Kiess, W., & Syrbe, S. (2014). Wide spectrum of clinical manifestations in children with tuberous sclerosis complex—Follow-up of 20 children. *Brain & Development, 36*(4), 306–314. https://doi.org/10.1016/j.braindev.2013.05.006

National Institute of Neurological Disorders and Stroke. (2022). *Tuberous sclerosis fact sheet.* https://www.ninds.nih.gov/Disorders/Patient-Caregiver-Education/Fact-Sheets/Tuberous-Sclerosis-Fact-Sheet

Northrup, H., Krueger, D. A., & the International Tuberous Sclerosis Complex Consensus Group. (2013). Tuberous sclerosis complex diagnostic criteria update: Recommendations of the 2012 International Tuberous Sclerosis Complex Consensus Conference. *Pediatric Neurology, 49*(4), 243–254. https://doi.org/10.1016/j.pediatrneurol.2013.08.001

Toldo, I., Brasson, V., Miscioscia, M., Pelizza, M. F., Manara, R., Sartori, S., Mantegazza, G., Vecchi, M., Nosadini, M., & Gatta, M. (2019). Tuberous sclerosis-associated neuropsychiatric disorders: A paediatric cohort study. *Developmental Medicine and Child Neurology, 61*(2), 168–173. https://doi.org/10.1111/dmcn.14055

Ullrich, N. J. (2016). Neurocutaneous syndromes and brain tumors. *Journal of Child Neurology, 31*(12), 1399–1411. https://doi.org/10.1177/0883073815604220

van Eeghen, A. M., Chu-Shore, C. J., Pulsifer, M. B., Camposano, S. E., & Thiele, E. A. (2012). Cognitive and adaptive development of patients with tuberous sclerosis complex: A retrospective, longitudinal investigation. *Epilepsy & Behavior, 23*(1), 10–15. https://doi.org/10.1016/j.yebeh.2011.10.005

Vignoli, A., La Briola, F., Peron, A., Turner, K., Vannicola, C., Saccani, M., Magnaghi, E., Scornavacca, G. F., & Canevini, M. P. (2015). Autism spectrum disorder in tuberous sclerosis complex: Searching for risk markers. *Orphanet Journal of Rare Diseases, 10*(1), Article 154. https://doi.org/10.1186/s13023-015-0371-1

Volpi, A., Sala, G., Lesma, E., Labriola, F., Righetti, M., Alfano, R. M., & Cozzolino, M. (2019). Tuberous sclerosis complex: New insights into clinical and therapeutic approach. *Nephrology, 32*(3), 355–363. https://doi.org/10.1007/s40620-018-0547-6

Wilde, L., Wade, K., Eden, K., Moss, J., de Vries, P. J., & Oliver, C. (2018). Persistence of self-injury, aggression and property destruction in children and adults with tuberous sclerosis complex. *Journal of Intellectual Disability Research, 62*(12), 1058–1071. https://doi.org/10.1111/jir.12472

Zaroff, C. M., Devinsky, O., Miles, D., & Barr, W. B. (2004). Topical review: Cognitive and behavioral correlates of tuberous sclerosis complex. *Journal of Child Neurology, 19*(11), 847–852. https://doi.org/10.1177/08830738040190110101

64

Conclusion: Looking Back and Looking Forward

Melissa A. Bray, Michelle M. Perfect, and Cynthia A. Riccio

This volume provides critical information for a multitude of disorders affecting different body systems with potentially long-term effects on child outcomes. Although there are obvious differences across disorders and for the individuals who are affected, some considerations cut across various health-related disorders. The goal of this chapter is to synthesize the knowledge base accumulated here, as well as what is known about the more frequent disorders not covered (e.g., attention-deficit/hyperactivity disorder). This synthesis is intended to aid in generalization of knowledge across currently identified disorders and new disorders or complications (e.g., those that may present as aftereffects of the COVID-19 pandemic).

Regardless of the disorder, medical, cognitive/academic, and social/behavioral factors should be considered in meeting the needs of those with any health-related condition. At the same time, the effects on a given individual may range from minimal to severe in one or all of those functional domains, with variability as the child develops. A theme emerged across disorders, that for most of these conditions, there is vast variability in skill acquisition and execution of those skills on a daily basis. This variability increases with consideration of multiple body system effects, availability of resources within health and educational systems, and impacts on the family system.

A gap persists in the consideration of educational and psychosocial needs for these children and youth by medical professionals, many of whom lack fundamental knowledge of the education system and how it operates in providing services to students with health care needs. Similarly, educators and school-based

https://doi.org/10.1037/0000349-064
Health-Related Disorders in Children and Adolescents: A Guidebook for Educators and Service Providers, Second Edition, M. M. Perfect, C. A. Riccio, and M. A. Bray (Editors)

service providers may not have access to the most critical information regarding the impact of the medical condition and treatment effects on cognitive/academic and social–emotional/behavioral functioning. Finally, parents may not understand the synergy that needs to be in place to fully support their child's changing needs over time. An integrated perspective is needed to create a flexible, adaptive, and targeted educational framework for these students. This final chapter seeks to incite school psychology professionals, educators, health care providers, and families to consider and act toward improving the outcomes of students with health-related conditions.

The guiding framework centers on common elements that emerged across disorders in meeting the needs of youth with health-related disorders and their families and the need for coordinated care (i.e., a multidisciplinary approach to identification and treatment). An ecological and multisystemic approach (M. S. Harris, 2009; Wallander & Koot, 2016) that begins when the disorder manifests and is identified is one approach to coordinated care. The emergence of behavioral health services in medical settings is a major step in advancing coordinated care for the children and families affected.

COMMUNICATION

Communication is a critical component of any model of coordinated care and should be ongoing from the time it is known that the child has a health-related disorder (Hay et al., 2015; Power et al., 2003). This is facilitated by documentation that allows for open communication among parents, medical personnel, school staff, and any others providing services (M. S. Harris, 2009; Power et al., 2003). Unfortunately, communication is the critical piece across systems that often falls short (Canto et al., 2014). To facilitate communication across systems providing services (i.e., physical and mental health systems, educational systems), appointing a liaison or coordinator from the medical and school settings to work with teams of individuals across settings has been recommended. The liaisons would serve as the conduit of information between the family, medical staff, school staff, and community resources. They would help identify training and support needs for the child, family, teachers, and peers with medical input. By virtue of their training in intervention, assessment, and consultation, school psychologists have the capacity to serve as the liaison of the school-based team. While school psychologists have knowledge of resources in schools that oftentimes are not known or prioritized by medical personnel (Grandinette, 2014), medical personnel have knowledge of community resources and medical management not necessarily known to school personnel.

COLLABORATION

Medical personnel, mental health professionals, educators, and parents need to work together. Parents cannot assume that school personnel are aware of their child's medical needs, their current health status, and all the circumstances that surround the student's health that might interfere with making progress. Similarly, it is not appropriate to presume that medical personnel have familiarity with the demands and expectations of the school or home environment. Although it seems intuitive, a useful strategy often overlooked is the inclusion of a nurse or someone qualified to understand medical information at multidisciplinary school-based meetings and a school representative at medical team meetings. Given time constraints, this may not always be realistic; however, liaisons can communicate and provide a conduit for information sharing at such meetings and review proposed programs or interventions to avoid conflict and contradictory information. Collaboration requires all parties to communicate interdisciplinary knowledge that together promotes optimal problem solving.

CONTINUITY OF CARE AND PROFESSIONAL DEVELOPMENT

In consideration of continuity of care, a multidisciplinary systems-level plan with emphasis on self-care, healthy behaviors, emotional well-being, and education provides the foundation. At this level, there is a need for bidirectional professional development efforts. The American School Health Association recommended that schools target communications throughout their programming as well as via social media, newsletters, clubs, and community service. This would address the need to inform others in schools and across various settings about medical conditions and to dispel myths as part of professional development activities. On the other hand, medical personnel and community mental health personnel need to be targeted with regard to how their patients can access services in the schools. Continuing education efforts by school personnel delivered to these professionals with general guidelines may increase their awareness of the mechanisms involved and requirements for school services. This is particularly important when the child with a chronic health-related disorder requires hospitalization or cannot attend school for some period of time (Riccio et al., 2022).

School Reintegration

Students with chronic illness miss 5 times the number of days healthy children do (McDougall et al., 2004), with a strong positive correlation between high absenteeism and poor academic performance (French et al., 2013). These absences may be sporadic or extensive. As is evident from the concerns and issues faced with remote education during the pandemic, absenteeism from the physical school environment yields additional complications. For those hospitalized and homebound for longer periods of time, research suggests reintegration often is not orchestrated smoothly and subsequently negatively affects all aspects of functioning and quality of life (B. Harris et al., 2016). The critical component is for communication to begin early, preferably in advance of the recurrent absences or inability to attend due to health reasons, in order for the school to establish an individualized plan. This could be a 504 plan or through the special education process. The key is that any plan should address not only the academic components of school attendance but also the social–emotional learning and relationships fostered by school engagement.

Training in the school setting needs to incorporate additional knowledge about the medical condition for school personnel, parents, and other students to dispel fears and myths. Canter and Roberts (2012) reported increased positive attitudes toward the returning student associated with increased illness-specific knowledge. A school reentry meeting with all involved parties is necessary prior to the student's return in order to prepare and coordinate services. For example, in some cases, changes in student functioning may necessitate physical changes to the child's desk. Access and ease of mobility need to be considered among other variables. In the school setting, arrangements for dealing with fatigue (e.g., a place to rest, shortened school day) may be needed as well.

Programming

Medical management will establish a plan focused on symptom management and treatment of the disorder. Their planning process incorporates medical treatment options, with ongoing monitoring and change as needed. Similarly, educational and mental health programs select curricular materials, programs, and intervention approaches, with identified goals specific to academic and social/behavioral health. As with medical checkups, those providing academic supports (i.e., teachers, tutors, parents) and those providing mental health services (i.e., school psychologists, counseling psychologists, other mental health professionals, parents) need to be monitoring progress in reaching identified goals. All professionals involved with the individual child and family need to be identifying obstacles as well as ways to move forward via consultation. From a coordinated care or behavioral health perspective, the personnel involved in the provision of services (i.e., medical personnel, educators, mental health personnel) and outcome monitoring need to be communicating with each other and with the parents. For the purposes of this text, the focus is on school-based interventions, which may apply to hospital-based schools, home school, homebound instruction, remote instruction, or the classroom.

Technology Use

Today's technology allows for continuous engagement of students with teachers, peers, and mental health. The pandemic has demonstrated both the ease with which students can access educational and mental health supports in this crisis situation, as well as limitations of this access. These same mechanisms can be used with chronic illness without teachers or peers having to visit the hospital or home. For instance, youth who are hospitalized or recuperating at home can interact via audio or video with teachers and peers in real time (Battles & Wiener, 2002). Connections with peers can be maintained by encouraging and facilitating the sending of cards, as well as by utilizing peers to take notes, tutor, and bring home schoolwork as appropriate (Root et al., 2016). The extent of engagement may vary with consideration of the student's fatigue and the desire to minimize disruption throughout the school day; however, even when all other children are in the classroom, maintaining some interaction for the child at home is important. In addition to the problems encountered with technology support and access in the pandemic, for the child with health-related disorders, medical and school personnel need to identify approaches for child engagement that are responsive to the child's illness and prevent feelings of isolation, depression, and anxiety. With the pandemic, there has been a burgeoning of telepsychology means to provide counseling that is consistent with confidentiality laws. Moving forward, the technology and skill sets developed during the pandemic can be implemented for students who are not able to attend school or in-person sessions.

School-Based Research-Based Interventions for Academic Success

The basic tenets of academic intervention apply when selecting intervention approaches. A system of measurement is necessary to establish the student's present levels of functioning in all cognitive/academic areas to establish areas that are at or above expectancy and skill sets that should be targeted for improvement. Similar to creating an individualized education program, goals and objectives should be reasonable and operationally defined, with expectations over time articulated and progress monitored.

Once objectives are defined, intervention programs need to be identified that address the targeted skill set(s), considered in conjunction with the child's limitations (e.g., fatigue), parent acceptability, and teacher buy-in. Obstacles to implementation (e.g., cost, time, evidence base, training of the person who will be implementing) should be considered, and a program or programs should be selected jointly by parents and teachers. The individuals implementing the program in the school setting, the means (remote or in person), the frequency and time commitment, and how and when progress is monitored need to be clearly identified. At the same time, any accommodations and modifications (e.g., extended time, notetaker, text-to-speech options for reading material, use of a calculator, oral examinations) should be consistently implemented and readily accessible to the student. Outcomes must be measured consistently and with sufficient frequency to determine if the intervention selected yields the intended outcome. If the intervention is not working, then the choice of intervention needs to be reconsidered.

School-Based Research-Based Interventions for Social/Behavioral Growth

The same problem-solving principles apply in this context as in academic areas. The first task is to identify the child's strengths and difficulties in social–emotional and behavioral areas. Goals and objectives that can be operationally defined and measured need to be established and prioritized, most often initially focusing on aggression, self-harm, and suicidal ideation if present. Once the goals to be targeted are defined, potential intervention approaches can be identified. Cultural considerations play a more prominent role in social/behavioral domains and must be considered in light of parental values, teacher values, and school culture. This discussion of obstacles, potential risk factors, and acceptability of the approach should include the parents, any involved teachers, and the mental health professional, with the goal of successfully selecting and implementing a program or programs and accurately collecting and reviewing outcome data. A behavior plan implemented at home and at school to address aggressive behavior may be one component, and another may be the development of alternative means of communicating feelings. Mindfulness is an additional approach to address depression and anxiety, with many apps now available for free. As with medical management and academic interventions, regular monitoring of outcome data is paramount. As noted with academic interventions, if the selected program is not yielding the desired outcomes, alternatives need to be considered.

POLICY AND REGULATIONS

Although the focus of this book is on individualized needs, systems-level considerations for integrated or coordinated care require modifications to policies at state levels. Federal and state statutes are influential in setting parameters for accessibility and accountability for service provision in the schools. For example, the limitations on homebound instruction in many states and the sense that special education services should not be considered until the child has demonstrated a lack of response to intervention often obstruct the accessibility of services for children with health-related disorders and those who are injured as a result of an accident. For the child with a chronic illness who just had brain surgery, their memory deficits are not the same as typical delays that will respond to increasingly intensive use of the same intervention. As another example, one systemic barrier for high school students is a strict attendance policy; for students requiring repeat medical intervention, these strict regulations may hinder their ability to earn credits toward graduation. At the school level, there may be inappropriate school rules and disciplinary policies. Examples include restricting access to the restroom, tardy notices if the student cannot get from one room to the other in a set amount of time, contacting the truant officer if a child is out ill for multiple days, and so forth.

SUMMARY

As the COVID-19 pandemic has shown us, it is not possible to know or predict health-related disorders or their impact. This text provides the most salient information available on an extensive number of health-related disorders that most often manifest in developmental years, with a focus on those that did not have an exhaustive research base. Although not considered rare, some of these disorders and variants are not seen as frequently as others. Still, professionals working with a pediatric population in a medical setting, the community, or schools will come in contact with children and youth with these disorders. Unfortunately, this is not an exhaustive compilation and does not consider the effects of neurotoxins (e.g., pollution) or traumatic brain injury that may similarly disrupt physical health, educational progress, and social/behavioral functioning. This underscores the need for ongoing professional continuing education.

The past 10 years have given rise to increased consideration of integrated behavioral health and coordinated care. Still, in many instances, although mental health professionals are brought to the table, school personnel are not. Concentrated efforts need to be made to seek that invitation and educate medical professionals on better communication and collaboration to meet the needs of children with health-related disorders. Together, professionals in medicine, mental health, and education may be able to make strides in addressing the policies that obstruct service delivery for these children and others.

REFERENCES

Battles, H. B., & Wiener, L. S. (2002). STARBRIGHT world: Effects of an electronic network on the social environment of children with life-threatening illnesses. *Children's Health Care, 31*(1), 47–68. https://doi.org/10.1207/S15326888CHC3101_4

Canter, K. S., & Roberts, M. C. (2012). A systematic and quantitative review of interventions to facilitate school reentry for children with chronic health conditions. *Journal of Pediatric Psychology, 37*(10), 1065–1075. https://doi.org/10.1093/jpepsy/jss071

Canto, A. I., Chesire, D. J., Buckley, V. A., Andrews, T. W., & Roehrig, A. D. (2014). Barriers to meeting the needs of students with traumatic brain injury. *Educational Psychology in Practice, 30*(1), 88–103. https://doi.org/10.1080/02667363.2014.883498

French, A. E., Tsangaris, E., Barrera, M., Guger, S., Brown, R., Urbach, S., Stephens, D., & Nathan, P. C. (2013). School attendance in childhood cancer survivors and their siblings. *The Journal of Pediatrics, 162*(1), 160–165. https://doi.org/10.1016/j.jpeds.2012.06.066

Grandinette, S. (2014). Supporting students with brain tumors in obtaining school intervention services: The clinician's role from an educator's perspective. *Journal of Pediatric Rehabilitation Medicine*, 7(4), 307–321. https://doi.org/10.3233/PRM-140301

Harris, B., Shaw, B., Lawson, H., & Sherman, B. (2016). Barriers to addressing adolescent substance use: Perceptions of New York school-based health center providers. *Journal of School Health, 86*(2), 96–104. https://doi.org/10.1111/josh.12358

Harris, M. S. (2009). School reintegration for children and adolescents with cancer: The role of school psychologists. *Psychology in the Schools, 46*(7), 579–592. https://doi.org/10.1002/pits.20399

Hay, G. H., Nabors, M., Sullivan, A., & Zigmund, A. (2015). Students with pediatric cancer: A prescription for school success. *Physical Disabilities: Education and Related Services, 34*(2), 1–13. https://doi.org/10.14434/pders.v34i2.19643

McDougall, J., King, G., de Wit, D. J., Miller, L. T., Hong, S., Offord, D. R., LaPorta, J., & Meyer, K. (2004). Chronic physical health conditions and disability among Canadian school-aged children: A national profile. *Disability and Rehabilitation, 26*(1), 35–45. https://doi.org/10.1080/09638280410001645076

Power, T. J., DuPaul, G. J., Shapiro, E. S., & Kazak, A. E. (2003). *Promoting children's health: Integrating health, school, family, and community systems.* Guilford Press.

Riccio, C. A., Maykel, C., Bray, M. A., Perdue, E., & Frye, S. (2022). School reintegration for youth with health-related conditions. *Contemporary School Psychology, 26*(2), 200–208. https://doi.org/10.1007/s40688-021-00376-3

Root, M. M., Bray, M. A., Maykel, C., Cross, K., Shankar, N., & Theodore, L. (2016). Students with cancer: Presenting issues and effective solutions. *International Journal of School & Educational Psychology, 4*(1), 25–33. https://doi.org/10.1080/21683603.2016.1130549

Wallander, J. L., & Koot, H. M. (2016). Quality of life in children: A critical examination of concepts, approaches, issues, and education. *Clinical Psychology Review, 45*, 131–143. https://doi.org/10.1016/j.cpr.2015.11.007

APPENDIX

Checklist for Developing Plans for Students With Health-Related Conditions

The following are suggested best practices to consider for all students with health-related conditions. Using these items as a reference point may help to reduce errors of omission and provide a framework for all teams of educators to address students' needs in a systematic and consistent way (U.S. Department of Education, 2020).

- ❑ Evaluation information
    - ❑ Unique evaluation considerations address functioning based on health status and in light of potential treatment impacts
- ❑ Present levels of academic achievement
    - ❑ Address any variability in performance
    - ❑ If student's final performance is meeting standards/expectations in light of their circumstances, include mitigating circumstances involved to understand factors that contributed to performance
    - ❑ If a student is struggling academically, describe progress (or setbacks)
- ❑ Functional performance
- ❑ Accommodations
    - ❑ Class schedule
    - ❑ Access to notes
        - ❑ Modality
            - ❑ Recording (only if no undue burden of repeating class, and with proper labeling)
            - ❑ Notetaker (familiar adult, peer)
            - ❑ Cloze or outlined notes

- ❑ Frequency
  - ❑ Ongoing, in advance
  - ❑ As needed or missed
  - ❑ As requested (student should not have to request accommodations, but record circumstances in which notes would be provided)

- ❑ Planned breaks
  - ❑ Shortened school day
  - ❑ Timing of services (adjusted schedule to allow time for therapy)
  - ❑ Extra time between classes
- ❑ Workload
  - ❑ Reduction of items to avoid fatigue (not level of difficulty)
  - ❑ Extended time to complete assignments
  - ❑ Grading effort versus accuracy, or quality (i.e., accuracy) over quantity
  - ❑ Work exemption for assignment during service time
  - ❑ Work reprieve or relief during noncore or study hall time (consider time for student to practice skills in between classes and giving other students the privilege of using that time to complete work)
  - ❑ Prioritizing assignments across all classes (consider exemption if outstanding assignments accumulate)
  - ❑ Modifications needed to provide work commensurate with present levels of academic functioning
- ❑ Testing formats
  - ❑ Oral, typed, written, scribed, dictated
  - ❑ Extension to begin
  - ❑ Breaks in between
  - ❑ Reduced number of items

❑ Assistive technologies

- ❑ Electronic
- ❑ Telepresence/virtual connection

- ❑ Amplifier
- ❑ Computer or keyboard for typing

❑ Occupational therapy

❑ Positive behavior supports

- ❑ Functional behavior assessment needed
- ❑ Behavior intervention plan
- ❑ Written into individualized education program
- ❑ Specially designed instruction
    - ❑ Addressing goals
    - ❑ Scientifically based instructional practices
    - ❑ Peer-reviewed research for special education and related services and supplementary aids and services

❑ Parental involvement

- ❑ Input (verbatim)

❑ Supports for school personnel

- ❑ Training needs
    - ❑ Regular education teachers
    - ❑ Paraprofessionals
    - ❑ Special education teacher
    - ❑ Parents
- ❑ Modality
    - ❑ Prerecorded videos
    - ❑ Synchronous in-person or telepresence
    - ❑ Consultations with health care providers or experts on condition
    - ❑ Written materials
- ❑ Frequency
- ❑ Paraprofessional support

❑ Communication between school and parents

❑ Crisis or emergency plan

- ❑ Health
- ❑ Behavioral

REFERENCE

U.S. Department of Education. (2020, January 10). *The civil rights of students with hidden disabilities under Section 504 of the Rehabilitation Act of 1973*. https://www2.ed.gov/about/offices/list/ocr/docs/hq5269.html

INDEX

B

D

G

H

M

T

U

V

W

X

Y

Z

ABOUT THE EDITORS

Michelle M. Perfect, PhD, is a professor in the School Psychology Program at the University of Arizona. Dr. Perfect received her doctorate in educational psychology (with a specialization in school psychology) from the University of Texas at Austin and her master's degree in psychology from New York University. She completed her American Psychological Association (APA)-accredited predoctoral psychology internship at the University of Medicine and Dentistry in Newark, New Jersey. Afterward, she completed postdoctoral fellowships in pediatric psychology at the University of Texas Medical Branch in Galveston, Texas, and in health psychology and biostatistics at Scott & White Memorial Hospital in Temple, Texas. Dr. Perfect is licensed in the state of Arizona; is an elected member of the Society for the Study of School Psychology; and has been active in American Psychological Association Division 16: School Psychology, serving as convention chair, vice president of publications and communications (2016–2021), and president (2023). She is also currently on the APA Committee on Professional Practice Standards. Dr. Perfect has secured over $6.5 million in external funding, including from the National Institutes of Health, National Science Foundation, Institute of Education Sciences, and American Diabetes Association. Her interdisciplinary research team's critical scholarly activities aim to (a) elucidate the role of health behaviors and traumatic event exposure and symptoms in academic and health (physical and mental) outcomes for diverse students; (b) design and examine the benefit of sleep, behavioral medicine, and mind–body interventions to improve school-related, neurobehavioral (cognitive, behavioral, and social–emotional functioning), and physical health outcomes; (c) examine and strengthen the essential and collaborative roles of multiple systems of care (school, family, health care, foster care, policy) in youths' lives; and (d) increase educational access and success for culturally and economically diverse students to mitigate effects of adversities. Dr. Perfect's teaching interests are in development, research methods, clinical supervision, therapy, evidence-based interventions, and school-community mental health.

Cynthia A. Riccio, PhD, is a professor emerita of the School Psychology Program at Texas A&M University; she also has emerita faculty status at the Texas A&M Institute of Neuroscience. Dr. Riccio's primary research interests include learning disabilities, attention-deficit/hyperactivity disorder, neuropsychology, and individual assessment. She has authored or coauthored more than 60 articles, 26 book chapters, two texts, and two edited texts, as well as one test instrument. Dr. Riccio is an active member in many professional organizations, such as the American Psychological Association (Divisions 16: School Psychology, 40: Society for Clinical Neuropsychology, 54: Society of Pediatric Psychology), National Association of School Psychologists, Society for the Study of School Psychology, National Academy of Neuropsychologists, and International Neuropsychological Society. Dr. Riccio is a fellow of both the American Psychological Association and the National Academy of Neuropsychology.

Melissa A. Bray, PhD, is a professor and the director of the School Psychology program within the Neag School of Education at the University of Connecticut. She is a fellow of both the American Psychological Association (APA) and the American Psychological Society. Dr. Bray is an elected member of the Society for the Study of School Psychology. She is licensed as a psychologist in the state of Connecticut and holds national certification in school psychology, state certification in school psychology, and licensure in speech–language pathology. Since receiving her doctorate in 1997, she has published or has in press over 200 articles, chapters, and reviews in the professional literature along with many books; further, she has presented over 150 scholarly papers at national and international conferences. In several studies on faculty productivity, it was determined that Dr. Bray was the first or second most prolific contributor to the five primary journals in school psychology. She serves as associate editor of the *International Journal of School and Educational Psychology* and has served as an associate editor of *School Psychology Quarterly*. She is the coeditor of the first *Oxford Handbook of School Psychology*. She has also guest edited numerous issues of *Psychology in the Schools,* including topics on video self-modeling, behavior disorders, positive psychology, statistical reform, childhood obesity, counseling, social–emotional disorders, equity-based practice, and autism spectrum disorder. As coprincipal investigator, she has secured over $2 million in student training contracts. Dr. Bray was the 2003 recipient of the prestigious APA Division 16's (School Psychology) Lightner Witmer Award, the division's highest honor given to young scholars. She has also been involved in state, national, and international professional associations, including service as vice president for social, ethical responsibility, and ethnic minority affairs and as president of the APA Division 16 (School Psychology) Executive Committee. Dr. Bray has also served as Division 16's convention chair, hospitality suite coordinator, chair of the publications committee, and member of the conversation webinar series. She is currently the division's vice president for membership. Her research interests are in the area of interventions for communication disorders, mainly stuttering and selective mutism, mind–body health, integrated behavioral health care, and physical health and wellness, especially in the areas of asthma and cancer.